Renal Failure: Latest Findings

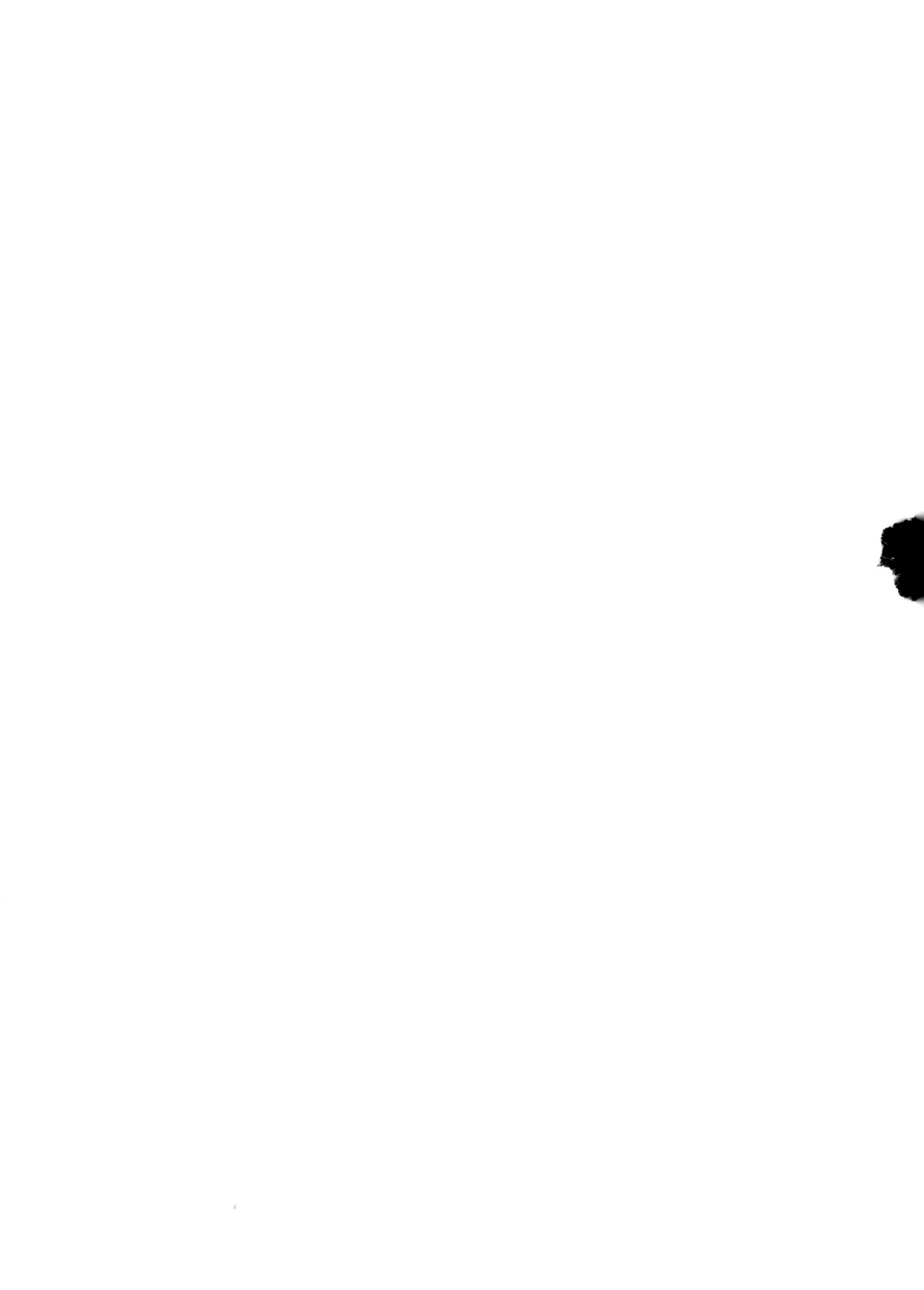

Renal Failure: Latest Findings

Edited by Hugh Colley

hayle
medical

New York

Hayle Medical,
750 Third Avenue, 9th Floor,
New York, NY 10017, USA

Visit us on the World Wide Web at:
www.haylemedical.com

ISBN: 978-1-63241-811-1

Cataloging-in-Publication Data

Renal failure : latest findings / edited by Hugh Colley.
   p. cm.
Includes bibliographical references and index.
ISBN 978-1-63241-811-1
1. Kidneys--Diseases. 2. Acute renal failure. 3. Chronic renal failure.
4. Kidneys--Diseases--Diagnosis. 5. Kidneys--Diseases--Treatment. I. Colley, Hugh.
RC902 .R46 2019
616.61--dc23

Table of Contents

Preface.. IX

Chapter 1   **A Comparison of the Long-Term Effects of Lanthanum Carbonate and Calcium
             Carbonate on the Course of Chronic Renal Failure in Rats with
             Adriamycin-Induced Nephropathy** 1
             Tsuyoshi Takashima, Toru Sanai, Motoaki Miyazono, Makoto Fukuda,
             Tomoya Kishi, Yasunori Nonaka, Mai Yoshizaki, Sae Sato and Yuji Ikeda

Chapter 2   **Shedding Light on the Chemical Diversity of Ectopic Calcifications in Kidney
             Tissues: Diagnostic and Research Aspects** 8
             Arnaud Dessombz, Dominique Bazin, Paul Dumas, Christophe Sandt,
             Josep Sule-Suso and Michel Daudon

Chapter 3   **Circulating Progenitor Cell Count for Cardiovascular Risk Stratification: A Pooled
             Analysis** 14
             Gian Paolo Fadini, Shoichi Maruyama, Takenori Ozaki, Akihiko Taguchi,
             James Meigs, Stefanie Dimmeler, Andreas M. Zeiher, Saula de Kreutzenberg,
             Angelo Avogaro, Georg Nickenig, Caroline Schmidt-Lucke and Nikos Werner

Chapter 4   **Elimination of Endogenous Toxin, Creatinine from Blood Plasma Depends on
             Albumin Conformation: Site Specific Uremic Toxicity & Impaired Drug Binding** 23
             Ankita Varshney, Mohd Rehan, Naidu Subbarao, Gulam Rabbani
             and Rizwan Hasan Khan

Chapter 5   **Management of Metformin-Associated Lactic Acidosis by Continuous Renal
             Replacement Therapy** 38
             Geoffray Keller, Martin Cour, Romain Hernu, Julien Illinger,
             Dominique Robert and Laurent Argaud

Chapter 6   **Salt-Induced Changes in Cardiac Phosphoproteome in a Rat Model of Chronic
             Renal Failure** 44
             Zhengxiu Su, Hongguo Zhu, Menghuan Zhang, Liangliang Wang, Hanchang He,
             Shaoling Jiang, Fan Fan Hou and Aiqing Li

Chapter 7   **Effects of Preoperative Aspirin on Cardiocerebral and Renal Complications in
             Non-Emergent Cardiac Surgery Patients: A Sub-Group and Cohort Study** 55
             Longhui Cao, Scott Silvestry, Ning Zhao, James Diehl and Jianzhong Sun

Chapter 8   **Mitochondrial DNA Backgrounds Might Modulate Diabetes Complications Rather
             than T2DM as a Whole** 61
             Alessandro Achilli, Anna Olivieri, Maria Pala, Baharak Hooshiar Kashani,
             Valeria Carossa, Ugo A. Perego, Francesca Gandini, Aurelia Santoro,
             Vincenza Battaglia, Viola Grugni, Hovirag Lancioni, Cristina Sirolla,
             Anna Rita Bonfigli, Antonella Cormio, Massimo Boemi, Ivano Testa,
             Ornella Semino, Antonio Ceriello, Liana Spazzafumo, Maria Nicola Gadaleta,
             Maurizio Marra, Roberto Testa, Claudio Franceschi and Antonio Torroni

Chapter 9   **Indicators of Acute and Persistent Renal Damage in Adult Thrombotic Microangiopathy** 73
Firuseh Dierkes, Nikolaos Andriopoulos, Christoph Sucker, Kathrin Kuhr,
Markus Hollenbeck, Gerd R. Hetzel, Volker Burst, Sven Teschner, Lars C. Rump,
Thomas Benzing, Bernd Grabensee and Christine E. Kurschat

Chapter 10   **Inhibition of the Soluble Epoxide Hydrolase Promotes Albuminuria in Mice with Progressive Renal Disease** 80
Oliver Jung, Felix Jansen, Anja Mieth, Eduardo Barbosa-Sicard, Rainer U. Pliquett,
Andrea Babelova, Christophe Morisseau, Sung H. Hwang, Cindy Tsai,
Bruce D. Hammock, Liliana Schaefer, Gerd Geisslinger,
Kerstin Amann and Ralf P. Brandes

Chapter 11   **Potassium and the Excitability Properties of Normal Human Motor Axons** *In Vivo* 90
Delphine Boëri, Hugh Bostock, Romana Spescha and Werner J. Z'Graggen

Chapter 12   **Geldanamycin Derivative Ameliorates High Fat Diet-Induced Renal Failure in Diabetes** 98
Hong-Mei Zhang, Howard Dang, Amrita Kamat, Chih-Ko Yeh and Bin-Xian Zhang

Chapter 13   **High-Dose Enalapril Treatment Reverses Myocardial Fibrosis in Experimental Uremic Cardiomyopathy** 107
Karin Tyralla, Marcin Adamczak, Kerstin Benz, Valentina Campean,
Marie-Luise Gross, Karl F. Hilgers, Eberhard Ritz and Kerstin Amann

Chapter 14   **Treatment of Cryptococcal Meningitis in KwaZulu-Natal** 118
Josephine V. J. Lightowler, Graham S. Cooke, Portia Mutevedzi, Richard J. Lessells,
Marie-Louise Newell and Martin Dedicoat

Chapter 15   **Postoperative Adverse Outcomes in Intellectually Disabled Surgical Patients** 123
Jui-An Lin, Chien-Chang Liao, Chuen-Chau Chang,
Hang Chang and Ta-Liang Chen

Chapter 16   **Vitamin C: Intravenous use by Complementary and Alternative Medicine Practitioners and Adverse Effects** 128
Sebastian J. Padayatty, Andrew Y. Sun, Qi Chen, Michael Graham Espey,
Jeanne Drisko and Mark Levine

Chapter 17   **Efficacy of Short-Term High-Dose Statin in Preventing Contrast-Induced Nephropathy** 136
Yongchuan Li, Yawei Liu, Lili Fu, Changlin Mei and Bing Dai

Chapter 18   **Scoring Systems for Predicting Mortality after Liver Transplantation** 146
Heng-Chih Pan, Chang-Chyi Jenq, Wei-Chen Lee, Ming-Hung Tsai, Pei-Chun Fan,
Chih-Hsiang Chang, Ming-Yang Chang, Ya-Chung Tian, Cheng-Chieh Hung,
Ji-Tseng Fang, Chih-Wei Yang and Yung-Chang Chen

Chapter 19   **Intravascular Administration of Mannitol for Acute Kidney Injury Prevention** 156
Bo Yang, Jing Xu, Fengying Xu, Zui Zou, Chaoyang Ye,
Changlin Mei and Zhiguo Mao

Chapter 20   **Ischemic Acute Kidney Injury Perturbs Homeostasis of Serine Enantiomers in the Body Fluid in Mice: Early Detection of Renal Dysfunction Using the Ratio of Serine Enantiomers** 165
Jumpei Sasabe, Masataka Suzuki, Yurika Miyoshi, Yosuke Tojo, Chieko Okamura, Sonomi Ito, Ryuichi Konno, Masashi Mita, Kenji Hamase and Sadakazu Aiso

Chapter 21   **The Association between Contrast Dose and Renal Complications Post PCI across the Continuum of Procedural Estimated Risk** 174
Judith Kooiman, Milan Seth, David Share, Simon Dixon and Hitinder S. Gurm

Chapter 22   **Persistent Catheter-Related *Staphylococcus aureus* Bacteremia after Catheter Removal and Initiation of Antimicrobial Therapy** 180
Ki-Ho Park, Yu-Mi Lee, Hyo-Lim Hong, Tark Kim, Hyun Jung Park, So-Youn Park, Song Mi Moon, Yong Pil Chong, Sung-Han Kim, Sang-Oh Lee, Sang-Ho Choi, Jin-Yong Jeong, Mi-Na Kim, Jun Hee Woo and Yang Soo Kim

Chapter 23   **Terlipressin versus Norepinephrine in the Treatment of Hepatorenal Syndrome** 189
Antonio Paulo Nassar Junior, Alberto Queiroz Farias, Luiz Augusto Carneiro d' Albuquerque, Flair José Carrilho and Luiz Marcelo Sá Malbouisson

Permissions

List of Contributors

Index

Preface

Over the recent decade, advancements and applications have progressed exponentially. This has led to the increased interest in this field and projects are being conducted to enhance knowledge. The main objective of this book is to present some of the critical challenges and provide insights into possible solutions. This book will answer the varied questions that arise in the field and also provide an increased scope for furthering studies.

Renal failure refers to the medical condition in which the kidneys are no longer able to function. It is also called end-stage kidney disease. It can be classified into two types, namely, acute kidney failure and chronic kidney failure. Some of its common symptoms include vomiting, nocturia, more frequent urination or less frequent urination, difficulty in urination, blood in the urine, muscle cramps and foamy or bubbly urine. Acute kidney injury is usually caused by injuries, accidents, and drug overdoses. Some of the common causes of chronic kidney disease include high blood pressure, diabetes mellitus and polycystic kidney disease. Assessment of glomerular filtration rate is helpful in diagnosing renal failure. This book provides significant information about renal failure to help develop a good understanding of its causes, symptoms, diagnosis and treatment. It will also provide interesting topics for research, which interested readers can take up. For all those who are interested in renal failure, this book can prove to be an essential guide.

I hope that this book, with its visionary approach, will be a valuable addition and will promote interest among readers. Each of the authors has provided their extraordinary competence in their specific fields by providing different perspectives as they come from diverse nations and regions. I thank them for their contributions.

Editor

A Comparison of the Long-Term Effects of Lanthanum Carbonate and Calcium Carbonate on the Course of Chronic Renal Failure in Rats with Adriamycin-Induced Nephropathy

Tsuyoshi Takashima[1]*, Toru Sanai[2], Motoaki Miyazono[1], Makoto Fukuda[1], Tomoya Kishi[1], Yasunori Nonaka[3], Mai Yoshizaki[1], Sae Sato[1], Yuji Ikeda[1]

1 Department of Nephrology, Faculty of Medicine, Saga University, Saga, Japan, 2 Department of Nephrology, Fukumitsu Hospital, Fukuoka, Japan, 3 Department of Nephrology, Ureshino Medical Center, Ureshino, Japan

Abstract

Lanthanum carbonate (LA) is an effective phosphate binder. Previous study showed the phosphate-binding potency of LA was twice that of calcium carbonate (CA). No study in which LA and CA were given at an equivalent phosphate-binding potency to rats or humans with chronic renal failure for a long period has been reported to date. The objective of this study was to compare the phosphate level in serum and urine and suppression of renal deterioration during long-term LA and CA treatment when they were given at an equivalent phosphate-binding potency in rats with adriamycin (ADR)-induced nephropathy. Rats were divided into three groups: an untreated group (ADR group), a CA-treated (ADR-CA) group and a LA-treated (ADR-LA) group. The daily oral dose of LA was 1.0 g/kg/day and CA was 2.0 g/kg/day for 24 weeks. The serum phosphate was lower in the ADR-CA or ADR-LA group than in the ADR group and significantly lower in the ADR-CA group than in the ADR group at each point, but there were no significant differences between the ADR and ADR-LA groups. The serum phosphate was also lower in the ADR-CA group than in the ADR-LA group, and there was significant difference at week 8. The urinary phosphate was significantly lower in the ADR-CA group than in the ADR or ADR-LA group at each point. The urinary phosphate was also lower in the ADR-LA group than in the ADR group at each point, and significant difference at week 8. There were no significant differences in the serum creatinine or blood urea nitrogen among the three groups. In conclusion, this study indicated the phosphate-binding potency of LA isn't twice as strong as CA, and neither LA nor CA suppressed the progression of chronic renal failure in the serum creatinine and blood urea nitrogen, compared to the untreated group.

Editor: Cecilia Zazueta, Instituto Nacional de Cardiologia I. Ch., Mexico

Funding: This study was supported by a grant from Bayer Yakuhin, Ltd. (Osaka, Japan). The funder had no role in the study design, data collection and analysis, decision to publish or preparation of the manuscript.

Competing Interests: This study was supported by a grant from Bayer Yakuhin, Ltd. (Osaka, Japan). This does not alter the authors' adherence to all the PLOS ONE policies on sharing data and materials.

* E-mail: takashim@cc.saga-u.ac.jp

Introduction

Effective control of the phosphate overload in patients with chronic kidney disease (CKD) is now recognized as an important target for reducing the high mortality rate associated with this condition [1,2], and current practice guidelines recommend aggressive treatment of hyperphosphatemia to achieve lower serum phosphorus targets.

A low-phosphate diet has been shown to prevent the progression of experimental renal disease [3–5]. However, the administration of a low-phosphate diet is consistently associated with a decreased intake of protein, calories and other nutrients, the absence of which results in nutritional deficits, especially in cases of progressive renal disease with massive proteinuria.

Phosphate binders are administered in order to decrease the serum phosphate levels by adsorbing phosphate in the intestine. They bind phosphate, form insoluble products, and selectively suppress the intestinal absorption of phosphate without leading to a deficiency of other nutritional elements. Therefore, oral administration of the phosphate-binders may be utilized to prevent renal deterioration, without causing subsequent malnutrition. Lumlertgul et al. reported that a phosphate binder (dihydroxyaluminum aminoacetate) suppressed the progression of chronic renal failure (CRF) in rats with 5/6 nephrectomy [6]. Sanai et al. reported that calcium carbonate (CA) and aluminum hydroxide suppressed the progression of CRF in rats with adriamycin (ADR)-induced nephropathy [7]. ADR-induced nephropathy in rats is a commonly used model of chronic renal disease, characterized by persistent proteinuria and progressive reduction in renal function leading to terminal renal failure [8]. Morphological lesions resemble focal glomerular sclerosis. Epithelial degeneration develops as an initial lesion in the kidney, and progresses to irreversible glomerular sclerosis and tubulointerstitial changes [9].

Lanthanum carbonate (LA) is a calcium-free oral phosphate binder that can control hyperphosphatemia without adding to the patient's calcium load [10]. Previous studies have shown a high phosphate binding capacity of LA [11]. According to the study by Hutchison et al. of 800 hemodialysis patients who were randomized to receive either LA or CA, where the dose was titrated to achieve control of the serum phosphate level [12], the phosphate-binding potency of LA was twice as strong as that of CA at the same weight [13]. Hutchison et al. also reported that at a dose of 1.0 g/kg/day of LA rapidly reduced the mean urinary phosphate excretion and sustained the reduction to the end of the six-week treatment period much better than a dose of 1.0 g/kg/day of CA in rats with 5/6 nephrectomy [14].

To the best of our knowledge, no study in which LA and CA were given at an equivalent phosphate-binding potency in rats or humans with CRF for a long period has been reported to date. The objective of this study was to compare the long-term effects of equivalent doses (in terms of potency) of LA and CA in terms of controlling the serum phosphate level and suppressing the renal deterioration in rats with ADR-induced nephropathy.

Materials and Methods

Ethics Statement

All experiments were approved by the Animal Experimental Ethical Committee of Saga University (Permit Number: 24-042-0), and were conducted in compliance with our institutional guidelines and with international standards for the manipulation and care of laboratory animals. All of the surgeries were performed under diethyl ether anesthesia, and all efforts were made to minimize suffering.

Animal Model

ADR (2.5 mg/kg) was intravenously administered to male Sprague-Dawley rats (Charles River Breeding, Kanagawa, Japan). The rats, aged 10 weeks and weighing 330–400 g, were treated with ADR twice at a 20-day interval according to the method reported previously [8] (Figure 1). The rats were then randomly divided into three groups: a group without a phosphate binder (ADR group, n = 18), an ADR-CA-treated group (ADR-CA group, n = 18) and an ADR-LA-treated group (ADR-LA group, n = 18). LA (FOSRENOL, Bayer Yakuhin, Ltd., Osaka, Japan) or CA (precipitated calcium carbonate, Asahi Kasei Pharma Corp., Tokyo, Japan) was mixed with standard chow (MF, Oriental Yeast

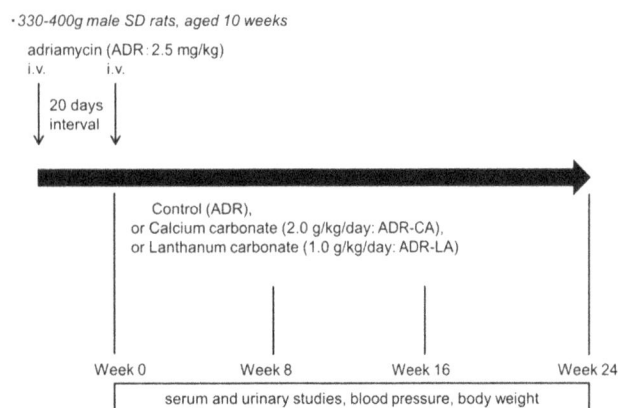

Figure 1. An outline of the experimental protocol. i.v.: intravenous injection.

Co., Ltd., Tokyo, Japan), containing 23.1% protein, 0.19% sodium, 1.07% calcium and 0.83% phosphorus, and 359 Cal/100 g. There were no significant differences among the groups. The phosphate binder treatments were started after the second administration of ADR (week 0). The daily dose of LA was 1.0 g/kg/day and that of CA was 2.0 g/kg/day throughout the experiment. The diet was adjusted to match that of the group with minimal ingestion, as determined at weekly intervals according to the consumption, in order to maintain the same calorie and protein intake in all groups. All groups had free access to tap water. The body weight, blood pressure, blood chemistry parameters and a 24-hour urinary collection were examined every eight weeks until week 24 after the second administration of ADR. The serum fibroblast growth factor (FGF)-23 levels and the serum parathyroid hormone (PTH) levels were determined at weeks 0, 8 and 24. The serum $1,25-(OH)_2$ vitamin D levels were determined at weeks 0 and 24. All surviving rats were sacrificed at week 24 and expression levels of Klotho in renal tissue were analyzed by real-time PCR.

Biochemical Analysis

The urinary protein from a 24-hour collection was measured using the pyrogallol red method. The urinary phosphate from the 24-hour collection was measured using the molybdate direct method, and the urinary calcium from a 24-hour collection was measured using the arsenazo III method. The systolic blood pressure was measured in the conscious state by the tail cuff method. Blood samples were drawn from a tail vein for determinations of the serum creatinine, phosphate, blood urea nitrogen (BUN) and total cholesterol level by enzymatic methods, the calcium level by use of orthocresolphthalein complex one, the total protein by the Biuret reaction, and albumin was detected by bromcresol green staining. The level of FGF-23 was determined by an ELISA kit (Kainos Laboratories, Inc., Tokyo, Japan). The level of serum PTH was measured with the rat PTH-EIA kit (Peninsula Laboratories, LLC., San Carlos, CA, USA). A radioimmunoassay kit (TFB, Inc., Tokyo, Japan) was used for the measurement of the serum $1,25-(OH)_2$ vitamin D.

Kidney

Kidneys were harvested and total RNA was isolated as earlier by RNeasy Protect Mini kit (QIAGEN K. K., Tokyo, Japan) using the manufacturer's protocol. Expression levels of Klotho were analyzed by real-time PCR using the manufacturer's protocol (Applied BioSystems, Inc.) and commercially available primers from Applied BioSystems, Inc. Glyceraldehyde 3-phosphate dehydrogenase (GAPDH) served as an internal control, and all results are expressed as the ratio of Klotho RNA/GAPDH. TaqMan Gene Expression Master Mix (Applied Biosystems, Inc., Carlsbad, CA, USA) was used to perform quantitative PCR. PCR conditions for all experiments were 2 minutes at $50°C$, 10 minutes at $95°C$, followed by 40 cycles of 15 seconds at $95°C$ and 1 minute at $60°C$. The data were collected and analyzed by the Step One Plus Real Time PCR System and software (Applied BioSystems). All primer sets were tested for specific amplification of mRNA by parallel analyses of controls that included omitting RT and resulted in no fluorescent signal detection. The $2^{-\Delta\Delta Ct}$ method described by Livak was used to analyze the data.

Statistical Analysis

Differences between multiple time points for each study group were determined by the Friedman test, followed by a Wilcoxon signed-rank test with Bonferroni correction. Comparisons between the study groups for each time point were assessed using a

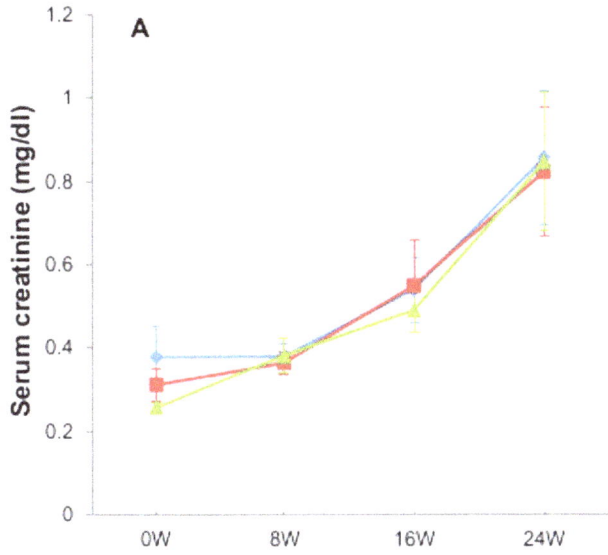

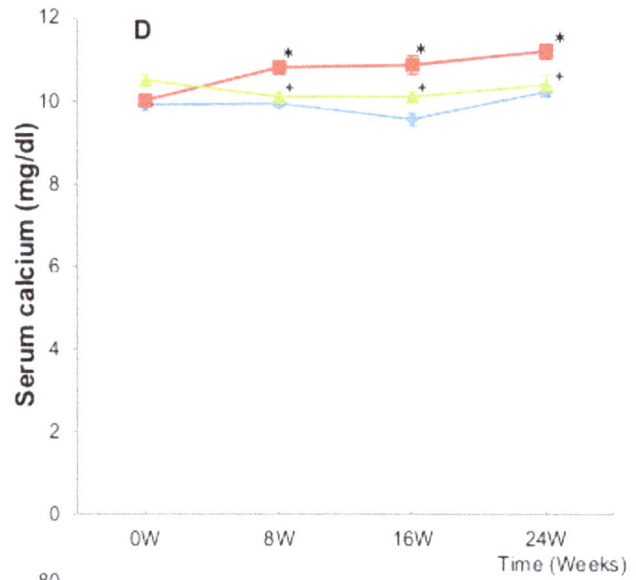

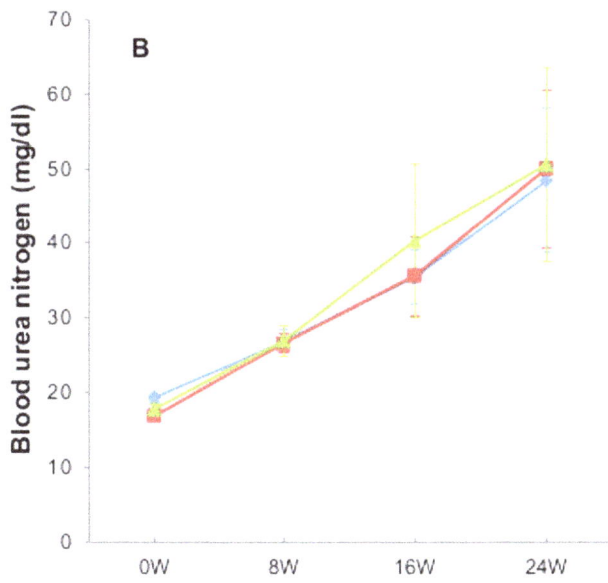

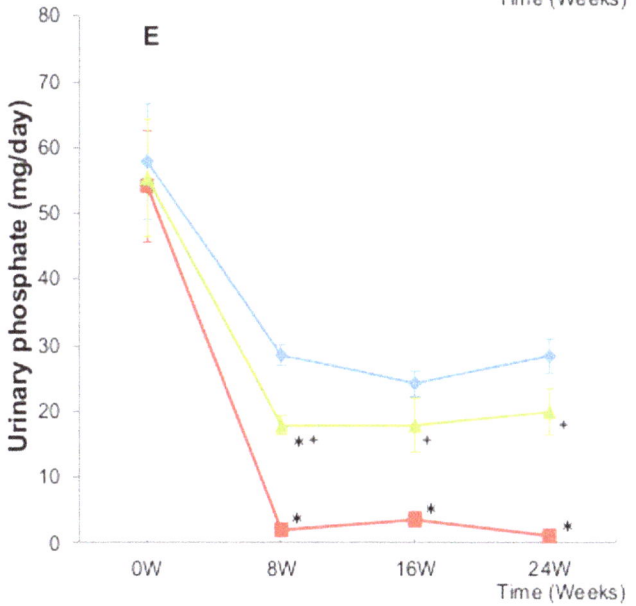

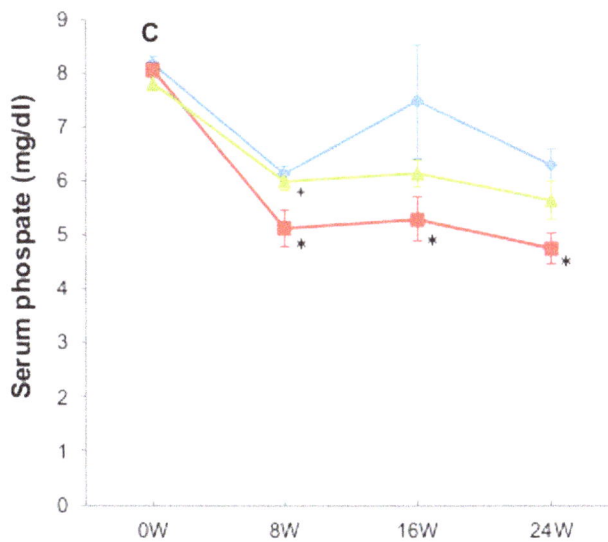

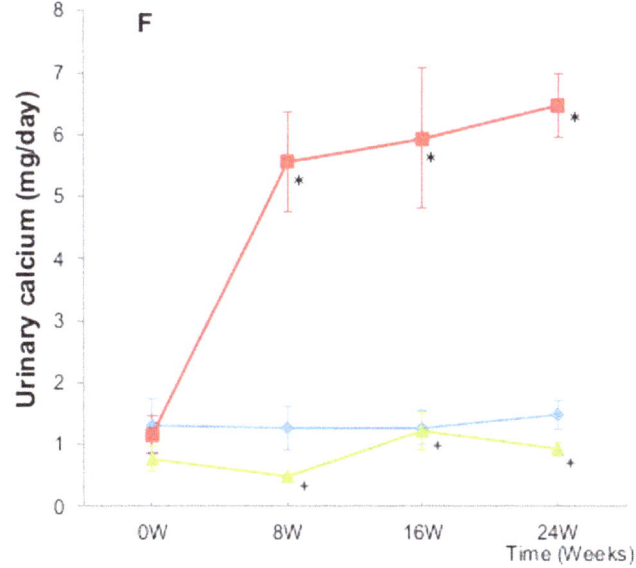

Figure 2. The serum and urine data. A: serum creatinine, B: blood urea nitrogen, C: serum phosphate, D: serum calcium, E: urinary phosphate, F: urinary calcium. The data are expressed as the means ± SEM. ◆ = ADR group, ■ = ADR-CA group, ▲ = ADR-LA group. *p<0.05 or less, vs. ADR group at the same time point, +p<0.05 or less vs. ADR-CA group at the same time point.

Kruskal-Wallis test, followed by a Mann-Witney U-test in combination with Bonferroni correction. A two-sided P-value was considered to be significant for values <0.05. The data are expressed as the means ± SD. All analyses were done using the SPSS 22.0 (IBM Japan, Tokyo, Japan).

Results

One of the eighteen rats died between weeks 8 and 16, and five rats died between weeks 16 and 24 in the ADR group. Five of the eighteen rats in the ADR-CA group died between weeks 16 and 24. Three of the eighteen rats died between weeks 8 and 16, and four rats died between weeks 16 and 24 in the ADR-LA group. All of the rats were considered to have died of uremia, because the daily food intake and body weight gradually decreased, and the serum creatinine level increased.

The serum creatinine and BUN levels increased progressively, but there were no significant differences among the three groups at any of the time points (Figures 2A, 2B).

The serum phosphate level was lower in the ADR-CA group and in the ADR-LA group compared to the ADR group at each point (Figure 2C). The serum phosphate level was significantly lower in the ADR-CA group than that in the ADR group at each point (p<0.05). However, while there were some differences in the serum phosphate level at some points in the ADR and ADR-LA groups, none of these differences was significant. The serum phosphate level was lower in the ADR-CA group compared to the ADR-LA group at each point, and there was significant difference at week 8 (p<0.05).

The serum calcium level in the ADR-CA group was significantly higher than that in the ADR group (p<0.01) or in the ADR-LA group (p<0.05) at each point (Figure 2D). In addition, there were no significant differences in the serum calcium level at any point between the ADR and ADR-LA groups.

The urinary phosphate excretion decreased to a negligible level in the ADR-CA group (Figure 2E). The urinary phosphate level was significantly lower in the ADR-CA group than that in the ADR group or in the ADR-LA group at each point (p<0.01). The urinary phosphate level was lower in the ADR-LA group than in the ADR group at each point, and there was significant difference at week 8 (p<0.01).

The urinary calcium level was significantly higher in the ADR-CA group than that in the ADR group or in the ADR-LA group at each point (p<0.01) (Figure 2F). There were no significant differences in the urinary calcium level at any point between the ADR and ADR-LA groups.

The other data are shown in Table 1. The body weight gradually increased in all of the groups, but there were no significant differences in body weight among the three groups at each point. A mild to moderate elevation in the systolic blood pressure was observed in all three groups, but there were no significant differences in the systolic blood pressure among the three groups at each point. In terms of the serum biochemical data (total protein, albumin, total cholesterol, PTH, and 1,25-$(OH)_2$ vitamin D), there were no significant differences among the three groups at each point. The serum FGF-23 level was lower in the ADR-CA group at weeks 8 and 24 than that in the ADR group or in the ADR-LA group, and was significantly lower in the ADR-CA group at week 8 than that in the ADR group (p<0.05). The

proteinuria increased in all three groups, but there were no significant differences among the three groups at any of the time points.

Expression level of Klotho in renal tissue was higher in the ADR-LA group than that in the ADR or in the ADR-CA group at week 24, and was 1.26±0.81 in the ADR group, 1.37±0.64 in the ADR-CA group and 2.48±0.88 in the ADR-LA group (Table 2). However, there were no significant differences in expression level of Klotho among the three groups (p = 0.059).

Discussion

This animal study directly compared the long-term effects of LA and CA at an equivalent phosphate binding potency for controlling the serum phosphate level and suppressing the renal deterioration in rats with ADR-induced nephropathy.

Patients who are pre-dialysis without end-stage renal disease maintain their urine output and the ability to excrete a proportion of any phosphate that is absorbed. In the "steady-state" condition, the amount excreted in the urine is proportional to the amount absorbed. As a result, the measurement of the urinary phosphate excretion can be used as a marker of intestinal phosphate absorption, and thus, as an indicator of the phosphate binding efficacy, even when there is no change in the serum phosphate level [15–19].

The results of the serum and urinary phosphate in this study suggest that the phosphate binding potency of LA is not twice as strong as that CA at the same weight. As mentioned above, Hutchison et al. compared LA and CA in 800 hemodialysis patients [12], and estimated that the phosphate-binding potency of LA is twice as strong as CA at the same weight [13]. However, D'Haese et al. compared LA and CA in 98 hemodialysis patients [20], and estimated that the phosphate-binding potency of LA was 1.6 times as strong as CA at the same weight [13]. The present study supports the latter of a lower potency for LA. There may also be differences in potency between humans and rats.

This study did not indicate that either of the phosphate-binders, LA and CA, could suppress the progression of CRF, based on the serum creatinine, BUN levels, and the other parameters compared to the untreated group. As mentioned above, Sanai et al. reported in a study that used a similar protocol to the present study that CA suppressed the progression of CRF in rats with ADR-induced nephropathy [7], but the daily dose of CA was 6.0 g/kg/day throughout their experiment, and they first noted a significant difference in serum creatinine compared to the ADR group at week 34, which was longer than the duration of the present study. We believe that if we administered a higher concentration of CA or LA to rats for a longer period, they might suppress the progression of CRF, as detected by changes in the serum creatinine, BUN levels, and the other parameters compared to the ADR group.

A possible mechanism for the decrease in renal deterioration resulting from phosphate restriction may be either the prevention of metastatic calcification or a decreased energy requirement in renal tissue. Nephrocalcinosis with chronic interstitial inflammation is known to accelerate the deterioration of renal function and the progression of renal disease [21,22]. The renal calcium content increases concomitantly with decreased renal function, a fact which has been demonstrated in biopsy materials from a wide

Table 1. The body weight, blood pressure, and biochemical data in the different groups.

Index	Group	Week 0	Week 8	Week 16	Week 24
Body weight (g)	**ADR**	445.3±40.9	520.3±64.0[a]	521.7±91.3[a]	578.0±81.8[a, c]
	ADR-CA	437.1±37.5	485.4±55.0[a]	491.1±66.8[a, b]	508.9±58.2[a, c]
	ADR-LA	440.2±28.4	495.9±48.0[a]	510.7±57.6[a, b]	537.3±49.3[a]
Systolic blood pressure (mmHg)	**ADR**	119.0±16.5	140.4±17.6	147.3±12.8[a]	140.3±18.5
	ADR-CA	124.0±15.5	139.2±16.9	144.1±20.2	153.5±16.4[a]
	ADR-LA	121.2±19.8	142.5±18.3	137.8±18.5	146.1±21.0
Serum creatinine (mg/dL)	**ADR**	0.38±0.36	0.38±0.14[a]	0.54±0.31[a]	0.86±0.56[a, b, c]
	ADR-CA	0.31±0.19	0.37±0.14	0.55±0.44	0.82±0.54[a, b, c]
	ADR-LA	0.26±0.04	0.38±0.20	0.49±0.20[a]	0.85±0.50[a, b]
Blood urea nitrogen (mg/dL)	**ADR**	19.4±2.6	26.9±7.6	35.4±13.8[a, b]	48.4±33.4[a, b]
	ADR-CA	16.9±2.1	26.6±6.1[a]	35.7±21.7[a]	50.0±38.1[a, c]
	ADR-LA	17.8±0.5	27.0±10.2	40.3±39.8[a]	50.5±43.0[a, b]
Serum phosphate (mg/dL)	**ADR**	8.17±0.74	6.13±0.64[a]	7.49±4.20[a]	6.30±1.04[a]
	ADR-CA	8.06±0.52	5.13±1.62*, a	5.29±1.70*, a	4.75±1.00*, a
	ADR-LA	7.81±0.65	6.00±0.79+, a	6.14±0.99[a]	5.64±1.16[a]
Serum calcium (mg/dL)	**ADR**	9.90±0.64	9.93±0.32	9.55±0.67	10.21±0.47
	ADR-CA	10.0±0.68	10.80±0.77*	10.86±0.93*	11.19±0.73*
	ADR-LA	10.50±0.68	10.09±0.52+	10.08±0.59+	10.38±0.89+
Serum total protein (g/dL)	**ADR**	6.66±0.59	8.37±2.67	7.23±1.15[a]	6.81±0.43
	ADR-CA	6.83±0.62	8.10±1.70	8.01±2.00	6.94±0.51
	ADR-LA	6.65±0.46	7.81±1.51	7.97±1.98	7.21±2.52
Serum albumin (g/dL)	**ADR**	4.35±0.24	2.92±0.35[a]	2.95±0.32[a]	2.95±0.23[a]
	ADR-CA	4.34±0.30	2.90±0.49[a]	2.82±0.35[a]	2.99±0.53[a]
	ADR-LA	4.42±0.23	2.85±0.31[a]	2.89±0.35[a]	2.95±0.37[a]
Serum total cholesterol (mg/dL)	**ADR**	69.8±10.0	402.1±184.1[a]	373.6±169.5[a]	357.0±143.1[a]
	ADR-CA	71.3±11.1	422.1±216.1[a]	454.5±173.0[a]	377.2±88.1[a]
	ADR-LA	71.1±11.0	442.1±208.6[a]	457.9±240.8[a]	348.4±171.7[a]
Serum FGF-23 (pg/mL)	**ADR**	403.2±107.2	620.5±117.9[a]	-	777.6±69.0[a, b]
	ADR-CA	416.4±90.4	444.2±123.5*	-	629.2±293.8[a, b]
	ADR-LA	371.9±111.6	544.0±190.5	-	780.0±128.4[a, b]
Serum PTH (pg/mL)	**ADR**	20.5±0.6	56.8±80.1	-	92.2±42.5
	ADR-CA	49.5±58.3	75.3±37.9	-	117.2±102.2
	ADR-LA	20.5±0.6	68.8±58.1	-	102.3±106.7
Serum 1,25-(OH)2 vitamin D (pg/mL)	**ADR**	275.9±119.3	-	-	81.9±55.3[a]
	ADR-CA	211.7±72.9	-	-	67.5±13.0[a]
	ADR-LA	334.1±132.5	-	-	103.1±52.3[a]
Urinary phosphate (mg/day)	**ADR**	57.9±42.9	28.5±4.4	24.2±7.5	28.4±9.4
	ADR-CA	54.2±41.5	1.97±2.69*, a	3.54±4.93*, a	1.12±1.78*, a
	ADR-LA	55.4±43.3	17.8±7.2*, +	17.9±16.2+	19.9±11.7+
Urinary calcium (mg/day)	**ADR**	1.32±1.46	1.27±1.22	1.27±0.96	1.49±0.82*, a
	ADR-CA	1.16±1.11	5.56±2.89*, a	5.93±4.07*, a	6.47±1.89*, a
	ADR-LA	0.77±0.68	0.49±0.11+	1.22±1.06+	0.94±0.37+, b
Urinary protein (mg/day)	**ADR**	52.1±75.3	491.4±163.1[a]	443.1±241.2[a]	504.5±111.3[a]
	ADR-CA	58.2±82.9	400.4±146.5[a]	404.4±123.5[a]	439.6±122.9[a]
	ADR-LA	49.6±62.4	459.3±191.9[a]	515.7±191.7[a]	456.1±118.3[a]

The data are expressed as the means ± SD.
*$p < 0.05$ vs. ADR group at the same time point,
+$p < 0.05$ vs. ADR-CA group at the same time point.
[a]$p < 0.05$ vs. Week 0 values of the same group, [b]$p < 0.05$ vs. Week 8 values of the same group, [c]$p < 0.05$ vs. Week 16 values of the same group.
Abbreviations: FGF-23, fibroblast growth factor-23; PTH, parathyroid hormone.

Table 2. Klotho expression in the kidney at week 24.

	Group	Week 24
Klotho (RNA/GAPDH)	**ADR**	1.26±0.81
	ADR-CA	1.37±0.64
	ADR-LA	2.48±0.88

The data are expressed as the means ± SD.
There were no significant differences among the three groups.
Abbreviations: GAPDH, Glyceraldehyde 3-phosphate dehydrogenase.

variety of renal diseases [23]. Elevated serum phosphate seems to be the most important factor for initiating the sequence necessary for the development of nephrocalcinosis. Under these conditions, preventing phosphate retention can ameliorate the metastatic calcification through the suppression of secondary hyperparathyroidism and reduction in the calcium-phosphate product [3,4]. The energy requirement increases in the remnant nephrons in rats with renal mass reduction, a fact which was considered to be a cause of renal injury [24]. Israel et al. also suggested that the elevation of energy metabolism was closely related to the destruction of damaged cells [25]. Prolonged phosphate depletion is known to change the renal energy metabolism. By reducing the energy requirement, the phosphate binder might exert beneficial effects on the damaged epithelial cells.

LA and CA are both commonly used to reduce the serum phosphate level during the treatment of CRF. However, CA is associated with a risk of hypercalcemia. In this study, the serum calcium level in the ADR-CA group was significantly higher than that in the ADR group or in the ADR-LA group at each point. Hypercalcemia initially leads to impaired urinary concentration [26], then to reduced renal plasma flow and glomerular filtration rates, and finally results in multiple functional and structural derangements of the kidneys. Calcium deposition in renal tissue is also a factor stimulating renal damage [27]. In addition, mineral and bone disorders in CKD patients, along with the use of calcium-based phosphate binders, may result in vascular calcification and an associated increase in mortality due to cardiovascular diseases. On the other hand, LA is associated with reduced hypercalcemic adverse events compared to calcium-based binders, although no superior effects with regard to the cardiovascular diseases have been reported so far that can justify further widespread utilization of this agent over CA [28]. In this study,

expression level of Klotho in renal tissue was higher in the ADR-LA group than that in the ADR or in the ADR-CA group at week 24, but there were no significant differences among the three groups. We think there are possibilities that if we administered a higher concentration of LA (at equivalent phosphate-binding doses of LA and CA) to rats, there might be significant differences between the ADR-LA group and the other groups in expression level of Klotho, and keeping the high levels of Klotho expression in the ADR-LA group compared to the other groups suggests that LA without adding to the calcium load has a good influence on decreasing mortality.

In conclusion, this study indicated that the phosphate binding potency of LA is less than twice as strong as CA at the same weight, and neither LA nor CA suppressed the progression of CRF, as determined by the serum creatinine and BUN levels, compared to untreated rats with ADR-induced nephropathy. However, LC is a very effective phosphate binder, and previous studies have shown a very high phosphate-binding capacity (> 97%) [11,13] (Table 3), as well as low gastrointestinal absorption of LA, without serious toxic side effects [29–33]. Clinicians should consider the dose-response relationship for the different phosphate binders when reviewing the doses or choices of binders. A direct comparison of the binding capacities of the currently available phosphate-binders would be useful to guide clinical practice.

Author Contributions

Conceived and designed the experiments: TT TS MM TK YI. Performed the experiments: TT MM MF YN MY SS YI. Analyzed the data: TT TS MM YI. Contributed reagents/materials/analysis tools: TT TS MM YI. Wrote the paper: TT.

Table 3. The relative phosphate-binding coefficients for various phosphate binders.

Phosphate binder	Relative phosphate-binding coefficient per gram of compound
Calcium carbonate (index value)	1.0
Calcium acetate	1.0
Magnesium carbonate (anhydrous weight)	1.7
"Heavy" magnesium carbonate (hydrated weight)	1.3
Aluminum hydroxide	1.5
Aluminum carbonate	1.9
Sevelamer (carbonate or hydrochloride)	0.75
Lanthanum carbonate	2.0

Reproduced from Daugirdas JT et al. [13].

References

1. Block GA, Klassen PS, Lazarus JM, Ofsthun N, Lowrie EG, et al. (2004) Mineral metabolism, mortality, and morbidity in maintenance hemodialysis. J Am Soc Nephrol 15: 2208–2218.
2. Danese MD, Belozeroff V, Smirnakis K, Rothman KJ (2008) Consistent control of mineral and bone disorder in incident hemodialysis patients. Clin J Am Soc Nephrol 3: 1423–1429.
3. Ibels LS, Alfrey AC, Haut L, Huffer WE (1978) Preservation of function in experimental renal disease by dietary restriction of phosphate. N Engl J Med 298: 122–126.
4. Karlinsky ML, Haut L, Buddington B, Schrier NA, Alfrey AC (1980) Preservation of renal function in experimental glomerulonephritis. Kidney Int 17: 293–302.
5. Laouari D, Kleinknecht C, Cournot-Witmer G, Habib R, Mounier F, et al. (1982) Beneficial effect of low phosphorus diet in uraemic rats: a reappraisal. Clin Sci (Lond) 63: 539–548.
6. Lumlertgul D, Burke TJ, Gillum DM, Alfrey AC, Harris DC, et al. (1986) Phosphate depletion arrests progression of chronic renal failure independent of protein intake. Kidney Int 29: 658–666.
7. Sanai T, Okuda S, Motomura K, Onoyama K, Fujishima M (1989) Effect of phosphate binders on the course of chronic renal failure in rats with focal glomerular sclerosis. Nephron 51: 530–535.
8. Okuda S, Oh Y, Tsuruda H, Onoyama K, Fujimi S, et al. (1986) Adriamycin-induced nephropathy as a model of chronic progressive glomerular disease. Kidney Int 29: 502–510.
9. Bertani T, Cutillo F, Zoja C, Broggini M, Remuzzi G (1986) Tubulo-interstitial lesions mediate renal damage in adriamycin glomerulopathy. Kidney Int 30: 488–496.
10. Persy VP, Behets GJ, Bervoets AR, De Broe ME, D'Haese PC (2006) Lanthanum: a safe phosphate binder. Semin Dial 19: 195–199.
11. Behets GJ, Dams G, Vercauteren SR, Damment SJ, Bouillon R, et al. (2004) Does the phosphate binder lanthanum carbonate affect bone in rats with chronic renal failure? J Am Soc Nephrol 15: 2219–2228.
12. Hutchison AJ, Maes B, Vanwalleghem J, Asmus G, Mohamed E, et al. (2005) Efficacy, tolerability, and safety of lanthanum carbonate in hyperphosphatemia: a 6-month, randomized, comparative trial versus calcium carbonate. Nephron Clin Pract 100: c8–19.
13. Daugirdas JT, Finn WF, Emmett M, Chertow GM (2011) The phosphate binder equivalent dose. Semin Dial 24: 41–49.
14. Hutchison AJ (2004) Improving phosphate-binder therapy as a way forward. Nephrol Dial Transplant 19 Suppl 1: i19–24.
15. Russo D, Miranda I, Ruocco C, Battaglia Y, Buonanno E, et al. (2007) The progression of coronary artery calcification in predialysis patients on calcium carbonate or sevelamer. Kidney Int 72: 1255–1261.
16. Burke SK, Slatopolsky EA, Goldberg DI (1997) RenaGel, a novel calcium- and aluminium-free phosphate binder, inhibits phosphate absorption in normal volunteers. Nephrol Dial Transplant 12: 1640–1644.
17. Sprague SM, Abboud H, Qiu P, Dauphin M, Zhang P, et al. (2009) Lanthanum carbonate reduces phosphorus burden in patients with CKD stages 3 and 4: a randomized trial. Clin J Am Soc Nephrol 4: 178–185.
18. Gonzalez-Parra E, Gonzalez-Casaus ML, Galan A, Martinez-Calero A, Navas V, et al. (2011) Lanthanum carbonate reduces FGF23 in chronic kidney disease Stage 3 patients. Nephrol Dial Transplant 26: 2567–2571.
19. Pennick M, Poole L, Dennis K, Smyth M (2012) Lanthanum carbonate reduces urine phosphorus excretion: evidence of high-capacity phosphate binding. Ren Fail 34: 263–270.
20. D'Haese PC, Spasovski GB, Sikole A, Hutchison A, Freemont TJ, et al. (2003) A multicenter study on the effects of lanthanum carbonate (Fosrenol) and calcium carbonate on renal bone disease in dialysis patients. Kidney Int Suppl: S73–78.
21. Klahr S, Buerkert J, Purkerson ML (1983) Role of dietary factors in the progression of chronic renal disease. Kidney Int 24: 579–587.
22. Walser M, Mitch WE, Collier VU (1979) The effect of nutritional therapy on the course of chronic renal failure. Clin Nephrol 11: 66–70.
23. Gimenez LF, Solez K, Walker WG (1987) Relation between renal calcium content and renal impairment in 246 human renal biopsies. Kidney Int 31: 93–99.
24. Katz AI, Epstein FH (1968) Physiologic role of sodium-potassium-activated adenosine triphosphatase in the transport of cations across biologic membranes. N Engl J Med 278: 253–261.
25. Israel Y, Videla L, Fernandez-Videla V, Bernstein J (1975) Effects of chronic ethanol treatment and thyroxine administration on ethanol metabolism and liver oxidative capacity. J Pharmacol Exp Ther 192: 565–574.
26. Serros ER, Kirschenbaum MA (1981) Prostaglandin-dependent polyuria in hypercalcemia. Am J Physiol 241: F224–230.
27. Lins LE (1978) Reversible renal failure caused by hypercalcemia. A retrospective study. Acta Med Scand 203: 309–314.
28. Spasovski G (2008) New strategies in treatment of mineral and bone disorders and associated cardiovascular disease in patients with chronic kidney disease. Recent Pat Cardiovasc Drug Discov 3: 222–228.
29. Damment SJ (2011) Pharmacology of the phosphate binder, lanthanum carbonate. Ren Fail 33: 217–224.
30. Chiang SS, Chen JB, Yang WC (2005) Lanthanum carbonate (Fosrenol) efficacy and tolerability in the treatment of hyperphosphatemic patients with end-stage renal disease. Clin Nephrol 63: 461–470.
31. Hutchison AJ, Maes B, Vanwalleghem J, Asmus G, Mohamed E, et al. (2006) Long-term efficacy and tolerability of lanthanum carbonate: results from a 3-year study. Nephron Clin Pract 102: c61–71.
32. Finn WF (2006) Lanthanum carbonate versus standard therapy for the treatment of hyperphosphatemia: safety and efficacy in chronic maintenance hemodialysis patients. Clin Nephrol 65: 191–202.
33. Hutchison AJ, Barnett ME, Krause R, Kwan JT, Siami GA (2008) Long-term efficacy and safety profile of lanthanum carbonate: results for up to 6 years of treatment. Nephron Clin Pract 110: c15–23.

Shedding Light on the Chemical Diversity of Ectopic Calcifications in Kidney Tissues: Diagnostic and Research Aspects

Arnaud Dessombz[1]*, Dominique Bazin[1], Paul Dumas[2], Christophe Sandt[2], Josep Sule-Suso[3], Michel Daudon[4]

1 Laboratoire de Physique des Solides, Bat. 510, Université Paris Sud, Orsay, France, 2 Synchrotron SOLEIL, L'Orme des Merisiers, Saint-Aubin - BP 48, Gif-sur-Yvette, France, 3 Cancer Centre, University Hospital of North Staffordshire, Newcastle Road, Stoke-on-Trent, Staffordshire, United Kingdom, 4 AP-HP, Hôpital Tenon, Service d'Exploration Fonctionnelle, Paris, France

Abstract

In most industrialized countries, different epidemiologic studies show that chronic renal failure is dramatically increasing. Such major public health problem is a consequence of acquired systemic diseases such as type II diabetes, which is now the first cause for end stage renal failure. Furthermore, lithogenic diseases may also induce intratubular crystallization, which may finally result in end-stage renal failure (ESRF). Up to now, such rare diseases are often misdiagnosed. In this study, based on twenty four biopsies, we show that SR µFTIR (Synchrotron Radiation-µFourier transform infrared) spectroscopy constitutes a significant opportunity to characterize such pathological µcalcifications giving not only their chemical composition but also their spatial distribution in the tissues. This experimental approach offers new opportunities to the clinicians to describe at the cell level the physico-chemical processes leading to the formation of the pathological calcifications which lead to ESRF.

Editor: Niels Olsen Saraiva Câmara, Universidade de Sao Paulo, Brazil

Funding: This work was supported by proposal 20100039 for Synchrotron experiments. This proposal was provided by Synchrotron SOLEIL. It was also supported by the physic and chemistry institutes of CNRS (Centre National de la Recherche Scientifique) and by an Agence Nationale de la Recheche contract (grant number: ANR-09-BLAN-0120-02). The funders had no role in study design, data collection and analysis, decision to publish, or preparation of the manuscript. All the supporters have no commercial interests.

Competing Interests: The authors have declared that no competing interests exist.

* E-mail: arnaud.dessombz@u-psud.fr

Introduction

Chronic renal failure is increasing in most industrialized countries as a consequence of acquired systemic diseases such as type II diabetes, which is now the first cause for end stage renal failure [1]. A number of other causes may be responsible for the loss of kidney function and tubular interstitial nephritis, but they are less frequent [2,3]. Among them, lithogenic diseases may induce intratubular crystallization, which may finally result in end-stage renal failure (ESRF). The diagnosis of such pathological conditions is of a prime importance before kidney transplantation in order to treat efficiently the disease and protect the grafted kidney against recurrence of crystallization. Unfortunately, such rare diseases are often misdiagnosed. The main consequence in affected patients is the progressive degradation of the kidney function which ends up in dialysis [4]. Often, crystals are found in kidney biopsies performed in order to understand the mechanism of the loss of renal function. However, only few histochemical tests are available to attempt an identification of the crystals. Moreover, in some cases, common crystals such as calcium oxalate monohydrate may be present as a consequence of renal failure, but they are not involved in the kidney loss. For these reasons, it is of clinical importance to accurately identify crystals found in the tissue as they can help to early characterization of a disease, which may be efficiently treated by specific drugs. To the best of our knowledge, very few papers have focussed on such subject and only few crystalline phases have been already reported [5,6].

The aim of this work is to emphasize the chemical diversity of ectopic calcifications present in kidney tissue. In some cases, crystals in tissues are very tiny and classical FTIR microscopy is not sensitive enough to identify their chemical composition. In those cases, Synchrotron Radiation–Fourier Transform Infrared microspectroscopy (µSR-FTIR) can be performed, such technique being able to collect infrared spectra on microscopic-sized minerals present in biopsies. Combined with optical microscopic and raster scanning, chemical cartography obtained with SR-spectroscopy can be associated to an optical image. This experimental configuration allowed us to study different biopsies. Such information regarding the chemical composition of ectopic calcifications will provide insight into the mechanisms leading to the loss of the kidney function.

Materials and Methods

Samples

Twenty-four kidney biopsies were investigated. The biological samples came from Necker Hospital (Paris- France). Five microns slices of the biopsies were deposited on low-e microscope slides (MirrIR, Kevley Technologies, Tienta Sciences, Indianapolis). For tissue embedded in paraffin, the paraffin was chemically removed

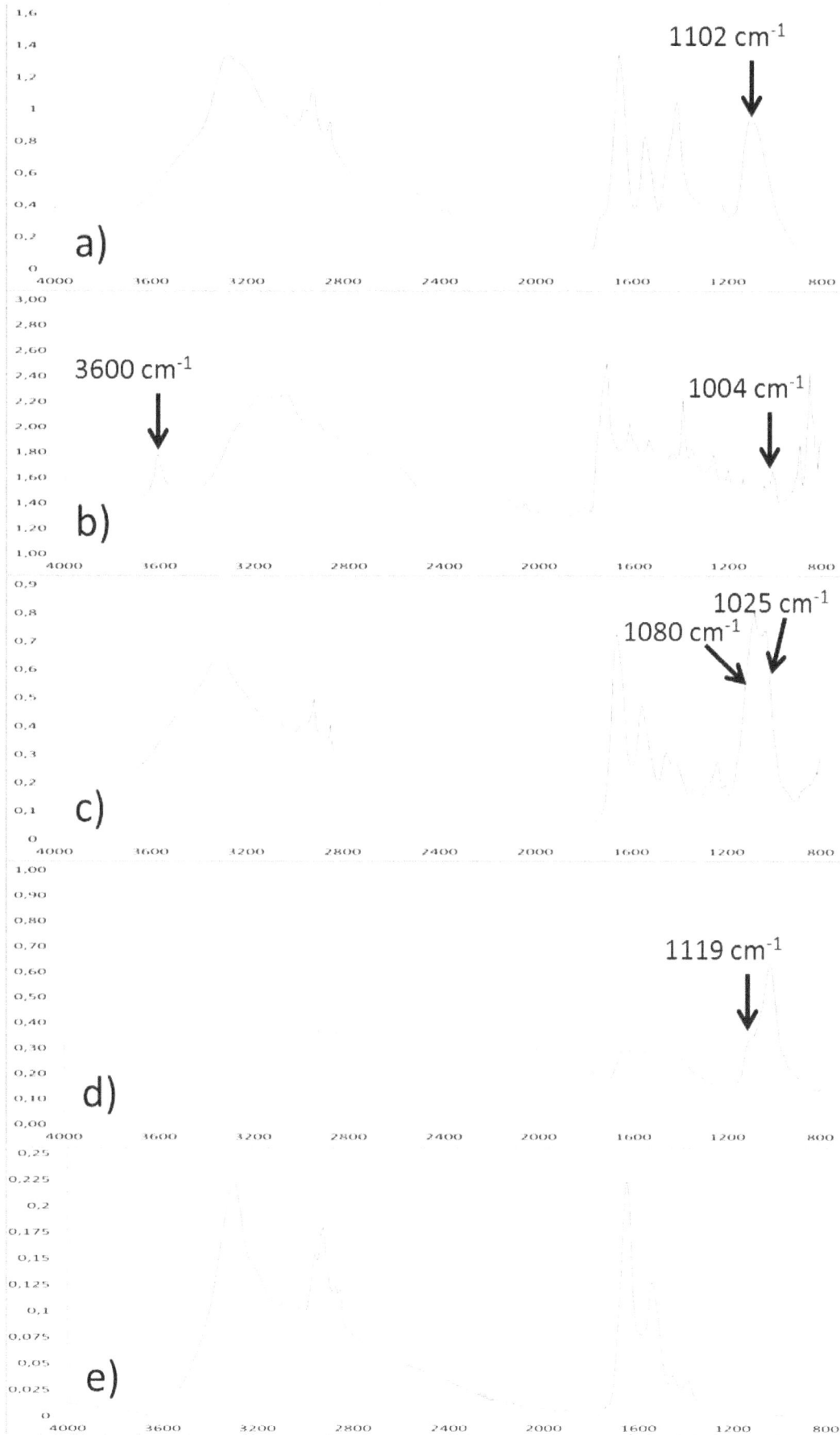

Figure 1. Selected examples of infrared spectra from biopsies. a) Amorphous silica identified by a band at 1102 cm^{-1}, b) sodium hydrogen urate monohydrate identified by specific bands at 3600 and 1004 cm^{-1}, c) several calcium phosphates including whitlockite (peaks at 1080, 1025 cm^{-1} and associated shoulders, d) octacalcium phosphate and carbapatite, identified by a shoulder at 1119 cm^{-1}, e) normal tissue, with signal of water (3300 cm^{-1} and peaks around 1600 cm^{-1}) and proteins (peaks at 2900 cm^{-1}).

in order to improve the crystal detection under the microscope. Ethical approval was obtained by the ethical committee of Necker Hospital for this study. Each sample was only named by a study number, without indication of the name of the patient or potential identification data. The ethical committee of Necker Hospital had approved this consent procedure.

Synchrotron FTIR microspectroscopy

The FTIR measurements were carried out at SOLEIL-Synchrotron (St Aubin-Gif sur Yvette, France) on the SMIS beamline [7]. The IR microspectroscopic mappings were collected in reflection mode using an Infrared microscope (Nicplan-Thermo Nicolet) coupled to a FTIR spectrometer (Magma 550-Thermo-Nicolet). The IR microscope is equipped with a motorized sample stage (precision 1 μm) and a liquid nitrogen cooled mercury cadmium telluride (MCT- 250 μm) detector. Most of the analysis and maps presented here were achieved with a projected area on the sample of 6×6 μm^2 and a step size of 6 μm, and each spectrum was acquired after 64 accumulations at 8 cm^{-1}

spectral resolution. Data acquisition and processing was performed using Omnic software (Version 7.4, Thermo-Scientific). The compounds were identified by comparing them to reference spectra [8].

Results

Selected examples of infrared spectra from biopsies are presented in Figure 1. Due to the high brilliance of the synchrotron source, the signal to noise ratio is excellent. Taking advantage of the small size of the probe, it was possible to select a small area of the biopsy for infrared spectra collection and thus to obtain a high quality spectrum of the crystals. Several chemical phases have been identified including amorphous silica through its infrared band at 1102 cm^{-1} (Figure 1a), sodium hydrogen urate monohydrate through its specific bands at 3600 and 1004 cm^{-1} (Figure 1b), and several calcium phosphates including whitlockite (peaks at 1080, 1025 cm^{-1} and associated shoulders, Figure 1c), octacalcium phosphate and carbapatite (Figure 1d).

Table 1. Different chemical phases identified in this study.

Samples	Sex–age (years)	Clinical data	Chemical phase identified
B85	M - 33	Acute renal failure (ARF)	Methyl-1 uric acid
B162	M - 72	Chronic renal failure (CRF)	Whewellite >>Weddellite
B163	M - 72	End stage renal failure (ESRF)	Whewellite
B164	M	Renal papilla	Carbapatite >> amorphous carbonated calcium phosphate (ACCP)
B165	M	Renal papilla	Sodium hydrogen urate monohydrate, Carbapatite and Whitlockite
B166	F - 53	CRF	Dihydroxyadenine
B167	M	ARF	Whewellite
B170	F - 39	CRF	Proteins (amylose)
B171	M - 58	CRF	Whewellite
B173	M - 48	CRF	Carbapatite+whewellite
B174	M - 50	ARF	Proteins
B175	M - 73	CRF, hypercalcemia	Octacalcium phosphate pentahydrate
B176	M - 66	CRF	Whewellite
B177	F - 39	Diabetes - CRF	Silicium dioxide (amorphous Silica)
B178	M - 55	ARF	Dihydroxyadenine
B179	M - 48	ESRF => Kidney transplantation (KT) => CRF	Dihydroxyadenine
B180*	M – 51	ESRF => KT => CRF	Dihydroxyadenine
B181**	M - 51	ESRF => KT => CRF	Dihydroxyadenine
B182	M - 26	ESRF => KT => CRF	Carbapatite and octacalcium phosphate pentahydrate
B183	F - 52	Diabetes => ESRF => KT => CMV infection =>ARF	Foscarnet and carbapatite
B184	M - 40	ESRF => KT	Whewellite
B189	F	Diabetes => ESRF => KT => CRF	Whewellite
B191	M - 74	ESRF => KT => CRF	Calcite, whewellite
B192	F - 68	CRF, hypercalcemia	Carbapatite, amorphous calcium phosphate

*Two years after kidney transplantation.
**Five years after kidney transplantation; same patient as for B180. Both biopsies were received in the same time.

All the results are gathered in Table 1. Twelve crystalline species were identified and in two cases, precipitates of proteins in tubular lumens were observed. Among crystalline compounds, calcium oxalate was observed commonly as whewellite and in one case as weddellite, which was found as a minor phase in a biopsy containing large amounts of whewellite. Several calcium phosphates were identified: the most common phase was carbapatite. Amorphous carbonated calcium phosphate (ACCP), octacalcium phosphate pentahydrate (OCP) and whitlockite were observed more scarcely. In one sample, some crystals of calcite were observed in association with whewellite. Among the other crystalline species, several purines were identified: sodium hydrogen urate monohydrate, dihydroxyadenine and methyl-1 uric acid. Lastly, foscarnet, a drug used against cytomegalovirus infection, was found in glomeruli in one patient.

By performing infrared mapping of selected areas of the biopsy, we were able to identify at least 2 different crystalline species in the same sample for 7 biopsies (27%), example in Figure 2 shows a representative example and even three compounds in one case.

Finally, in Figure 3, an optical image of a kidney biopsy shows the glomerulus containing very refringent crystals and the proximal tubules close to the glomerulus, in which pathological deposits were also observed (Fig. 3a). The small size of the probe allowed us to characterize separately the phases deposited in the glomerulus and in the wall of the tubules. The crystals agglomerated in the glomerulus were identified as sodium foscarnet (Fig. 3b). In contrast, deposits within in the cells of the proximal tubules were made of apatite (Fig. 3c).

Discussion

Crystal deposits within the kidney tissue may occur as a consequence of genetic disorders such as primary hyperoxaluria, adenine phosphoribosyltransferase deficiency, distal renal tubular acidosis, Dent's disease, acquired diseases such as primary hyperparathyroidism, Sjögren's syndrome or intoxication with ethylene glycol which leads to renal failure due to calcium salts deposition.

Classical characterisation of intratissular calcification performed at the hospital is based on tissue coloration with von Kossa and alizarin dyes. These methods help to identified Ca^{2+} oxalate and Ca^{2+} phosphate deposits but are not able to separate whewellite and weddellite or the different Ca^{2+} phosphates namely whitlockite, brushite or apatite.

Through classical FTIR investigation of 25 biopsies, Estepa-Maurice, et al. have underlined the presence of seven chemical phases (whewellite, weddellite, carbapatite, anhydrous uric acid, brushite, dihydroxyadenine and 4′-hydroxytriamterene sulfate) [6]. Thanks to the high flux of synchrotron radiation, micrometer scale calcifications have been characterized. This technique was especially required for analysis of very small crystals (less than 10 μm). Previous experiments [6] were performed on larger crystals (more than 15 μm). Another advantage of synchrotron radiation was its very high signal-to-noise ratio, since such measurements could be the base for a medical diagnosis. Samples could be sent to synchrotrons and that once specific markers are found, then benchtop spectrometers can be used for next measurements. A striking point of our investigation comes from the fact that six new chemical phases have been identified including amorphous silica, sodium hydrogen urate, methyl-1 uric acid and three different Ca^{2+} phosphates namely whitlockite, OCP and ACCP. Moreover, for the first time, mappings with a 10×10 μm^2 probe have allowed us to underline the chemical heterogeneity of intratissular calcifications. Among the 24 samples which corresponded to 23 patients (B180 and B181 samples correspond to two successive biopsies for the same patient performed two and five years after kidney transplantation), 8 samples contained two to three different crystalline phases.

For the Ca^{2+} phosphates we have already underlined the clinical interest to distinguish the different crystalline species in kidney

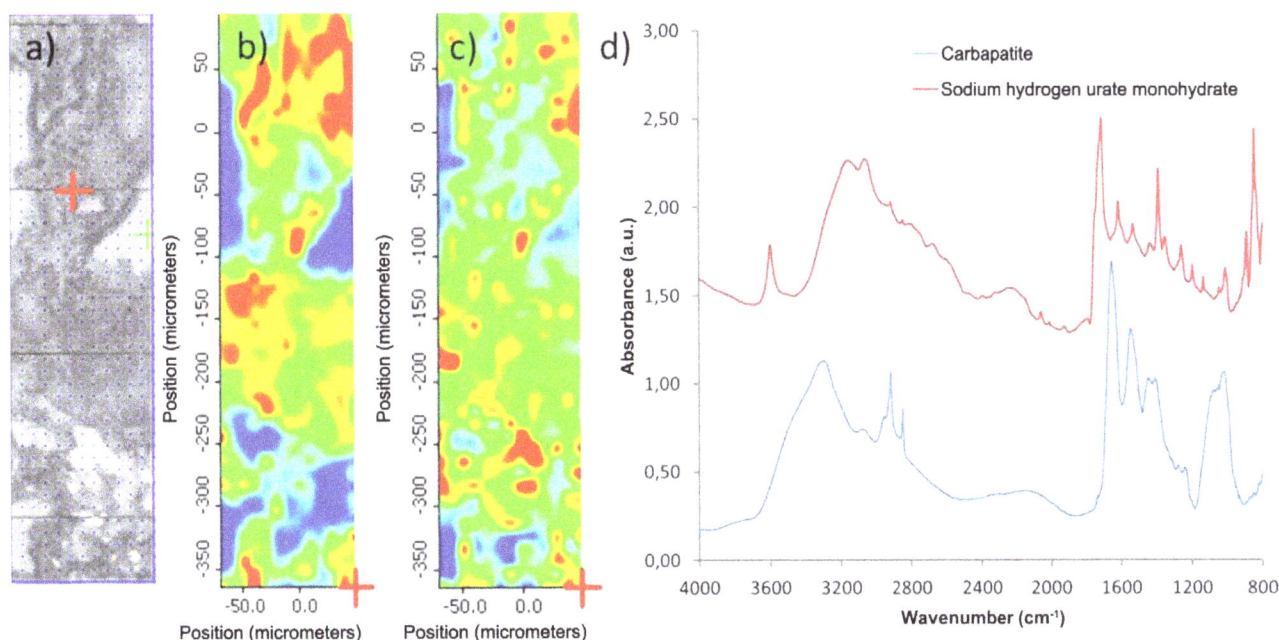

Figure 2. Optical image and mapping of BR165 biopsy (scale from blue to red with increasing concentration), and FT-IR spectra of crystals. a) Optical image of BR165, b) carbapatite map (done at 1030 cm^{-1}), c) sodium hydrogen urate monohydrate map (done at 3600 cm^{-1}), d) FT-IR spectra of those compounds.

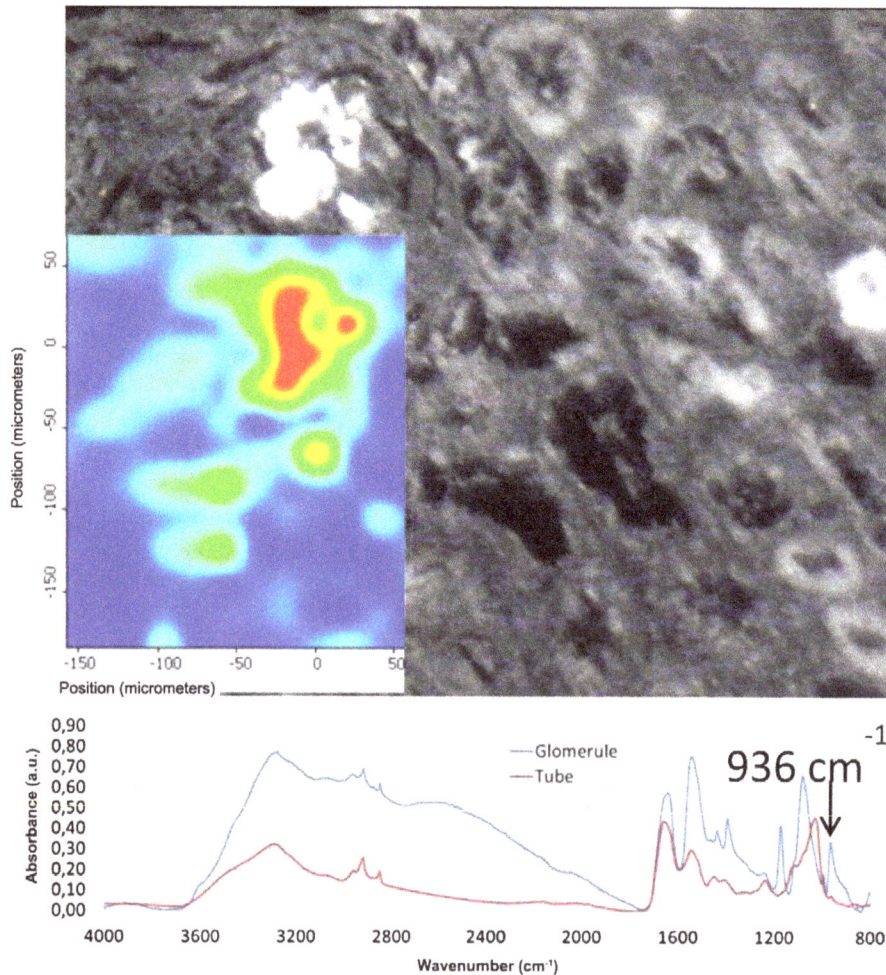

Figure 3. Mapping and optical image of a birefringent structure. The poorly soluble foscarnet can be detected and quantified after a mapping of the biopsy thanks to the characteristic peak at 936 cm[-1].

stones. For example, whitlockite in kidney stones is an infrequent component and has been associated with chronic urinary tract infection in most calculi in women [9]. In contrast, brushite was often associated with hypercalciuria [10] and primary hyperparathyroidism [11]. The presence of OCP is quite interesting. OCP is a thermodynamically metastable phase and it transforms to apatite spontaneously [12]. From a physiological point of view, this compound has been proposed to participate as a precursor of biological apatites. Also, regarding kidney stones, this compound has been found in pregnant women for which the metabolism of Ca^{2+} is modified in order to build the bone network of the foetus [13]. For these reasons, it seems of primary importance to distinguish these different Ca^{2+} phosphates in the tissues.

Another original aspect of our study comes from the opportunity to use SR µFTIR spectroscopy for indirect diagnosis of a genetic disease. Dihydroxyadenine crystals were found in four patients (five biopsies in Table 1). Such crystals deposits in parenchyma are pathognomonic of a rare disease, adenine phosphoribosyltransferase deficiency, an inherited disease able to induce recurrent kidney stones and/or kidney failure. Dihydroxyadenine is often too late identified in patients who have developed renal insufficiency and sometimes after the crystal-induced destruction of a kidney transplant. As recently emphasized, these data suggest this disease could be less rare than commonly

reported [14]. In our series, two patients were diagnosed using synchrotron examination of biopsies after renal impairment of the grafted kidney. They were treated with allopurinol and they recovered a large part of their kidney function. Such observations underline the clinical interest of early identification of crystals in the tissue.

Finally, high spatial resolution infrared mapping is a powerful tool to study the kidney distribution of some poorly soluble drugs and metabolites. It is well known that foscarnet crystallizes in glomeruli [15]. Foscarnet (phosphonoformic acid) is a pyrophosphate analogue that inhibits the DNA polymerase of all herpes viruses, which is commonly used in immuno-suppressed patients (AIDS, grafted patients) who developed CMV infection. Through SR-µ FTIR, spectroscopy we observed sodium foscarnet crystals in glomeruli in line with a previous study [16]. In addition, we found in the cells of the proximal tubule an accumulation of apatite crystals suggesting that the drug is locally metabolized by splitting the bond between the two phosphate residues of foscarnet. To the best of our knowledge, no data has been reported about associated crystalline phases deposited within the cells of the tubules.

In conclusion, here, we give the first structural evidence of a chemical diversity for mineral deposits in the kidney tissue. New crystalline phases were described such as amorphous silica, sodium hydrogen urate, methyl-1 uric acid and three different Ca^{2+}

phosphates namely whitlockite, OCP and ACCP. Moreover, for the first time, we underline the chemical heterogeneity of intratissular calcifications.

Other striking results of this study concern the opportunity to establish early medical diagnosis. Such approach should be generalized when the usual techniques at the hospital are not able to identify accurately pathological intratissular deposits. The relatively high number of APRT deficiency cases identified from dihydroxyadenine crystals, a disease easily treated with allopurinol when correctly diagnosed, underlined the utmost clinical impor-

tance of identifying crystals in kidney biopsies in order to improve the etiologic diagnosis of some renal impairments.

Author Contributions

Conceived and designed the experiments: AD DB PD CS MD. Performed the experiments: AD DB PD CS MD. Analyzed the data: AD DB PD CS MD. Contributed reagents/materials/analysis tools: AD DB PD CS MD. Wrote the paper: AD DB PD CS JS-S MD.

References

1. Atkins RC (2005) The epidemiology of chronic kidney disease. Kidney Int 67: s14–s18.
2. Perazella MA (1999) Crystal-induced acute renal failure. Am J Med 106: 459–465.
3. Hassan I, Juncos LA, Milliner DS, Sarmiento JM, Sarr MG (2001) Chronic renal failure secondary to oxalate nephropathy: a preventable complication after jejunoileal bypass. Mayo Clinic Proceed 76: 758–760.
4. Eller P, Rosenkranz AR, Mark W, Theurl I, Laufer J, et al. (2004) Four consecutive renal transplantations in a patient with adenine phosphoribosyl-transferase deficiency. Clin Nephrol 61: 217–221.
5. Parasuramain R, Venkat KK (2010) Crystal-induced kidney disease in two kidney transplant recipients. Am J Kidney Dis 55: 192–197.
6. Estepa-Maurice L, Hennequin C, Marfisi C, Bader C, Lacour B, et al. (1996) Fourier Transform infra red microscopy identification of crystal deposits in tissues. Am J Clin Path 105: 576–582.
7. Dumas P, Polack F, Lagarde B, Chubar O, Giorgetta JL, et al. (2006) Synchrotron infrared microscopy at the French Synchrotron Facility SOLEIL. Infrared Physics & Technology 49: 152–160.
8. Quy-Dao N, Daudon M (1997) Infrared and Raman Spectra of Calculi. Elsevier.
9. Maurice-Estepa L, Levilain P, Lacour B, Daudon M (1999) Crystalline phase differentiation in urinary calcium phosphate and magnesium phosphate calculi. Scan J. Urol Nephrol 33:299–305.
10. Daudon M, Bouzidi H, Bazin D (2010) Composition and morphology of phosphate stones and their relation with etiology. Urol Res 38: 459–467.
11. Bouzidi H, Hayek D, Nasr D, Daudon M, Fadhel Najjar M (2011) Inherited tubular renal acidosis. Annales Biol. Clin. 69: 405–410.
12. Iijima M, Kamemizu H, Wakamatsu N, Goto T, Doi Y, et al. (1998) Effects of Ca addition on the formation of octacalcium phosphate and apatite in solution at pH 7.4 and at 37°C. J. of Crystal Growth 193: 182–188.
13. Méria P, Hadjadj H, Jungers P, Daudon M and Members of the Urolithiasis Committee of the French Urological Association (2010) Stone formation and pregnancy: pathophysiological insights gained from morphoconstitutional stone analysis. J Urol 183: 1412–1416.
14. Bollée G, Dollinger C, Boutaud L, Guillemot D, Bensman A, et al. (2010) Phenotype and genotype characterization of adenine phosphoribosyltransferase deficiency. J Am Soc Nephrol 21: 679–688.
15. Beaufils H, Deray G, Katlama C, Dohin E, Henin D, et al. (1990) Foscarnet and crystals in glomerular capillary lumens. Lancet 336: 755.
16. Maurice-Estepa L, Daudon M, Katlama C, Jouanneau C, Sazdovitch V, et al. (1998) Identification of crystals in kidneys of AIDS patients treated with foscarnet. Am J Kidney Dis 32: 392–400.

Circulating Progenitor Cell Count for Cardiovascular Risk Stratification: A Pooled Analysis

Gian Paolo Fadini[1]*, Shoichi Maruyama[2], Takenori Ozaki[2], Akihiko Taguchi[3], James Meigs[4], Stefanie Dimmeler[5], Andreas M. Zeiher[5], Saula de Kreutzenberg[1], Angelo Avogaro[1], Georg Nickenig[6], Caroline Schmidt-Lucke[7], Nikos Werner[6]

1 Department of Clinical and Experimental Medicine, University of Padova Medical School, Padova, Italy, 2 Department of Nephrology, Nagoya University Graduate School of Medicine, Nagoya, Japan, 3 Department of Cerebrovascular Disease, National Cardiovascular Center, Osaka, Japan, 4 Harvard Medical School and General Medicine Division, Massachusetts General Hospital, Boston, Massachusetts, United States of America, 5 Molecular Cardiology and Internal Medicine III, Wolfgang Goethe University, Frankfurt, Germany, 6 Department of Internal Medicine II, Division of Cardiology, Pneumology, and Angiology, University Hospital Bonn, Bonn, Germany, 7 Department of Cardiology and Pneumology, Charité, Universitätsmedizin Berlin, Campus Benjamin Franklin, Berlin, Germany

Abstract

Background: Circulating progenitor cells (CPC) contribute to the homeostasis of the vessel wall, and a reduced CPC count predicts cardiovascular morbidity and mortality. We tested the hypothesis that CPC count improves cardiovascular risk stratification and that this is modulated by low-grade inflammation.

Methodology/Principal Findings: We pooled data from 4 longitudinal studies, including a total of 1,057 patients having CPC determined and major adverse cardiovascular events (MACE) collected. We recorded cardiovascular risk factors and high-sensitive C-reactive protein (hsCRP) level. Risk estimates were derived from Cox proportional hazard analyses. CPC count and/or hsCRP level were added to a reference model including age, sex, cardiovascular risk factors, prevalent CVD, chronic renal failure (CRF) and medications. The sample was composed of high-risk individuals, as 76.3% had prevalent CVD and 31.6% had CRF. There were 331 (31.3%) incident MACE during an average 1.7 ± 1.1 year follow-up time. CPC count was independently associated with incident MACE even after correction for hsCRP. According to C-statistics, models including CPC yielded a non-significant improvement in accuracy of MACE prediction. However, the integrated discrimination improvement index (IDI) showed better performance of models including CPC compared to the reference model and models including hsCRP in identifying MACE. CPC count also yielded significant net reclassification improvements (NRI) for CV death, non-fatal AMI and other CV events. The effect of CPC was independent of hsCRP, but there was a significant more-than-additive interaction between low CPC count and raised hsCRP level in predicting incident MACE.

Conclusions/Significance: In high risk individuals, a reduced CPC count helps identifying more patients at higher risk of MACE over the short term, especially in combination with a raised hsCRP level.

Editor: Stefan Kiechl, Innsbruck Medical University, Austria

Funding: The authors have no support or funding to report.

Competing Interests: The authors have declared that no competing interests exist.

* E-mail: gianpaolofadini@hotmail.com

Introduction

Cardiovascular disease (CVD) is the leading cause of death in western countries. Thus, identification of patients at risk for future CVD must be pursued in order to implement preventive strategies. Traditional cardiovascular risk factors are commonly used for this purpose and many risk scores have been proposed based on various combinations of risk factors. However, a significant number of cardiovascular events still occur in subjects classified in the low or intermediate risk categories [1], thus reducing the chance to apply disease prevention in many subjects who would benefit from it. Identification of emerging risk factors and novel biomarkers of CVD has recently gained attention, in an attempt to improve the performance of risk prediction algorithms. A number of CVD biomarkers have been identified, many of which are independently associated with incident cardiovascular events in survival analyses

[2]. However, the usefulness of testing biomarkers in the clinical setting has been questioned, because there is no definite evidence that biomarkers, alone or in combination, improve cardiovascular risk stratification and identification of patients at risk for future CVD. Indeed, it is increasingly recognized that basic association measures are insufficient to assess prognostic utility of biomarkers while newer methods, that assess how well biomarkers assign patients to clinical risk categories [3], yielded rather disappointing results [4,5].

Inflammatory molecules are among the most extensively studied CVD biomarkers. For instance, a mildly raised C-reactive protein (CRP) reflects a condition of chronic low-grade inflammation that is considered one underlying cause of CVD development and progression [6]. However, inconsistency exists regarding the ability of CRP testing to improve risk assessment [7].

In the last decade, pathogenic models of CVD have moved to consider the role of circulating cells potentially involved in cardiovascular repair [8]. Endothelial progenitor cells (EPCs) are bone marrow-derived cells able to migrate into the bloodstream and participate in endothelial regeneration and angiogenesis [9,10,11]. Many animal models confirm the protective effects of EPCs on the cardiovascular system, and clinical studies show that low levels of circulating EPCs associate with prevalent and incident CVD [12,13,14]. Different phenotypes of circulating progenitor cells (CPC), including EPCs, are thus emerging as novel CVD biomarkers, which are also involved in disease pathogenesis [15]. In survival analyses of longitudinal studies, a reduced CPC count has been shown to independently predict cardiovascular events in patients with CVD [13,16], chronic renal failure [17] or metabolic syndrome [18], but it is still not clear if CPC count is useful in the clinical setting for cardiovascular risk stratification. Re-analysis of individual data from relevant prospective studies of cardiovascular outcomes is emerging as a mean to address this uncertainty in a rapid and cost-effective manner [19].

This study, resulting from the collaboration of 4 independent research groups, tested the hypothesis that: i) adding CPC count to a standard risk model for cardiovascular risk stratification of high-risk individuals has a significant incremental predictive value; ii) the relationship between CPC and incident cardiovascular events is modified by inflammation and there is an interaction between CPC and CRP levels in cardiovascular event prediction.

Methods

Participants

This study was conceived as a post-hoc re-analysis of crude data from 4 previously published cohorts [13,16,17,18]. The individual studies used for this pooled analysis were approved by the respective local Institutional Ethical committees (University of Saarland, J.W. Goethe University of Frankfurt, University Hospital of Padova and Nagoya Kyoritsu Hospital), and written informed consent was obtained from all subjects at time of the study. Investigators of each source study provided patients' data on the basis of an agreed protocol and data scheme. The following data were recorded for all patients: age, sex, smoking habit, presence of cardiovascular risk factors, chronic renal failure (CRF), prevalent CVD, and use of drugs. Twelve patients were excluded because of missing at least one the above-mentioned parameters. Shared definitions of cardiovascular risk factors were used: diabetes mellitus was defined by fasting plasma glucose ≥ 126 mg/dL or self-reported diabetes; smoking status was defined as habitual smoking of ≥ 1 cigarette per day; hypertension was defined as systolic blood pressure ≥ 140 mmHg or a diastolic blood pressure ≥ 90 mmHg, or the use of anti-hypertensive drugs; dyslipidemia was defined as either a total cholesterol concentration ≥ 200 mg/dL or a triglycerides concentration ≥ 200 mg/dl or a HDL cholesterol concentration of less than 40 mg/dl in men and 50 mg/dl in women or the use of statin/fibrates. CRF was defined as serum creatinine >1.3 mg/dL for at least 6 months or if the patient was on dialysis. CVD was defined as any of the following: a history of previous myocardial infarction or stable angina, a significant coronary artery diseases at angiography, peripheral arterial disease (claudication, rest pain or ischemic foot ulcers), cerebro-vascular disease (a history of stroke or carotid atherosclerosis), presence of abdominal aortic aneurysm.

We also collected data on high sensitive C-reactive protein (hsCRP) concentrations, which were categorized as high and low according to an established cut-off (≤ 3.0 mg/L or >3.0 mg/L) [20]. hsCRP was measured using the turbidimetric method of Roche Diagnostics [13,21] or Behring's ultrasensitive LatexCRP

monotest [16], or the latex-enhanced high-sensitive CRP immu-noassay (Nittobo Medical Co. Ltd) [22].

Circulating progenitor cell count

CPC were defined as circulating CD34+KDR+ cells in 2 studies [13,16], or as circulating CD34+ cells in the other 2 studies [17,18]. Given the different definitions and measures of CPC, we adopted a strategy to render CPC count as much comparable as possible, by expressing CPC as belonging to a tertile of the normal distribution within each cohort. Thus, CPC count in the pooled sample could be reported as high (3rd tertile), intermediate (2nd tertile) or low (1st tertile). A review of previous data suggest that CD34+ cell level is more stable over time than CD34+KDR+ cell level, which is more influenced by pharmacological treatment [23,24].

Follow-up and definition of the endpoint

In all source studies, follow-up was conducted by telephone contact, ambulatory visit or consultation of death registry. Potential events were verified by analysis of medical records, such as hospital charts and discharge letters. The main outcome measure of this pooled study was a modified definition of major adverse cardiovascular event (MACE). An incident MACE was recorded if the patient matched one of the following conditions during the follow-up period: cardiovascular (CV) death; non-fatal acute myocardial infarction (AMI); hospitalization for unstable angina or congestive heart failure (according to Framingham criteria [25]); coronary or peripheral revascularization procedure; angiographic evidence of restenosis after coronary revasculariza-tion; major amputation due to peripheral ischemia, stroke or transient ischemic attack. Event-free survival analyses were also performed separately for CV death, non-fatal AMI, non-fatal stroke and other CV events.

Statistical methods

Continuous data were reported as mean $\pm$ standard error of the mean (SEM), and categorical data as percentage. Event-free survival was assessed with Cox proportional hazard analyses. Four different sets of variables were constructed, to be entered into 4 models, respectively. In model 1 (reference model), sex, age, cardiovascular risk factors, CRF, prevalent CVD and use of statins and ACE inhibitors/ARBs were forced into the model. This reference model was built to include all standard predictors of cardiovascular events that could be retrieved from all source studies. We included only those medications that were supposed to influence both outcome and CPC, to be controlled for. In model 2, variables of model 1 plus CPC were entered; in model 3, variables of model 1 plus hsCRP were entered; in model 4, variables of model 1 plus CPC and hsCRP were entered simultaneously. Estimated risk functions were calculated using beta coefficients from survival analyses and exponential transformation, similarly to what described for generating the Framingham risk equation. Risks estimated by Cox regressions were used to compare the performance of the 4 models. Average C-statistics was calculated as the area under ROC curve using either the logistic approach, which ignores time-to-event, or Chambless and Diao's method [26] and Harrell's method [27], which add time component to area under curve estimation. Confidence intervals for $\hat{C}$ were calculated based on Kendall's τ approximation as proposed by Pencina et al.[28]. P-values for comparison between $\hat{C}$ were computed from approximation to a normal distribution. Improvement in model performance with addition of CPC and/or hsCRP was also assessed by calculating the net reclassification improve-ment (NRI) with pre-specified tertile categories of risk and the

Table 1. Characteristics of study patients.

Characteristic	Value
Age (years, mean ± SEM)	63.1±0.4
Male gender (%)	64.2
Smoking (%)	24.3
Diabetes (%)	32.0
Hypertension (%)	70.7
Dyslipidemia (%)	56.8
hsCRP >3.0 mg/L (%)	39.1
Chronic renal failure/dialysis (%)	31.7
Prevalent CVD (%)	76.3
Statin use (%)	33.3
ACE inhibitor/ARB use (%)	51.4

integrated discrimination improvement (IDI), as previously described [3].

To explore the interaction between CPC and hsCRP levels in relation to incident MACE, we divided patients into 6 groups according to CPC tertiles and hsCRP<>3.0 mg/L. We then compared unadjusted event rates using χ^2 and adjusted relative risks (RR) derived from Cox regression analysis of model 1 in these categories of subjects. Rothman's synergy index, a measure of interaction as departure from additivity, was calculated as previously described using adjusted RRs [29]. Confidence interval of synergy index was calculated as suggested by Zou [30]. SPSS versions 13.0 was used and statistical significance was accepted at p<0.05.

Results

Patients' characteristics

Clinical characteristics of the study patients are summarized in Table 1. The study sample was representative of a high risk population, as 76.3% of patients had CVD at baseline and 31.7% had chronic renal failure. This is in compliance with a relatively high incidence of MACE (331 events; 31.3% of subjects) over a relatively short follow-up time (1.7±1.1 years). Events were distributed as follows: 48 CV deaths, 19 non-fatal AMI, 19 non-fatal stroke, and 245 other CV events.

Survival analysis

Cox proportional hazard analyses were performed to derive different prediction models (Table 2). In model 1 (reference model), hypertension, dyslipidemia, and prevalent CVD were significant predictors of incident MACE. Both low CPC and raised hsCRP (>3.0 mg/L), that were added respectively in models 2 and 3 were significant event predictors besides hypertension, dyslipidemia and CVD. CPC count was a significant predictor of incident MACE also in model 4, independently of hsCRP, dyslipidemia and CVD. Patients were then divided into 2 groups according to the presence/absence of prevalent CVD at baseline and model 4 was run for both: CPC tertile was a significant inverse event predictor in the CVD group, while there was a non-significant trend for a higher event rate with decreasing CPC tertile in the non-CVD group. Regarding event type, higher CPC tertile in model 4 was an independent inverse predictor of CV death (RR = 0.59; p = 0.007), non-fatal AMI (RR = 0.50; p = 0.037) and other CV events (RR = 0.81; p = 0.009), while it was not significantly associated with incident stroke/TIA (RR = 0.78; p = 0.404). Figure 1 shows Kaplan-Meier curves of incident events according to CPC tertiles (model 4) in the different groups.

Linear risk functions were then calculated for each model using regression coefficients of survival analyses and exponential transformation, similarly to the equation used to derive the Framingham 10-year risk. Discrimination and performance of the risk estimates based on the 4 models were then assessed.

Effects of CPC on discrimination of survival models

Average C ($\hat{C}$) was calculated using 3 methods. Logistic $\hat{C}$, which ignores time-to-event, was not significantly increased in models 2, 3 and 4 as compared to model 1 (Figure 2A). Figure 2B

Table 2. Results of the Cox hazard-proportional analyses.

Variable	Model 1 (reference)		Model 2 (+CPC)		Model 3 (+hsCRP)		Model 4 (+CPC+hsCRP)	
	RR	p	RR	p	RR	P	RR	p
Male gender	1.17	0.207	1.19	0.159	1.15	0.254	1.17	0.206
Age (for 10 yrs)	1.03	0.577	1.02	0.672	1.02	0.773	1.01	0.861
Smoke	0.94	0.668	0.92	0.551	0.93	0.611	0.92	0.512
Diabetes	1.18	0.151	1.14	0.266	1.18	0.154	1.13	0.290
Hypertension	1.45	0.022	1.38	0.046	1.45	0.023	1.36	0.061
Dyslipidemia	1.50	0.003	1.46	0.006	1.48	0.005	1.44	0.008
Chronic renal failure	0.98	0.894	0.97	0.814	0.96	0.782	0.95	0.708
Prevalent CVD	10.90	<0.001	10.48	<0.001	10.05	<0.001	9.57	<0.001
Use of statin	1.17	0.210	1.20	0.144	1.15	0.270	1.19	0.174
Use of ACEI/ARBs	0.96	0.767	0.97	0.817	0.98	0.838	0.98	0.900
CPC tertiles	-	-	0.77	<0.001	-	-	0.76	<0.001
hsCRP>3.0 mg/L	-	-	-	-	1.52	<0.001	1.57	<0.001

All explanatory variables were entered simultaneously in the model. CPC was entered as a continuous variable and relative risk (RR) expressed per tertile increase. RR for age is reported for each 10 yrs increase. ACEI, angiotensin converting enzyme inhibitors; ARB, angiotensin receptor blockers.

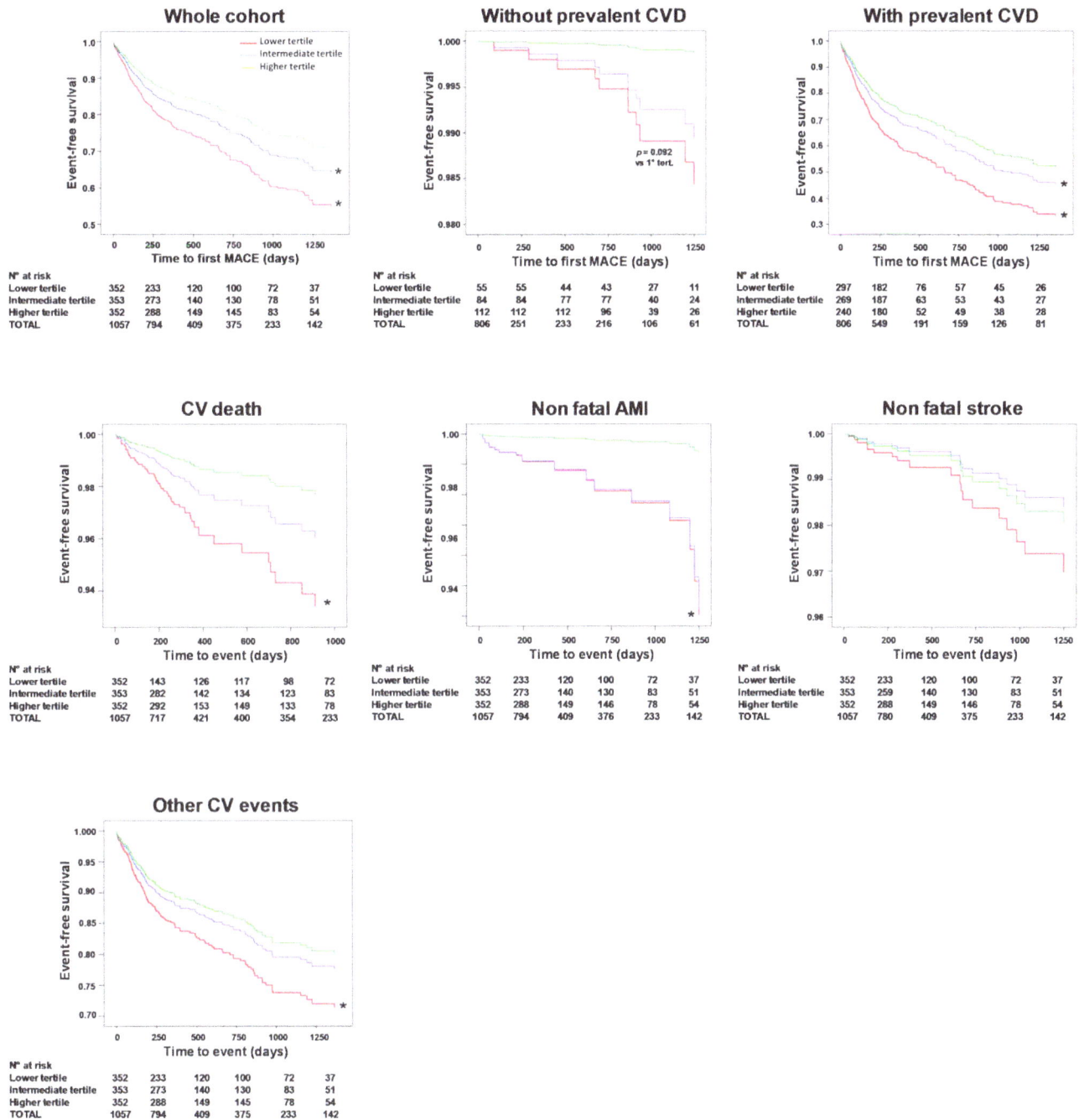

Figure 1. Kaplan-Meier Curves. Different curves are plotted for patients belonging to the different CPC tertiles in the whole cohort, and in groups of patients with or without prevalent CVD at baseline. Separate curves are also shown according to event type in whole cohort. Survival is corrected for confounders entered in model 4. *significantly different versus the higher CPC tertile group.

shows that AUCs from logistic $\hat{C}$ increased not significantly also when CV death, non-fatal AMI and other CV events were considered separately. Similarly, Chambless and Diao's $\hat{C}$, which adds time component to the area under ROC curve estimation, was not significantly higher when CPC count was entered in the model, with our without hsCRP, as compared to model 1. Harrell's $\hat{C}$, which is independent of calibration, showed no significance discrimination improvement in model 2, 3 and 4, as well. As expected [3], $\hat{C}$ was highest with the logistic approach and lowest with Harrell's method for all models (Table 3). These results indicate that, on the basis of C-statistics, the addition of CPC did

not significantly improve discrimination of the new survival model in comparison with a standard reference model.

Effects of CPC on improvement in model performance

We then assessed whether the models including CPC with or without hsCRP yielded a better reclassification of patients in terms of MACE prediction. To this end, the NRI was calculated based on reclassification across tertiles of risk categories yielded by new models in comparison to the reference model. Movement of patients with incident MACE in higher risk categories and

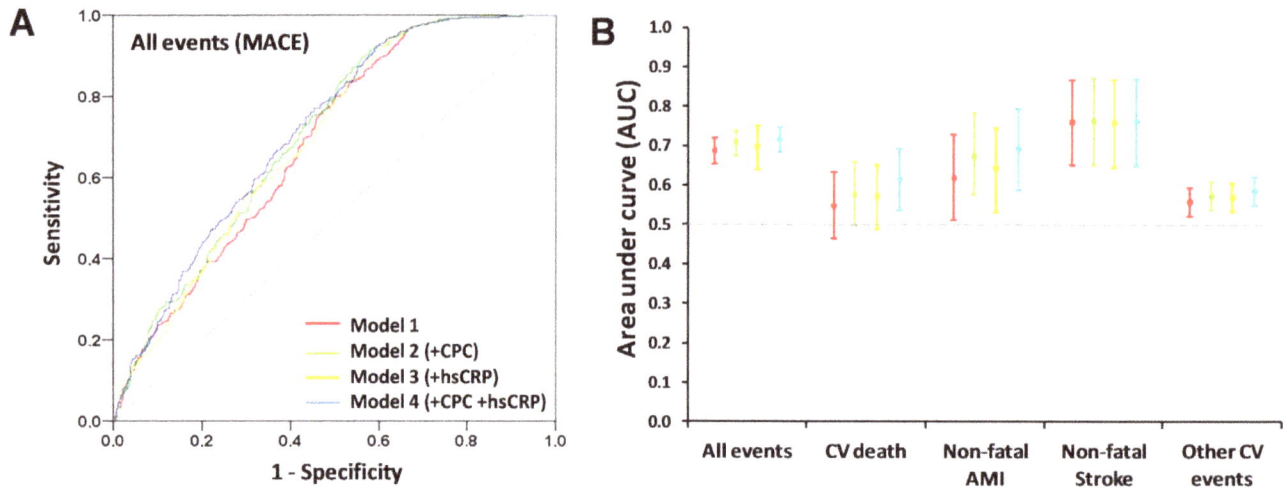

Figure 2. Discrimination analysis. Panel A shows ROC curves: logistic Ĉ is shown for each model. Panel B shows AUCs of logistic Ĉ with 95% confidence intervals (bars) according to event type and model 1 to 4.

movement of patients without incident MACE in lower risk categories were considered as correct reclassifications. As shown in Table 4, in comparison to the reference model, inclusion of either CPC or hsCRP was not associated with a statistically significant NRI. Inclusion of both CPC and hsCRP in the model yielded better reclassification of 6.5%, but still was not statistically significant (p = 0.13). Re-analysis by event type indicated that inclusion of CPC measurement provided significant NRI for CV death (model 2 vs model 1: NRI = 18.6%, p = 0.034; model 4 vs model 1: NRI = 22.7%, p = 0.014), non-fatal AMI (model 2 vs model 1: NRI = 21.5%, p = 0.043), and other CV events (model 2 vs model 1: NRI = 6.5%, p = 0.015; model 4 vs model 1: NRI = 11.9%, p<0.001), but not for non-fatal stroke.

Given that the NRI is highly dependent upon the pre-specified categories of risk, we also calculated the integrated discrimination improvement (IDI), which is a continuous assessment of reclassification improvement, not based on risk categories. IDI showed significant better discrimination by the models including CPC with or without hsCRP as compared to the reference model. Interestingly, there also was a significant IDI in the comparison of model 4 with models 2 and 3, suggesting that the inclusion of both CPC and hsCRP improved discrimination over the inclusion of either CPC alone or hsCRP alone. Then, an interaction between CPC and hsCRP was looked for.

Interaction between CPC and hsCRP

Patients were divided into groups according to their concentration of hsCRP (<>3.0 mg/L) and their belonging tertile of CPC count. As shown in Figure 3, the risk of incident MACE across CPC tertiles was different in the high versus low hsCRP

population: unadjusted event rates were significantly higher in patients with a hsCRP>3.0 mg/L across all CPC tertiles. After adjusting for age, sex, cardiovascular risk factors, CRF, prevalent CVD and medications (model 1), a high hsCRP was significantly associated with a higher relative risk (RR) of events in patients in the lowest CPC tertile. The slope of the relationship between CPC tertiles and RR of MACE was significantly higher in the high than in the low hsCRP group (8.81 [95% C.I. 8.12–9.51] versus 12.70 [95% C.I. 12.07–13.33]; p<0.001). This trend was suggestive of an interaction between CPC and hsCRP in relation to incident MACE. Rothman's synergy index, calculated as the excess risk in patients with both low CPC and high hsCRP divided by the sum of excess risk in patients either low CPC or high hsCRP, was significantly different from zero (= 1.709/[0.450+0.589] = 1.64 [95% C.I. 1.04–2.60]; p = 0.032), indicating a more-than-additive interaction between CPC in the lower tertile and hsCRP >3.0 mg/L in determining incident MACE.

Subsidiary analyses

Calibration analyses, performed using the Hosmer-Lemeshow test, indicated no significant differences between observed and expected event rates in all models and the χ^2 value was lower in models including CPC (model 2 an 4). Accordingly, observed event rates across deciles of risk almost always fall within the 95% confidence interval of expected event rates (calculated according to the Poisson distribution), indicating good calibration (Figure 4).

Since the phenotype of CPC was inconsistent among studies (CD34+KDR+ in 2 studies and CD34+ in 2 studies), we performed distinct Cox regression analyses for subjects with CD34+ or CD34+KDR+ cell counts. We found that both CPC

Table 3. Performance of MACE prediction models using average C (Ĉ).

	Model 1 (reference)	Model 2 (+CPC)	Model 3 (+hsCRP)	Model 4 (+hsCRP+CPC)
Logistic Ĉ	0.687 (0.655–0.719)	0.707 (0.676–0.738)	0.695 (0.663–0.727)	0.716 (0.685–0.747)
Chambless and Diao's Ĉ	0.691 (0.642–0.731)	0.707 (0.663–0.750)	0.695 (0.651–0.739)	0.716 (0.673–0.759)
Harrell's Ĉ	0.631 (0.596–0.666)	0.635 (0.600–0.671)	0.644 (0.609–0.677)	0.648 (0.614–0.683)

95% confidence intervals reported in brackets.

Table 4. Improvement of model performance.

	NRI	IDI
Model 2 vs Model 1	1.5% (p = 0.71)	0.017 (p = 0.0003)
Model 3 vs Model 1	−3.4% (p = 0.40)	0.011 (p = 0.013)
Model 4 vs Model 1	6.3% (p = 0.13)	0.029 (p<0.0001)
Model 3 vs Model 2	6.1% (p = 0.16)	−0.006 (p = 0.38)
Model 4 vs Model 2	5.1% (p = 0.17)	0.012 (p = 0.008)
Model 4 vs Model 3	10.0% (p = 0.008)	0.018 (p = 0.0002)

Net reclassification improvement (NRI) is reported as the net percentage of patients correctly reclassified by the new model across tertiles of MACE risk categories. The integrated discrimination improvement (IDI), which can be interpreted as a continuous version of NRI, is reported as absolute value.

phenotypes were independent event predictors besides hsCRP in model 4 (not shown), re-assuring us on the possibility to merge together the cohorts. Further, when available data on CD34+KDR+ cells of the Italian cohort [18] were merged to data of the other 2 studies using CD34+KDR+ cell count (making a total of 842 patients with a homogenous CPC definition), CPC count was still an independent event predictor besides hsCRP in model 4 (not shown), but improvement in C-statistics was minimal (Logistic Ĉ: 0.730 [95% C.I.: 0.696–0.764] versus 0.729 [95% C.I.: 0.695–0.763]; p = 0.96. Chambless Ĉ: 0.718 [95% C.I.: 0.671–0.765] versus 0.715 [95% C.I.: 0.668–0.762]; p = 0.93). In 2 studies data on CD34+ and CD34+KDR+ cells could be retrieved. Thus, we compared categorization in tertiles using either CD34+ or CD34+KDR+ cells and found that 61.2% of patients were categorized in the same tertile by both definitions. Moreover, only 5% of these patients were categorized in the lowest tertile by one definition and in the higher tertile by the other definition, suggesting a good correspondence between CPC categorization in pooled cohorts.

Discussion

This pooled analysis represents the first attempt to determine the ability of CPC count to improve cardiovascular risk stratification.

Based on C-statistics, inclusion of CPC in the risk equation provided limited and non-significant improvement over and beyond a standard model based on classic risk factors. However, a less restrictive metric (the IDI) showed that the model including CPC outperformed the reference model in terms of accuracy of even prediction, independently and beyond the effect of hsCRP inclusion.

In each of the cohorts that compose the present study population, CPC count was a significant independent predictor of cardiovascular events [13,16,17,18], but none of the source studies were well-powered to perform analysis of discrimination improvement. Indeed, large clinical studies on CPC are not available, because multicenter projects are hampered by the lack of standardized methods for CPC quantification, and because fresh blood samples for CPC determination must be processed within a few hours, thus limiting the possibility to analyze stored samples [31]. We tried to overcome these limitations by pooling crude data from distinct yet similar studies. Our results show that a low CPC count helps in identifying more patients at risk for future MACE, for the first time providing some evidence in support of a potential application of CPC count for cardiovascular risk stratification in the clinical practice. CPC are protective against the onset of CVD because they are involved in maintenance of a healthy endothelial layer, by means of promoting re-endothelialization of injured arteries [9]. Further, CPC are also protective against CVD progression as they promote compensatory angiogenesis in ischemic syndromes, thus limiting the extent of residual ischemia [11]. Therefore, it is expected that a paucity of these cells predispose to CVD onset or progression. Indeed, a reduced CPC count is linearly associated with severity of CVD involvement [12]. Furthermore, low CPC were found to predict incident events suggestive of CVD onset or progression in survival analyses of different cohorts of patients [13,16,17,18]. Thus, CPC count is revealing as a novel prototype of surrogate biomarkers for cardiovascular risk, supported by both pathophysiological and epidemiological evidence. In the present study, we addressed the next important step in the evaluation pipeline of a putative biomarker, that is the incremental value in quantitative risk assessment over traditional risk factors [3]. Studying a high-risk population, we first confirm that CPC count is independently associated with incident events, and then looked at reclassification improvement yielded by addition of CPC measure beyond

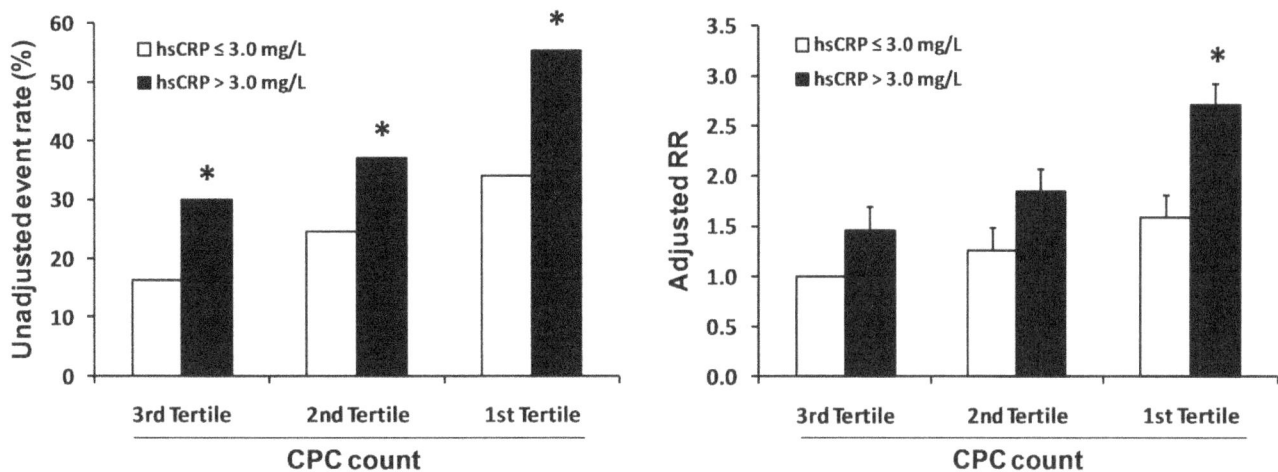

Figure 3. Interaction between CPC and hsCRP levels. Patients were divided into 6 groups according to CPC tertiles and high/low hsCRP. Left panel shows unadjusted events rates (* significantly different in χ^2 analysis versus hsCRP≤3.0 mg/L). Right panel shows adjusted relative risks (RR) from model 1 (Bars = SE; * significantly different versus hsCRP≤3.0 mg/L).

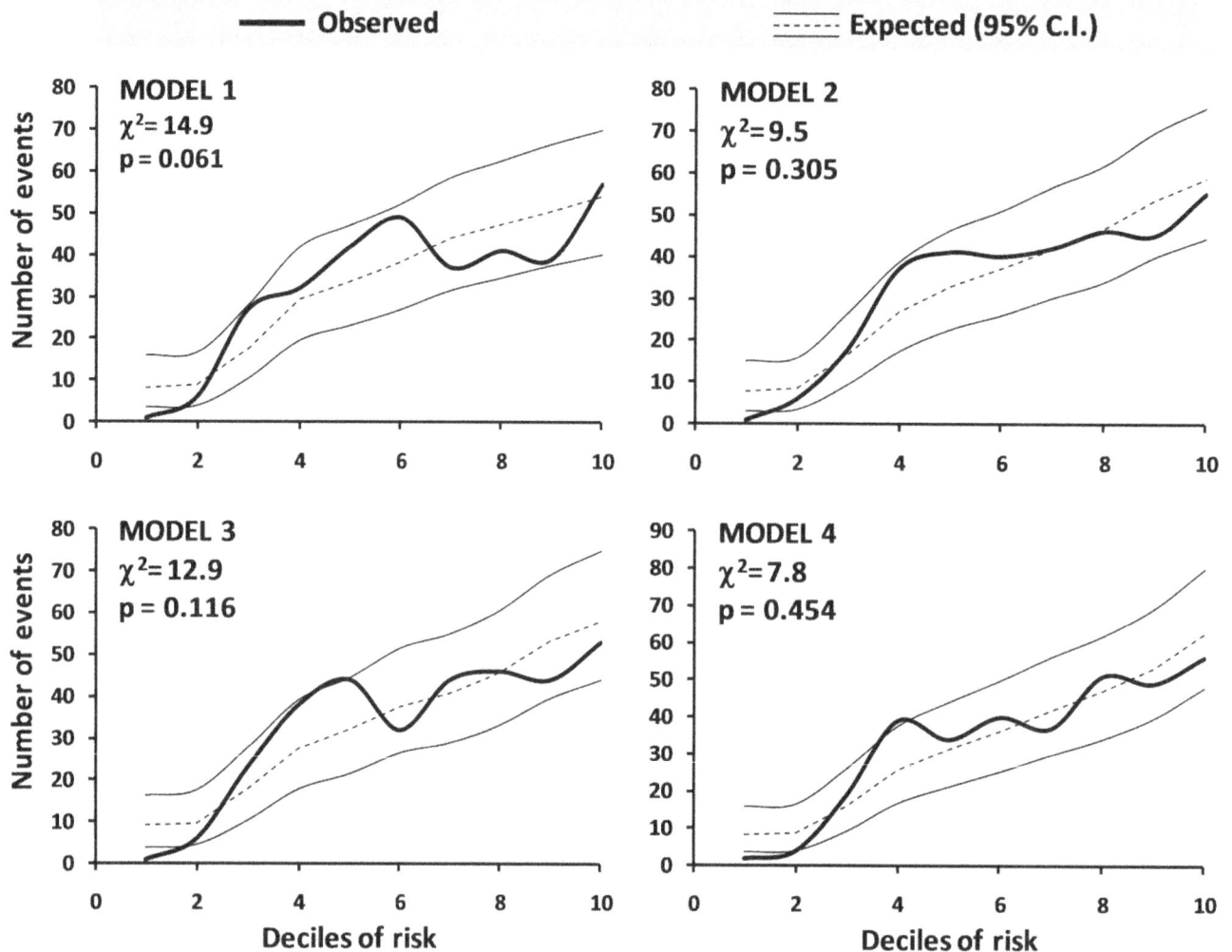

Figure 4. Calibration of predictive models. Deciles of risk were calculated for each model. Observed and expected even rates are plotted against deciles of risk. 95% confidence intervals (C.I.) for expected data according to the respective model were calculated according to the Poisson distribution. Results of the Hosmer-Lemeshow χ^2 test is shown for each model.

traditional demographics and risk factors. To this end, we used metrics specifically designed to assess the clinical utility of one or more biomarker(s) under scrutiny. Addition of CPC to a risk model built on conventional risk factors had marginal and non-significant effects on C statistics calculated using both the logistic method and methods that take into account time to event. This is not surprising, because C statistic is poorly sensitive to small changes in predictive accuracy, such that even established risk factors could be discarded as non-significant is some circumstances [32]. Indeed, it is very uncommon that a single surrogate biomarker improves C statistics when added to a well-fitted reference model; notably, in previous studies, even combinations of several biomarkers yielded modest changes in Ĉ when added to a standard risk assessment [5,33]. Given the limitations of C statistics, we also calculated the IDI, a newer metric that improves when novel markers correctly assign individuals to higher or lower probabilities of having events. The IDI for MACE prediction improved significantly when either CPC or hsCRP were added to the reference model, and improved further when both were added together (Table 4). The NRI, a discrete version of IDI based on upward or downward movement across pre-specified risk categories, was significant for CV death, non-fatal AMI and other

CV risk, but not for the combined MACE. We used risk tertiles to calculate the NRI given the impossibility to translate risk estimates in the present population into the clinically-relevant standard 10-year risk estimate. This might have affected results, since the NRI is highly sensitive to pre-specified categories.

Cumulatively, our data suggest that CPC measure may add incremental predictive value to standard risk assessment and that this effect might be modulated by hsCRP levels. Accordingly, we found a significant interaction between low CPC and high hsCRP levels in predicting incident events. After statistical adjustment, the excess risk of MACE in patients with both CPC in the lower tertile and hsCRP>3.0 mg/L was higher than the sum of excess risks in patients with either low CPC or high hsCRP, indicating a more-than-additive interaction between the two risk biomarkers in determining incident MACE. Biologically, this observation suggests that reduced vascular repair and inflammation are two distinct pathways of cardiovascular disease that synergize to increase the likelihood of adverse outcomes.

Limitations

This study has limitations inherent to the pooling of data coming from 4 different cohorts. First, the definition of CPC in the source studies was different. The exact definition and cellular progeny of circulating (endothelial) progenitor cells is debated [34]. In this pooled analysis, by transforming CPC counts into tertiles, we could make data comparable and poolable, but potential biological differences between CD34+ cells (measured in 2 studies [17,18]; n = 430) and CD34+KDR+ cells (measured in the other 2 studies [13,16]; n = 627) might confound results. There is evidence that CD34+ and CD34+KDR+ cell counts are correlated each other and are subjected to consistent variations [35], but the CD34+ cells form a more generic population of progenitor cells, while CD34+KDR+ cells are primed to the endothelial lineage and can be considered EPC [31,35]. Thus, future studies should focus on a single CPC phenotype, but our separated analyses for CD34+ and CD34+KDR+ cells showed consistent results, suggesting that there is no definite evidence that one phenotype is superior to the other(s) in terms of risk prediction. Our analyses are limited by the need to categorize CPC count to pool together the source studies; assessment of this surrogate biomarker along the continuous scale may provide better results and may offer the opportunity to define cutoffs. A second limitation is that methods for hsCRP measurement were not standardized among centers, and we simply could categorize hsCRP levels as high or low according to the standard 3.0 mg/L cutoff. Third, the original populations of patients are heterogeneous and the pooled cohort is mainly composed of high risk individuals in primary and secondary prevention. It is generally agreed that biomarkers perform better in high-risk than in low-risk populations [36] and, in the present study, more significant results were obtained in patients with baseline CVD. In addition, even if we tried to harmonize the endpoint by using a modified definition of MACE, event adjudication was not centralized.

Future directions

Results of the present study need to be replicated in a more homogenous group of patients, yet large enough to allow statistical power in the analysis of discrimination improvement. Finally, to establish a definite causal link between reduced CPC and CVD onset or progression, studies with a pathophysiology-focused

design are needed, such as mendelian randomization studies and/or biomarker-guided targeted treatment studies [37,38]. Mendelian randomization studies could address polymorphisms in the cd34 gene itself [39] or in the cxcl12 gene, encoding the progenitor cell-regulating chemokine SDF-1α [40]. Interestingly, CPC levels are also potentially modifiable and amenable to pharmacological and non-pharmacological interventions. Many drugs currently used in the treatment of CVD, including statins and RAS blockers, have been shown to favorably modulate CPC [9,41,42]. Lifestyle interventions, such as diet [43], weight loss [44], exercise [45], and smoke cessation [46], have beneficial effects on CPC, as well. Therefore, besides being a pathogenetic actor, a disease biomarker and a prognostic indicator, CPC also appear to be a potential therapeutic target. It remains to be determined to what extent a therapeutic increase in CPC will translate into an improvement of event-free survival.

Conclusions

Our data confirm that low CPC counts predicts adverse cardiovascular outcomes independently of chronic low grade inflammation, but synergistically with raised hsCRP levels. Analysis of this pooled cohort also supports the potential use of CPC count in cardiovascular risk stratification of high-risk individuals, especially in combination with the measure of hsCRP. A simplified CPC assessment by isolated CD34 expression analysis may be a simple and cheap way of measuring this new surrogate CV risk biomarker. Larger epidemiological and intervention studies are needed to understand the causal relationships between low CPC and CVD as well as the potential therapeutic implications.

Author Contributions

Conceived and designed the experiments: GPF SdK AA. Performed the experiments: SM TO AT SD AMZ GN CSL NW. Analyzed the data: GPF AT JBM. Contributed reagents/materials/analysis tools: SM TO SD AMZ AA GN CSL NW. Wrote the paper: GPF SdK AA NW. Contributed to discussion: JBM.

References

1. Khot UN, Khot MB, Bajzer CT, Sapp SK, Ohman EM, et al. (2003) Prevalence of conventional risk factors in patients with coronary heart disease. Jama 290: 898–904.
2. Hackam DG, Anand SS (2003) Emerging risk factors for atherosclerotic vascular disease: a critical review of the evidence. Jama 290: 932–940.
3. Pencina MJ, D'Agostino RB Sr, D'Agostino RB, Jr., Vasan RS (2008) Evaluating the added predictive ability of a new marker: from area under the ROC curve to reclassification and beyond. Stat Med 27: 157–172; discussion 207–112.
4. Melander O, Newton-Cheh C, Almgren P, Hedblad B, Berglund G, et al. (2009) Novel and conventional biomarkers for prediction of incident cardiovascular events in the community. Jama 302: 49–57.
5. Wang TJ, Gona P, Larson MG, Tofler GH, Levy D, et al. (2006) Multiple biomarkers for the prediction of first major cardiovascular events and death. N Engl J Med 355: 2631–2639.
6. Libby P (2002) Inflammation in atherosclerosis. Nature 420: 868–874.
7. Shah SH, de Lemos JA (2009) Biomarkers and cardiovascular disease: determining causality and quantifying contribution to risk assessment. Jama 302: 92–93.
8. Dimmeler S, Zeiher AM (2004) Vascular repair by circulating endothelial progenitor cells: the missing link in atherosclerosis? J Mol Med 82: 671–677.
9. Werner N, Priller J, Laufs U, Endres M, Bohm M, et al. (2002) Bone marrow-derived progenitor cells modulate vascular reendothelialization and neointimal formation: effect of 3-hydroxy-3-methylglutaryl coenzyme a reductase inhibition. Arterioscler Thromb Vasc Biol 22: 1567–1572.
10. Losordo DW, Dimmeler S (2004) Therapeutic angiogenesis and vasculogenesis for ischemic disease: part II: cell-based therapies. Circulation 109: 2692–2697.
11. Asahara T, Murohara T, Sullivan A, Silver M, van der Zee R, et al. (1997) Isolation of putative progenitor endothelial cells for angiogenesis. Science 275: 964–967.

12. Fadini GP, Agostini C, Sartore S, Avogaro A (2007) Endothelial progenitor cells in the natural history of atherosclerosis. Atherosclerosis 194: 46–54.
13. Werner N, Kosiol S, Schiegl T, Ahlers P, Walenta K, et al. (2005) Circulating endothelial progenitor cells and cardiovascular outcomes. N Engl J Med 353: 999–1007.
14. Taguchi A, Matsuyama T, Moriwaki H, Hayashi T, Hayashida K, et al. (2004) Circulating CD34-positive cells provide an index of cerebrovascular function. Circulation 109: 2972–2975.
15. Rosenzweig A (2005) Circulating endothelial progenitors—cells as biomarkers. N Engl J Med 353: 1055–1057.
16. Schmidt-Lucke C, Rossig L, Fichtlscherer S, Vasa M, Britten M, et al. (2005) Reduced number of circulating endothelial progenitor cells predicts future cardiovascular events: proof of concept for the clinical importance of endogenous vascular repair. Circulation 111: 2981–2987.
17. Maruyama S, Taguchi A, Iwashima S, Ozaki T, Yasuda K, et al. (2008) Low circulating CD34(+) cell count is associated with poor prognosis in chronic hemodialysis patients. Kidney Int.
18. Fadini GP, de Kreutzenberg S, Agostini C, Boscaro E, Tiengo A, et al. (2009) Low CD34+ cell count and metabolic syndrome synergistically increase the risk of adverse outcomes. Atherosclerosis in press.
19. Danesh J, Erqou S, Walker M, Thompson SG, Tipping R, et al. (2007) The Emerging Risk Factors Collaboration: analysis of individual data on lipid, inflammatory and other markers in over 1.1 million participants in 104 prospective studies of cardiovascular diseases. Eur J Epidemiol 22: 839–869.
20. Ridker PM, Buring JE, Cook NR, Rifai N (2003) C-reactive protein, the metabolic syndrome, and risk of incident cardiovascular events: an 8-year follow-up of 14,719 initially healthy American women. Circulation. pp 391–397.
21. Fadini GP, de Kreutzenberg S, Agostini C, Boscaro E, Tiengo A, et al. (2009) Low CD34+ cell count and metabolic syndrome synergistically increase the risk of adverse outcomes. Atherosclerosis 207: 213–219.

22. Maruyama S, Taguchi A, Iwashima S, Ozaki T, Yasuda K, et al. (2008) Low circulating CD34+ cell count is associated with poor prognosis in chronic hemodialysis patients. Kidney Int 74: 1603–1609.

23. Fadini GP, Boscaro E, de Kreutzenberg S, Agostini C, Seeger F, et al. (2010) Time course and mechanisms of circulating progenitor cell reduction in the natural history of type 2 diabetes. Diabetes Care 33: 1097–1102.

24. Fadini GP, Boscaro E, Albiero M, Menegazzo L, Frison V, et al. The oral dipeptidyl peptidase-4 inhibitor sitagliptin increases circulating endothelial progenitor cells in patients with type 2 diabetes mellitus. Possible role of stromal derived factor-1{alpha}. Diabetes Care.

25. McKee PA, Castelli WP, McNamara PM, Kannel WB (1971) The natural history of congestive heart failure: the Framingham study. N Engl J Med 285: 1441–1446.

26. Chambless LE, Diao G (2006) Estimation of time-dependent area under the ROC curve for long-term risk prediction. Stat Med 25: 3474–3486.

27. Harrell FE, Jr., Lee KL, Mark DB (1996) Multivariable prognostic models: issues in developing models, evaluating assumptions and adequacy, and measuring and reducing errors. Stat Med 15: 361–387.

28. Pencina MJ, D'Agostino RB (2004) Overall C as a measure of discrimination in survival analysis: model specific population value and confidence interval estimation. Stat Med 23: 2109–2123.

29. Rothman KJ (1976) The estimation of synergy or antagonism. Am J Epidemiol 103: 506–511.

30. Zou GY (2008) On the estimation of additive interaction by use of the four-by-two table and beyond. Am J Epidemiol 168: 212–224.

31. Fadini GP, Baesso I, Albiero M, Sartore S, Agostini C, et al. (2008) Technical notes on endothelial progenitor cells: ways to escape from the knowledge plateau. Atherosclerosis 197: 496–503.

32. Cook NR (2007) Use and misuse of the receiver operating characteristic curve in risk prediction. Circulation 115: 928–935.

33. Blankenberg S, McQueen MJ, Smieja M, Pogue J, Balion C, et al. (2006) Comparative Impact of Multiple Biomarkers and N-Terminal Pro-Brain Natriuretic Peptide for the Prediction of Recurrent Cardiovascular Events in the Heart Outcomes Prevention Evaluation (HOPE) Study. Circulation 114: 201–208.

34. Prokopi M, Pula G, Mayr U, Devue C, Gallagher J, et al. (2009) Proteomic analysis reveals presence of platelet microparticles in endothelial progenitor cell cultures. Blood 114: 723–732.

35. Fadini GP, de Kreutzenberg SV, Coracina A, Baesso I, Agostini C, et al. (2006) Circulating CD34+ cells, metabolic syndrome, and cardiovascular risk. Eur Heart J 27: 2247–2255.

36. Zethelius B, Berglund L, Sundstrom J, Ingelsson E, Basu S, et al. (2008) Use of multiple biomarkers to improve the prediction of death from cardiovascular causes. N Engl J Med 358: 2107–2116.

37. Smith GD, Ebrahim S (2004) Mendelian randomization: prospects, potentials, and limitations. Int J Epidemiol 33: 30–42.

38. Ridker PM, Danielson E, Fonseca FA, Genest J, Gotto AM, Jr., et al. (2008) Rosuvastatin to prevent vascular events in men and women with elevated C-reactive protein. N Engl J Med 359: 2195–2207.

39. Sakurai M, Furusawa T, Ikeda M, Hikono H, Shimizu S, et al. (2006) Anti-bovine CD34 monoclonal antibody reveals polymorphisms within coding region of the CD34 gene. Exp Hematol 34: 905–913.

40. Bogunia-Kubik K, Gieryng A, Dlubek D, Lange A (2009) The CXCL12-3′A allele is associated with a higher mobilization yield of CD34 progenitors to the peripheral blood of healthy donors for allogeneic transplantation. Bone Marrow Transplant 44: 273–278.

41. Dimmeler S, Aicher A, Vasa M, Mildner-Rihm C, Adler K, et al. (2001) HMG-CoA reductase inhibitors (statins) increase endothelial progenitor cells via the PI 3-kinase/Akt pathway. J Clin Invest 108: 391–397.

42. Bahlmann FH, de Groot K, Mueller O, Hertel B, Haller H, et al. (2005) Stimulation of endothelial progenitor cells: a new putative therapeutic effect of angiotensin II receptor antagonists. Hypertension 45: 526–529.

43. Croce G, Passacquale G, Necozione S, Ferri C, Desideri G (2006) Nonpharmacological treatment of hypercholesterolemia increases circulating endothelial progenitor cell population in adults. Arterioscler Thromb Vasc Biol 26: e38–39.

44. Muller-Ehmsen J, Braun D, Schneider T, Pfister R, Worm N, et al. (2008) Decreased number of circulating progenitor cells in obesity: beneficial effects of weight reduction. Eur Heart J 29: 1560–1568.

45. Adams V, Lenk K, Linke A, Lenz D, Erbs S, et al. (2004) Increase of circulating endothelial progenitor cells in patients with coronary artery disease after exercise-induced ischemia. Arterioscler Thromb Vasc Biol 24: 684–690.

46. Kondo T, Hayashi M, Takeshita K, Numaguchi Y, Kobayashi K, et al. (2004) Smoking cessation rapidly increases circulating progenitor cells in peripheral blood in chronic smokers. Arterioscler Thromb Vasc Biol 24: 1442–1447.

4

Elimination of Endogenous Toxin, Creatinine from Blood Plasma Depends on Albumin Conformation: Site Specific Uremic Toxicity & Impaired Drug Binding

Ankita Varshney[1], Mohd Rehan[2], Naidu Subbarao[2], Gulam Rabbani[1], Rizwan Hasan Khan[1]*

1 Interdisciplinary Biotechnology Unit, Aligarh Muslim University, Aligarh, India, 2 School of Information Technology, Centre for Computational Biology and Bioinformatics, Jawaharlal Nehru University, New Delhi, India

Abstract

Uremic syndrome results from malfunctioning of various organ systems due to the retention of uremic toxins which, under normal conditions, would be excreted into the urine and/or metabolized by the kidneys. The aim of this study was to elucidate the mechanisms underlying the renal elimination of uremic toxin creatinine that accumulate in chronic renal failure. Quantitative investigation of the plausible correlations was performed by spectroscopy, calorimetry, molecular docking and accessibility of surface area. Alkalinization of normal plasma from pH 7.0 to 9.0 modifies the distribution of toxin in the body and therefore may affect both the accumulation and the rate of toxin elimination. The ligand loading of HSA with uremic toxin predicts several key side chain interactions of site I that presumably have the potential to impact the specificity and impaired drug binding. These findings provide useful information for elucidating the complicated mechanism of toxin disposition in renal disease state.

Editor: Collin Stultz, Massachusetts Institute of Technology, United States of America

Funding: This work was supported by Council of Scientific and Industrial Research, New Delhi [37/1278/06 EMR-II]. The funders had no role in study design, data collection and analysis, decision to publish, or preparation of the manuscript.

Competing Interests: The authors have declared that no competing interests exist.

* E-mail: rizwanhkhan@hotmail.com

Introduction

The uremic syndrome is attributed to the progressive retention of a large number of biologically/biochemically active endogenous solutes called "uremic toxins", which under normal conditions are excreted by the healthy kidneys [1,2]. The accumulation of these human metabolic products in blood has been implicated in a number of toxic effects in uremic patients, including cardiovascular damage, progressive loss of glomerular filtration, bleeding tendencies from platelet dysfunction, hypertension, neuropathy, irregularities in thyroid function, and defective protein binding of medicinal preparations [3–5].

Among the highly increased uremic guanidino compounds (GCs), creatinine (CTN; 2-Amino-1-methyl-5H-imidazol-4-one, $C_4H_7N_3O$), is the most typical example of small water-soluble breakdown waste product generated from muscle metabolism which can easily be removed by any dialysis strategy [6,7]. CTN have been used as a conventional biomarker that predicts several important health outcomes, to diagnose acute kidney injury involving the measurement of levels of serum creatinine, blood urea nitrogen, and urinary enzymes, all of which are elevated after substantial kidney function is lost [8]. Its concentration for a healthy person is in the range of 35–106 µM whereas for a person with uremia reaches upto µM [6]. The normal level of albumin-to-creatinine ratio (ACR) in blood depends highly on sex, body muscle mass, age, racial/ethnic groups [9] and diseased states. ACR predicts several health outcomes such as neurotoxicity [10], hypertension [11,12], and vascular damage due to leukocyte activation [13], kidney failure [14], cardiovascular events, [15] and microalbuminuria [16]. In renal diseases, the pharmacokinetics of many drugs are altered even when the primary route of elimination is not renal, due to changes in protein binding, volume of distribution, and/or acid-base disturbance [17].

We elucidate the interaction of CTN during the pH dependent structural transition, often referred to as the Neutral (N) – Basic (B) transition [18,19] of Human serum albumin (HSA) which regulates the volume of circulating plasma; therefore, albumin must be conserved by the body [20]. The structural transitions and toxin binding properties were evaluated by means of calorimetric and, spectroscopic approaches using typical site-specific bound drugs (warfarin, phenylbutazone, ibuprofen and diazepam). The competitive binding of a toxin affects the transport of endogenous as well as exogenous substances especially site specific drugs targeted to the focus of disease for therapeutic effect [20]. The elimination of such toxins from the blood stream of patients suffering from chronic renal failure which was an important therapeutic goal was found to be dependent on albumin conformation. We determine the high affinity binding site of CTN on HSA using displacement, molecular docking and surface accessibility. The major amino acid residue being involved in the interaction was Arg257 which provides the guanidino group to the toxin. The primary binding site of toxin was located in the vicinity of Arg257 or near to loop 4 and 6 in subdomain IIA which corresponds approximately to amino acid position of 190–300, one of the two principal sites on HSA for small ligands [20]. Thus, binding of CTN to its high affinity (site I) and low affinity (site II) sites indirectly displaces drugs from albumin and increases the transiently liberated toxin molecules leading to impaired drug binding.

Materials and Methods

Materials

Human serum albumin (lot No. A1887; essentially fatty acid free and globulin), creatinine (lot No. C4255), warfarin (lot No. A2250), ibuprofen (lot No. I4883) and phenylbutazone (lot No. P8386) were purchased from Sigma. Diazepam was a product from Ranbaxy Laboratories Ltd., India. All of the other reagents were of analytical grade.

Preparation of HSA Isomers and creatinine solutions

The protein and toxin solutions were prepared in pH 7.0 (60 mM sodium phosphate) and pH 9.0 (10 mM glycine-NaOH) buffer solutions. The protein concentration used was similar to that of albumin concentration present in blood i.e. 500 μM and was determined spectrophotometrically using $E_{1cm}^{1\%}$ of 5.31 [21] at 279 nm on a Hitachi spectrophotometer, model U-1500. The concentration of creatinine ($M_w = 113.12$) used varies accordingly from normal serum creatinine (106 μM) to uremic conditions (2000 μM) as previously analyzed in a survey of patients suffering from uremic disorders [6]. For all measurements we have used three form of protein preparations as 'free HSA' not complexed with toxin; 'normal condition' describes the solution of HSA complexed with minimal craetinine concentration and 'uHSA' describes the term used for the protein/toxin complex responsible for maximal uremic conditions. In all of these preparations, we have used HSA/CTN ratio similar to that of in-vivo conditions i.e. ACR = 5 (normal condition) and ACR = 0.25 (maximal uremic condition).

Differential Scanning Calorimetry (DSC)

The thermal denaturation of the proteins was carried out on a VP-DSC microcalorimeter (MicroCal Inc., Northampton, MA). The thermograms were obtained in the temperature range of 30–90°C at a scanning rate of 0.5 K/min. Before being loaded into the cells, the sample (HSA or HSA-CTN) and the reference (buffer or buffer-CTN) solutions were degassed by stirring in an evacuated chamber at room temperature. The solution with the vial was weighed before and after degassing, and the appropriate amount of degassed deionized water was added to make up for any loss of water thus evaporated. The solutions were then immediately loaded into the respective cells. The calorimetric reversibility of the thermal transitions was determined by heating the sample to a temperature that was a little over the transition maximum, cooling immediately, and then reheating. The reversible non-two-state denaturation model provides the temperature where the area under the transition curve is half complete (ΔT_m), van't Hoff (ΔH_{VH}) and calorimetric (ΔH_m) enthalpies depicting actual heat absorption during protein unfolding. The cooperative unit is defined by the ratio $\Delta H_m/\Delta H_{VH}$ [22].

Isothermal Titration Calorimetry (ITC)

The energetic of the binding of creatinine to HSA were measured using a VP-ITC titration microcalorimeter (MicroCal Inc., Northampton, MA). All the solutions were thoroughly degassed before loading, and the consequent water loss was compensated using degassed deionized water. The reactant (500 μM protein solution) was placed in the sample cell (1.4 ml) and the injectant (2000 μM creatinine solution) was introduced into the calorimeter in 8 μl increments spaced 400 sec apart. The

injection syringe rotated at a speed of 300 rpm throughout the experiment to facilitate mixing of the reaction components. Sequential titrations were performed to ensure full occupancy of the binding sites by loading and titrating with the same ligand without removing the samples from the cell until the titration signal was essentially constant. To correct for the dilution effect by the injection of toxin solution, two controls were obtained: titration of HSA solution by the buffer to account for HSA dilution and titration of buffer solution by creatinine solution to account for toxin dilution effect. Experiments were repeated two or more times to get a reproducibility of better than 3%. The generated were integrated using the single set of identical binding sites model of Origin 7 software provided by MicroCal. The experimental data were best fitted to a binding model depending upon the least chi-square values obtained. The enthalpy change for each injection was calculated by integrating the area under the peaks of the recorded time course of change of power and then subtracted with the control titrations. The other thermodynamic parameters were calculated according to the formulas [23,24]:

$$\Delta G = -RT \ln K_a = \Delta H - T \Delta S \dots \dots \dots \quad (i)$$

Where T is the absolute temperature (298K) and R = 8.3151 J mol^{-1} K^{-1}.

Fluorescence Measurements

The intrinsic fluorescence properties of the protein were studied on a Hitachi spectrophotometer, model F-4500. The fluorescence spectra were measured at 25 ± 0.1°C with a 1 cm path length cell. The excitation and emission slits were set at 10 and 20 nm, respectively. Intrinsic fluorescence was measured by exciting the protein solution at 280 and 295 nm to selectively excite the chromophoric molecules, and the emission spectra were monitored in the wavelength range 300–500 nm. The emission spectra of the protein-toxin solutions were subtracted from the buffer-toxin blanks, and an average of three accumulated scans was recorded as the final graph. The fluorescence data were analyzed according to linear and modified stern-volmer equations as [21,25]:

$$\frac{F_0}{F} = 1 + K_{sv}[Q] \dots \dots \dots \quad (ii)$$

$$\log\left[\frac{(F_o - F)}{F}\right] = \log K + n\log[Q] \dots \dots \dots \quad (iii)$$

FT-IR Spectroscopic Measurements

Infrared spectra were recorded on a Nicolet Magna 750 FT-IR spectrophotometer (DTGS detector, Ni-chrome source and KBr beamsplitter) with a total of 100 scans and resolution of 16 cm^{-1}, using AgBr windows at room temperature. The concentration of HSA was 500 μM. The difference spectra [(protein solution) - (protein solution + ligand solution)] were collected after 1 h of incubation of HSA. The protein FT-IR spectra were processed as the procedures as reported by Kang et al. [26].

Determination of the Protein Secondary Structure

The secondary structure content of HSA and the HSA complexed with toxin under normal and maximal uremic conditions was determined from the shape of the amide I band, located around 1650–1660 cm^{-1}. The FT-IR spectra were

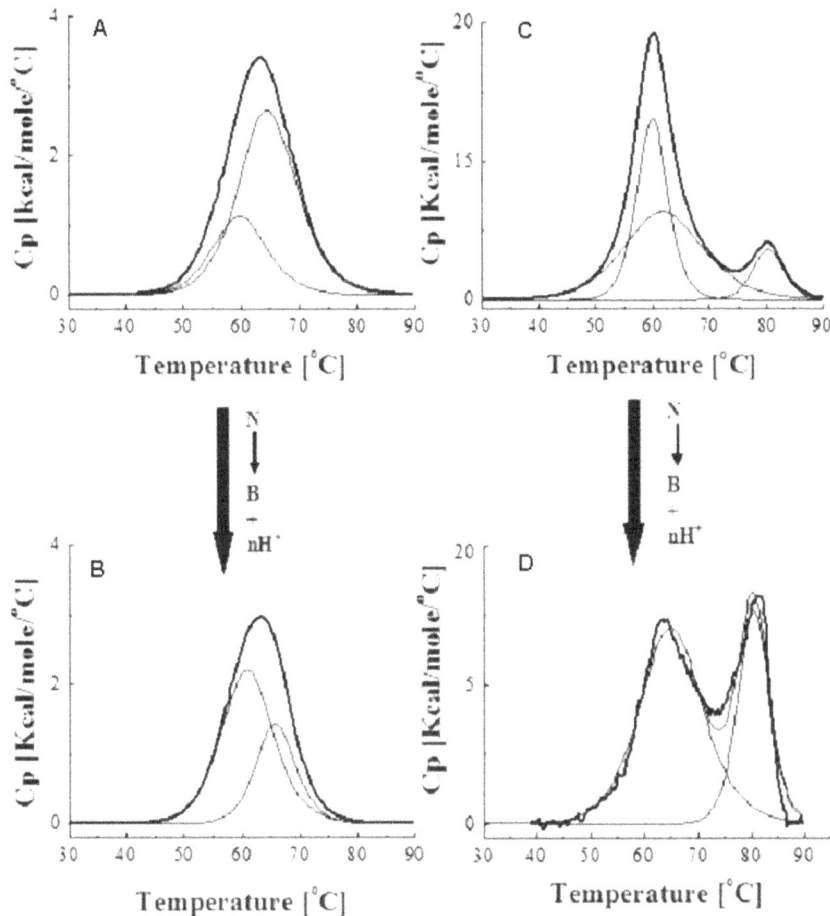

Figure 1. Differential scanning calorimetry of HSA in absence and presence of creatinine. Melting thermograms of Human Serum Albumin under normal (A and B) and uremic (C and D) conditions at pH 7.0 (A and C) and pH 9.0 (B and D).

smoothed, and their baselines were corrected automatically using the built-in software of the spectrophotometer (OMNIC version 3.1). Each Lorentzian band was assigned to a secondary structure according to the frequency of its maximum; α-helix (1656–1658 cm^{-1}), β-sheet (1614–1638 cm^{-1}), turn (1660–1677 cm^{-1}), random coil (1640–1648 cm^{-1}), and β-antiparallel (1680–1692 cm^{-1}) were adjusted and the area was measured with the Gaussian function. The relative percentage of the secondary structural elements was obtained from the area under the Gaussian curve [27].

CD and UV spectroscopic Measurements

CD and UV spectra were recorded on a Jasco J-815 spectropolarimeter, equipped at $25\pm0.2°$C in a rectangular cuvette with 1 cm pathlength under a constant nitrogen flow. Each spectrum was signal-averaged at least two times with a bandwidth of 1.0 nm and resolution of 0.2 nm, at a scan speed of 20 nm/min. Temperature control was provided by a Peltier thermostat equipped with magnetic stirring. Stock solutions of the site specific markers 6.8×10^3 µM warfarin, 6.8×10^3 µM phenylbutazone, 1.2×10^4 µM ibuprofen, 8×10^3 µM diazepam were prepared and added stepwise in µl volumes to the creatinine–HSA solutions both at pH 7.0 and 9.0. These solutions were prepared by dissolving in ethanol such as its concentration never exceeded 13% and the effects of the organic solvent on the CD measurements were undetectable. Induced CD spectra resulting

from the interaction of the toxin with HSA were obtained by subtracting the CD spectrum of the protein from that of the protein-toxin complex. Ellipticities values were converted to 'Δε' values using the equation $\Delta\varepsilon = \theta/(33982cl)$ where, Δε is the molar

Table 1. Thermodynamic parameters accompanying thermal unfolding of HSA complexes with creatinine at a scan rate of 0.5 K/min.

Condition	T_m [K]		ΔH_m [Kcal/mol]	
	$T_m^{1\,a}$	$T_m^{2\,a}$	$\Delta H_m^{1\,b}$	$\Delta H_m^{2\,b}$
A	59.84±0.63	64.59±0.28	14.2±0.52	35.2±0.54
B	61.01±0.51	65.83±0.35	26.2±0.38	13.2±0.38
C	59.93±0.02	80.27±0.05	143.00±0.52	39.31±0.09
D	65.06±0.12	80.31±0.07	110.30±0.96	58.69±0.15

Condition A: N Isomer of HSA at pH 7.0.
Condition B: B Isomer of HSA at pH 9.0.
Condition C: N Isomer of HSA at pH 7.0+ CTN.
Condition D: B Isomer of HSA at pH 9.0+ CTN.
[a]Midpoint of thermal denaturation.
[b]Calorimetric enthalpy.
Superscripts 1 and 2 refer to the low and high unfolding transition, respectively (see text for details).

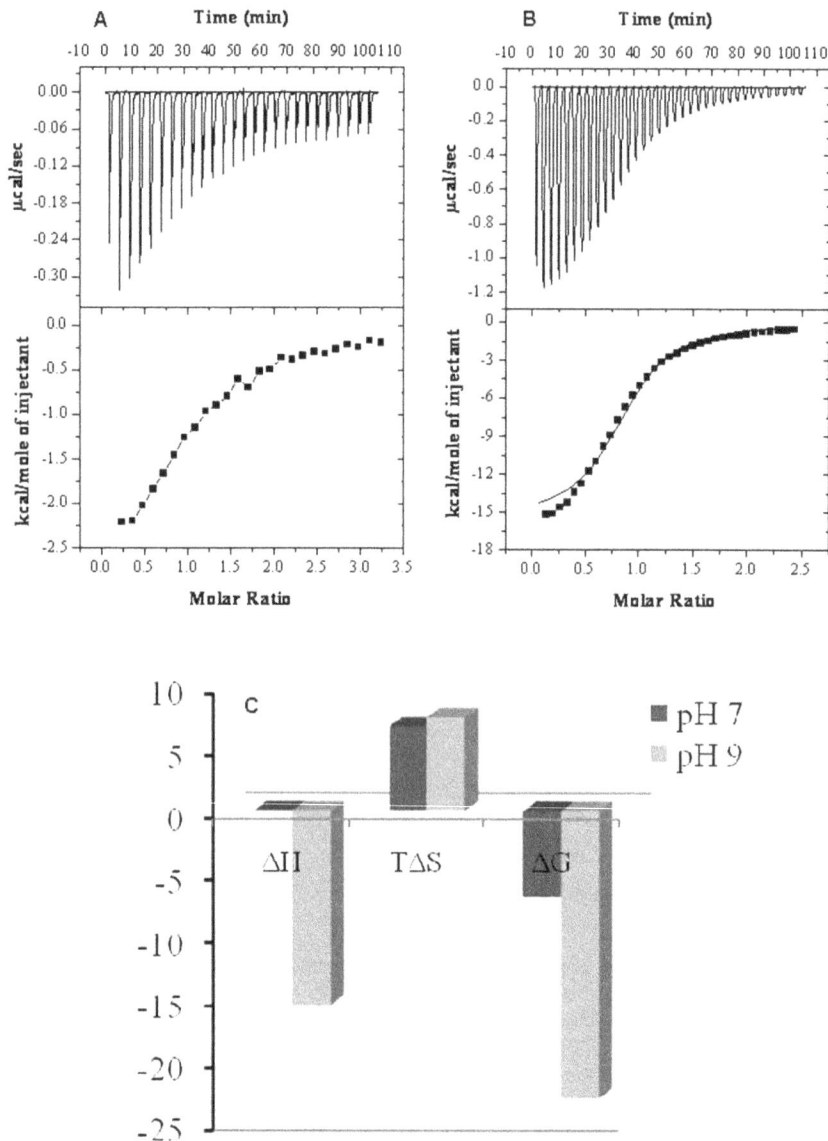

Figure 2. Isothermal titration calorimetry of HSA complexed with creatinine. The ITC experiments of N and B isomers of Human serum albumin at pH 7.0 (A) and 9.0(B) respectively were performed at 25°C. In the top panels, the heat released per unit time (μcal/sec) was plotted vs time where each peak corresponds to the injection of an aliquot of ligand. In the bottom panels, the heat of reaction per injection (kcal/mole) was determined by integration of the area under each peak, plotted vs [CTN]/[HSA], and fit using the software provided by Microcal. (C) Comparative distribution of ΔH, TΔS and ΔG at pH 7.0 (dark grey) and pH 9.0 (light grey).

Table 2. Association constants and thermodynamic data for binding of creatinine to HSA.

Condition	$K_a[M^{-1}]$		n		ΔG^a [Kcal/mol]	ΔH^a [Kcal/mol]	ΔS^a [cal/mol/K]
	ITC^a	Spec^b	ITC^a	Spec^b			
A	8.92×10^4	*1.15×10^4 #2.92×10^4	0.98	*0.94 #1.07	−6.75	−0.017±0.91	22.6
B	2.69×10^5	*9.76×10^5 #1.36×10^5	0.94	*1.29 #1.17	−23.03	−15.53±0.79	−25.2

Condition A: N Isomer of HSA at pH 7.0+ CTN.
Condition B: B Isomer of HSA at pH 9.0+ CTN.
^{a}Constants determined by Isothermal Titration Calorimetry.
^{b}Constants determined by Fluorescence spectroscopy ($^*\lambda_{excitation}=280$ nm; $^{\#}\lambda_{excitation}=295$ nm).

circular dichroic absorption coefficient expressed in $M^{-1}cm^{-1}$, c is the concentration of the sample expressed in mol/L, and l is the pathlength through the cell expressed in cm.

Molecular Docking Studies

The crystal structure of HSA site I markers (warfarin, PDB ID: 1H9Z; phenylbutazone, PDB ID: 2BXC) and the site II markers (diazepam, PDB ID: 2BXF; ibuprofen, PDB ID: 2BXG) were derived from Protein Data Bank. The residues falling within 5 Å distance of the marker were extracted and combined to define the binding site. The two dimensional (2D) structures of ligands were extracted from Pubchem database in SDF (Structure Data File) format. The three dimensional structures were generated with CORINA version 2.6 [28]. Molecular docking simulations of uremic toxin and site specific probes were carried out using the GOLD version 3.1.4 program (Genetic Optimization Ligand Docking) [29] software which uses a genetic algorithm to calculate the possible conformations of the toxin that binds to the protein. The ligands were docked to active site of HSA using standard set parameters of GOLD throughout the simulations. For each of the 100 independent genetic algorithm runs, a selection pressure of operations were set to terminate after a maximum of 2,500,000 energy evaluations. Lowest energy complex geometries and the corresponding free energy of binding

were calculated. Top 20 poses were saved for each ligand and best score values were used to correlate with experimental data. The binding energies of docked molecules were also calculated using X-score [30]. The hydrogen bonding (cutoff distance of 2.8–3.2 Å between donor and acceptor) and hydrophobic interactions between ligand and protein were calculated using Getneares, a program available with DOCK version 3.1.4 [31]. PyMol version 0.99 [32] and chimera version 1.3 [33] were used for visualization and measurement of distances between the ligand and the receptor.

The Accessible Surface Area (ASA) of uncomplexed HSA and complexes of ligands with HSA were calculated using NACCESS version 2.1.1 [34]. The structure of the ligands corresponding to the final docked conformation was chosen and composite coordinates were generated to form the docked complex. The change in ASA (ΔASA) of the ith residue was calculated using the expression:

$$\Delta ASA_i = ASA_i^{HSA} - ASA_i^{HSA\text{-}Ligand} \quad\dots\dots\dots \quad (iv)$$

If a residue lost more than 10 Å^2 ASA on going from the uncomplexed to the complexed state, it was considered as being involved in interaction [35].

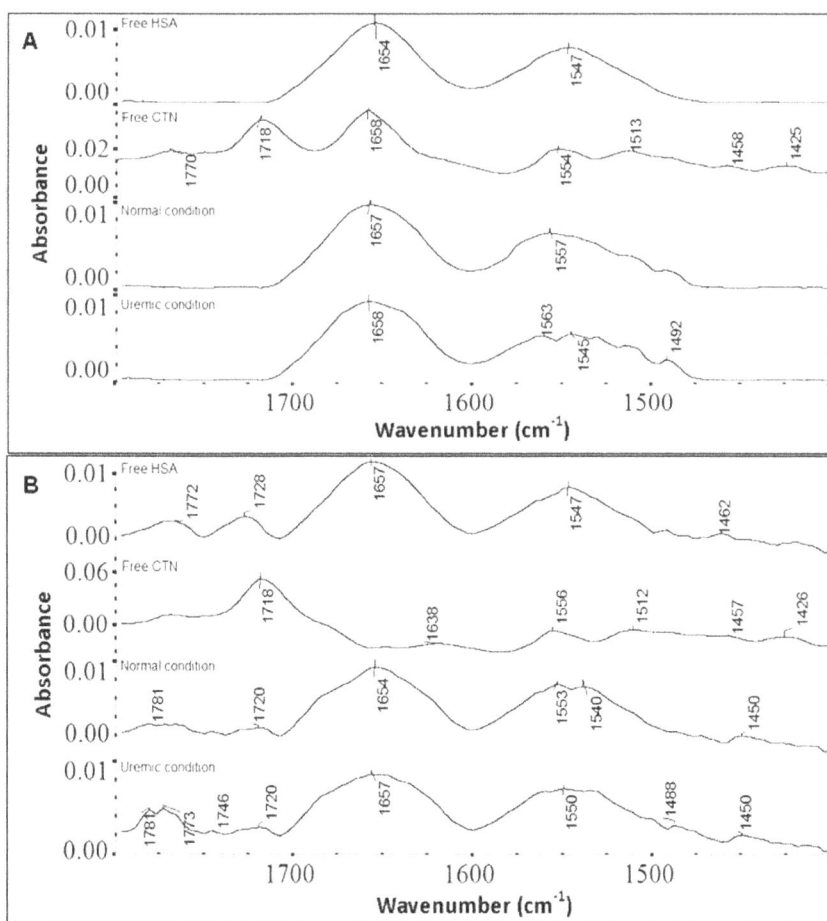

Figure 3. Fourier transform infrared (FTIR) measurements of HSA in absence and presence of creatinine. Infrared spectra were recorded on a FTIR spectrometer in the region 1800–1400 cm^{-1} at pH 7.0 (A) and pH 9.0 (B) for the free HSA, free CTN and difference spectra of HSA-CTN complexes (bottom two curves) obtained under normal serum (ACR = 5) to uremic condition (ACR = 0.25) (indicated in the figure).

Results

Thermal Denaturation of N and B isomer of HSA in presence of creatinine

The representative differential scanning calorimetric profiles of thermal denaturation of N and B isomers of HSA in absence and presence of creatinine were performed under normal and uremic condition as shown in Figure 1 (for simplicity we have only shown data for native protein at pH 7.0 (A) pH 9.0 (B) and maximal uremic conditions at pH 7.0 (C) and 9.0 (D) respectively. The corresponding thermodynamic parameters accompanying the transitions were reported in Table 1. In the absence of toxin, N isomer of HSA unfolds with reversible endotherm at transition temperatures of 59–64°C and an average calorimetric enthalpy of 14.2–35.2 kcal/mol. Almost similar value of the transition temperature of N and B isomeric forms (in absence of toxin) indicates the extent of the binding interactions of positive charge of amino acid residues participating in the molecular mechanism of this equilibrium. However, a little difference in the cooperativity ratio

β was found to be 1.02 ± 0.01 (data not shown), indicating that the thermal unfolding of the protein in the presence of toxin even at higher concentrations was a reversible process. These values were in concurrence with those reported in the literature [36]. The melting curve of uremic plasma (albumin complexed with creatinine) shows a different shape without any reversal in amplitude of the two peaks but a slight shift to the right at higher temperature. The toxin renders the strongest influence on the endotherms (more pronounce for basic isomer of HSA, Figure 1D) by transforming the unimodal curve of its melting to a bimodal one. As it follows from Figure 1, on reaching from normal to maximal uremic condition, the melting curve was practically identical to that for the complex "albumin-nonconjugated bilirubin" [37].

Isothermal Titration Calorimetry of N and B isomer of HSA in presence of creatinine

In order to determine thermodynamic parameters for binding we performed isothermal titration calorimetry of creatinine with

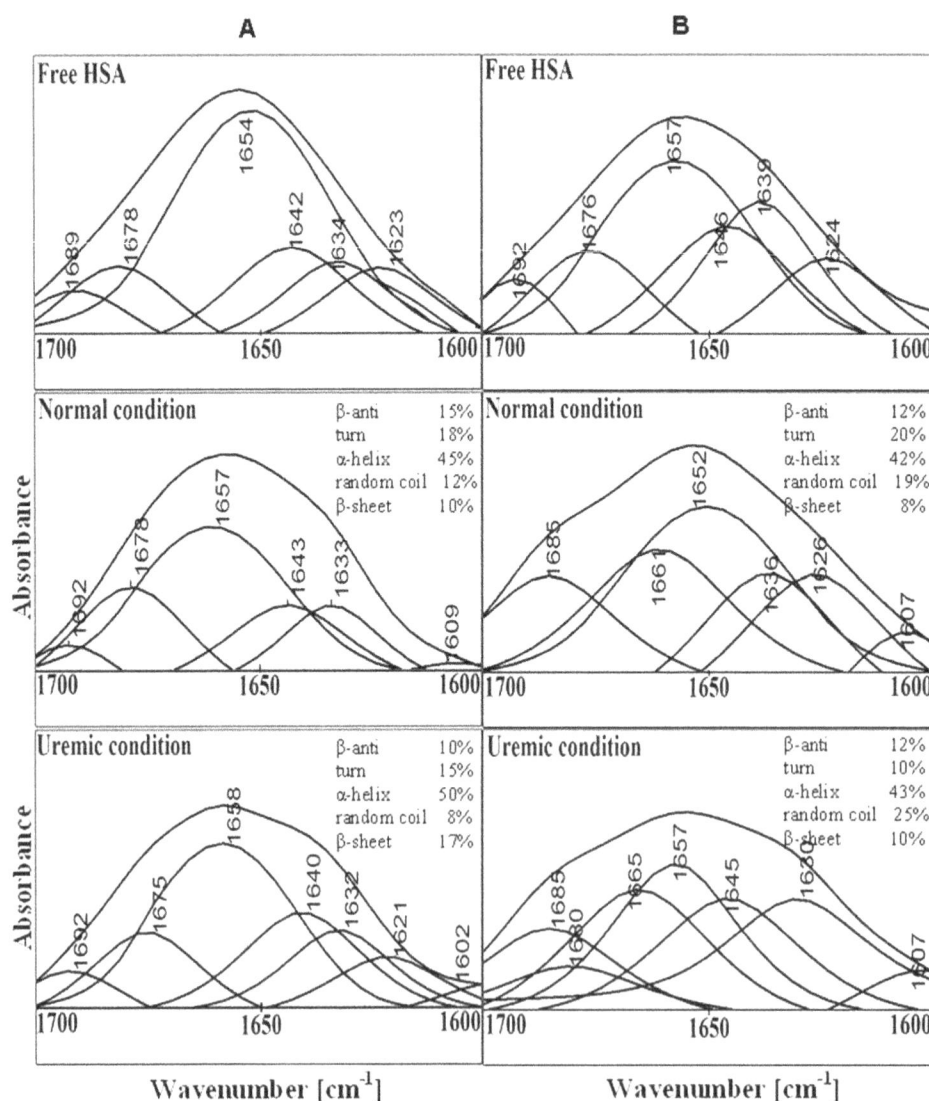

Figure 4. Determination of protein secondary structure complexed with creatinine. Curve fitted amide I region (1700–1600 cm^{-1}) with secondary structure determination of the free HSA and its toxin adducts in aqueous solution with varying ACR molar ratios and 500 μM protein concentrations at pH 7.0 (A) and pH 9.0 (B).

neutral and basic isomer of HSA. A representative calorimetric titration profile of ACR at molar ratio of 1:4 (HSA in normal serum: HSA complexed with creatinine under uremic conditions) at pH 7.0 (A) and pH 9.0 (B) were shown in Figure 2. Each peak in the binding isotherms (Figure 2, upper panels) represents a single injection of creatinine. The negative deflections from the baseline on addition of creatinine indicate that heat was evolved (an exothermic process). The enthalpy change associated with each injection of ligand was plotted versus the [CTN]/[HSA] molar ratio (Figure 2, lower panel), and the ΔH, K_a, the free energy change (ΔG) associated with binding were determined from the plots. The thermodynamic data derived from the model fitting were summarized in Table 1. The 1:4 binding stoichiometry of CTN to basic isomer of HSA with a binding constant of 2.69×10^5 M^{-1} indicates a strong and specific interaction. This binding constant was of larger order of magnitude than that of neutral form (8.92×10^4 M^{-1}) as shown in Table 2. Furthermore, the heat released during the CTN-HSA reaction increases with increasing pH, i.e., the ion pair attraction and H-bonds between CTN and HSA were weakened. This indicates that the number of H-bonds formed by CTN was lower at pH 7.0. In contrast, ΔS become more negative with increasing pH. This indicates that CTN binding destroyed the internal hydrophobic interactions in HSA at pH 9.0, replacing them with ion pair attraction and H-bonds. Comparison of the ΔG, ΔH, and $T\Delta S$ values suggests that the CTN-HSA interaction was amphipathic and H-bonds and ion pair binding were both major contributors, i.e., the interaction of CTN with HSA depends on a combination of ion pair attraction and H-bonds (Figure 2C).

Analysis of secondary structure of N and B isomer of HSA in presence of creatinine

To investigate the effects of the uremic toxin creatinine on the secondary structure of albumin, we analyzed regions of IR spectra caused by vibrations of polypeptide backbone, viz., the amide I (1700–1600 cm^{-1}, mainly C=O stretch) band and the amide II (1500–1600 cm^{-1}, C-N stretching coupled with N-H bending modes) band. The amide I band of free HSA (Figure 3) had a major maximum around 1654 cm^{-1} for native and 1657 cm^{-1} for basic isomer, characteristic of the α-helical conformation [34]. Similarly, the infrared self-deconvulation and curve fitting

procedures were used to determine the protein secondary structure under normal and uremic conditions both at pH 7.0 and 9.0 (Figure 4, Table 3).

Positions and relative intensities of the components in presence of toxin (i.e. uremic condition) did not differ significantly from those of normal HSA (free HSA without toxin). Though quantitative analysis of the amide I (Table 3) revealed a substantial decrease in the amount of α-helical conformation and an increase in β-sheets and or/extended chains in uremic HSA. The decrease in the intensity of amide I and amide II bands, mainly C=O and C-N vibrations, compared to low toxin concentration (normal condition) suggests major protein conformational changes upon HSA-toxin interaction possibly caused by a reorganization of intra- and intermolecular hydrogen bonding. The toxin-HSA complexation suggests partial protein unfolding more pronounced at higher molar ratio (uremic condition) i.e. similar to uremic diseased state and for basic isomeric form of HSA. The IR spectra of uremic HSA (HSA complexed with toxin) at higher molar ratios for both isomers showed appearance of some new components for amide II band (Figure 3). This band was caused by vibrations of the peptide N-H groups and by motions of Glu, Asp, Tyr, Lys and His side chains. We observed main alterations in the range 1652–1695 cm^{-1} that were basically associated with that of Arg environment. Because the appearance of this component in the IR spectra of uHSA was accompanied by no changes in the peptide C=O absorption, it likely reflects alterations in the environment of Glu and Asp side chains in uHSA molecules [38].

Fluorescence spectroscopy of N and B isomer of HSA in presence of creatinine

Both the intensity and the position of the fluorescence emission spectrum of tryptophan were sensitive to changes in the fluorescence environment and consequently to the protein conformation. Hence, to understand the influence of creatinine binding on the neutral and basic form of HSA we studied the changes in the intrinsic fluorescence of the protein. Figure 5 shows the fluorescence spectra of HSA in the presence of increasing concentration of creatinine. The fluorescence quenching data were analyzed according to the Linear (Figure 5A and C) and modified Stern-Volmer equation (Figure 5B and D) [21,35] after

Table 3. FT-IR/ATR determination of secondary structure percentages of N and B isomers of HSA and its uremic complexes.

Amide I components	N isomer			B isomer		
	Free HSA (%)	Normal[a] (%)	Uremic[b] (%)	Free HSA (%)	Normal[a] (%)	Uremic[b] (%)
β-antiparallel (1675–1695 cm^{-1})	8±2	15±1	10±1	10±2	12±2	12±1
Turns (1666–1673 cm^{-1})	15±1	18±1	15±1	15±2	20±1	10±2
α-helix (1650–1658 cm^{-1})	54±2	45±1	50±2	53±1	42±2	43±2
Random coil (1637–1645 cm^{-1})	6±1	12±1	8±1	15±2	19±2	25±1
β-sheets (1613–1625 cm^{-1})	17±1	10±1	17±1	7±2	8±2	10±2

[a]Normal condition: HSA complexed with creatinine under normal serum condition.
[b]Uremic condition: HSA complexed with creatinine under maximal uremic condition.
These complexes were obtained incubating uremic toxin with 500 µM of HSA for 1 hr at room temperature. Data represent average obtained from two independent replicates, standard error is indicated.

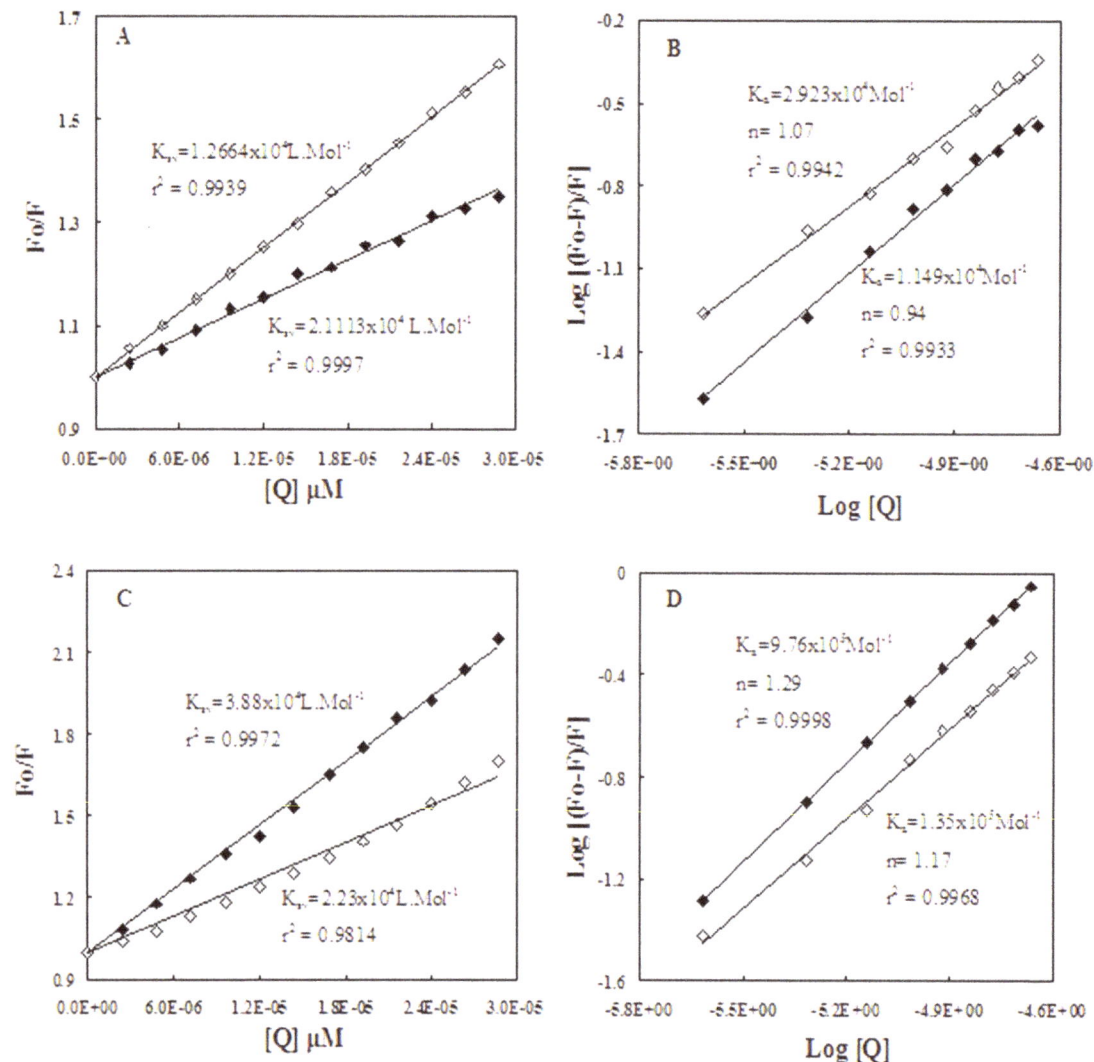

Figure 5. Fluorescence quenching of HSA with creatinine at different ligand/protein ratios. Stern-Volmer (A&C) and modified Stern-Volmer (B&D) plots of N (A&B) and B (C&D) isomeric conformations of HSA with uremic toxin creatinine. Each data point was the mean of 3 independent observations (S.D. ranging 0.03–0.4%). The Protein was excited at 280 (◆) and 295 nm (◇).

exciting the protein at 280 and 295 nm. We observed that, quenching of albumin fluorescence was not affecting the binding strength of tryptophan fluorescence. This may be so because binding of uremic toxin was not exactly at the site where tryptophan resides but it could be somewhere near to it as it mainly affects tyrosine fluorescence. These results are comparable with that of our ITC results and are presented in Table 2 further confirming that association constant K_a of uremic toxin depends on conformation of HSA underwent N-B transitions.

Dependence on alkalization of the Optical properties of creatinine-HSA solution

The conjugated double bond system of creatinine constitutes the light absorbing chromophore that has no element of chirality; it does not show CD activity. The toxin gives the weak absorption band associated with an electronic dipole allowed $\Lambda-\Lambda^*$ transition which becomes optically active upon binding to the asymmetric environment of HSA and an induced CD spectrum emerges a weak positive $\Lambda-\Lambda^*$ CD band between 250–350 nm (Figure 6).

Regarding the interaction of toxin with the albumin binding site, it has to be noted that dissociated ligand molecules lose their hydrogen donor properties but at the same time, they become more powerful proton acceptors ready to form H bonds with basic residues of HSA. Upon increasing pH value, the CD signals and absorption curves of HSA-CTN complex enhances; triggered by the protonation of histidine residues, toxin flips away at neutral and alkaline pH values and the cavity becomes accessible for the ligand molecule. The spectra obtained by toxin titration experiment (Figure 6A) clearly demonstrate that the protein microenvironment at pH 7.0 was less favourable to accommodate toxin as a chiral conformer.

Probing the binding site of Creatinine on HSA by Ligand Displacement experiments

Further spectroscopic experiments were undertaken to obtain information on the potential location of the HSA binding site of CTN. Albumin possesses two main drug binding sites, site I and II, which are located in hydrophobic cavities of subdomains IIA and

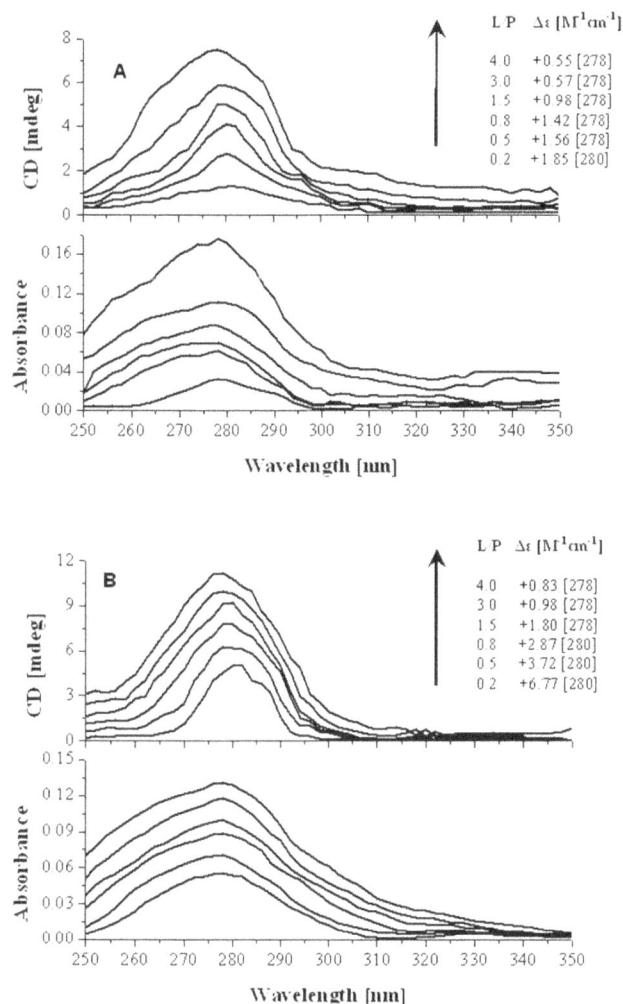

Figure 6. Induced circular dichroism and UV/vis spectra of creatinine-HSA complex. Representative CD and UV spectra obtained following the titration of the buffer solution of HSA with creatinine at (A) pH 7.0 and (B) pH 9.0. Spectral contributions of the protein alone were subtracted from the spectra of the toxin–protein mixture ([HSA] = 100 μM, T = 25°C). $\Delta\varepsilon_{max}$ values calculated on the basis of the total ligand concentrations are displayed at the different molar ratios (L/P). Arrows denote increasing concentration of uremic toxin CTN.

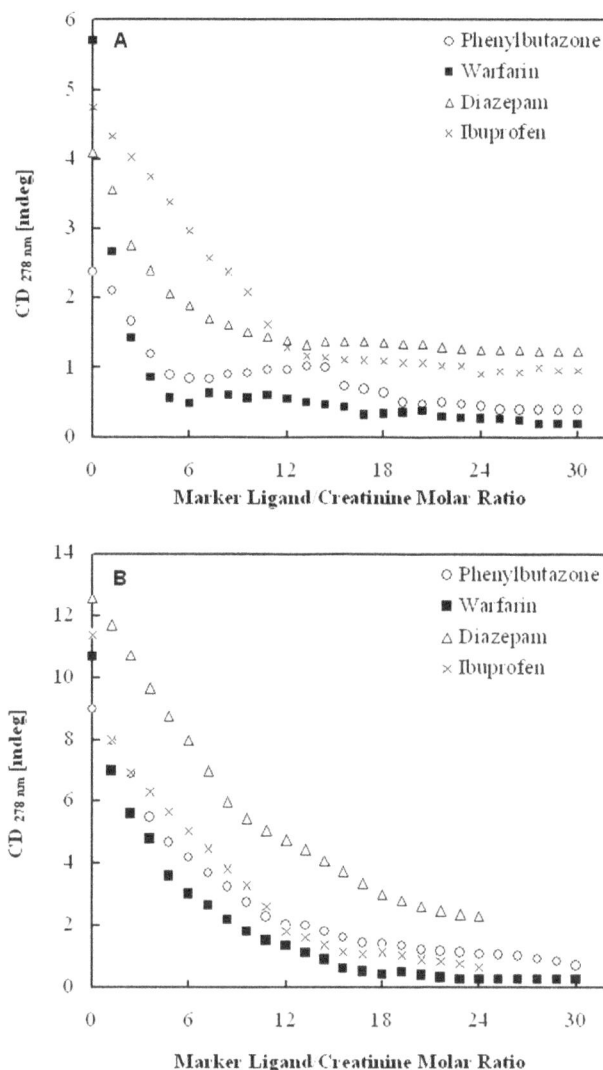

Figure 7. Displacing effect of HSA site specific markers on the ICD signal of creatinine-HSA complex. Results of CD displacement experiments performed with warfarin, phenylbutazone, ibuprofen and diazepam on HSA-CTN complex at (A) pH 7.0 and (B) pH 9.0 (l = 1 cm, T = 25°C). Displacers were added as μl aliquots of stock solutions. Positive induced CD values measured at 278 nm are plotted against displacer/creatinine molar ratios (for further details see Materials and methods).

IIIA, respectively [20]. In the presence of a compound having the same binding site as creatinine, amplitudes of the induced cotton effects should decrease due to competition. Therefore, CD displacement experiments were performed using four marker ligands warfarin and phenylbutazone for site I whereas ibuprofen and the benzodiazepine agent diazepam for site II. Monitoring the induced CD spectrum of creatinine during the titration showed a rapid extinction of extrinsic CD activity for both isomers of HSA but this extinction was found to be more steep at pH 9.0 (Figure 7). Especially the site I markers, phenylbutazone followed by warfarin were found to be responsible for reducing the CD signal of the protein-toxin complex to almost zero. Thereby, suggesting the direct competitive interaction between site I markers and creatinine for the binding site I. Notably, nearly complete extinction of the CD signal was achieved for both isomeric forms of HSA suggesting that the binding site was not affected by the protonation of albumin molecules.

Molecular docking study of uremic toxin creatinine–HSA interaction

The locations of uremic toxin creatinine in the active sites (site I and site II) of HSA was explored by conducting docking simulations using GOLD [29] as presented in Figure 8 and 9. The principal regions of ligand binding to HSA were located in hydrophobic cavities in subdomains IIA and IIIA, which are consistent with site I and site II, respectively [20]. The creatinine, site I markers (phenylbutazone and warfarin) were docked to HSA and the results have been shown in Table 4 and 5. The Gold Fitness Score, measure of binding affinity was found to be low for CTN at both of the sites when compared to respective markers used in this study; however specificity was higher for site I as evident from the presence of hydrogen bond and hydrophobic interactions. The spectroscopic experimental

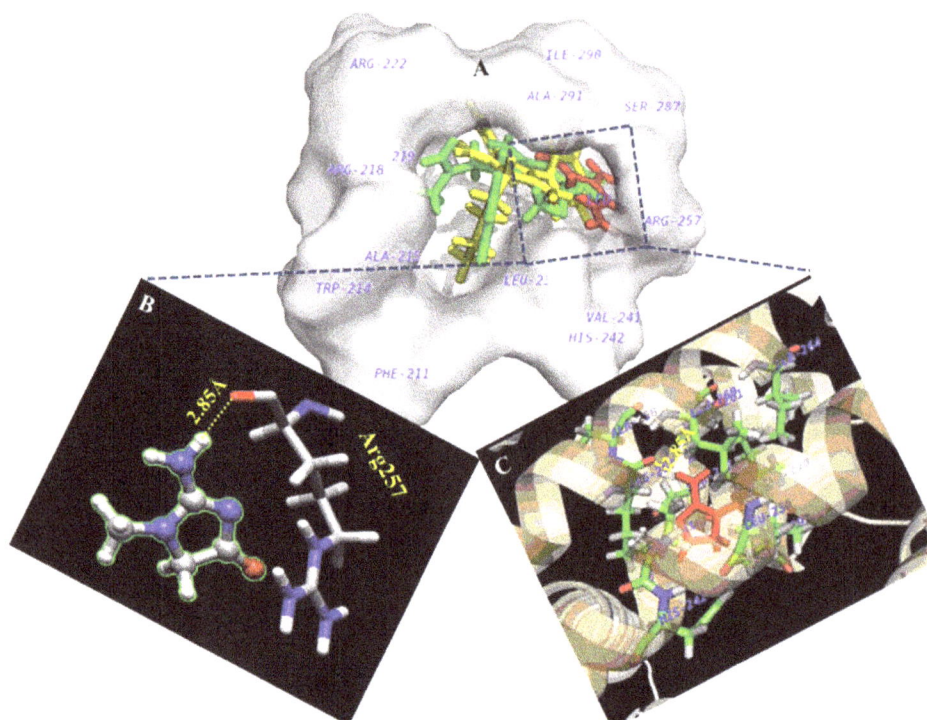

Figure 8. Molecular docking of HSA complexed with site I specific markers. (A) Molecular surface representations of HSA showing site I specific markers [warfarin (limegreen); phenylbutazone (yellow)] and the toxin CTN (red) at binding site I. (B) One hydrogen bond (as highlighted by the yellow dashed line) was formed between CTN and Arg257 of HSA. The hydrogen bond length was represented in yellow colour (C) Other site I amino acid residues of HSA interacting with CTN within 5 Å distance.

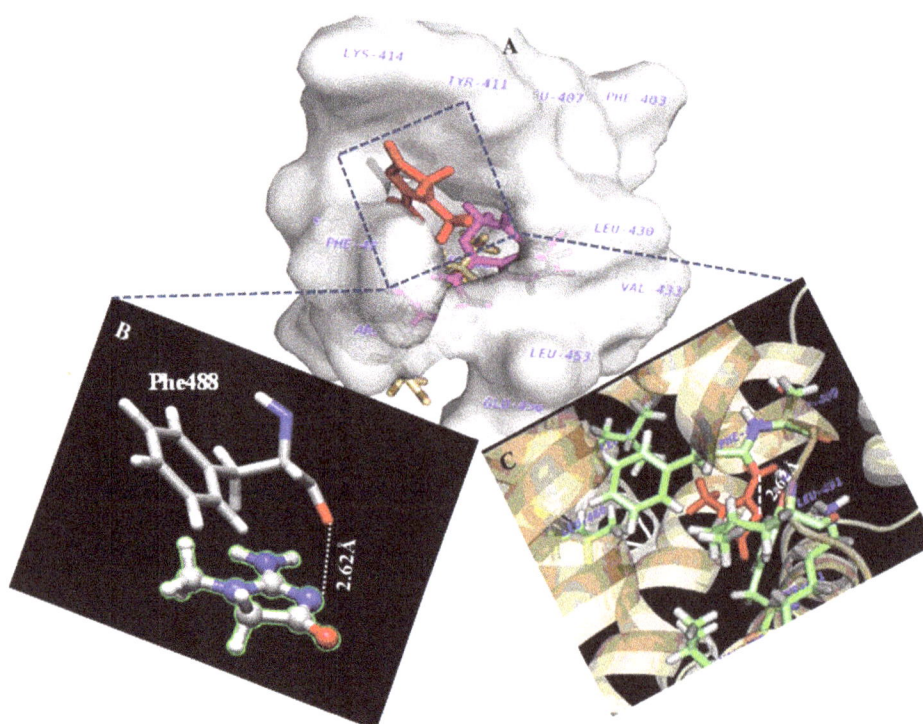

Figure 9. Molecular docking of HSA complexed with site II specific markers. (A) Molecular surface representations of HSA showing site II specific markers [ibuprofen (light orange); diazepam (magenta)] and the toxin CTN (red) at binding site II. (B) The toxin molecule forming repulsive interaction (white colour) with Phe488 of HSA (as highlighted by the white dashed line). (C) Other site II amino acid residues of HSA interacting with CTN within 5 Å distance.

Table 4. Change in Accessible surface area and binding interactions of the site I amino acid residues of HSA with uremic toxin creatinine.

Ligands	Amino acidresidue	ΔASA (Å^2)	Location	Electrostatic Interaction	Number of other interacting residues (5 Å)	GOLD Fitness score	X-score
Creatinine	Arg257	17.96	IIa-h4	Hydrogen bond $\overline{C=O...H^2N}$ Arg257(2.85 Å)	10	28.16	−5.68
	Leu238	17.08	IIa-h6				
	Ala291	16.05	IIa-h3				
	Ser287	12.02	IIa h6				
	Leu260	10.58	IIa-h4				
Phenyl-butazone	Ala 291	42.9	IIa-h6		15	47.82	−8.49
	Leu238	41.79	IIa-h3				
	Leu242	33.66	IIa-h3				
	Trp214	22.61	IIa-h2				
	Arg257	18.95	IIa-h4				
	Ile264	13.04	IIa-h4				
	Arg222	12.82	IIa-h2				
	Leu219	12.69	IIa-h2				
	Ser287	12.02	IIa-h6				
	Ile290	11.48	IIa-h6				
	Leu260	11.17	IIa-h4				
Warfarin	Leu238	39.03	IIa-h3		15	41.62	−8.05
	Ala291	38.6	IIa-h6				
	Leu242	35.6	IIa-h3				
	Trp214	28.93	IIa-h2				
	Arg257	16.4	IIa-h4				
	Arg222	14.05	IIa-h2				
	Leu219	12.25	IIa-h2				
	Ser287	12.02	IIa-h6				
	Ile290	11.48	IIa-h6				
	Phe211	11.26	IIa-h2				
	Leu260	10.72	IIa-h4				

results were substantiated by docking results which shows that high and low affinity binding sites of toxin on plasma protein are located within the binding pocket of subdomain IIA and IIIA. The creatinine binds deep inside the cavity at site I (Figure 8) whereas in site II (Figure 9), it binds at peripheral side of the cavity. The inside wall of the pocket was lined by hydrophobic side chains whereas the entrance to the pocket was surrounded by several non-polar residues (Leu238, Val241, Ala258, Leu260, Ala261, Ile264, Ile290, Ala291); one polar (Ser287) and few charged residues (His242, Arg257) in the proximity distance of 5 Å of the bound toxin (Figure 8, Table 4). Although the involvement of non polar residues makes the interactions to be

Table 5. Change in Accessible surface area and binding interactions of the site II amino acid residues of HSA with uremic toxin creatinine.

Ligands	Amino acid residue	ΔASA (Å^2)	Location	Electrostatic Interaction	Number of other interacting residues (5 Å)	GOLD Fitness score	X-score
Creatinine	Tyr 411	35.66	IIa-h2	Repulsive force $\overline{C=O...N^3}$ Phe488(2.62 Å)	7	29.14	−5.55
	Phe 488	26.38	IIIa-h6				
	Glu 489	10.27	IIIa-h4				
Diazepam	Leu 453	31.13	IIIa-h4		15	41.10	−8.43
	Asn 391	28.27	IIIa-h1				
	Ile 388	23.93	IIIa-h1				
	Leu 387	18.46	IIIa-h1				
	Leu 430	16.62	IIIa-h3				
	Arg 485	14.67	IIIa-h6				
	Ala 449	13.73	IIIa-h4				
Ibuprofen	Leu 453	28.22	IIIa-h4		13	42.74	−7.29
	Val 485	27.55	IIIa-h6				
	Asn 391	21.82	IIIa-h1				
	Leu 387	19.4	IIIa-h1				
	Ile 388	16.85	IIIa-h1				
	Pro 384	10.79	IIIa-h1				
	Glu 450	10.79	IIIa-h4				

hydrophobic in nature but the strong intermolecular hydrogen bond between carbonyl oxygen atom of Arg257 and N_2 atom of creatinine (2.85 Å, 124.36°), makes the electrostatic interaction as the primary binding force responsible for the retention of toxin in the plasma. The hydrogen bond residue of site I (Arg 257) was part of helix 4 and 6 of subdomain IIA (represented as IIa-h4 & IIa-h6, Table 4). While at site II, the complex was stabilized by hydrophobic interactions without involvement of any hydrogen bond. Additionally, electrostatic repulsive force between oxygen atom of Phe488 with N_3 of creatinine (2.62 Å) destabilizes the complex (Figure 9, Table 5). To further identify the residues taking part in the interaction, we have calculated the accessible surface area (ASA) of the amino acid residues. The changes in ASA of the interacting residues are presented in Table 4 and 5.

Discussion

The HSA solutions used in our preparations was approximately equivalent to that present in the blood i.e. 500 µM. Although under this condition the HSA solution was very concentrated but we have checked for the possibility of aggregation formation while performing the experiments. No evidence was found for aggregation/turbidity in solution provided by the Rayleigh light scattering (RLS) experiments (Figure S1) in scattering intensity after 1 hr. By RLS time dependent in solutions increase was in a concentration dependent manner. It appears that no aggregation was been reported when concentration was increased from 150 µM (10 mg/ml) to higher concentrations ~500 µM (33 mg/ml).

The melting thermograms for HSA were shown in Figure 1 attributes to an excessive load of hydrophobic uremic toxin bound to the albumin molecule. The uremic plasma under physiological conditions have a different shape with a shift to the right at higher temperatures and increase in the height above baseline which was also reflected in the values of the melting enthalpy (Table 1). This was attributed to a higher thermoresistance of the albumin component, most probably because of the binding of uremic toxin to HSA. An increase in the number of intramolecular bonds increases the thermal stability of the protein molecule and more pronounced at pH 9.0. Therefore, binding of toxin increases the cooperativity of the melting process and depends on its affinity for the albumin molecule. Comparison of thermodynamic parameters with the spectroscopic method (Table 2) shows that the two measurements yield similar 'n' values at both pHs. Because ΔH was much less than 60 Kcal/mol [39], the CTN-HSA interaction was non-covalent: it involves H-bonds, ion-pair attraction, hydrophobic interaction, and van der waals forces. It can be observed that, at physiological pH, the binding affinity decreases. This was reflected in the high negative values of enthalpy of binding, ΔH_{ITC}, and in a larger affinity binding constant, K_{ITC} (Table 2). Our finding that the secondary structure of serum albumin from conditions similar to uremic patients remains intact was consistent with circular dichroism data on the uHSA conformation in solution as determined previously [38]. Likewise, modification of IR spectra indicating alterations in structure of uHSA agrees well with published data about the physicochemical peculiarities of albumin in chronic uremia. We do not observe any significant changes in the secondary environment of protein on complexation with the toxin. On the other hand, number of binding sites 'n' remained almost unaffected. This indicates increased stability of B-CTN complex. Since under increased Ca^{2+} concentration in the blood plasma, the B isomer predominates, it is suggested that N-B conformational changes have physiological significance [20,18].

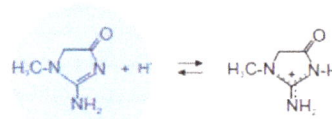

In aqueous solutions this tautomer exists

Figure 10. The acidic-basic equilibrium of creatinine. In aqueous solution creatinine exists in the form of a tautomer.

The question arises which binding sites on the albumin molecule were usually affected by creatinine? Data for the binding ability of albumin before and after its loading with uremic toxin with marker ligand specific for sites I and II were represented by displacement experiments as shown in Figure 7. The site I markers at pH 7 and 9 reduces the induced CD signal to almost zero. The association constant of phenylbutazone was K_a 7×10^5 M^{-1}, n = 1 and warfarin was $K_a = 3.3 \times 10^5$ M^{-1}, n = 1 [20] and that for CTN (after exciting the protein at 280 nm) was $K_a = 1.4 \times 10^5$ M^{-1}, n≈1 (Table 2) the site I markers can displace CTN from its binding site on albumin. The association constant for diazepam ($K_a = 3.8 \times 10^5$ M^{-1}, n = 1) and ibuprofen ($K_a = 2.7 \times 10^5$ M^{-1}, n = 1) [20] was higher than that for CTN and lower than that for site I markers. Site II markers were, therefore, likely to weak inhibitors of the binding of CTN. Thus, fluorescence quenching and induced CD spectrums were utilized to achieve three goals (i) calculating the association constant (K_a) (ii) determining the dependence of toxin binding on albumin conformation and (iii) probing the location of uremic toxin binding site on HSA. Furthermore, CTN possesses two pKa values of 4.88 for protonation [40] and 12.7–13.4 for deprotonation of the exocyclic amino group. This suggests that CTN predominantly occurs in aqueous solution and in blood plasma at pH 7.4 in neutral form. In aqueous solution it exists in the form of a tautomer, its acido–basic equilibrium has been shown in Figure 10. When analyzing the accessible surface area we found main involvement of arginine residues in the toxin complexation with albumin (Table 4). This change seemed to be caused by His residues because most of the pK_a values of His residues are within this pH region i.e. 6.4. Thus, during alkalization of HSA, the affinity of CTN increases. On the onset of pH 9.0, the Arg residues involved in binding protonate (pKa of Arg = 9.04 (NH^{3+}) and 12.04 (side chain)), and then may

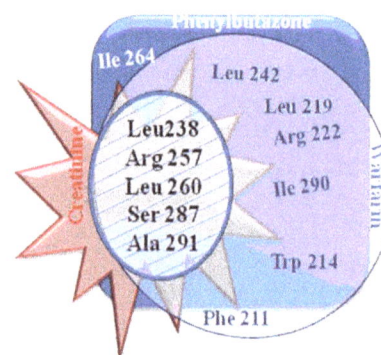

Figure 11. Common amino acid residues between creatinine and HSA. The shaded area depicts the common amino acid residues spanning uremic toxin creatinine and specific drug site I markers of HSA.

interact favorably with the toxin. Whilst at pH 7.0, deprotonation weakens the interaction with the cation.

What actually happens under in vivo conditions during chronic renal failure (CRF) when urine eliminates from the body? The glomerulus is a selective filtration membrane. The filtration barrier of body composed of three layers that allow for the filtration of solutes (eg. blood urea nitrogen, creatinine, electrolytes) and water, but prevent the loss of blood components and plasma proteins. Two mechanisms act to prevent albumin from being lost from the body by filtration through the glomerular membrane. The first relates to the glomerular membrane pore size, which is small compared to the size and shape of albumin. The second mechanism involves the negatively charged sialo-protein-rich electrical charge on the surface of endothelial cells covering the inner surface of the basement membrane. Since albumin has a net negative charge, it is electrostatically repulsed by the glomerular membrane. As a result, it has been estimated that only about 2 g of albumin was filtered each day across the glomerular capillary wall. Creatinine, on the other hand, lacks electrical charges at physiological pH and hence is able to escape across the muscle cell membrane. It is found that highly alkaline urine occurs in CRF. Our in vitro results could be correlated with this fact i.e. under alkaline conditions interaction of toxins enhances due to increased affinity with HSA. Thus, elimination of toxin would be more feasible at physiological pH.

Furthermore, the major changes in ASA occur for the residues (role in binding) belonging to the hydrophobic pocket of site I. These residues were overlapping to those of site I markers (Table 4) thereby again supporting the results of site I displacement (Figure 11). Whereas, the residues involved in binding of CTN to site II (Table 5) were non overlapping to those of respective markers, moreover the no. of such residues was less than that for site I.

Curry *et al.* have determined the crystal structure of HSA complexed with five molecules of fatty acid at 2.5 Å resolution [20]. Arg 257 was found to interact with myristate bound to subdomain IIA. Similar interaction we observed with HSA-CTN complexation. It was noteworthy that the single tryptophan residue of HSA (Trp 214) was not in the immediate environment of the docked toxin molecule as proved by our spectroscopic results and was further confirmed by computational mapping approaches. Guanidino compounds are generated *in vivo* as a result of protein and amino acid metabolism. In general the GCs acquire the guanidino group from arginine, with subsequent methylation to creatine and further metabolization to creatinine [41]. In patients with renal impairment, several-fold increases in specific guanidino compounds were observed due to the impaired renal function and altered metabolism [6]. Most drugs are bound to serum proteins to a various degree. Only unbound or free drug is pharmacologically active. There is equilibrium between bound and free drugs, and concentration of free drug can be predicted from total drug concentration. However, under uremic conditions this equilibrium is disturbed and the measured free drug concentration can be significantly higher than expected from total drug concentrations, especially for strongly protein-bound drugs. In such case a patient may experience drug toxicity (Figure 12).

Furthermore, creatinine is removed by hemodialytic strategies [42] but under diseased states uremic compounds of low molecular mass can displace strongly albumin-bound drugs from binding sites responsible for the binding defect of various drugs in uremic sera. To account for the mechanisms that govern such specificity in inhibitory potency, we carefully examined the relationship

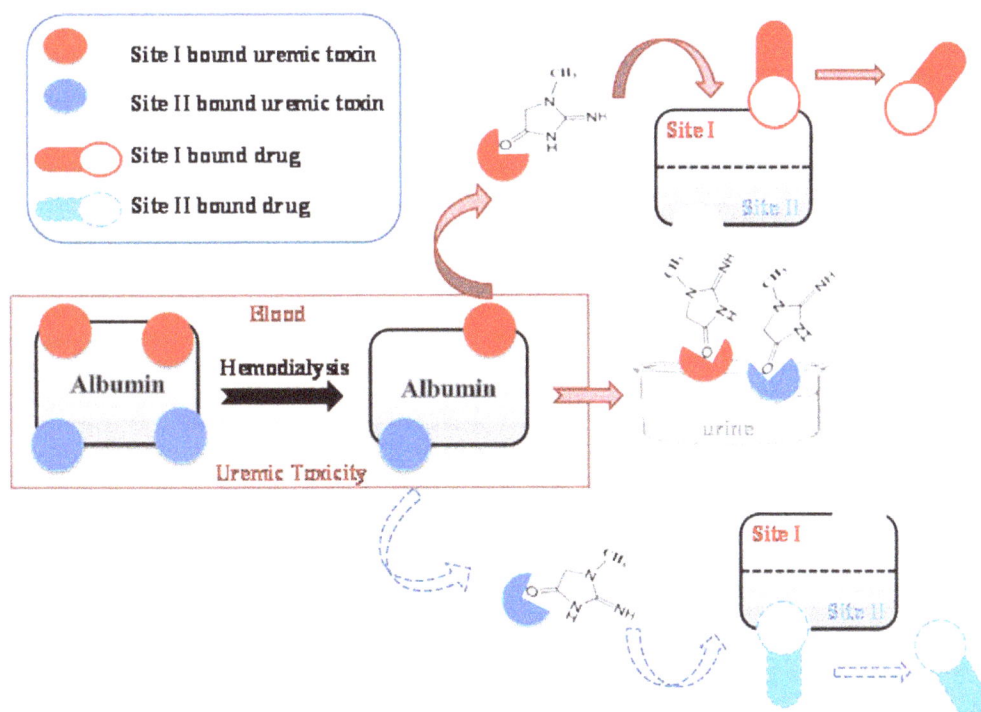

Figure 12. Correlation between uremic toxicity and impaired drug binding. Mechanism showing possible cascade displacement model in uremic toxin– drug system depicts allosteric effect of toxin when binding to site I and site II. Red colour: CTN binding to its high-affinity site, site I as shown by solid arrows; blue colour: CTN binding to its low-affinity site, site II as shown by dashed arrows. Hemodialytic reaction occurring within the blood plasma has been shown in red box.

between the drug binding site(s) and the uremic toxin binding sites. In summary, accumulation of creatinine in patients with renal failure appears to account for a substantial portion of the impaired serum protein binding of drug especially at site I. Consequently, interactions of toxin and drug with respect to serum protein binding and renal excretion may increase the free fraction of drug in serum of patients with renal insufficiency [43]. These findings lend further support to the hypothesis that a retained ligand(s) was responsible for impaired plasma binding associated with uremia and suggests a role for CTN known to accumulate in renal failure.

Renal failure not only alters the renal elimination but also the non renal elimination disposition of drugs that are extensively metabolized by the liver. Clearance of CTN from the blood depends on intramuscular CTN levels, hormone levels, muscle mass, and kidney function/glomerular filtration rate. Creatinine is representative for small uremic toxins, important in clinical analytic domain for it is used as a probe to evidence renal failure or muscular dysfunction. Consequently, accumulation of uremic toxin and slight increase of pH may cause increase of the free fraction of drug due to interaction of toxin in patients with renal failure. Thus, accumulation of uremic toxin in body can be due to conformational change caused by neutral to basic transition which in turn may affect the site–site interactions between domain IIA and domain IIIA such that site interactions between domains will disappear. The findings obtained here will provide useful information for elucidating the complicated mechanism of drug and toxin disposition in renal disease state. This is the current interest of the pharmaceutical companies. This is extremely important for various diseases such as muscular dystrophy and diabetes. Most of the future research and advances well be spun off of these clinical studies.

Acknowledgments

The authors would like to thank Prof. Rajiv Bhat (School of Biotechnology) and Dr. Andrew M. Lynn (School of Bioinformatics), Jawaharlal Nehru University, New Delhi for providing lab facilities for performing calorimetry (ITC and DSC), and computational studies respectively. RHK lab has published more than 100 research articles in high impact factor journals.

Author Contributions

Conceived and designed the experiments: AV MR NS GR RHK. Performed the experiments: AV MR GR. Analyzed the data: AV MR NS GR RHK. Contributed reagents/materials/analysis tools: AV MR NS GR RHK. Wrote the paper: AV MR NS RHK.

References

1. Vanholder R, De Smet R, Hsu C, Vogeleere P, Ringoir S (1994) Uremic toxicity: the middle molecule hypothesis revisited. Semin Nephrol 14: 205–218.

2. Vanholder R, Argiles A, Baurmeister U, Brunet P, Clark W, et al. (2001) Uremic toxicity: count when interpreting the results. Present state of the art. Int J Artif Organs 24: 695–725.

3. Vanholder R, Massy Z, Argiles A, Spasovski G, Verbeke F, et al. (2005) European Uremic Toxin Work Group (EUTox) Chronic kidney disease as cause of cardiovascular morbidity and mortality. Nephrol Dial Transplant 20: 1048–1056.

4. Van Biesen W, De Bacquer D, Verbeke F, Delanghe J, Lameire N, et al. (2007) The glomerular filtration rate in an apparently healthy population and its relation with cardiovascular mortality during 10 years. Eur Heart J 28: 478–483.

5. Mingrone G, Smet R, Greco A, Bertuzzi A, Gandel A, et al. (1997) Serum uremic toxins from patients with chronic renal failure displace the binding of L-tryptophan to HSA. Clin Chim Acta 260: 27–34.

6. Vanholder R, Smet R De, Glorieux G, Argile A, Baurmeister U, et al. (2003) Review on uremic toxins: Classification, concentration, and interindividual variability. Kidney Int 63: 1934–1943.

7. Vanholder R, De Smet R, Glorieux G, Dhondt A (2003) Survival of Hemodialysis Patients and Uremic Toxin Removal. Artif Organs 27: 218–223.

8. Vaidya VS, Ford GM, Waikar SS, Wang Y, Clement MB, et al. (2009) A rapid urine test for early detection of kidney injury. Kidney Int 76: 108–114.

9. Mattix HJ, Hsum CY, Shaykevichm S, Curhan G (2002) Use of the Albumin/Creatinine Ratio to Detect Microalbuminuria: Implications of Sex and Race. J Am Soc Nephrol 13: 1034–1039.

10. De Deyn PP, Vanholder R, Eloot S, Glorieux G (2009) Guanidino Compounds as Uremic (Neuro) Toxins. Semin Dialysis 22: 340–345.

11. Kestenbaum B, Rudser KD, De Boer IH, Peralta CA, Fried LF, et al. (2008) Differences in Kidney Function and Incident Hypertension: The Multi-Ethnic Study of Atherosclerosis. Ann Intern Med 148: 501–508.

12. Brantsm AH, Bakker SJ, De Zeeuw D, De Jong PE, Gansevoort RT (2006) Urinary albumin excretion as a predictor of the development of hypertension in the general population. J Am Soc Nephrol 17: 331–335.

13. Glorieux GL, Dhondt AW, Jacobs P, Van Langeraert J, Lameire NH, et al. (2004) In vitro study of the potential role of guanidines in leukocyte functions related to atherogenesis and infection. Kidney Int 65: 2184–2192.

14. Peterson JC, Adler S, Burkart JM, Greene T, Hebert LA, et al. (1995) Blood pressure control, proteinuria, and the progression of renal disease: the Modification of Diet in Renal Disease Study. Ann Intern Med 123: 754–762.

15. Gerstein HC, Mann JF, Yi Q, Zinman B, Dinneen SF, et al. (2001) Hope Study Investigators. Albuminuria and risk of cardiovascular events, death, and heart failure in diabetic and nondiabetic individuals. JAMA 286: 421–426.

16. Forman JP, Brenner BM (2006) 'Hypertension' and 'microalbuminuria': the bell tolls for thee. Kidney Int 69: 22–28.

17. Perna AF, Ingrosso D, Satta E, Lombardi C, Galletti P, et al. (2004) Plasma protein aspartyl damage is increased in hemodialysis patients: studies on causes and consequences. J Am Soc Nephrol 15: 2747–2754.

18. Ahmad B, Parveen S, Khan RH (2006) Effect of Albumin conformation on the Binding of Ciprofloxacin to Human Serum Albumin: A Novel Approach Directly Assigning Binding Site. Biomacromolecules 7: 1350–1356.

19. Kosa T, Nishi K, Maruyama T, Sakai N, Yonemura N, et al. (2007) Structural and ligand-binding properties of serum albumin species interacting with a biomembrane interface. J Pharm Sci 96: 3117–3124.

20. Varshney A, Sen P, Ahmad E, Rehan M, Subbarao N, et al. (2010) Ligand Binding Strategies on Human Serum Albumin: How Can the cargo be Utilized further? Chirality 22: 77–87.

21. Ahmad B, Ankita, Khan RH (2005) Urea induced unfolding of F isomer of human serum albumin: A case study using multiple probes. Arch Biochim Biophys 437: 159–167.

22. Celej MS, Dassie SA, Freire E, Bianconi ML, Fidelio GD (2005) Ligand-induced thermostability in proteins: Thermodynamic analysis of ANS–albumin interaction. Biochim Biophys Acta 1750: 122–133.

23. Cheema MA, Taboada P, Barbosa S, Castro E, Siddiq M, et al. (2007) Energetics and Conformational Changes upon Complexation of a Phenothiazine Drug with Human Serum Albumin. Biomacromolecules 8: 2576–2585.

24. Gao HW, Xu Q, Chen L, Wang SL, Wang Y, et al. (2008) Potential Protein Toxicity of Synthetic Pigments: Binding of Ponceau S to Human Serum Albumin. Biophys J 94: 906–917.

25. Varshney A, Ahmad B, Khan RH (2008) Comparative studies of unfolding and binding of ligands to human serum albumin in the presence of fatty acid: spectroscopic approach. Int J Biol Macromol 42: 483–490.

26. Kang J, Liu Y, Xie MX, Li S, Jiang M, et al. (2004) Interactions of human serum albumin with chlorogenic acid and ferulic acid. Biochim Biophys Acta 1674: 205–214.

27. Kanakis CD, Tarantilis PA, Tajmir-Riahi HA, Polissiou MG (2007) Crocetin, Dimethylcrocetin, and Safranal Bind Human Serum Albumin: Stability and Antioxidative Properties. J Agric Food Chem 55: 970–977.

28. Tetko IV, Gasteiger J, Todeschini R, Mauri A, Livingstone D, et al. (2005) Virtual computational chemistry laboratory-design and description. J Comput Aided Mol Des 19: 453–463.

29. Jones G, Willett P, Glen RC, Leach AR, Taylor R (1997) Development and validation of a genetic algorithm for flexible docking. J Mol Biol 267: 727–748.

30. Wang R, Lu Y, Wang S (2003) Comparative evaluation of 11 scoring functions for molecular docking. J Med Chem 46: 2287–2303.

31. Ewing TJ, Makino S, Skillman AG, Kuntz ID (2001) DOCK4.0: Search strategies for automated molecular docking of flexible molecule databases. J Comput Aided Mol Des 15: 411–428.

32. DeLano WL (2002) The PyMOL Molecular Graphics System DeLano Scientific. California, , USA: Palo Alto.

33. Pettersen EF, Goddard TD, Huang CC, Couch GS, Greenblatt DM, et al. (2004) UCSF Chimera–a visualization system for exploratory research and analysis. J Comput Chem 25: 1605–1612.

34. Hubbard SJ, Thornton JM (1993) *'Naccess', computer program. Technical report*: Department of Biochemistry and Molecular Biology, University College London.

35. Ghosh KS, Sen S, Sahoo BK, Dasgupta SA (2009) Spectroscopic Investigation into the Interactions of 3′-O-Carboxy Esters of Thymidine with Bovine Serum Albumin. Biopolymers 91: 737–744.

36. Sarnatskaya VV, Lindup WE, Niwa T, Ivanov A, Yushko LA, et al. (2002) Effect of protein bound ureamic toxins on the thermodynamic characteristics of human albumin. Biochem Pharmacol 63: 1287–1296.

37. Sarnatskaya VV, Yushko LA, Sakhno LA, Nikolaev VG, Nikolaev AV, et al. (2007) New Approaches to the Removal of Protein-Bound Toxins from Blood Plasma of Uremic Patients. Artif Cells Blood Substit Immobil Biotechnol 35: 287–308.

38. Ivanov AI, Korolenko EA, Korolik EV, Firsov SP, Zhbankov RG, et al. (2002) Chronic liver and renal diseases differently affect structure of human serum albumin. Arch Biochim Biophys 408: 69–77.

39. Yang M (1998) Molecular recognition of DNA targeting small molecule drugs. J Beijing Med Univ 30: 97–99.

40. Berge-Lefranc D, Pizzala H, Denoyel R, Hornebecq V, Berge-Lefranc J, et al. (2009) Mechanism of creatinine adsorption from physiological solutions onto mordenite. Micro Meso Mate 119: 186–192.

41. Taes YEC, Marescau B, De Vriese A, De Deyn PP, Schepers E, et al. (2008) Guanidino compounds after creatine supplementation in renal failure patients and their relation to inflammatory status. Nephrol Dial Transplant 23: 1330–1335.

42. Sarnatskaya V, Ivanov AI, Nikolaev VG, Rotellar E, Von Appen K, et al. (1998) Structure and binding properties of serum albumin in uremic patients at different periods of hemodialysis. Artif Organs 22: 107–115.

43. Sun H, Frassetto L, Benet LZ (2006) Effects of renal failure on drug transport and metabolism. Pharm & Therap 109: 1–11.

Management of Metformin-Associated Lactic Acidosis by Continuous Renal Replacement Therapy

Geoffray Keller[1,2], Martin Cour[1,2], Romain Hernu[1], Julien Illinger[1], Dominique Robert[1,2], Laurent Argaud[1,2]*

1 Hospices Civils de Lyon, Groupement Hospitalier Edouard Herriot, Service de Réanimation Médicale, Lyon, France, 2 Université de Lyon, Université Lyon 1, Faculté de médecine Lyon-Est, Lyon, France

Abstract

Background: Metformin-associated lactic acidosis (MALA) is a severe metabolic failure with high related mortality. Although its use is controversial, intermittent hemodialysis is reported to be the most frequently used treatment in conjunction with nonspecific supportive measures. Our aim was to report the evolution and outcome of cases managed by continuous renal replacement therapy (CRRT).

Methodology and Principal Findings: Over a 3-year period, we retrospectively identified patients admitted to the intensive care unit for severe lactic acidosis caused by metformin. We included patients in our study who were treated with CRRT because of shock. We describe their clinical and biological features at admission and during renal support, as well as their evolution. We enrolled six patients with severe lactic acidosis; the mean pH and mean lactate was 6.92 ± 0.20 and 14.4 ± 5.1 mmol/l, respectively. Patients had high illness severity scores, including the Simplified Acute Physiology Score II (SAPS II) (average score 63 ± 12 points). Early CRRT comprised either venovenous hemofiltration ($n = 3$) or hemodiafiltration ($n = 3$) with a mean effluent flow rate of 34 ± 6 ml/kg/h. Metabolic acidosis control and metformin elimination was rapid and there was no rebound. Outcome was favorable in all cases.

Conclusions and Significance: Standard use of CRRT efficiently treated MALA in association with symptomatic organ supportive therapies.

Editor: Jeffrey A. Gold, Oregon Health and Science University, United States of America

Funding: The authors have no support or funding to report.

Competing Interests: The authors have declared that no competing interests exist.

* E-mail: laurent.argaud@chu-lyon.fr

Introduction

Metformin is the recommended first-line treatment for overweight patients with type 2 diabetes mellitus [1]. The incidence of metformin-associated lactic acidosis (MALA) is rare, estimated at 2–9 patients per 100,000 patients receiving metformin per year; MALA accounts for approximately 1% of total patients admitted to intensive care units (ICU) [2]. This life-threatening complication is usually associated with a mortality rate of 30%–50% [2,3]. The etiology of lactic acidosis is multifactorial and uncertain. Briefly, metformin increases the redox potential from aerobic to anaerobic metabolism, and inhibits gluconeogenesis by reducing hepatic lactate reuptake [4]. This situation is worsened by circulatory failure and altered tissue perfusion, both of which increase lactate production.

The optimal treatment modality for MALA is controversial and relies on nonspecific supportive measures. The use of intermittent hemodialysis may be protective, and it is recommended by many intensivists [2,5,6]. Despite potential advantages, continuous renal replacement therapy (CRRT) to treat MALA is poorly documented with only a few case reports available, and it has only been considered as a rescue therapy under exceptional circumstances [7–9]. We report on six cases of severe MALA that were successfully managed with CRRT and discuss the safety and effectiveness of CRRT when it is used for this purpose.

Materials and Methods

The ethics committee of the Hospices Civils de Lyon approved this retrospective noninterventional study. This institutional review board waived the need for consent given the retrospective design of the project. The study was performed in compliance with the ethical standard of the Helsinki Declaration and according to the French laws.

From November 2005 to October 2008, we identified all of the patients who were admitted to our ICU for severe MALA and treated with CRRT because of hemodynamic instability. Patients were included if they met the two following criteria: blood pH<7.20 and arterial lactate >5 mmol/l [10]. An abdominal ultrasound exploration and/or a computerized tomography scanner was systematically performed to eliminate mesenteric infarction.

The following clinical features were collected at admission: age, sex, MacCabe and Knaus scores (used to assess the severity of comorbidities and functional status, respectively), Charson index (to evaluate comorbidity), preexisting chronic renal failure, use of

Table 1. Patient characteristics.

	Case 1	Case 2	Case 3	Case 4	Case 5	Case 6	Mean ± SD
Demographics							
Age (years)	81	81	72	54	63	64	69±11
Gender	F	F	F	M	F	F	-
Coexisting medical conditions							
McCabe scale	0	0	0	1	0	0	-
Knaus score	B	B	B	C	D	A	-
Charlson comorbidity index	3	5	1	2	2	1	2.3±1.5
Chronic renal failure	No	No	Yes	Yes	No	No	-
Nephrotoxic drugs							
Diuretics	No	Yes	No	Yes	Yes	Yes	-
Angiotensin converter inhibitors	Yes	No	No	Yes	No	Yes	-
Nonsteroidal anti-inflammators	No	No	No	No	No	No	-
Aspirin	No	No	No	Yes	No	Yes	-
Metformin							
Daily dose (mg)	2250	3000	1700	1000	3000	3000	2375±842

F, female; M, male; McCabe scale (life expectancy), 0: none or nonfatal underlying disease, 1: ultimately fatal disease (death≤5 years), 2: rapidly fatal disease (death≤1 year); Knaus score (functional status), A: no daily activity limitation, the patient was in good health, B: moderate limitation of activity because of a chronic medical problem, C: strong limitation of activity due to disease, D: severe limitation and/or restriction of activity due to disease; Charlson comorbidity index, components (weights): myocardial infarct (1), congestive heart failure (1), peripheral vascular disease (1), cerebrovascular disease (1), dementia (1), chronic pulmonary disease (1), connective tissue disease (1), ulcer disease (1), mild liver disease (1), diabetes (1), hemiplegia (2), moderate or severe renal disease (2), diabetes with end-organ damage (2), any tumor (2), leukemia (2), lymphoma (2), moderate or severe liver disease (3), metastatic solid tumor (6), AIDS (6).

Table 2. Illness severity.

	Case 1	Case 2	Case 3	Case 4	Case 5	Case 6	Mean ± SD
Admission vitals							
Heart rate (beats/min)	104	101	83	82	78	120	95±16
Mean arterial blood pressure (mmHg)	44	41	48	38	55	54	47±7
Respiratory rate (breaths/min)	32	20	30	30	29	40	30±7
Body temperature (°C)	33.0	34.5	33.0	35.8	35.9	30.9	33.9±1.9
Diuresis (ml/h)	4	9	0	88	8	0	18±34
Glasgow coma score	15	11	8	15	11	12	12±3
Multiple organ failure							
Cardiovascular dysfunction	Yes	Yes	Yes	Yes	Yes	Yes	-
Renal dysfunction	Yes	Yes	Yes	Yes	Yes	Yes	-
Respiratory dysfunction	No	Yes	No	Yes	Yes	Yes	-
Neurological dysfunction	No	Yes	Yes	No	No	No	-
Hepatic dysfunction	No	No	Yes	No	No	No	-
Hematological dysfunction	No	No	No	No	No	No	-
Number of organ dysfunctions	2	4	4	3	3	3	3.2±0.8
SOFA score	9	14	15	8	12	14	12±3
Symptomatic intensive therapies							
Renal replacement therapy (days)	7	12	15	2	3	5	7±5
Mechanical ventilation (days)	0	19	0	5	15	9	8±8
Vasoactive drugs (days)	3	9	4	1	2	5	4±3
Norepinephrine (µg/kg/min)	0.3	1.3	0.8	0.2	0.2	0.9	0.6±0.5
SAPS II	66	74	73	51	46	66	63±12

SOFA, Sequential-related Organ Failure Assessment; SAPS II, Simplified Acute Physiology Score II.

medication potentially responsible for renal impairment, daily dose of metformin, Simplified Acute Physiology Score II (SAPS II), hemodynamics, body temperature, Glasgow coma score, number of organ failures according to Fagon *et al.*, Sequential-related Organ Failure Assessment (SOFA score), type and intensity of renal support, mechanical ventilation and vasopressor requirement, and ICU length of stay and outcome [11–17]. Biological data recorded at admission were pH and lactate, bicarbonate, partial oxygen pressure (PaO_2) and partial carbon dioxide pressure ($PaCO_2$) from arterial samples, and sodium, potassium, aminotransferase ALAT, creatine kinase, troponin I, creatinine, urea, glucose, hemoglobin and C-reactive protein (CRP) concentrations, as well as anion gap, prothrombin index, white blood cell and platelets counts from venous samples. The presence of metformin was identified, and both plasmatic and erythrocyte concentrations were quantified in a venous blood sample by high performance liquid chromatography (HPLC).

CRRT (i.e., continuous venovenous hemofiltration [CVVH] or hemodiafiltration [CVVHDF]) was performed with a Prismaflex device (Hospal, Meyzieu, France). We used polysulfone hollow-fiber hemofilters with a surface area of 1.2 m². Blood flow rate was maintained between 150 and 250 ml/min according to the targeted ultrafiltration rate. Bicarbonate-based replacement solutions to maintain fluid balance were infused so that the predilution was equal to 30%. Anticoagulation was performed with 5000 IU unfractionated heparin, added to the priming solution and followed by a continuous infusion, with a targeted systemic activated partial

thromboplastin (aPTT) at 1.5 time control. CRRT was discontinued as soon as clinical condition and renal function had improved.

Data are expressed as mean values and standard deviation (SD). Comparisons between time-based measurements were performed with two-way ANOVA with repeated measures on one factor using GraphPad Prism 5 (GraphPad Software, La Jolla, CA, USA). Statistical significance was defined at a value of $p < 0.05$.

Results

Patient clinical characteristics at admission are shown in both Table 1 and Table 2. There was one man and five women. In all cases, acute renal failure was present and associated with clinically and biologically profound extracellular dehydration. Patients 3 and 4 had previous chronic renal insufficiency without a requirement for renal replacement therapy. Except for patient 3, all of the patients took at least one of the following potentially nephrotoxic medications: diuretics, angiotensin converter enzyme inhibitors, nonsteroidal anti-inflammatory drugs, or aspirin (Table 1).

All of the patients presented with clinical nonspecific symptoms such as malaise, myalgia, drowsiness, or abdominal pain, as well as hemodynamic failure which required fluid challenge and vasopressive support (Table 2). Hypothermia was systematically present; four patients required mechanical ventilation (Table 2).

Biological characteristics at admission are presented in Table 3. None of the patients experienced severe hypoglycemia (Table 3). Inflammatory syndrome, if present, was minor since CRP level was always below 30 mg/l.

Table 3. Biological data at admission.

	Case 1	Case 2	Case 3	Case 4	Case 5	Case 6	Mean ± SD
Arterial blood gases							
Arterial pH	7.04	6.81	6.71	7.09	7.15	6.72	6.92±0.20
Arterial lactate (mmol/l)	16.2	19.1	15.6	9.8	6.6	19.0	14.4±5.1
Bicarbonate (mmol/l)	5	2	1	7	15	1	5±5
Anion gap (mmol/l)	51	42	51	52	36	54	48±7
$PaCO_2$ (mmHg)	16.5	15.0	24.8	23.3	43.5	9.0	21.8±12.0
PaO_2/FiO_2 (mmHg)	250	238	194	181	233	313	235±47
Standard biochemistry							
Sodium (mmol/l)	140	135	131	139	136	133	136±3
Potassium (mmol/l)	5.0	6.2	7.5	6.7	7.6	7.2	6.7±1.0
Glycemia (mmol/l)	12.5	2.2	9.3	13.0	8.7	6.3	8.7±4.0
Urea (mmol/l)	26	26	39	24	21	31	28±7
Creatinine (μmol/l)	670	416	841	585	372	723	601±181
Aminotransferase ALAT (IU/l)	12	29	128	40	13	15	39±45
Creatine kinase (IU/l)	150	63	554	124	43	484	236±224
Troponin I (ng/ml)	0.18	<0.1	1.33	<0.1	<0.1	1.14	0.9±0.6
Hematology							
Hemoglobin (g/l)	81	116	93	100	128	86	101±18
Platelets (10^9/l)	160	161	350	251	363	401	281±106
White blood cell (10^9/l)	18	25	27	17	13	39	23±9
Prothrombin index (%)	50	48	24	60	41	28	42±14
Metformin concentration							
Plasma (mg/l), N<1 mg/l	80.0	125	74.4	36.4	54.9	61.9	72.1±30.1
Erythrocyte (mg/l), N<0.81 mg/l	25.8	26.8	22.5	14.7	51.8	20.6	27.0±12.9

N, laboratory level limit; $PaCO_2$, partial carbon dioxide pressure in arterial blood; PaO_2, partial oxygen pressure in arterial blood; FiO_2, inspiratory fraction of oxygen.

Continuous renal replacement management, as well as outcomes, are shown in Table 4. CVVH and CVVHDF were each used in three patients. Metabolic acidosis, as well as metformin plasma concentrations, were dramatically reduced in the first 24 h and/or normalized on the second day in every case (Figure 1). There was no rebound in acidosis. The mean individual rates of metformin elimination, from the blood compartment, in the first 24 hours after admission was estimated from 1.5 to 4.0%/h (Table 4). CRRT was well tolerated in our patients. There was no occurrence of CRRT-associated complications such as bleeding. Renal replacement was not necessary after discharge for any of the patients, and kidney function recovered prior levels in each case. All of the patients were transferred to a medical ward before they were discharged to their homes.

Discussion

To our knowledge, this study represents the largest case series of MALA managed by early CRRT. All six patients had a favourable outcome despite severe initial metabolic disorders associated with multiple organ failure.

MALA is strictly defined by arterial lactate >5 mmol/l and blood pH<7.35 within the context of recent metformin exposure [10,18]. It is the most frequent pattern of lactic acidosis related to metformin use [10]. This confusing term of MALA, shared by many different nosologic entities, is caused by an acute metformin accumulation [10]. Because metformin normally undergoes rapid and unchanging glomerular filtration and tubular excretion, MALA occurs only if renal function is altered or in rare cases of

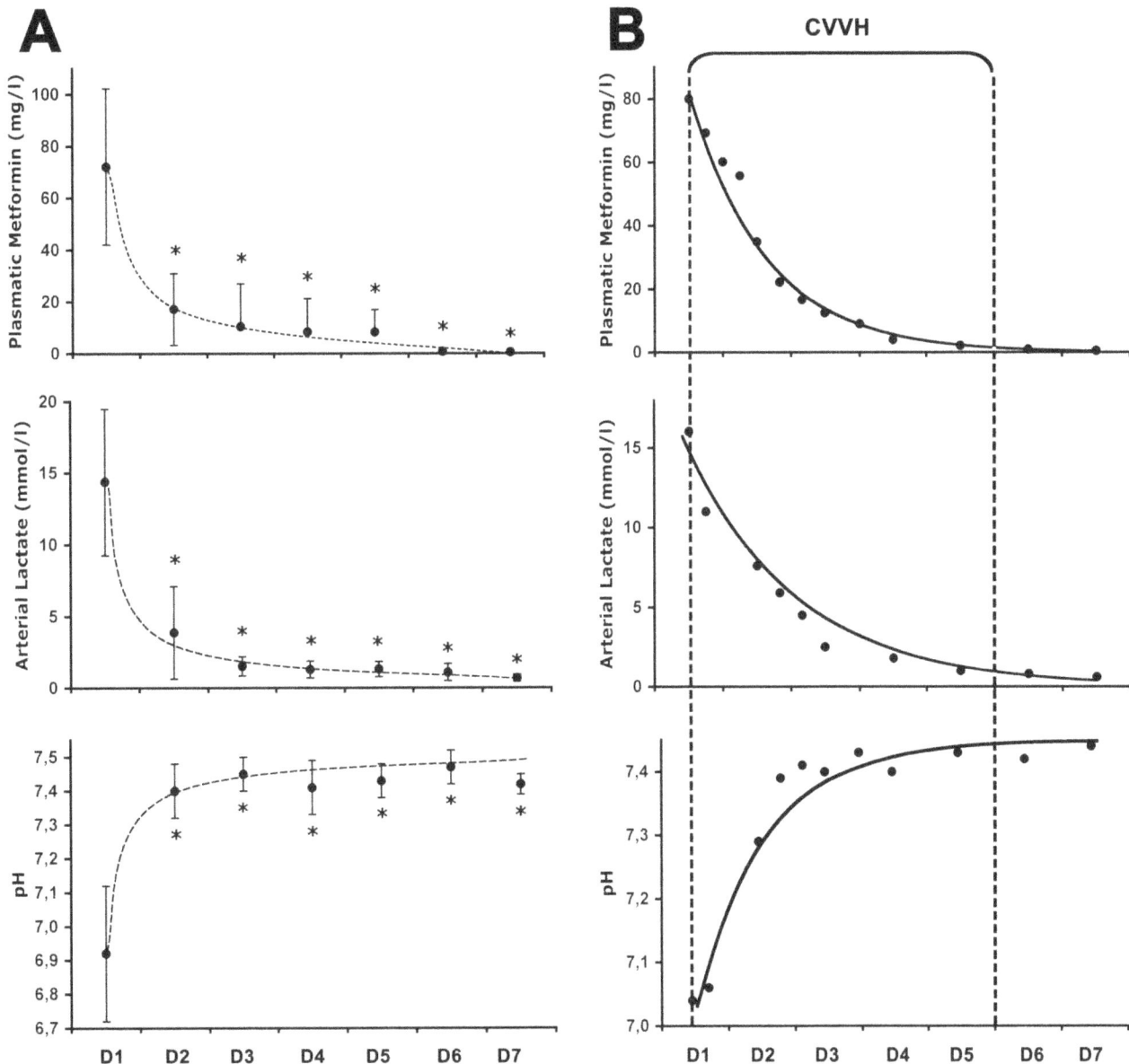

Figure 1. Acidosis, lactate and metformin levels under continuous renal replacement therapy. Panel A: Data from all patients, expressed as mean ± SD, showing that metabolic acidosis, as well as the excessive dose of metformin observed at admission (day 1, D1), were dramatically reduced from day 2 (D2). * p<0.01 versus D1. Panel B: Typical evolution in case patient 1 of both metformin plasma concentrations and metabolic disorders, which were controlled within 2 days of initiating continuous venovenous hemofiltration (CVVH), i.e. without dialysate.

Table 4. Continuous renal replacement therapy and outcomes.

	Case 1	Case 2	Case 3	Case 4	Case 5	Case 6	Mean ± SD
Type							
CVVH or CVVHDF	CVVH	CVVH	CVVHDF	CVVH	CVVHDF	CVVHDF	-
Therapy parameters							
Blood flow rate (ml/min)	200	180	150	200	180	250	193±33
Effluent rate (ml/kg/h)	34	33	39	22	38	36	34±6
Dialysate rate (ml/h)	0	0	2500	0	2000	500	1250±1215
Replacement fluid rate (ml/h)	1600	2500	2000	2500	2500	2800	2317±436
Filtration fraction (%)	13	30	22	29	17	19	22±7
Initial fluid removal (ml/h)	0	50	0	0	100	0	25±42
Length (days)	5	12	15	1	3	5	7±5
Metformin clearance							
Rate of elimination (%/h)	2.7	4.0	1.5	1.6	2.1	2.3	2.4±0.9
Outcomes							
ICU length of stay (days)	11	26	17	8	22	9	16±7
Survival to discharge	Yes	Yes	Yes	Yes	Yes	Yes	-
Discharge at home	Yes	Yes	Yes	Yes	Yes	Yes	-

CVVH, continuous venovenous hemofiltration; CVVHDF, continuous venovenous hemodiafiltration.

massive metformin ingestion [8,10]. Dehydration was the precipitating factor responsible for acute renal failure in our patients. In addition, the use of nephrotoxic drugs and/or chronic renal failure may have favoured the development of MALA.

Our patients presented with classical symptoms of MALA within a context that suggested metformin accumulation [2,10]. However, the diagnosis of MALA was made only once other causes of lactic acidosis (e.g., mesenteric infarction or septic shock) were excluded. Plasma metformin concentrations, ideally measured in the emergency room, helped us to ensure the correct diagnosis. These measurements are usually performed to eliminate metformin as the cause of lactic acidosis in patients with low plasma levels. However, the concentration of metformin in erythrocytes may be more useful, since it better reflects tissue accumulation [19]. Thus, as reported in this case series of metformin-treated patients, severe lactic acidosis associated with acute renal failure and/or other sepsis-like symptoms should systematically lead physicians to request metformin assays. Using this restrictive approach, we were able to generate a report on a rare, albeit small, series of MALA-only patients.

There are some concerns about using renal replacement therapy to manage MALA. For example, it is not certain whether rapid metformin elimination, either by intermittent hemodialysis or CRRT, is an appropriate endpoint in studies of MALA therapy [10]. Indeed, as previously reported by Lalau and Race, metformin (and also lactate) concentrations are not closely associated with prognosis [20]. In addition, increased levels of both metformin and lactate could even have beneficial cardiovascular, metabolic, and cytoprotective properties [21,22]. With regard to lactate management, it is now well established that lactate is not an acidogenic substance; the amount removed by replacement therapy with dialysis using bicarbonate-buffered fluids is negligible when compared to the overall plasma lactate clearance [23]. In the same way, the CRRT that was used in this case series is considered by some authors to be a supportive measure only to buffer metabolic acidosis and control volemia [10].

Even if there is also no consensus as to the best replacement therapy, hemodialysis appears to be the first-line treatment in association with symptomatic organ failure treatment [2,4–6,24]. In contrast, CRRT to manage MALA has only received attention in a few case reports [7–9,25,26]. Surprisingly, it usually appears to have been used as a rescue therapy either when high flow rates are set or in combination with hemodialysis [8,25,26]. In our practice, we began CRRT as early as possible after patients were admitted to the ICU. Using unfractionated heparin as anticoagulation, we did observe in the present study any of the classical CRRT-associated complications such as bleeding or extracorporeal circuit clotting [27]. We chose to use of CVVHDF, rather than CVVH, in cases of severe and threatening hyperkalemia. We used also a flow rate of the total effluent (the sum of the dialysate and ultrafiltrate) averaging 34±6 ml/kg/h; i.e., a "standard" dose of replacement solution when compared to the very high flow rates (50 to 80 ml/kg/h) sometimes proposed to treat MALA [25,26]. As classically reported, renal recovery (urine output increase and spontaneous urea/creatinine decrease), metabolic state improvement, fluid overload correction, as well as hemodynamic stability were the mean criteria to decide cessation of CRRT [28].

CRRT seems more physiologically appropriate than intermittent hemodialysis in this setting for several reasons. First, because of the drug's low molecular weight and lack of protein binding, conventional modalities of treatment (i.e., dialysis and/or ultrafiltration) can perform high plasma clearance of metformin [24]. Second, metformin has a large volume of distribution (3.1 l/kg) secondary to intracellular penetration [29]. Seidowsky et al. determined recently that 15 cumulative hours of hemodialysis were needed to return patients to therapeutic levels of metformin [5]. CRRT can be used for extended durations and maximizes metformin removal, with a rate of metformin elimination from the blood compartment averaging 2.4±0.9%/h. If prolonged renal therapy is required, initiation of CRRT upon patient admission may be a fast and convenient treatment. Third, all of our patients had circulatory failure upon admission. Because of this, we needed to avoid the detrimental impact of highly intermittent dialysis on hemodynamics, which is caused by major variations in solutes, bicarbonate, electrolytes, pH, and volemia. Thus, CRRT may be a superior choice for MALA, because it gradually removes solutes and places patients in a prolonged physiologically steady state [30].

The reported mortality in patients with MALA was initially very high, nearing 50% [3,18]. More recently, Peters *et al.* reported a 30% death rate in patients admitted to the ICU with MALA [2]. Awareness of metformin complications, as well as better organ failure treatment in ICUs may be the reasons for this decrease in mortality. Indeed, symptomatic management of organ failure (e.g., mechanical ventilation and/or vasoactive drugs) at admission was our priority even before ensuring diagnosis and starting CRRT as a specific treatment. Furthermore, in the present study, in addition to CRRT, we aggressively corrected both the precipitating and the underlying conditions of metformin accumulation by nonspecific therapeutic measures, which could also explain the favourable outcomes we observed.

In summary, early CRRT appears to be a safe and effective means of managing MALA in patients with hemodynamic instability and its use should become more widespread. This modality of replacement therapy, in conjunction with other symptomatic intensive therapies, rapidly corrects metabolic disorders and efficiently eliminates metformin when the standard guidelines for use are followed. However, further studies are needed to determine the most adequate ways of administering this CRRT in patients with MALA.

Author Contributions

Conceived and designed the experiments: LA DR GK. Performed the experiments: GK MC RH JI. Analyzed the data: GK. Contributed reagents/materials/analysis tools: GK LA. Wrote the paper: GK DR LA.

References

1. UK Prospective Diabetes Study (UKPDS) Group (1998) Effect of intensive blood-glucose control with metformin on complications in overweight patients with type 2 diabetes (UKPDS 34). Lancet 352: 854–865.
2. Peters N, Jay N, Barraud D, Cravoisy A, Nace L, et al. (2008) Metformin-associated lactic acidosis in an intensive care unit. Crit Care 12: R149.
3. Misbin RI, Green L, Stadel BV, Gueriguian JL, Gubbi A, Fleming GA (1998) Lactic acidosis in patients with diabetes treated with metformin. N Engl J Med 338: 265–6.
4. Kruse JA (2001) Metformin-associated lactic acidosis. J Emerg Medicine 20: 267–272.
5. Seidowsky A, Nseir S, Houdret N, Fourrier F (2009) Metformin-associated lactic acidosis: a prognostic and therapeutic study. Crit Care Med 37: 2191–2196.
6. Lalau JD, Westeel PF, Debussche X, Dkissi H, Tolani M, et al. (1987) Bicarbonate haemodialysis: an adequate treatment for lactic acidosis in diabetics treated by metformin. Intensive Care Med 13: 383–387.
7. Bruijstens LA, van Luin M, Buscher-Jungerhans PM, Bosch FH (2008) Reality of severe metformin-induced lactic acidosis in the absence of chronic renal impairement. Neth J Med 66: 185–190.
8. Galea M, Jelacin N, Bramham K, White I (2007) Severe lactic acidosis and rhabdomyolysis following metformin and ramipril overdose. Br J Anaesth 98: 213–215.
9. Arroyo AM, Walroth TA, Mowry JB, Kao LW (2010) The MALAdy of metformin poisoning: is CVVH the cure? Am J Ther 17: 96–100.
10. Lalau JD, Race JM (2000) Metformin and lactic acidosis in diabetic humans. Diabetes Obes Metab 2: 131–137.
11. Jackson GG, Arana Sialer JA, Andersen BR, Grieble HG, McCabe WR (1962) Profiles of pyelonephritis. Arch Intern Med 110: 63–75.
12. Knaus WA, Zimmerman JE, Wagner DP, Draper EA, Lawrence DE (1981) APACHE-acute physiology and chronic health evaluation: a physiologically based classification system. Crit Care Med 9: 591–597.
13. Charlson ME, Pompei P, Ales KL, MacKenzie CR (1987) A new method of classifying prognostic comorbidity in longitudinal studies: development and validation. J Chronic Dis 40: 373–383.
14. Le Gall JR, Lemeshow S, Saulnier F (1993) A new Simplified Acute Physiology Score (SAPS II) based on a European/North American multicenter study. JAMA 270: 2957–2963.
15. Teasdale G, Murray G, Parker L, Jennett B (1979) Adding up the Glasgow Coma Score. Acta Neurochir Suppl 28: 13–16.
16. Fagon JY, Chastre J, Novare A, Medioni P, Gibert C (1993) Characterization of intensive care unit patients using a model based on the presence or absence of organ dysfunctions and/or infection: the ODIN model. Intensive Care Med 19: 137–144.
17. Vincent JL, Moreno R, Takala J, Willatts S, De Mendonca A, et al. (1996) The SOFA (Sepsis-related Organ Failure Assessment) score to describe organ dysfunction/failure. On behalf of the Working Group on Sepsis-Related Problems of the European Society of Intensive Care Medicine. Intensive Care Med 22: 707–710.
18. Stades AM, Heikens JT, Erkelens DW, Hollememan F, Hoekstra JB (2004) Metformin and lactic acidosis: cause or coincidence? A review of case reports. J Intern Med 255: 179–187.
19. Lalau JD, Lacroix C (2003) Measurement of metformin concentration in erythrocytes: clinical implications. Diabetes Obes Metab 5: 93–98.
20. Lalau JD, Race JM (1999) Lactic acidosis in metformin-treated patients. Prognostic value of arterial lactate levels and plasma metformin concentrations. Drug Saf 20: 377–384.
21. Kirpichnikov D, McFarlane SI, Sowers JR (2002) Metformin: an update. Ann Intern Med 137: 25–33.
22. Leverve XM (2005) Lactate in the intensive care unit: pyromaniac, sentinel or fireman? Crit Care 9: 588–593.
23. Levraut J, Ciebiera JP, Jambou P, Ichai C, Labib Y, et al. (1997) Effect of continuous venovenous hemofiltration with dialysis on lactate clearance in critically ill patients. Crit Care Med 25: 58–62.
24. Guo PY, Storsley LJ, Finkle SN (2006) Severe lactic acidosis treated with prolonged hemodialysis: recovery after massive overdoses of metformin. Semin Dial 19: 80–83.
25. Pan LT, MacLaren G (2009) Continuous venovenous haemodiafiltration for metformin-induced lactic acidosis. Anaesth Intensive Care 37: 830–83.
26. Panzer U, Kluge S, Kreymann G, Wolf G (2004) Combination of intermittent haemodialysis and high-volume continuous haemofiltration for the treatment of severe metformin-induced lactic acidosis. Nephrol Dial Transplant 19: 2157–2158.
27. Finkel KW, Podoll AS (2009) Complications of continuous renal replacement therapy. Semin Dial 22: 155–159.
28. Uchino S, Bellomo R, Morimatsu H, Morgera S, Schetz M, et al. (2009) Discontinuation of continuous renal replacement therapy: a posthoc analysis of a prospective multicenter observational study. Crit Care Med 37: 2576–2582.
29. Sambol NC, Chiang J, O'Conner M, Liu CY, Lin ET, et al. (1996) Pharmacokinetics and pharmacodynamics of metformin in healthy subjects and patients with noninsulin-dependent diabetes mellitus. J Clin Pharmacol 36: 1012–1021.
30. Ronco C, Ricci Z (2008) Renal replacement therapies: physiological review. Intensive Care Med 34: 2139–2146.

Salt-Induced Changes in Cardiac Phosphoproteome in a Rat Model of Chronic Renal Failure

Zhengxiu Su, Hongguo Zhu, Menghuan Zhang, Liangliang Wang, Hanchang He, Shaoling Jiang, Fan Fan Hou*, Aiqing Li*

Division of Nephrology, Nanfang Hospital, Southern Medical University, State Key Laboratory of Organ Failure Research, National Clinical Research Center of Kidney Disease, Guangzhou, Guangdong, China

Abstract

Heart damage is widely present in patients with chronic kidney disease. Salt diet is the most important environmental factor affecting development of chronic renal failure and cardiovascular diseases. The proteins involved in chronic kidney disease - induced heart damage, especially their posttranslational modifications, remain largely unknown to date. Sprague-Dawley rats underwent 5/6 nephrectomy (chronic renal failure model) or sham operation were treated for 2 weeks with a normal- (0.4% NaCl), or high-salt (4% NaCl) diet. We employed TiO_2 enrichment, iTRAQ labeling and liquid-chromatography tandem mass spectrometry strategy for phosphoproteomic profiling of left ventricular free walls in these animals. A total of 1724 unique phosphopeptides representing 2551 non-redundant phosphorylation sites corresponding to 763 phosphoproteins were identified. During normal salt feeding, 89 (54%) phosphopeptides upregulated and 76 (46%) phosphopeptides downregulated in chronic renal failure rats relative to sham rats. In chronic renal failure rats, high salt intake induced upregulation of 84 (49%) phosphopeptides and downregulation of 88 (51%) phosphopeptides. Database searches revealed that most of the identified phospholproteins were important signaling molecules such as protein kinases, receptors and phosphatases. These phospholproteins were involved in energy metabolism, cell communication, cell differentiation, cell death and other biological processes. The Search Tool for the Retrieval of Interacting Genes analysis revealed functional links among 15 significantly regulated phosphoproteins in chronic renal failure rats compared to sham group, and 23 altered phosphoproteins induced by high salt intake. The altered phosphorylation levels of two proteins involved in heart damage, lamin A and phospholamban were validated. Expression of the downstream genes of these two proteins, desmin and SERCA2a, were also analyzed.

Editor: Dominique Guerrot, Rouen University Hospital, France

Funding: This study is supported by the Major State Basic Research Development Program of China (National 973 program) (Nos. 2012CB517703 & 2011CB504005) to Dr. Fan Fan Hou and National Nature and Science Grants (Nos. 81270825 & 31201751) to Dr. Ai Qing Li. The funders had no role in study design, data collection and analysis, decision to publish, or preparation of the manuscript.

Competing Interests: The authors have declared that no competing interests exist.

* Email: liaiqing@smu.edu.cn (AQL); ffhouguangzhou@163.com (FFH)

Introduction

Chronic kidney disease (CKD) is a global public health problem affecting over 10.8% or 13% of western [1] or Chinese population, respectively [2]. A large number of observational studies have demonstrated excess cardiovascular risks associated with CKD [3–5]. Rate of cardiovascular morbidity and mortality significantly increased in adults with CKD as compared with general population [3,6]. Conventional cardiovascular risk factors such as hypertension and diabetes are highly prevalent in patients with CKD and end-stage renal disease. Cardiovascular diseases occur in progressive stages of chronic renal failure[7], in which besides the conventional cardiovascular risk factors, many factors more specific to CKD, such as proteinuria, anaemia, left ventricular hypertrophy, arterial calcification, abnormal calcium/phosphate/vitamin D homeostasis and inflammation contribute to cardiovascular risk [8]. Heart damage is widely present in patients with CKD, but the mechanisms underlying CKD-induced heart damage remains unclear.

Numerous epidemiologic, clinical, and experimental studies demonstrate dietary salt intake has been related to blood pressure,

and salt restriction has been documented to lower blood pressure [9,10]. Patients with CKD often are salt sensitive and their blood pressure increased with increasing salt intake [11]. Hypertension is common in non-dialysis CKD patients and known as a major risk factor for CVD as well as progression of renal disease [12,13]. Cardiovascular events occurred more frequently in patients with salt-sensitive hypertension. Salt sensitivity has been demonstrated an independent cardiovascular risk factor in Japanese patients with essential hypertension [14]. In contrast, sodium reduction, may reduce long term risk of cardiovascular events [15]. In addition, left ventricular hypertrophy and pulse pressure were influenced by salt intake independent of blood pressure in humans [16–18]. Together, salt diet is the most important environmental factor affecting the development of chronic renal failure and cardiovascular diseases.

Protein phosphorylation is a ubiquitous post-translational modification involved in several key intracellular processes including metabolism, secretion, homeostasis, transcriptional and translational regulation, and cellular signaling [19]. There is overwhelming evidence that protein phosphorylation plays a critical role in cardiac remodeling process. First, a lot of serine–

threonine kinases and kinase signaling pathways, such as PI3K, Akt, GSK-3, TGF-β, CaMKII, PkA, MAPKs, PkC, etc., are involved in regulation of cardiovascular diseases [20–22]; Second, secretion and generation of vasoconstrictor peptides, such as angiotensin II, endothelin-1, norepinephrine, and Rho and Ras proteins, are increased through the activation of protein kinases [22,23] and play critical roles in hypertrophic response to nephrogenic hypertension; Third, protein phosphatase such as protein phosphatase 1 and calcineurin, and a number of phosphoproteins such as phospholamban and epidermal growth factor receptor, are also involved in the remodeling process [22–24]. Mass spectrometry (MS)-based proteomics in combination with phosphoprotein enrichment technique is to-date probably the most powerful tool to analyze large-scale protein phosphorylation events in a variety of biological samples without a prior knowledge of function or distribution [25]. However, there are so far no studies on heart phosphoproteomic change associated with CKD.

In this study, we performed large-scale phosphoproteomic analysis of left ventricular free walls in a salt-load rat model of chronic renal failure using tandem MS [liquid chromatography (LC)−MS/MS] methods used previously [26–28] along with TiO$_2$ enrichment. We identified a total of 1724 unique phosphopeptides, including 165 and 132 phosphopeptides differentially regulated in chronic renal failure and by high salt intake, respectively. This study provides a database resource for future studies of heart diseases. We hope that new scientific research ideas and therapeutic strategies deriving from phosphoproteins or phosphorylation sites reported in this study could be employed to antagonize heart diseases either with or without renal disease.

Materials and Methods

Ethics Statement

The care and use of the rats were approved by the Animal Experiment Ethics Committee of Southern Medical University.

Animals

Male Sprague-Dawley rats (initial weight 150 to 180 g; Southern Medical University Animal Experiment Center) were maintained under standardized conditions and fed a standard rodent diet that contained 16% protein. The rats were divided into three groups. Briefly, the rats were subjected either to five-sixths nephrectomy (5/6 Nx; $n = 12$; by performing a right nephrectomy with surgical resection of two thirds of the left kidney) or to sham operation (controls; $n = 6$). One week after the operation, the 5/6 Nx rats were randomized by the percent remnant kidney weight removed ([right kidney weight − weight of two poles of left kidney]/right kidney weight×100) and were divided into two subgroups (n = 6 in each group). At the end of 4, 8, and 10 wk after operation, the rats (n = 6 in each group at each time point) were anesthetized with sodium pentobarbital and Orbital venous blood was collected from the 5/6 Nx and sham rats for hemodynamic detection.

The experimental procedures are illustrated in Figure 1.

Salt Diet Treatment and Tissue Preparation

At the end of week 10 after operation, 5/6 nephrectomy rats and sham rats were randomly divided into 3 groups and treated as follows: (1) sham-operated rats with normal-salt diet (0.4% sodium chloride, wt/wt) (NS, n = 6); (2) 5/6 nephrectomy rats with normal-salt diet (0.4% sodium chloride, wt/wt) (NC, n = 6); (3) 5/6 nephrectomy rats with high-salt diet (4% sodium chloride, wt/wt) (HC, n = 6). The rats received commercially available rat chow containing different concentrations of salt (TROPHIC, Nantong,

China) for 2 weeks. After salt diet administration, the whole heart was harvested after perfusion with 200 ml of ice-cold normal saline and washed with normal saline. The harvested heart was then weighed, and the upper third part of the left ventricle was dissected for histological analysis. After removing the atria and right ventricle, the free wall of left ventricle was quickly placed in liquid nitrogen until protein or RNA extraction. The 24-h urine samples were collected in metabolic cages at end of the study period.

Renal Function and BP Measurement

Serum and urine creatinine levels were determined using commercial kits (sarcosine oxidase-peroxidase-antiperoxidase; Zixing, Shanghai, China). The creatinine clearance (Ccr) was calculated as described previously and factored for body weight [29]. The 24-hr urinary protein excretion was measured using the Coomassie Blue method [30].

Blood pressure was measured using tail cuff with a sphygmomanometer (BP-98A, softron, Japan) before and after salt diet treatment. Systolic blood pressure was measured 5–6 times and the values were averaged.

Protein Extraction

Approximately 2 g frozen, treated heart tissues from an equal amount of four biological replicates in the same subgroup were ground into a powder in liquid nitrogen and homogenized in extraction buffer [4% SDS, 1 mM DTT, 150 mM Tris-HCl, pH 8]. After 3 min incubation in boiling water, the homogenate was sonicated on ice. The crude extract was then incubated in boiling water again and clarified by centrifugation at 16,000 g at 25°C for 10 min. The protein content was determined by the Bicinchoninic acid protein assay kit (Beyotime, China).

Protein Digestion and iTRAQ Labeling

Protein digestion was performed according to the FASP procedure described by Wisniewski et al. [31] and the resulting peptide mixture was labeled using the 8-plex iTRAQ (isobaric tags for relative and absolute quantification) reagent according to the manufacturer's instructions (Applied Biosystems). Briefly, 200 μg of proteins for each sample were incorporated into 30 μl standard buffer (4% SDS, 100 mM DTT, 150 mM Tris-HCl pH 8.0). The detergent, DTT and other low-molecular-weight components were removed using uric acid (UA) buffer (8 M Urea, 150 mM Tris-HCl pH 8.0) by repeated ultrafiltration (Microcon units, 30 kD). Then 100 μl 0.05 M iodoacetamide in UA buffer was added to block reduced cysteine residues and the samples were incubated for 20 min in darkness. The filters were washed with 100 μl UA buffer three times and then 100 μl DS buffer (50 mM triethylammoniumbicarbonate at pH 8.5) twice. Finally, the protein suspensions were digested with 2 μg trypsin (Promega) in 40 μl DS buffer overnight at 37°C, and the resulting peptides were collected as a filtrate. The peptide content was estimated by UV light spectral density at 280 nm using an extinctions coefficient of 1.1 of 0.1% (g/l) solution that was calculated on the basis of the frequency of tryptophan and tyrosine in vertebrate proteins. For labeling, each iTRAQ reagent was dissolved in 70 μl of ethanol and added to the respective peptide mixture. The samples marked NS, NC and HC were labeled with iTRAQ tags 113, 114 and 115, respectively, multiplexed and vacuum dried.

Enrichment of Phosphorylated Peptiedes by the TiO$_2$ Beads

The final peptide mixture, which was concentrated by a vacuum concentrator, was resuspended in 500 μL loading buffer

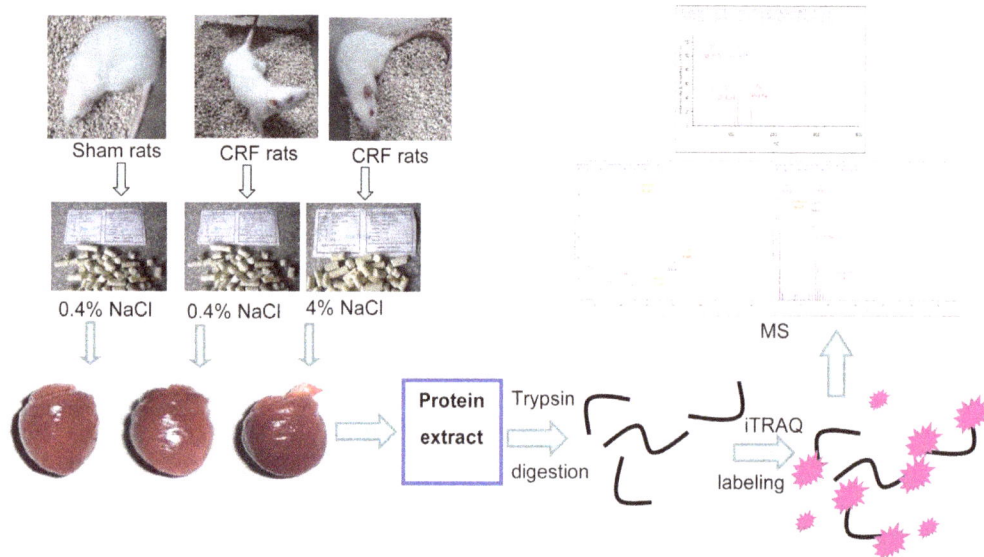

Figure 1. Flow chart of phosphoproteomic analysis of left ventricle free walls in sham and chronic renal failure rats. Male Sprague-Dawley rats were subjected either to five-sixths nephrectomy or to sham operation. Ten weeks after surgery, 5/6 nephrectomy induced chronic renal failure (CRF) rats were fed normal salt (0.04% NaCl) or high salt (4% NaCl) diet for 2 weeks. Sham group was maintained with normal salt diet. The whole heart was harvested and the free wall of left ventricle was dissected for protein extraction. The proteins were then digested with trypsin, labeled using the 8-plex isobaric tags for relative and absolute quantification (iTRAQ) reagent and multiplexed. The phosphorylated peptides enriched with TiO$_2$ beads were subjected for nano-liquid chromatography tandem mass spectrometry (MS) analysis using a Q Exactive MS equipped with easy nano-liquid chromatography.

(2% glutamic acid/65% ACN/2% TFA). Then, TiO$_2$ beads were added and then agitated for 40 min. The centrifugation was carried out for 1 min at 5000 g, resulting in the first beads. The supernatant from the first centrifugation were mixed with another TiO$_2$ beads, resulting in the second beads which collected as before. Both beads were combined and washed with 50 uL of washing buffer I (30% ACN/3% TFA) three times and then 50 μL of washing buffer II (80% ACN/0.3% TFA) three times to remove the remaining non-adsorbed material. Finally, the phosphopeptides were eluted with 50 uL of elution buffer (40% ACN/15% NH$_4$OH), followed by lyophilization and MS analysis.

Mass Spectrometry

Five microliters of the phosphopeptides solution mixed with 15 ul 0.1% (v/v) trifluoroacetic acid and then 10 ul of the solution mixture was injected for nanoLC-MS/MS analysis using an Q Exactive MS (Thermo Finnigan) equipped with Easy nLC (Proxeon Biosystems, now Thermo Fisher Scientific). The peptide mixture was loaded onto a C18-reversed phase column (15 cm long, 75 μm inner diameter, RP-C18 3 μm, packed in-house) in buffer A (0.1% formic acid) and separated with a linear gradient of buffer B (80% acetonitrile and 0.1% formic acid) at a flow rate of 250 nL/min controlled by IntelliFlow technology over 240 min. The peptides were eluted with a gradient of 0%–60% buffer B from 0 min to 200 min, 60% to 100% buffer B from 200 min to 216 min, 100% buffer B from 216 min to 240 min.

For MS analysis, peptides were analyzed in positive ion mode. MS spectra were acquired using a data-dependent top 10 method dynamically choosing the most abundant precursor ions from the survey scan (300–1800 m/z) for higher energy collisional (C-trap) dissociation (HCD) fragmentation. Determination of the target value is based on predictive Automatic Gain Control (pAGC). Dynamic exclusion duration was 40.0 s. Survey scans were acquired at a resolution of 70,000 at m/z 200 and resolution for HCD spectra was set to 17,500 at m/z 200. Normalized collision energy was 27 eV and the under fill ratio, which specifies the minimum percentage of the target value likely to be reached at maximum fill time, was defined as 0.1%. The instrument was run with peptide recognition mode enabled.

Data Analysis

MS/MS spectra were searched using Mascot 2.2 engine against the Uniprot database and the reversed database. For protein identification, the following options were used. Peptide mass tolerance = 20 ppm, MS/MS tolerance = 0.1 Da, Enzyme = Trypsin, Missed cleavage = 2, Fixed modification: Carbamidomethyl (C), Variable modification: Oxidation (M), Phosphorylation (S/T/Y), FDR≤0.01.

The phosphorylation peptides were analyzed using Proteome Discoverer 1.3 (Thermo Electron, San Jose, CA). pRS score above 50 indicate a good PSM (Peptide Spectrum Matches) and pRS probabilities above 75 percent indicate that a site is truly phosphorylated.

Western Blot Analysis

Western blot analyses were carried out as described previously [26]. Briefly, left ventricular free walls were lysed with the radioimmunoprecipitation assay buffer, and the lysates were separated by SDS-PAGE. The separated proteins were then transferred to Polyvinylidene fluoride membranes. The membrane blots were first probed with a primary antibody overnight at 4°C and then secondary antibody coupled to horseradish peroxidase. The proteins were visualized with the enhanced chemiluminescent system (Pierce, Rockford, IL) and the bands densitometry was analyzed. Phosphoprotein levels were normalized to total protein levels. The primary antibodies used included anti-Phospho-phospholamban (Ser16, Cell Signaling, Beverly, MA, USA), anti-phospholamban (Abcam, Cambridge, MA, USA), anti-

Phospho-lamin A (Ser22, Santa Cruz Biotechnology, Santa Cruz, CA, USA) and anti-lamin A (Abcam).

Real-time Reverse Transcriptase-polymerase Chain Reaction

Total RNA was extracted from left ventricular free walls in the animals using Trizol reagent (Invitrogen). Aliquots of each RNA extraction were reverse-transcribed simultaneously into cDNA using M-MLV reverse transcriptase according to the manufacturer's protocol (Invitrogen). Each quantitative real-time PCR was performed in a total volume of 25 µL in duplicate by using the Premix Ex Taq kit (TaKaRa, Kyoto, Japan) and the Fast Real-Time PCR system 7500 (Applied Biosystems, CA). The thermal cycling conditions comprised a 30-second step at 95°C, followed by 40 cycles with denaturation at 95°C for 5 seconds, annealing at 60°C (desmin, SERCA2) or 56°C (GAPDH)) for 30 seconds, and extension at 72°C for 60 seconds. The following sets of primers, which were designed using Primer Quest software, were used: desmin forward: 5′–GGG CGA GGA GAG CCG GAT CA–3′, reverse: 5′–TCC CCG TCC CGG GTC TCA ATG–3′; SERCA2 forward: 5′–AAG CAG TTC ATC CGC TAC CT–3′, reverse: 5′–AGA CCA TCC GTC ACC AGA TT–3′; GADPH forward: 5′–GGG TGT GAA CCA CGA GAA AT–3′, resverse: 5′–ACT GTG GTC ATG AGC CCT TC–3′. For normalization of differences in RNA amounts, the GAPDH RNA was coamplified. Relative quantification of each gene was calculated after normalization to GAPDH RNA by using the comparative Ct method. The results were shown as relative expression ratio with respect to NC group for all samples.

Result

Physiological Parameters

Ten weeks after 5/6 nephrectomy or sham operation, 5/6 Nx rats displayed substantially elevated systolic blood pressure (SBP), serum creatinine, blood urea nitrogen and 24-hour urinary protein excretion relative to sham rats, that demonstrated chronic renal failure (CRF) rats were successfully prepared. The rats were fed high or normal salt diets for 2 weeks (see Materials and Methods). As shown in Table 1, high salt intake induced a significant increase in SBP, urinary sodium excretion and urinary protein excretion in CRF rats relative to normal salt intake, suggesting that high salt intake aggravated kidney damage. Both the average heart weight and heart weight/body weight ratio of CRF rats with high salt diet was significantly greater than that with normal salt diet. These data demonstrated that high salt intake aggravated cardiac hypertrophy in CRF rats.

Identification of Phosphorylated Proteins and Sites

In this study, phosphopeptides were identified after manual confirmation of MS/MS spectra by combining phosphopeptide enrichment using titanium dioxide with LC−MS/MS quantitative proteomics using iTRAQ. These identified phosphopeptides (Table S1) were clustered into 1724 unique peptides representing 2551 non-redundant phosphorylation sites on 763 different proteins. To precisely assign phosphorylation sites within a peptide, we used posttranslational modification score to calculate probabilities of phosphorylation at each site as previously described [32]. We could localize 1002 phosphosites with high confidence as class I phosphorylation site, i.e., singly-phosphorylated. Around 58.1% of the phosphopeptides identified were found to be singly phosphorylated including 14 phosphotyrosine sites, 52 phosphothreonine sites, and 565 phosphoserine sites. The other peptides were doubly (36.4%), triply (4.8%), or more highly (0.6%)

phosphorylated (Figure 2 a and b). It is worth pointing out that most of proteins identified from the phosphopeptides are important signaling molecules such as protein kinases, receptors, phosphatases, and transcription regulators including transcription factors and repressors. They are involved in cell energy metabolism, signal transduction, apoptosis and other biological processes.

Among these differentially phosphorylated peptides (Table S2), we found that ~6.3% in NC versus NS group (NC/NS) (108 out of 1724 phosphopeptides) and ~6.7% in HC versus NC (HC/NC) group (115 out of 1724 phosphopeptides) were significantly altered using a cut-off value of 1.5-fold up- or down-regulation (Figure 2, c and d). Among these altered phosphopeptides, 58 phosphopeptides were found in common between NC/NS and HC/HS comparison groups, in which 12 have the same alteration trend (Figure 2 e and f).

Properties of Phosphorylated Proteins

To understand biological roles of these phosphoproteins in cardiac remodeling process, a Gene Ontology (GO) analysis with PANTHER classification system was utilized to analyze molecular functions and biological process of these differentially phosphorylated proteins. As shown in Figure 3, GO analysis for NC/NS comparison group demonstrated that the differentially expressed phosphoproteins were classified into 12 groups based on their molecular functions including protein binding, catalytic activity, nucleotide binding, metal ion binding, structural molecule activity, enzyme regulator activity, DNA binding, motor activity, transporter activity, RNA binding, signal transducer activity, and 16 groups according to their biological process such as energy metabolism, transport, cell growth, cell death, cell communication, cell differentiation cell organization and biogenesis and development, (Figure 3 a and b). Similarly, GO analysis demonstrated that the differentially expressed phosphoproteins for HC/NC comparison group were classified into 13 groups based on their molecular functions including catalytic activity, protein binding, nucleotide binding, metal ion binding, structural molecule activity, RNA binding, motor activity, DNA binding, transporter activity, signal transducer activity, enzyme regulator activity, receptor activity, and 16 groups according to their biological process such as energy metabolism, transport and cell differentiation (Figure 3 c and d). Here, energy metabolism means the chemical processes occurring within a living cell or organism that are necessary for the maintenance of life. Cell organization and biogenesis means a process that results in the biosynthesis of constituent macromolecules, assembly, arrangement of constituent parts, or disassembly of a cellular component. Cell communication includes any process that mediates interactions between a cell and its surroundings. Cell differentiation means the process in which relatively unspecialized cells, e.g. embryonic or regenerative cells, acquire specialized structural and/or functional features that characterize the cells, tissues, or organs of the mature organism or some other relatively stable phase of the organism's life history. Cell death includes any biological process that results in permanent cessation of all vital functions of a cell. Cellular homeostasis defines any process involved in the maintenance of an internal steady state at the level of the cell. Cell proliferation defines the multiplication or reproduction of cells, resulting in the expansion of a cell population. Cellular component movement means the directed, self-propelled movement of a cellular component without the involvement of an external agent such as a transporter or a pore. Cell growth defines the process in which a cell irreversibly increases in size over time by accretion and biosynthetic production of matter similar to that already present. Cell division

Table 1. Physiological and metabolic parameters in Sham and CRF rats at week 12 after surgery.[A]

	Sham	CRF	
	Normal salt	Normal salt	High salt
HW (mg)	1.6±0.1	1.9±0.1[B]	2.3±0.1[C]
HW/BW (*1000)	2.9±0.0	3.8±0.1[B]	4.2±0.2[C]
SBP (mmHg)	126.3±4.1	137.1±3.3[B]	153.1±3.5[C]
Serum Na+(mmol/l)	139.6±0.8	141.3±1.3	144.3±0.37[C]
Urine Na+ μmol/24 h)	871.0±67.9	747.0±69.3	11212.2±1012.2[C]
UPE (mg/24 h)	10.60±0.7	16.38±1.2[B]	40.29±3.1[C]

[A]Data from 3 independent experiments are expressed as mean ± SD (n=6 in each group);
[B]P<0.05 versus rats fed with normal salt in the sham group;
[C]P<0.05 versus CRF group fed with normal salt diet.
HW, heart weight, recorded for perfused hearts after removal of the atria and major blood vessels; HW/BW, heart weight/body weight; SBP, systolic blood pressure; UPE, urinary protein excretion.

means the process resulting in the physical partitioning and separation of a cell into daughter cells. Transport covers the processes involved in positioning a substance or cellular entity. Defense response means reactions, triggered in response to the presence of a foreign body or the occurrence of an injury, which

result in restriction of damage to the organism attacked or prevention/recovery from the infection caused by the attack. Development defines the process whose specific outcome is the progression of the cell over time, from its formation to the mature structure. Reproduction means a process, occurring at the cellular level, that is involved in the reproductive function of a multicellular or single-celled organism. Coagulation means the process in which a fluid solution, or part of it, changes into a solid or semisolid mass. In addition, we have listed some known proteins that are associated with heart damage (Table 2). The involved heart diseases included hypertrophic cardiomyopathy, arrhythmogenic right ventricular cardiomyopathy, dilated cardiomyopathy and viral myocarditis.

STRING Protein-protein Analysis of Differentially Expressed Heart Proteins

STRING (Search Tool for the Retrieval of Interacting Genes) is a protein-protein analysis database program generating a network of interactions from a variety of sources, including different interaction databases, text mining, genetic interactions, and shared pathway interactions [33]. This analysis provides an essential system-level understanding of cellular events in a functional heart. The networks formed by interacting proteins provided insights into the potential mechanisms of how salt and renal failure affects cardiac functions. In this study, the STRING analysis revealed functional links among 15 significantly regulated phosphoproteins in NC/NS comparison group (Figure 4) and 23 significantly regulated phosphoproteins in HC/NC comparison group (Figure 5).

Validation of Selected Proteins and Analysis of their Downstream Gene Expression

Given that one of the major goals of this project was to identify phosphoproteins that may be contributing to salt-induced heart damage, we examined expression of phospho-lamin A and phospho-phospholamban as well as their downstream genes desmin and SERCA2a, which altered significantly in response to high salt intake in CRF rats. We initially examined expression of phospho-lamin A by western blot. It has been shown that lamin A/C-deficient myoblasts showed a decrease in desmin protein and transcript [34]. Restoration of lamin A in cardiomyocytes improves cardiac function [35]. Consistent with our proteome analysis, we noted high salt-induced a marked increase in

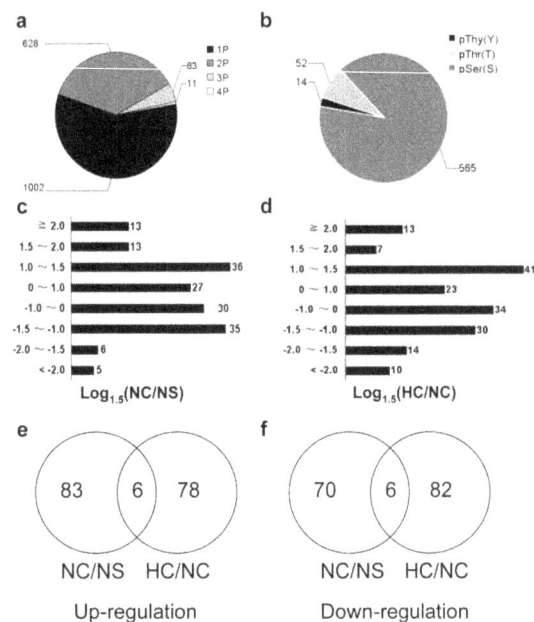

Figure 2. Characterization of phosphopeptides, phosphosites and phosphoproteins. (a) Distribution of singly, doubly, triply and quadruply phosphorylated peptides; (b) Distribution of the Ser, Thr, Tyr phosphosites in the heart phosphoproteome. Phosphopeptides were categorized into class I phosphosites by calculating the probabilities for phosphorylation at each site based on posttranslational modification scores. Here, only class I phosphosites (high probability) were used to analyze the distribution. (c, d) Phosphopeptide Log 1.5 (NC/NS) and Log 1.5 (HC/NC) ratio after different salt intake. (e, f) Venn diagram of differentially phosphorylated peptides in NC/NS and HC/NC comparison groups. HC represents CRF rats with high salt intake, NC represents CRF rats with normal salt intake. NS represents sham rats with normal salt intake. 1P, 2P, 3P and 4P represent singly, doubly, triply and quadruply phosphorylated peptides, respectively. NS, sham-operated rats fed with normal-salt diet; NC, 5/6 nephrectomized rats fed with normal-salt diet; HC, 5/6 nephrectomized rats fed with high-salt diet.

Table 2. List of some identified proteins and their known associated heart disease.

Gene name	ID	Heart disease
phospholamban	IPI00195376	Dilated cardiomyopathy
desmin	IPI00421517	Hypertrophic cardiomyopathy; Arrhythmogenic right ventricular cardiomyopathy; Dilated cardiomyopathy
myosin, heavy chain 9, non-muscle	IPI00209113	Viral myocarditis
lamin A	IPI00454367	Hypertrophic cardiomyopathy; Arrhythmogenic right ventricular cardiomyopathy; Dilated cardiomyopathy
junctophilin-2	IPI00199887	hypertrophic cardiomyopathy
catenin, alpha 1	IPI00358406	Arrhythmogenic right ventricular cardiomyopathy
desmoplakin	IPI00366081	Arrhythmogenic right ventricular cardiomyopathy
desmoglein 2	IPI00951246	Arrhythmogenic right ventricular cardiomyopathy
plakophilin 2	IPI00763527	Arrhythmogenic right ventricular cardiomyopathy
myosin binding protein C, cardiac	IPI00870316	Hypertrophic cardiomyopathy; Dilated cardiomyopathy
myosin, heavy chain 6, cardiac muscle, alpha	IPI00189809	Hypertrophic cardiomyopathy; Dilated cardiomyopathy; Viral myocarditis
myosin, heavy chain 7, cardiac muscle, beta	IPI00189811	Hypertrophic cardiomyopathy; Dilated cardiomyopathy; Viral myocarditis
troponin I type 3 (cardiac)	IPI00231689	Hypertrophic cardiomyopathy; Dilated cardiomyopathy

NC/NS

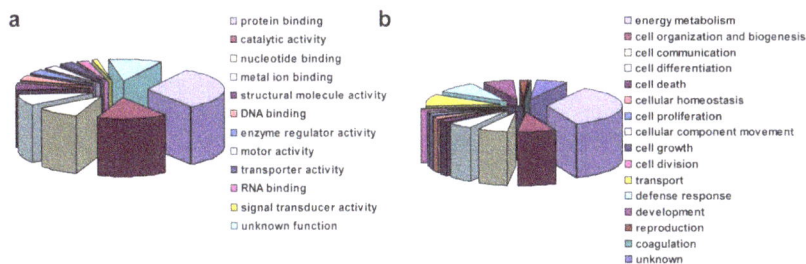

HC/NC

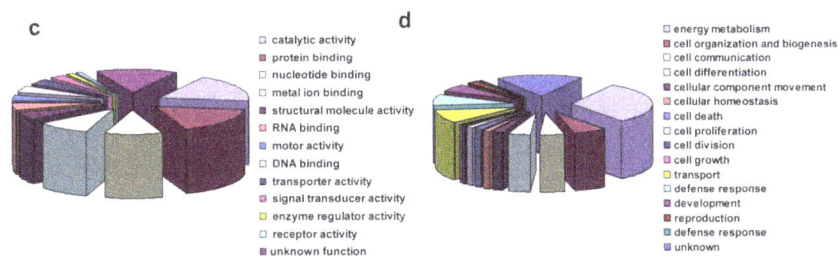

Figure 3. GO analysis of the phosphoproteins differentially expressed in NC/NS and HC/NC comparison groups based on their molecular function (a, c) and biological process (b, d) using PANTHER classification, respectively.

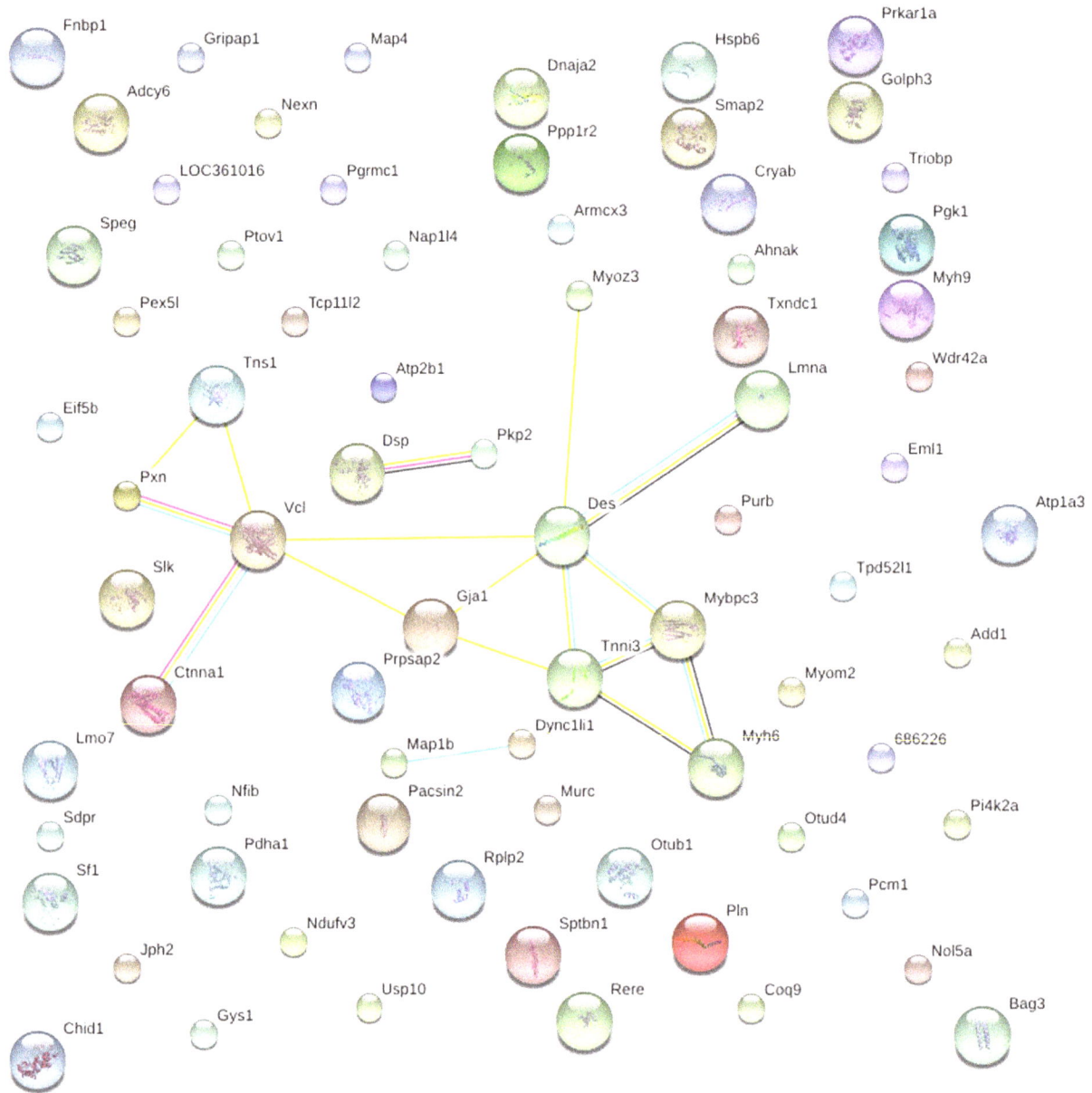

Figure 4. STRING analysis reveals protein interaction networks in heart phosphoproteome in NC/NS comparison group. Interactions of the identified phosphoproteins were mapped by searching the STRING (Search Tool for the Retrieval of Interacting Genes/Proteins) database version 9.0 with a confidence cutoff of 0.6. In the resulting protein association network, proteins are presented as nodes which are connected by lines whose thickness represents the confidence level (0.6–0.9).

phospho-lamin A in CRF animals (Figure 6a). Further, a significant increase in desmin mRNA level was observed in high salt-fed CRF rats (Figure 6c), which corresponded with increased phospho-lamin A expression.

We then examined expression of phospho-phospholamban in left ventricular free walls. SERCA/phospholamban complex regulates cardiac muscle contractility by controlling Ca2+ transport in cariomyocytes. Phosphorylation of phospholamban increases SERCA expression [36]. Western analysis of left ventricular free walls revealed a significant decrease in phosphor-phospholamban expression in CRF rats (Figure 6b). High salt intake resulted in a further reduction of phosphorylated phospholamban in CRF rats (Figure 6b). Consistently, mRNA levels of its downstream gene SERCA were thus decreased in NC

and HC groups (Figure 6d). Together, these data lend support to our proteomic analysis.

Discussion

Previous studies have suggested significant changes of phosphorylated heart proteins in animal models such as spontaneously hypertensive rats [21,37–39], Dahl rats [40] and heart failure model [41] or cardiac cell line [42]. Protein phosphorylation plays a critical role in regulation of cardiac function. It must be noted that we were the first to investigate the phosphorylated proteins of the heart as well as characterize the variations induced by high salt intake in the remnant kidney model.

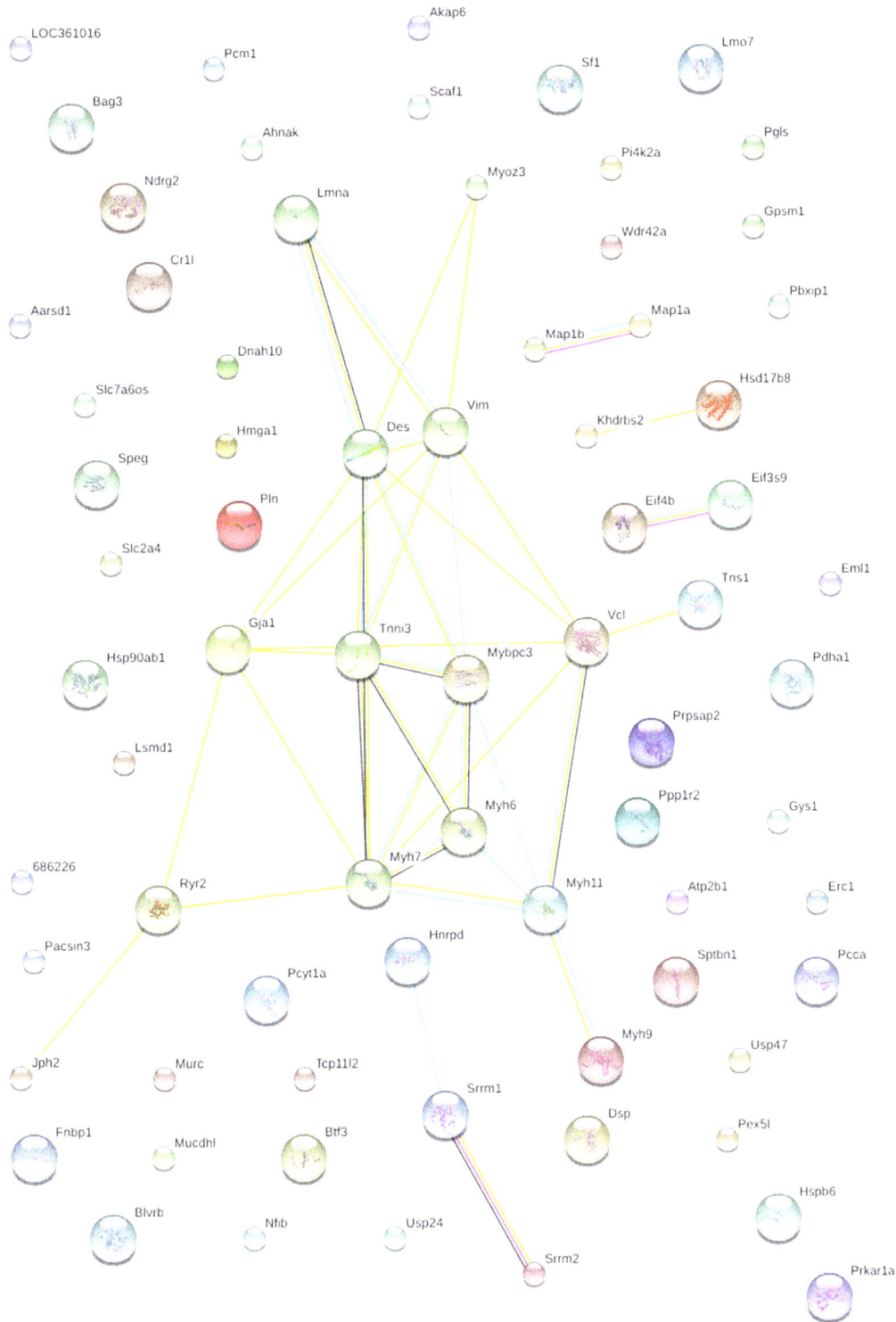

Figure 5. STRING analysis reveals protein interaction networks in heart phosphoproteome in HC/NC comparison group. Interactions of the identified phosphoproteins were mapped by searching the STRING database version 9.0 with a confidence cutoff of 0.6. In the resulting protein association network, proteins are presented as nodes which are connected by lines whose thickness represents the confidence level (0.6–0.9).

We have identified 763 phosphorylated proteins and 1724 phosphopeptides by iTRAQ along with LC-MS/MS. Here we have demonstrated that quantitative iTRAQ-based LC MS/MS is a robust protein discovery technique, and has the potential to uncover proteins as yet unknown to function in pathogenesis of cardiovascular changes caused by CRF. Our investigation focused on identifying as many post-translational modification alterations as possible. Phosphorylation is the most prevalent post-translational modification. Titanium dioxide enrichment was performed, which has been proved highly efficient and selective for phospho-

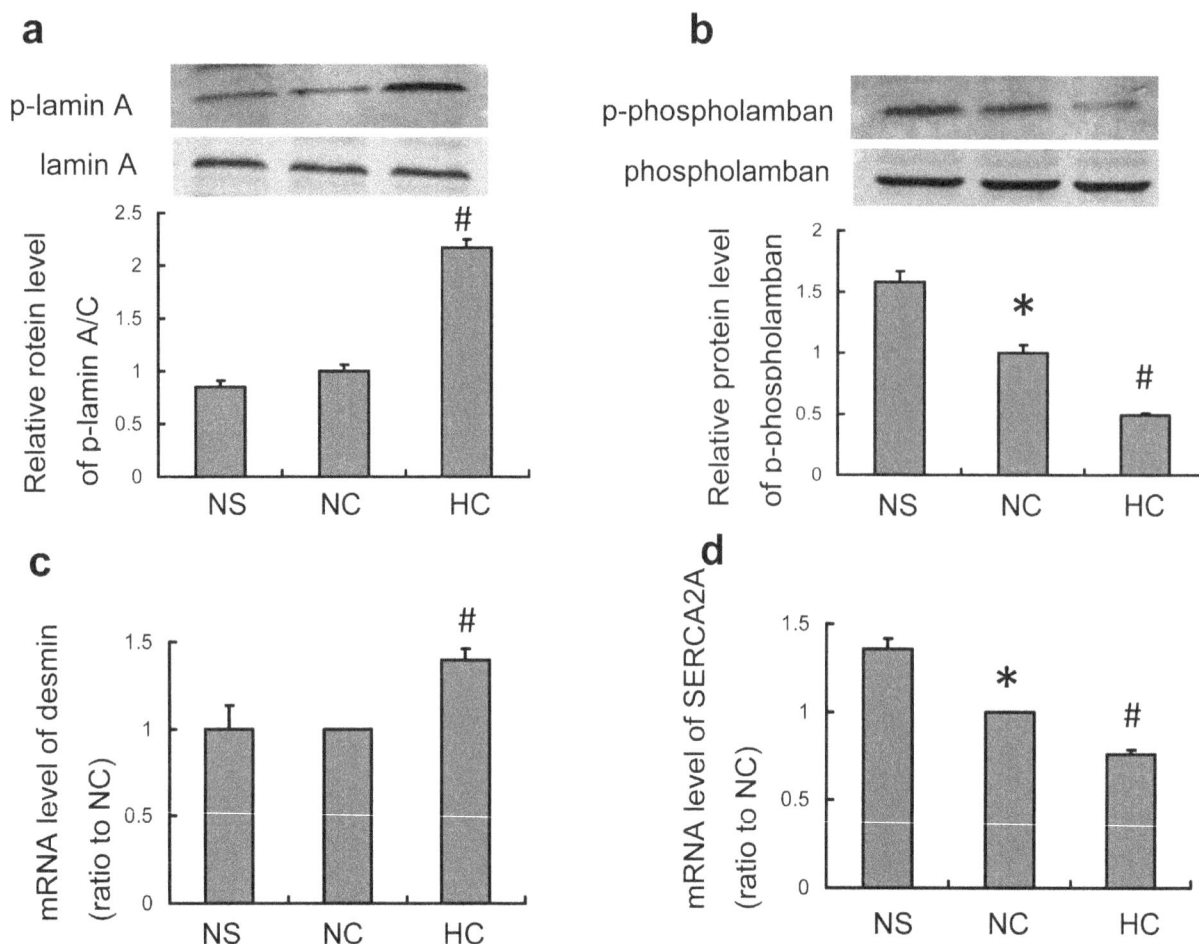

Figure 6. High salt intake induced significant expression changes of p-lamin A and p-phospholamban as well as their downstream genes desmin and SERCA2a. High salt intake increased protein level of p-lamin A (a) and mRNA level of its downstream gene desmin (c). Phosphorylation level of phospholamban decreased (b) and that resulted in decrease of mRNA level of the downstream gene SERCA2a (d) in NC and HC groups. $P < 0.05$ vs. NS (*) and vs. NC group (#).

enrichment [43], as phosphosignals are frequently restrained to such an extent that they are lost to their more abundant unmodified counterparts without any enrichment methods. Therefore, post-translational modifications were specifically searched for.

We have identified many molecules associated with cardiac function. For instance, cMyBP-C, cardiac myosin-binding protein-C, is an important regulator of cardiac contractility, and its phosphorylation by PKA contributes to increased cardiac output in response to β-adrenergic stimulation [44]. cMyBP-C phosphorylation level is markedly decreased in human and animals with heart failure [45]. Similarly, we have observed cMyBP-C phosphorylation levels in high salt-fed CRF rats, suggesting an important maladaption to salt-reduced cardiac damage in CRF rats.

Phospholamban is a member of calcium signaling pathway and small transmembrane protein that is located in the cardiac sarcoplasmic reticulum. Phospholamban binds to and regulates the activity of a Ca2+ pump SERCA2a through altering its phosphorylation state. There is evidence that dilated cardiomyopathy in humans can result from chronic inhibition of SERCA2a by the prevention of phosphorylation of phospholamban by PKA [46]. In our study, proteomic data revealed that phospholamban phosphorylation level decreased significantly in CRF rat hearts,

that were aggravated by salt loading. Change of phospholamban phosphorylation was validated by secondary method western blot. Importantly, a marked decrease in SERCA2a transcript was also observed here. These data may suggest dysregulation of Ca2+ pump activity and signaling. This may reveal a mechanism underlining dilated cardiomyopathy in CRF.

Junctophilin-2, a unique subtype rich in the heart, is a membrane-binding protein that plays a key role in organization of junctional membrane complexes in cardiac myocytes. It is essential for cellular Ca^{2+} homeostasis and cardiac excitation-contraction coupling. Junctophilin-2 decreased in cardiac diseases such as hypertrophic cardiomyopathy [47,48], dilated cardiomyopathy and heart failure [47,49], thus contributing to defective excitation-contraction coupling. In this study, phosphorylation level of junctophilin-2 was observed to decrease significantly in salt-fed CRF group, suggesting that phosphorylation of junctophilin-2 may play an important role in salt-induced cardiac injury associated with CRF.

To reveal potential signaling pathways represented by the heart phosphoproteome, we searched the identified phosphoproteins based on the widely used pathway database, Kyoto Encyclopedia of Genes and Genomes (KEGG) [50,51]. Many fundamental biological pathways were highlighted by phosphoproteins differentially expressed in NC/NS and HC/NC comparison groups, as shown in Table S3 and S4, which included calcium signaling pathway, hypertrophic cardiomyopathy, dilated cardiomyopathy, Arrhythmogenic right ventricular cardiomyopathy, cardiac muscle contraction, MAPK signaling pathway, adherens junction, tight junction, etc. These signaling pathways may be related to differences in heart phosphoproteome of 5/6 Nx rats with different salt intake. Therefore, our phosphoproteomics data provided a deeper understanding of phosphorylation regulation and laid a foundation for future dissection of the phosphorylation network in damaged hearts due to renal failure and salt load.

Conclusions

Our global phosphoprotein analysis based on iTRAQ identified 1724 unique phosphopeptides representing 2551 non-redundant phosphorylation sites corresponding to 763 phosphoproteins in left ventricular free walls of CRF rats. Among these phosphopeptides, 89 upregulated and 76 downregulated in CRF animals relative to sham group. Compared to normal salt intake, salt load induced upregulation of 84 phosphopeptides and downregulation of 88 phosphopeptides in CRF rats. The differentially expressed phospholproteins are important signaling molecules, receptors, phosphatases, and transcription regulators involved in energy metabolism, transport, cell organization and biogenesis, cell communication, cell differentiation, cell death and other biological processes. Although the pathological significance of differentially phosohorylated peptides remains to be tested, identification of phosphopeptide profiles involved in CRF and salt load will

advance our understanding of chronic kidney disease -induced heart damage and help identify new potential therapeutic target.

Author Contributions

Conceived and designed the experiments: ZXS FFH AQL. Performed the experiments: ZXS HGZ MHZ LLW HCH SLJ. Analyzed the data: ZXS HGZ MHZ LLW. Contributed reagents/materials/analysis tools: FFH. Wrote the paper: ZXS AQL.

References

1. Coresh J, Selvin E, Stevens LA, Manzi J, Kusek JW, et al. (2007) Prevalence of chronic kidney disease in the United States. JAMA 298: 2038–2047.
2. Zhang L, Wang F, Wang L, Wang W, Liu B, et al. (2012) Prevalence of chronic kidney disease in China: a cross-sectional survey. Lancet 379: 815–822.
3. Mataradzija A, Resic H, Rasic S, Kukavica N, Masnic F (2010) Risk factors for development of cardiovascular complications in patients with chronic renal disease and diabetic nephropathy. Bosn J Basic Med Sci 10 Suppl 1: S44–S50.
4. Matsushita K, van der Velde M, Astor BC, Woodward M, Levey AS, et al. (2010) Association of estimated glomerular filtration rate and albuminuria with all-cause and cardiovascular mortality in general population cohorts: a collaborative meta-analysis. Lancet 375: 2073–2081.
5. Van Biesen W, De Bacquer D, Verbeke F, Delanghe J, Lameire N, et al. (2007) The glomerular filtration rate in an apparently healthy population and its relation with cardiovascular mortality during 10 years. Eur Heart J 28: 478–483.
6. Muntner P, He J, Astor BC, Folsom AR, Coresh J (2005) Traditional and nontraditional risk factors predict coronary heart disease in chronic kidney disease: results from the atherosclerosis risk in communities study. J Am Soc Nephrol 16: 529–538.
7. Shiba N, Shimokawa H (2011) Chronic kidney disease and heart failure–Bidirectional close link and common therapeutic goal. J Cardiol 57: 8–17.
8. Ross L, Banerjee D (2013) Cardiovascular complications of chronic kidney disease. Int J Clin Pract 67: 4–5.
9. Frisoli TM, Schmieder RE, Grodzicki T, Messerli FH (2012) Salt and hypertension: is salt dietary reduction worth the effort? Am J Med 125: 433–439.
10. Aviv A (2001) Salt and hypertension: the debate that begs the bigger question. Arch Intern Med 161: 507–510.
11. Weir MR, Fink JC (2005) Salt intake and progression of chronic kidney disease: an overlooked modifiable exposure? A commentary. Am J Kidney Dis 45: 176–188.
12. Mensah GA, Croft JB, Giles WH (2002) The heart, kidney, and brain as target organs in hypertension. Cardiol Clin 20: 225–247.
13. Mensah GA, Croft JB, Giles WH (2003) The heart, kidney, and brain as target organs in hypertension. Curr Probl Cardiol 28: 156–193.
14. Morimoto A, Uzu T, Fujii T, Nishimura M, Kuroda S, et al. (1997) Sodium sensitivity and cardiovascular events in patients with essential hypertension. Lancet 350: 1734–1737.
15. Cook NR, Cutler JA, Obarzanek E, Buring JE, Rexrode KM, et al. (2007) Long term effects of dietary sodium reduction on cardiovascular disease outcomes: observational follow-up of the trials of hypertension prevention (TOHP). BMJ 334: 885–888.
16. du Cailar G RJDJ (1992) Sodium and left ventricular mass in untreated hypertensive and normotensive subjects. Am J Physiol Heart Circ Physiol 263: 177–181.
17. du Cailar G MA (1995) Sodium and left ventricular hypertrophy in patients with hypertension. Arch Mal Coeur 88: 15–19.
18. du Cailar G MAFP (2004) Dietary sodium and pulse pressure in normotensive and essential hypertensive subjects. J Hypertens 22: 693–697.
19. Delom F, Chevet E (2006) Phosphoprotein analysis: from proteins to proteomes. Proteome Sci 4: 15.
20. Rizzi E, Ceron CS, Guimaraes DA, Prado CM, Rossi MA, et al. (2013) Temporal changes in cardiac matrix metalloproteinase activity, oxidative stress, and TGF-beta in renovascular hypertension-induced cardiac hypertrophy. Exp Mol Pathol 94: 1–9.
21. Sun Z, Hamilton KL, Reardon KF (2012) Phosphoproteomics and molecular cardiology: techniques, applications and challenges. J Mol Cell Cardiol 53: 354–368.
22. Kotlo K, Johnson KR, Grillon JM, Geenen DL, DeTombe P, et al. (2012) Phosphoprotein abundance changes in hypertensive cardiac remodeling. J Proteomics 77: 1–13.
23. Cacciapuoti F (2011) Molecular mechanisms of left ventricular hypertrophy (LVH) in systemic hypertension (SH)-possible therapeutic perspectives. J Am Soc Hypertens 5: 449–455.
24. Stenvinkel P, Carrero JJ, Axelsson J, Lindholm B, Heimburger O, et al. (2008) Emerging biomarkers for evaluating cardiovascular risk in the chronic kidney disease patient: how do new pieces fit into the uremic puzzle? Clin J Am Soc Nephrol 3: 505–521.
25. Engholm-Keller K, Martin R. Larsen MR (2013) Technologies and challenges in large-scale phosphoproteomics. Proteomics 13: 910–931.
26. Li A, Choi YS, Dziema H, Cao R, Cho HY, Jung YY, Obreitan K (2010) Proteomic profiling of the epileptic dentate gyrus. Brain Pathol 20: 1077–1089.
27. Li A, Benoit JB, Lopez-Martinez G, Elnitsky MA, Lee RE, Denlinger DL (2009) Distinct contractile and cytoskeletal protein patterns in the Antarctic midge are elicited by desiccation and rehydration. Proteomics 9: 2788–2798.
28. Li A, Michaud MR, Denlinger DL (2009) Rapid elevation of Inos and decreases in abundance of other brain proteins at pupal diapause termination in the flesh fly Sarcophaga crassipalpis. BBA- Proteins & Proteom 1794: 663–668.
29. Levey AS: Clinical evaluation of renal function. In: Primer on Kidney Diseases, Ed., edited by Greenberg A, San Diego, Academic Press, 1998, 20–26.
30. Lott JA, Stephan VA, Pritchard KJ (1983) Evaluation of the Coomassie Brilliant Blue G-250 method for urinary protein. Clin Chem 29: 1946–1950.
31. Wisniewski JR, Zougman A, Nagaraj N, Mann M (2009) Universal sample preparation method for proteome analysis. Nat Methods 6: 359–362.
32. Beausoleil SA, Villen J, Gerber SA, Rush J, Gygi SP (2006) A probability-based approach for high-throughput protein phosphorylation analysis and site localization. Nature Biotech. 24: 1285–1292.

33. Szklarczyk D, Franceschini A, Kuhn M, Simonovic M, Roth A, Minguez P, et al. (2011) The STRING database in 2011: functional interaction networks of proteins, globally integrated and scored. Nucleic Acids Res 39: D561–568.

34. Frock RL, Kudlow BA, Evans AM, Jameson SA, Hauschka SD, et al. (2006) Lamin A/C and emerin are critical for skeletal muscle satellite cell differentiation. Genes Dev 20: 486–500.

35. Frock RL, Chen SC, Da D-F, Frett E, Lau C, et al. (2012) Cardiomyocyte-Specific Expression of Lamin A Improves Cardiac Function in Lmna2/2 Mice. PLoS ONE 7(8): e42918. doi:10.1371/journal.pone.0042918.

36. Gustavsson M, Verardi R, Mullen DG, Mote KR, Traaseth NJ, et al. (2013) Allosteric regulation of SERCA by phosphorylation-mediated conformational shift of phospholamban. Proc Natl Acad Sci USA 110: 17338–17343.

37. Meng C, Jin X, Xia L, Shen SM, Wang XL, et al. (2009) Alterations of mitochondrial enzymes contribute to cardiac hypertrophy before hypertension development in spontaneously hypertensive rats. J Proteome Res 8: 2463–2475.

38. Jin X, Xia L, Wang LS, Shi JZ, Zheng Y, et al. (2006) Differential protein expression in hypertrophic heart with and without hypertension in spontaneously hypertensive rats. Proteomics 6: 1948–1956.

39. Zamorano-Leon JJ, Modrego J, Mateos-Caceres PJ, Macaya C, Martin-Fernandez B, et al. (2010) A proteomic approach to determine changes in proteins involved in the myocardial metabolism in left ventricles of spontaneously hypertensive rats. Cell Physiol Biochem 25: 347–358.

40. Grussenmeyer T, Meili-Butz S, Roth V, Dieterle T, Brink M, et al. (2011) Proteome analysis in cardiovascular pathophysiology using Dahl rat model. J Proteomics 74: 672–682.

41. Bugger H, Schwarzer M, Chen D, Schrepper A, Amorim PA, et al. (2010) Proteomic remodelling of mitochondrial oxidative pathways in pressure overload-induced heart failure. Cardiovasc Res 85: 376–384.

42. Aggeli IK, Beis I, Gaitanaki C (2008) Oxidative stress and calpain inhibition induce alpha B-crystallin phosphorylation via p38-MAPK and calcium signalling pathways in H9c2 cells. Cell Signal 20: 1292–1302.

43. Thingholm TE, Jorgensen TJD, Jensen ON, Larsen MR (2006) Highly selective enrichment of phosphorylated peptides using titanium dioxide. Nat Protocols 1: 1929–1935.

44. Gupta MP (2007) Factors controlling cardiac myosin-isoform shift during hypertrophy and heart failure. J Mol Cell Cardiol 43: 388–403.

45. El-Armouche A, Pohlmann L, Schlossarek S, et al. (2007) Decreased phosphorylation levels of cardiac myosin-binding protein-C in human and experimental heart failure. J Mol Cell Cardiol 43: 223–229.

46. Maclennan DH, Kranias EG (2003) Phospholamban: a crucial regulator of cardiac contractility. Nat Rev Mol Cell Biol 4: 566–577.

47. Garbino A, Wehrens X H (2010) Emerging role of junctophilin-2 as a regulator of calcium handling in the heart. Acta Pharmacol Sin 31: 1019–1021.

48. Landstrom AP, Weisleder N, Batalden K B, et al. (2007) Mutations in JPH2-encoded junctophilin-2 associated with hypertrophic cardiomyopathy in humans. J Mol Cell Cardiol 42: 1026–1035.

49. Minamisawa S, Oshikawa J, Takeshima H, et al. (2004) Junctophilin type 2 is associated with caveolin-3 and is down-regulated in the hypertrophic and dilated cardiomyopathies. Biochem Biophys Res Commun 325: 852–856.

50. Kanehisa M, Goto S, Furumichi M, Tanabe M, Hirakawa M (2010) KEGG for representation and analysis of molecular networks involving diseases and drugs Nucleic Acids Res 38: D355–D360.

51. Kanehisa M, Goto S, Sato Y, Furumichi M, Tanabe M (2012) KEGG for integration and interpretation of large-scale molecular data sets. Nucleic Acids Res 40: D109–D114.

Effects of Preoperative Aspirin on Cardiocerebral and Renal Complications in Non-Emergent Cardiac Surgery Patients: A Sub-Group and Cohort Study

Longhui Cao[1,3], Scott Silvestry[2], Ning Zhao[4], James Diehl[2], Jianzhong Sun[1]*

1 Department of Anesthesiology, Jefferson Medical College, Thomas Jefferson University, Philadelphia, Pennsylvania, United States of America, 2 Division of Cardiothoracic Surgery, Jefferson Medical College, Thomas Jefferson University, Philadelphia, Pennsylvania, United States of America, 3 Anesthesiology Department, Sun Yat-Sen University Cancer Center, Guangzhou, People's Republic of China, 4 Department of Psychiatry, University of Pennsylvania Health System, Philadelphia, Pennsylvania, United States of America

Abstract

Background and Objective: Postoperative cardiocerebral and renal complications are a major threat for patients undergoing cardiac surgery. This study was aimed to examine the effect of preoperative aspirin use on patients undergoing cardiac surgery.

Methods: An observational cohort study was performed on consecutive patients (n = 1879) receiving cardiac surgery at this institution. The patients excluded from the study were those with preoperative anticoagulants, unknown aspirin use, or underwent emergent cardiac surgery. Outcome events included were 30-day mortality, renal failure, readmission and a composite outcome - major adverse cardiocerebral events (MACE) that include permanent or transient stroke, coma, perioperative myocardial infarction (MI), heart block and cardiac arrest.

Results: Of all patients, 1145 patients met the inclusion criteria and were divided into two groups: those taking (n = 858) or not taking (n = 287) aspirin within 5 days preceding surgery. Patients with aspirin presented significantly more with history of hypertension, diabetes, peripheral arterial disease, previous MI, angina and older age. With propensity scores adjusted and multivariate logistic regression, however, this study showed that preoperative aspirin therapy (vs. no aspirin) significantly reduced the risk of MACE (8.4% vs. 12.5%, odds ratio [OR] 0.585, 95% CI 0.355–0.964, P = 0.035), postoperative renal failure (2.6% vs. 5.2%, OR 0.438, CI 0.203–0.945, P = 0.035) and dialysis required (0.8% vs. 3.1%, OR 0.230, CI 0.071–0.742, P = 0.014), but did not significantly reduce 30-day mortality (4.1% vs. 5.8%, OR 0.744, CI 0.376–1.472, P = 0.396) nor it increased readmissions in the patients undergoing cardiac surgery.

Conclusions: Preoperative aspirin therapy is associated with a significant decrease in the risk of MACE and renal failure and did not increase readmissions in patients undergoing non-emergent cardiac surgery.

Editor: Giuseppe Biondi-Zoccai, University of Modena and Reggio Emilia, Italy

Funding: The authors have no funding or support to report.

Competing Interests: The authors have declared that no competing interests exist.

* E-mail: jian-zhong.sun@jefferson.edu

Introduction

Although tremendous progress has been made in the field of cardiac surgery over the past four decades, major cerebral, cardiac and renal complications associated with cardiac surgery remain common and significant [1]–[3]. According to the Society of Thoracic Surgeons (STS) data reports (2009), the 30-day operative death and major complication rates for valve plus coronary artery bypass graft (CABG) procedure were 6.8% and 30.1%, respectively, including stroke (2.9%), renal failure (9.0%), reoperation (11.9%), prolonged ventilation (21.2%), and sternal infection (0.7%) [3].

Importantly, there is still lacking of an effective clinical therapy to prevent these major cardiocerebral and renal complications. Nonetheless, aspirin as an antiplatelet and antiinflammatory agent has been one of major medicines in prevention and treatment of cardiovascular disease (CVD). Accumulating evidence has demonstrated that aspirin significantly reduces all-cause mortality, MI and stroke in patients with risk of CVD [4]–[7]. Meanwhile, early postoperative aspirin therapy has been applied to improve postoperative outcomes in patients undergoing CABG, including improved graft patency, a reduced risk of death and ischemic complications [8]–[13]. However, it remains to be determined about whether preoperative aspirin therapy can reduce major adverse cardiocerebral (MACE) and renal events in patients undergoing cardiac surgery [14]–[16].

Based on the finding of aspirin's overall beneficial effects in patients with CVD from previous large clinical trials and meta-analysis [4–7], we hypothesized that preoperative use of aspirin, mainly through its antiinflammatory and antithrombotic effects, would provide cardiovascular protection against major cardiocerebral and renal complications in patients undergoing cardiac surgery. Thus, the present study aimed to test the overall effects of preoperative aspirin use on cardiocerebral and renal outcomes in patients undergoing non-emergent cardiac surgery.

Methods

Study Design

This study was an observational cohort study involving consecutive patients (n = 1879) receiving cardiac surgery (84% patients were for CABG or/and valve surgery) at this university hospital from August 2003 to December 2009. The study was in compliance with Declaration of Helsinki and reviewed and approved by Thomas Jefferson University Institutional Review Board, and individual consent was waived in compliance with the HIPAA regulations and the waiver criteria. The patients excluded from the study were those with preoperative anticoagulants, unknown aspirin use, or underwent emergent cardiac surgery, i.e., the patient's clinical status includes any of the following: ischemic dysfunction, mechanical dysfunction (such as acute evolving MI or shock with circulatory support) or emergent salvage (see details at: http://www.sts.org/documents/pdf/trainingmanuals/Tab9-SectionIOPERATIVE.pdf. [accessed at July 9, 2010]). Of all patients, 1145 patients met the inclusion criteria and were divided into two groups: using (n = 858) or not using (n = 287) preoperative (within 5 days preceding surgery) aspirin (Fig. 1).

Data Collection

The patient data were collected and organized to follow the template of the STS national database, including demographics, patient history, medical record information, preoperative risk factors, preoperative medications, intraoperative data, postoperative MACE, renal failure and 30-day all cause mortality. Independent investigators prospectively collected the data on each patient during the course of hospitalization for cardiac surgery. Missing data values for dichotomous variables were assigned the most frequent value, while continuous variables were assigned the median value, except for body surface area, which was assigned the sex-specific median value [17]. Preoperative use of aspirin indicates use of aspirin in the patient within 5 days preceding surgery.

MACE included permanent or transient stroke, coma, perioperative MI, heart block and cardiac arrest. Based on the STS national criteria, permanent stroke is defined as a new-onset cerebrovascular accident persisting >24 h; transient stroke as a

transient episode of neurological dysfunction caused by focal brain, spinal cord, or retinal ischemia, without acute infarction; coma, the patient had a new postoperative coma that persists for at least 24 hrs secondary to anoxic/ischemic and or/metabolic encephalopathy, thromboembolic event or cerebral bleed; perioperative MI as patient as documented by the following criteria (<24 hours post-op): The CK-MB (or CK if MB not available) must be greater than or equal to 5 times the upper limit of normal, with or without new Q waves present in two or more contiguous ECG leads, no symptoms required; or as documented by at least one of the following criteria (>24 hours post-op): 1) Evolutionary ST- segment elevations, 2) Development of new Q- waves in two or more contiguous ECG leads, 3) New or presumably new LBBB pattern on the ECG, 4) The CK-MB (or CK if MB not available) must be greater than or equal to 3 times the upper limit of normal; heart block as a new heart block requiring the implantation of a permanent pacemaker of any type prior to discharge; postoperative renal failure as acute or worsening renal failure resulting in one or more of the followings: increase in serum creatinine >2.0 mg/dL and 2× most recent preoperative creatinine level over baseline or new requirement for dialysis postoperatively; and readmission as the patient was readmitted as an in-patient within 30-days from the date of initial surgery for any reason. This includes readmissions to acute care, primary care institutions only, not to rehabilitation hospital or nursing home. The remaining definitions are available at http://www.sts.org/documents/pdf/trainingmanuals/adult2.61/V-c-AdultCVDataSpecifications2.61.pdf (accessed at July 27, 2010).

Statistical Analysis

Continuous and categorical variables were reported as mean ± SD or percentages, and compared with a 2-sample t tests or a chi-square test (two tailed), respectively. Univariate and multivariate logistic regression were performed to assess associations of demographic, therapeutic and clinical outcome variables.

As described previously [18], because this was an observational study, a propensity score-adjusted analysis was performed to control for selection bias as result of nonrandom assignment to the two groups. A propensity score was derived, reflecting the probability that a patient would receive preoperative aspirin. This was accomplished by performing a multivariable logistic regression analysis using preoperative aspirin as the dependent variable and entering all baseline (preoperative) variables as in table 1 that clinically would likely affect the probability of using preoperative aspirin.

In this study, the propensity score was used in regression (covariance) adjustment [19], i.e., using large set of preoperative variables as above to estimate the propensity score, and then the propensity score was subsequently regressed as an independent covariate in the multivariate logistic regression analysis, which was performed by using all relevant variables to identify independent predictors or risk factors for postoperative MACE, renal failure, and mortality.

Potential preoperative confounding factors considered in this analysis were selected on the basis of a literature review, clinical plausibility and variables collected in the database. These variables included (1) demographic characteristics such as age, gender, and body mass index (BMI); (2) patient history such as diabetes, hypertension, peripheral vascular disease, cerebrovascular disease, chronic lung disease, family History of coronary artery disease (CAD); (3) preoperative risk factors such as angina, congestive heart failure, previous MI, multiple CAD, left main CAD, and preoperative medications such as β-blockers, digitalis, diuretics and rennin-angiotensin system inhibitors (RAS inhibitors includ-

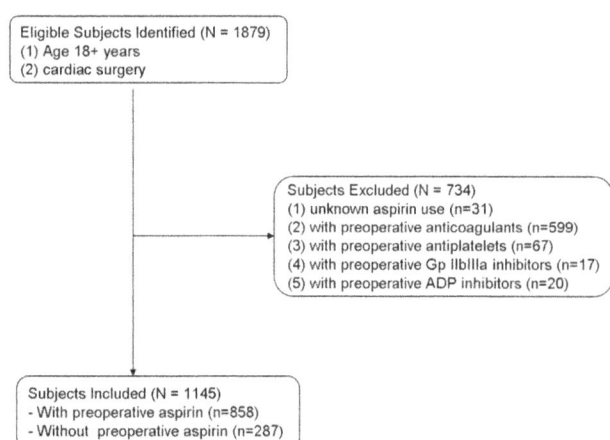

Eligible Subjects Identified (N = 1879)
(1) Age 18+ years
(2) cardiac surgery

Subjects Excluded (N = 734)
(1) unknown aspirin use (n=31)
(2) with preoperative anticoagulants (n=599)
(3) with preoperative antiplatelets (n=67)
(4) with preoperative Gp IIbIIIa inhibitors (n=17)
(5) with preoperative ADP inhibitors (n=20)

Subjects Included (N = 1145)
- With preoperative aspirin (n=858)
- Without preoperative aspirin (n=287)

Figure 1. Selection of study sample.

Table 1. Demographic and clinical characteristics.

Characteristics	Aspirin		P value
	Yes	No	
	n = 858	n = 287	
Age, yrs	65.3±12.0	59.1±15.3	<0.001
Male gender, %	602(70.2)	167(58.2)	<0.001
Body mass index, kg/m2	29.6±9.3	29.8±15.0	0.774
Past medical history			
Diabetes	300(35.0)	68(23.7)	<0.001
Hypertension	724(84.4)	198(69.0)	<0.001
Smoker	163(19.0)	63(22.0)	0.276
Cerebrovascular disease	116(13.5)	30(10.5)	0.178
Peripheral vascular disease	94(11.0)	12(4.2)	0.001
Chronic lung disease	256(29.8)	78(27.2)	0.391
Family History CAD	500(58.3)	123(42.9)	<0.001
Clinical pattern			
Angina	248(28.9)	50(17.4)	<0.001
Congestive heart failure	104(12.1)	43(15.0)	0.210
Previous MI	222(25.9)	42(14.6)	<0.001
Multiple CAD	661(77.0)	108(37.6)	<0.001
Left main CAD	167(19.5)	18(6.3)	<0.001
Medical therapy			
Beta-blockers	662(77.2)	140(48.8)	<0.001
Diuretics	253(29.5)	80(27.9)	0.603
Digitalis	35(4.1)	11(3.8)	0.854
ACE or ARB Inhibitors	357(41.6)	83(28.9)	<0.001
Perfusion time (min)	104.3±46.9	120.2±56.2	<0.001
Cross-clamp time (min)	82.6±41.3	95.3±49.5	<0.001

Values are n (%) for categorical variables and mean±SD for continuous variables.

ing angiotensin-converting enzyme [ACE] Inhibitors or angiotensin-II receptor blockers [ARB]) in addition to aspirin and (4) intraoperative factors including perfusion time and cross-clamp time.

Models fit analysis was evaluated with the Hosmer-Lemeshow goodness-of-fit statistic. The C statistic was reported as a measure of predictive power. Results are reported as percentages and odds ratios (OR) and with 95% confidence intervals (CI). All reported p values were 2-sided, and p values<0.05 were considered to be statistically significant. Statistical analysis was performed with SPSS 17.0 software for Windows (SPSS Inc., Chicago, IL).

Results

Baseline and intraoperative parameters

Of 1879 patients in the database, 1145 patients met the inclusion criteria and were divided into two groups: using (n = 858) or not using (n = 287) preoperative (within 5 days preceding surgery) aspirin (Fig. 1). Demographic and clinical data of the patients who did and did not receive preoperative aspirin therapy are presented in Table 1. No significant differences were evident between two groups in body mass index (BMI), medical history (smoking, cerebrovascular disease, chronic lung disease), clinical pattern (congestive heart failure, cardiogenic shock), and preop-

erative medical therapy (digitalis, diuretics use). However, the patients with aspirin presented more with history of hypertension (84.4% vs. 69.0%, P<0.001), diabetes (35.0% vs. 23.7%, P<0.001), peripheral vascular disease (11.0% vs. 4.2%, P<0.001), previous MI (25.9% vs. 14.6%, P<0.001), angina (28.9% vs. 17.4%, P<0.001) and family history of coronary artery disease (CAD) (58.3% vs. 43.9%, P<0.001). And the patients with aspirin also presented more with preoperative using beta-blockers and rennin-angiotensin system (RAS) inhibitors. Meanwhile, the procedural characteristics, including perfusion time (120.2±56.2 vs. 104.3±46.9, P<0.001) and aortic cross-clamp time (95.3±49.5 vs. 82.6±41.3, P<0.001), were significantly longer in the patients without aspirin.

Postoperative cardiocerebral and renal complications and mortality

Among 1145 patients undergoing cardiac surgery, a total of 9.5% of all patients experienced at least one of cardiocerebral complications, including permanent or transient stroke, coma, perioperative MI, heart block and cardiac arrest. The incidence of MACE in patients who received preoperative aspirin was 8.4% compared with 12.5% for patients who did not receive aspirin (P = 0.035), indicating preoperative use of aspirin significantly decreased the risk of a composite outcome - cardiocerebral complications (by 33.3%) in patients undergoing cardiac surgery (Fig. 2).

Among other complications, compared with no aspirin preoperatively, preoperative use of aspirin also significantly reduced the risk of postoperative renal failure (2.6% vs. 5.2%, P = 0.035) and dialysis required (0.8% vs. 3.1%, P = 0.014). Importantly there was no difference in incidence of readmission (Fig. 2), which was most due to such as pericardial effusion and/or tamponade, deep stern infection, pneumonia or respiratory complication, arrhythmia and etc, indicating that an obvious increase in postoperative bleeding that needs to be admitted did not occur in patients taking preoperative aspirin.

Overall, the 30-day all cause mortality rate was 50 of 1145 (4.4%). The 30-day mortality was 4.1% for patients with preoperative aspirin and 5.8% for patients without one (P = 0.396). The 30-day mortality rate was 9.3% (10/107) for patients with postoperative cardiocerebral events compared with 4.0% (40/988) for patients without postoperative cardiocerebral events (P = 0.013), indicating postoperative cardiocerebral complications significantly contributing to the death associated with cardiac surgery.

Independent risk factors for MACE

The unadjusted univariate analysis showed that risk factors related with MACE were age, male sex, diabetes, hypertension, angina, congestive heart failure, multiple CAD, preoperative aspirin, diuretics and digitalis therapy, perfusion time and cross-clamp time (Table 2).

Figure 2 (3 columns on the right) presents the multivariate analysis to assess independent risk factors for postoperative complications, including cardiocerebral (MACE) and renal complications and 30-day all-cause mortality. After adjusting for propensity score and covariates, preoperative aspirin did not show a significant effect on readmission (12.6% vs. 14.3%) and 30-days all cause mortality (4.1% vs. 5.8%), also individual adverse cardiocerebral events including periopeative MI (1.5% vs. 1.7%), coma (1.6% vs. 1.4%), heart block (3.4% vs. 5.6%) and cardiac arrest (1.2% vs. 2.4%).

Using multivariable logistic regression adjusted with propensity scores, however, patients who took preoperative aspirin compared

No. of patients	Outcome No.(% of incidence)		univariate OR	P value	Adjusted OR	95% CI	P value	Adjusted Odd Ratio (95% CI)
	Pre-operative aspirin							
	Yes	No						
	858	287						
Cardiocerebral complication	72(8.4)	36(12.5)	0.635	0.037	0.585	0.355-0.964	0.035	
Perioperative MI	13(1.5)	5(1.7)	0.868	0.789	0.364	0.114-1.163	0.088	
Permanent stroke	19(2.2)	11(3.8)	0.568	0.137	0.406	0.170-0.969	0.042	
TIA	3(0.3)	0		0.316				
Coma	14(1.6)	4(1.4)	1.174	0.779	1.068	0.309-3.693	0.918	
Heart block	29(3.4)	16(5.6)	0.593	0.098	0.751	0.368-1.532	0.431	
Cardiac arrest	10(1.2)	7(2.4)	0.472	0.123	0.502	0.194-1.867	0.379	
Renal failure	22(2.6)	18(5.2)	0.477	0.027	0.458	0.223-0.945	0.035	
Dialysis required	7(0.8)	9(3.1)	0.254	0.004	0.230	0.071-0.742	0.014	
30-day mortality	34(4.1)	16(5.8)	0.686	0.224	0.744	0.376-1.472	0.396	
Readmission	108(12.6)	41(14.3)	0.864	0.459	0.896	0.572-1.404	0.633	

Forest plot axis: 0.5 · 1 · 1.5 · 2 · 2.5 — Preoperative aspirin better / Preoperative aspirin worse

Values are n (%) for categorical variables and mean±SD for continuous variables. OR, odd ratio; CI, confidence interval; MI, myocardial infarction; TIA, transient ischemic attack.

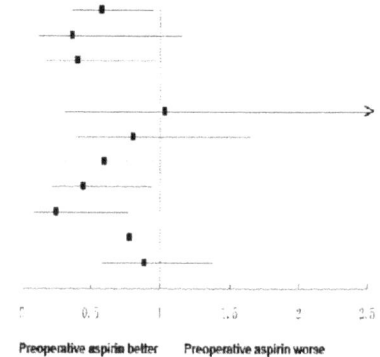

Figure 2. Effects of aspirin on postoperative complications and mortality in patients undergoing cardiac surgery. Values are n (%) for categorical variables and mean±SD for continuous variables. OR, odd ratio; CI, confidence interval; MACE, major adverse cardiocerebral events; MI, myocardial infarction; TIA, transient ischemic attack.

with without one were associated with a significant decrease in the risk of postoperative MACE, permanent stroke, renal failure and dialysis required (Fig. 2).

The multivariate model significantly predicted the occurrence of postoperative cardiocerebral complications (model χ^2, 90.48; $P<0.001$). The discriminatory ability of the logistic model was acceptable (C statistic, 0.749; 95% CI, 0.697 to 0.801; $P<0.001$). The model was well calibrated among deciles of observed and expected risk (Hosmer-Lemeshow χ^2, 8.60; $P=0.38$).

Discussion

The major findings from this observational cohort study are that preoperative use of aspirin is associated with a significant decrease in the risk of postoperative MACE (8.4% vs. 12.5%), renal failure (2.6% vs. 5.2%) and dialysis required (0.8% vs. 3.1%), meanwhile it is not associated with increased risk of readmissions in patients undergoing non-emergent cardiac surgery. However, preoperative use of aspirin did not show a significant effect on postoperative mortality in this sub-group study.

Cardiocerebral events are still common postoperative complications for patients undergoing cardiac surgery, including stroke (1.4%–4.6%), cardiac arrest (5.0%), MI (3.1%–9.1%) [1]–[3], [20–22]. Although there has been lacking of the effective therapy to prevent these complications, several lines of evidence have demonstrated the effectiveness of aspirin, as an antiplatelet and antiinflammatory medicine, in the prevention and treatment of CVD. First, the Antiplatelet Trialists' Collaboration, a meta-analysis, has shown that among the high risk patients for CVD, aspirin significantly reduced rates of MI, stroke and death [5]. Second, in the setting acute MI and stroke, aspirin therapy reduced cardiovascular morbidity and mortality, including recurrent ischemic stroke [23] and myocardial reinfarction [24]. Third, the antiplatelet therapy with aspirin and clopidogrel (plavix) has been recommended to be started before and continuously in percutaneous coronary intervention [25].

In the setting of cardiac surgery, in 2002, Mangano et al [8] in a prospective multicenter study (n = 5065) showed that among patients who received aspirin within 48 hours after revascularization (CABG), subsequent mortality was 1.3%, as compared with 4.0% among those who did not receive aspirin during this period (OR 0.41, 95% CI 0.27–0.62, P<0.001). In addition, aspirin therapy was associated with a 48% reduction in the incidence of MI (2.8% vs. 5.4%, P<0.001), a 50% reduction in the incidence of stroke (1.3% vs. 2.6%, P = 0.01), a 74% reduction in the incidence of renal failure (0.9% vs. 3.4%, P<0.001), and a 62% reduction in the incidence of bowel infarction (0.3% vs. 0.8%, P = 0.01). The risk of hemorrhage, gastritis, infection, or impaired wound healing was not increased with aspirin use (OR for these adverse events, 0.63; 95% CI 0.54 to 0.74).

Although the strong evidence supporting aspirin treatment in the non-surgical setting and even in the surgical setting, such as immediate postoperative use of aspirin in patients undergoing CABG as described above [8], preoperative use of aspirin is still controversial. A major concern of preoperative use of aspirin is its increasing risk of bleeding and transfusion [10], [15]. As a matter of fact, AHA/ACC [26] the Society of Thoracic Surgeons (STS) [27] and the European Association for Cardio-Thoracic Surgery [28] recommended that patients should stop aspirin several days (ranged from 2–10 days) before elective cardiac surgery, mainly due to concerns of perioperative bleeding.

With these controversies, in 2005, Bybee et al [29] performed a retrospective study on preoperative aspirin therapy and postoperative outcomes in patients (n = 1636) undergoing first-time isolated CABG at a single institution. Major findings of this study are 1) preoperative aspirin significantly lowered postoperative in-hospital mortality compared with those not receiving preoperative aspirin (1.7% vs. 4.4%, adjusted OR 0.34, 95% CI 0.15–0.75, P = 0.007). 2) Rates of postoperative cerebrovascular events including cerebral vascular accident or transient ischemic attack were similar between groups (2.7% vs. 3.8%, adjusted OR 0.67, 95% CI

Table 2. Univariate Logistic Regression Analysis for Risk Factor Associated with Postoperative Cardiocerebral Events.

Characteristics	Cardiocerebral Events		P value
	Yes	No	
	n = 108	n = 1037	
Age, yrs	61.4±14.1	64.0±13.0	0.043
Male gender, %	84(72.5)	685(66.1)	0.014
Body mass index, kg/m2	29.0±7.6	29.7±11.3	0.510
Past medical history			
Diabetes	46(42.6)	322(31.1)	0.015
Hypertension	96(88.9)	826(79.7)	0.021
Smoker	27(25.0)	199(19.2)	0.149
Cerebrovascular disease	12(11.1)	134(12.9)	0.591
Peripheral vascular disease	11(10.2)	95(9.2)	0.727
Chronic lung disease	27(25.0)	307(29.6)	0.316
Family History CAD	50(46.3)	573(55.3)	0.075
Clinical pattern			
Angina	38(35.2)	260(25.1)	0.023
Congestive heart failure	43(39.8)	104(10.0)	<0.001
Previous MI	31(28.7)	233(22.5)	0.143
Multiple CAD	61(56.5)	708(68.3)	0.013
Left main CAD	22(20.4)	163(15.7)	0.211
Medical therapy			
Beta-blockers	82(75.9)	720(69.4)	0.161
Diuretics	49(45.4)	284(27.4)	<0.001
Digitalis	9(8.3)	37(3.6)	0.016
ACE or ARB Inhibitors	47(43.5)	393(37.9)	0.253
Aspirin	72(66.7)	786(75.8)	0.037
Perfusion time (min)	131.4±71.3	105.8±46.3	<0.001
Cross-clamp time (min)	103.2±61.1	84.0±41.2	<0.001

Values are n (%) for categorical variables and mean±SD for continuous variables.

0.32–1.50, P = 0.31), and 3) Preoperative aspirin therapy was not associated with an increased risk of reoperation for bleeding (3.5% vs. 3.4%, P = 0.96) or requirement for postoperative blood product transfusion (adjusted OR, 1.17, 95% CI, 0.88–1.54, P = 0.28).

Recently, Jacob et al [30] reported in an observational single institution study that among patients undergoing non-emergent isolated CABG, late (within 5 days of the surgery) use of aspirin (vs. discontinued aspirin ≥6 days before surgery) was associated with no significant difference in a composite outcome of in-hospital mortality, MI and stroke (1.8% vs. 1.7%, P = 0.80) and reoperations for bleeding (3.4% vs. 2.4%, P = 0.10) but more intraoperative transfusions (23% vs. 20%, P = 0.03) and postoperative transfusions (30% vs. 26%, P = 0.009). Although the study of Jacob et al showed that preoperative aspirin was associated with a small increase in transfusion requirements (23% vs. 20%), the patients with preoperative aspirin use (vs. nonaspirin) were associated with increased anticoagulant use (49% vs. 30%, P<0.0001), which may cause/contribute to the increase in transfusion requirements.

Compared with these earlier studies, this study showed that preoperative use of aspirin was associated with a decrease of a composite outcome - MACE by 33% in patients undergoing cardiac surgery; it was also associated with reduced the risk of postoperative renal failure and dialysis required. The renal protective effect by aspirin was unexpected when starting this study, though a previous report also showed that preoperative aspirin had beneficial effects on renal function in patients with renal insufficiency undergoing CABG [31]. Potential mechanism(s) for this renoprotection remains to be investigated and probably are more related to anti-inflammatory (than anti-platelet) effects of aspirin in the setting of cardiac surgery.

The present study did show a trend to decrease the death (4.1% vs. 5.8%; OR 0.744, 95% CI 0.376–1.472 P = 0.396). The authors recognized, however, that a sample size larger than the present one would be needed to determine the effect of aspirin on postoperative mortality (to detect a statistical difference), which has been demonstrated in our recent study [32]. Noticeably, the patients with preoperative aspirin were older and sicker, such as more with history of hypertension, diabetes, peripheral vascular disease, previous MI, angina, left main and multiple CAD (as seen in Table 1). Nevertheless, this study provided additional evidence (to a recent study [32]) that aspirin protects the heart, brain and kidneys against those major risk factors in a sub-group (non-emergent) of patients, indicating its efficacy and potential application to these high-risk patients.

Limitations of this study. This is an observational cohort study. Although multivariate regression in combination with the propensity score adjustment was used in this study to reduce overt biases, the potential flaws of a non-randomized study may remain. Second, this is a separate and sub-group study on preoperative aspirin and cardiac surgery, which excluded the patients undergoing emergent cardiac surgery; multicenter, larger (than the present one in the sample size) and cohort studies are needed to investigate this subject step-by-step, as showed in our recent study [32]. Third, cardiac surgery patients share the common risk of postoperative complications involving the brain, heart and kidneys, despite of undergoing different cardiac surgeries. While aspirin, mainly through its antiinflammatory and antithrombotic effects, may break common final pathways responsible for these complications. Thus, although this study provided an overall analysis on effects of preoperative aspirin on outcomes in patients undergoing cardiac surgery (mainly CABG and/or valve surgery), further studies to dissect different types of cardiac surgery (CABG, valve, emergent or elective alone or/and combinations) are needed and probably would provide more detail information about aspirin and cardiac surgery. As indicated before, nonetheless, "the overall result of the clinical study (trial) is usually a better guide to the direction of effect in subgroups than the apparent effect observed from the individual subgroups" [33]. Finally, this study did not provide detailed information about perioperative bleeding, and further studies are still needed to examine this potential side effect carefully (on a case by case base).

In conclusion, the results of this study showed that preoperative use of aspirin is associated with a significant decrease in the risk of MACE and renal complications in patients undergoing non-emergent cardiac surgery; these beneficial effects were not associated with increased risk of readmissions. Further clinical studies including randomized or (large) observational studies are needed to elucidate the role of preoperative aspirin in cardiac surgery.

Acknowledgments

The authors thank Margaret Lusardi, RN, for her contribution to data entry and collection.

Author Contributions

Conceived and designed the experiments: LC SS JD JS. Performed the experiments: LC JS. Analyzed the data: LC NZ JS. Contributed reagents/materials/analysis tools: SS JD JS. Wrote the paper: LC SS JD JS.

References

1. Brown PP, Kugelmass AD, Cohen DJ, Reynolds MR, Culler SD, et al. (2008) The frequency and cost of complications associated with coronary artery bypass grafting surgery: results from the United States Medicare program. Ann Thorac Surg 85: 1980–6.

2. Shroyer AL, Coombs LP, Peterson ED, Eiken MC, DeLong ER, et al. (2003) The Society of Thoracic Surgeons: 30-day operative mortality and morbidity risk models. Ann Thorac Surg 75: 1856–64.

3. Shahian DM, O'Brien SM, Filardo G, Ferraris VA, Haan CK, et al. (2009) The Society of Thoracic Surgeons 2008 cardiac surgery risk models: part 3–valve plus coronary artery bypass grafting surgery. Ann Thorac Surg 88(1 Suppl): S43–S62.

4. Berger JS, Brown DL, Becker RC (2008) Low-dose aspirin in patients with stable cardiovascular disease: a meta-analysis. Am J Med 121: 43–9.

5. (2002) Collaborative meta-analysis of randomised trials of antiplatelet therapy for prevention of death, myocardial infarction, and stroke in high risk patients. BMJ 324: 71–86.

6. Awtry EH, Loscalzo J (2000) Aspirin. Circulation 101: 1206–18.

7. Tran H, Anand SS (2004) Oral antiplatelet therapy in cerebrovascular disease, coronary artery disease, and peripheral arterial disease. JAMA 292: 1867–74.

8. Mangano DT (2002) Aspirin and mortality from coronary bypass surgery. N Engl J Med 347: 1309–17.

9. Chesebro JH, Clements IP, Fuster V, Elveback LR, Smith HC, et al. (1982) A platelet-inhibitor-drug trial in coronary-artery bypass operations: benefit of perioperative dipyridamole and aspirin therapy on early postoperative vein-graft patency. N Engl J Med 307: 73–8.

10. Kim DH, Daskalakis C, Silvestry SC, Sheth MP, Lee AN, et al. (2009) Aspirin and clopidogrel use in the early postoperative period following on-pump and off-pump coronary artery bypass grafting. J Thorac Cardiovasc Surg 138: 1377–84.

11. Goldman S, Copeland J, Moritz T, Henderson W, Zadina K, et al. (1988) Improvement in early saphenous vein graft patency after coronary artery bypass surgery with antiplatelet therapy: results of a Veterans Administration Cooperative Study. Circulation 77: 1324–32.

12. Goldman S, Copeland J, Moritz T, Henderson W, Zadina K, et al. (1989) Saphenous vein graft patency 1 year after coronary artery bypass surgery and effects of antiplatelet therapy. Results of a Veterans Administration Cooperative Study. Circulation 80: 1190–7.

13. Fremes SE, Levinton C, Naylor CD, Chen E, Christakis GT, et al. (1993) Optimal antithrombotic therapy following aortocoronary bypass: a meta-analysis. Eur J Cardiothorac Surg 7: 169–80.

14. Berger JS (2009) Platelet-directed therapies and coronary artery bypass grafting. Am J Cardiol 104(5 Suppl): 44C–8C.

15. Sun JC, Teoh KH, Lamy A, Sheth T, Ellins ML, et al. (2010) Randomized trial of aspirin and clopidogrel versus aspirin alone for the prevention of coronary artery bypass graft occlusion: the Preoperative Aspirin and Postoperative Antiplatelets in Coronary Artery Bypass Grafting study. Am Heart J 160: 1178–84.

16. Kulik A, Chan V, Ruel M (2009) Antiplatelet therapy and coronary artery bypass graft surgery: perioperative safety and efficacy. Expert Opin Drug Saf 8: 169–82.

17. Ferguson TB, Jr., Coombs LP, Peterson ED (2002) Preoperative beta-blocker use and mortality and morbidity following CABG surgery in North America. JAMA 287: 2221–7.

18. Barodka V, Silvestry S, Zhao N, Jiao X, Whellan DJ, et al. (2011) Preoperative renin-angiotensin system inhibitors protect renal function in aging patients undergoing cardiac surgery. J Surg Res 167: e63–e69.

19. D'Agostino RB (2007) Propensity scores in cardiovascular research. Circulation 115: 2340–3.

20. Bucerius J, Gummert JF, Borger MA, Walther T, Doll N, et al. (2003) Stroke after cardiac surgery: a risk factor analysis of 16,184 consecutive adult patients. Ann Thorac Surg 75: 472–8.

21. Chen JC, Kaul P, Levy JH, Haverich A, Menasche P, et al. (2007) Myocardial infarction following coronary artery bypass graft surgery increases healthcare resource utilization. Crit Care Med 35: 1296–301.

22. Tolpin DA, Collard CD, Lee VV, Elayda MA, Pan W (2009) Obesity is associated with increased morbidity after coronary artery bypass graft surgery in patients with renal insufficiency. J Thorac Cardiovasc Surg 2009 138: 873–9.

23. (1997) The International Stroke Trial (IST): a randomised trial of aspirin, subcutaneous heparin, both, or neither among 19435 patients with acute ischaemic stroke. International Stroke Trial Collaborative Group. Lancet 349: 1569–81.

24. (1988) Randomised trial of intravenous streptokinase, oral aspirin, both, or neither among 17,187 cases of suspected acute myocardial infarction: ISIS-2. ISIS-2 (Second International Study of Infarct Survival) Collaborative Group. Lancet 2: 349–60.

25. King SB, Smith SC, Hirshfeld JW, Jacobs AK, Morrison DA, et al. (2008) 2007 Focused Update of the ACC/AHA/SCAI 2005 Guideline Update for Percutaneous Coronary Intervention: a report of the American College of Cardiology/American Heart Association Task Force on Practice Guidelines: 2007 Writing Group to Review New Evidence and Update the ACC/AHA/SCAI 2005 Guideline Update for Percutaneous Coronary Intervention, Writing on Behalf of the 2005 Writing Committee. Circulation 117: 261–95.

26. Eagle KA, Guyton RA, Davidoff R, Edwards FH, Ewy GA, et al. (2004) ACC/AHA 2004 guideline update for coronary artery bypass graft surgery: summary article: a report of the American College of Cardiology/American Heart Association Task Force on Practice Guidelines (Committee to Update the 1999 Guidelines for Coronary Artery Bypass Graft Surgery). Circulation 110: 1168–76.

27. Ferraris VA, Ferraris SP, Moliterno DJ, Camp P, Walenga JM, et al. (2005) The Society of Thoracic Surgeons practice guideline series: aspirin and other antiplatelet agents during operative coronary revascularization (executive summary). Ann Thorac Surg 79: 1454–61.

28. Dunning J, Versteegh M, Fabbri A, Pavie A, Kolh P, et al. (2008) Guideline on antiplatelet and anticoagulation management in cardiac surgery. Eur J Cardiothorac Surg 34: 73–92.

29. Bybee KA, Powell BD, Valeti U, Rosales AG, Kopecky SL, et al. (2005) Preoperative aspirin therapy is associated with improved postoperative outcomes in patients undergoing coronary artery bypass grafting. Circulation 112(9 Suppl): I286–I292.

30. Jacob M, Smedira N, Blackstone E, Williams S, Cho L (2011) Effect of timing of chronic preoperative aspirin discontinuation on morbidity and mortality in coronary artery bypass surgery. Circulation 123: 577–83.

31. Gerrah R, Ehrlich S, Tshori S, Sahar G (2004) Beneficial effect of aspirin on renal function in patients with renal insufficiency postcardiac surgery. J Cardiovasc Surg (Torino) 45: 545–50.

32. Cao LH, Young N, Liu H, Silvestry S, Sun W, et al. (2011) Preoperative aspirin use and outcomes in cardiac surgery patients. Ann Surg [Oct 12, Epub ahead of print]. PMID 21997805.

33. Yusuf S, Wittes J, Probstfield J, Tyroler HA (1991) Analysis and interpretation of treatment effects in subgroups of patients in randomized clinical trials. JAMA 266: 93–8.

Mitochondrial DNA Backgrounds Might Modulate Diabetes Complications Rather than T2DM as a Whole

Alessandro Achilli[1 ꙮ], Anna Olivieri[2 ꙮ], Maria Pala[2], Baharak Hooshiar Kashani[2], Valeria Carossa[2], Ugo A. Perego[2,3], Francesca Gandini[2], Aurelia Santoro[4,5], Vincenza Battaglia[2], Viola Grugni[2], Hovirag Lancioni[1], Cristina Sirolla[6], Anna Rita Bonfigli[7], Antonella Cormio[8], Massimo Boemi[7], Ivano Testa[7], Ornella Semino[2,9], Antonio Ceriello[10], Liana Spazzafumo[6], Maria Nicola Gadaleta[8], Maurizio Marra[7], Roberto Testa[7], Claudio Franceschi[4,5], Antonio Torroni[2*]

1 Dipartimento di Biologia Cellulare e Ambientale, Università di Perugia, Perugia, Italy, 2 Dipartimento di Genetica e Microbiologia, Università di Pavia, Pavia, Italy, 3 Sorenson Molecular Genealogy Foundation, Salt Lake City, Utah, United States of America, 4 Dipartimento di Patologia Sperimentale, Università di Bologna, Bologna, Italy, 5 CIG-Interdepartmental Center for Biophysics and Biocomplexity Studies, Università di Bologna, Bologna, Italy, 6 Department of Gerontology Research, Statistic and Biometry Center, Italian National Research Center on Aging (INRCA), Ancona, Italy, 7 Metabolic and Nutrition Research Center on Diabetes, Italian National Research Center on Aging, INRCA-IRCCS, Ancona, Italy, 8 Dipartimento di Biochimica e Biologia Molecolare "E. Quagliariello", Università di Bari, Bari, Italy, 9 Centro Interdipartimentale "Studi di Genere", Università di Pavia, Pavia, Italy, 10 Institut d'Investigacions Biomèdiques August Pi Sunyer (IDIBAPS) and Centro de Investigacion Biomedica en Red de Diabetes y Enfermedades Metabolicas Asociadis (CIBERDEM), Barcelona, Spain

Abstract

Mitochondrial dysfunction has been implicated in rare and common forms of type 2 diabetes (T2DM). Additionally, rare mitochondrial DNA (mtDNA) mutations have been shown to be causal for T2DM pathogenesis. So far, many studies have investigated the possibility that mtDNA variation might affect the risk of T2DM, however, when found, haplogroup association has been rarely replicated, even in related populations, possibly due to an inadequate level of haplogroup resolution. Effects of mtDNA variation on diabetes complications have also been proposed. However, additional studies evaluating the mitochondrial role on both T2DM and related complications are badly needed. To test the hypothesis of a mitochondrial genome effect on diabetes and its complications, we genotyped the mtDNAs of 466 T2DM patients and 438 controls from a regional population of central Italy (Marche). Based on the most updated mtDNA phylogeny, all 904 samples were classified into 57 different mitochondrial sub-haplogroups, thus reaching an unprecedented level of resolution. We then evaluated whether the susceptibility of developing T2DM or its complications differed among the identified haplogroups, considering also the potential effects of phenotypical and clinical variables. MtDNA backgrounds, even when based on a refined haplogroup classification, do not appear to play a role in developing T2DM despite a possible protective effect for the common European haplogroup H1, which harbors the G3010A transition in the MTRNR2 gene. In contrast, our data indicate that different mitochondrial haplogroups are significantly associated with an increased risk of specific diabetes complications: H (the most frequent European haplogroup) with retinopathy, H3 with neuropathy, U3 with nephropathy, and V with renal failure.

Editor: Doron M. Behar, Rambam Health Care Campus, Israel

Funding: This research received support from Fondazione Alma Mater Ticinensis (to AT and OS), Roberto and Cornelia Pallotti Legacy for Cancer Research (to CF), and the Italian Ministry of the University: Progetti Ricerca Interesse Nazionale 2007 (to AT), FIRB 2001 Protocol RBNE018AAP (to CF and AT), FIRB-Futuro in Ricerca 2008 (to AA and AO). The funders had no role in study design, data collection and analysis, decision to publish, or preparation of the manuscript.

Competing Interests: The authors have declared that no competing interests exist.

* E-mail: antonio.torroni@unipv.it

ꙮ These authors contributed equally to this work.

Introduction

The etiology of type 2, or non-insulin-dependent, diabetes mellitus (T2DM), the most common metabolic disease in the Western hemisphere, is the result of an interaction of environmental factors with a combination of genetic variants, most of which are still unknown. Case-control studies can be used to predict and quantify the association of genetic factors and lifestyle with some common diseases, thus contributing to the body of knowledge of primary prevention for these conditions. Different genome-wide association studies have led to recent discoveries of novel diabetes-related nuclear loci [1–3], which often fail to be replicated and confirmed in different populations, possibly because of population-specific susceptibility patterns [4]. This may reflect differences in the genetic structure of human populations, each with its peculiar evolutionary history, for instance turning minor alleles in a certain population to prevalent ones in another population, and thus deeply affecting the frequencies of allele combinations.

Obviously, the possibility of obtaining false positive/negative results is greatly decreased when patients and controls come from the same population and/or geographic area where the genetic background should be more homogenous. This is particularly true when association studies involve a genetic system such as the maternally transmitted mitochondrial DNA (mtDNA), whose worldwide "natural" sequence variation is geographically and ethnically differentiated. MtDNA haplotypes and haplogroups (groups of mtDNA haplotypes sharing the same mutational motifs by descent from a common female ancestor) are extremely common in one continent or even a single geographic area/population group, but completely absent in all others [5,6].

Mitochondrial involvement in the pathogenesis of major common metabolic disorders, including T2DM, stems from the observation of dysfunctions in the mitochondrial energy production machinery (OXPHOS) of many patients [7–10]. Single mtDNA mutations, including both major rearrangements and point mutations, and/or mitochondrial haplogroups have been associated with conditions of type 2 diabetes. For instance a protective role has been attributed to the Asian haplogroup N9a [11,12] and to the Western Eurasian haplogroup J1 [13], while the super-haplogroup J/T and the T haplogroup alone have been associated with an increased risk of diabetes in Europeans [14]. Yet, most studies either failed to report definitive associations between T2DM and variation in the mitochondrial genome, or even conflicting results have been observed [15–17]. Thus, all associations reported so far between mtDNA mutations (or haplogroups) and diabetes, with the exception of the rare mutations associated with Maternally Inherited Diabetes and Deafness (MIDD, [MIM #520000]), remain provisional (see Mitomap for a review http://www.mitomap.org/MITOMAP). This is not a feature restricted to T2DM. Indeed, with the exception of Leber Hereditary Optic Neuropathy (LHON), the association between disorders and mtDNA haplogroups has rarely been replicated by studies in other populations [18,19]. Association studies can be confounded if patients and controls are poorly characterized or not well matched. However, mtDNA association studies are probably affected also by another major specific problem: the level of resolution employed in the classification of mtDNA haplogroups has been generally very low. Recent studies confirm that mtDNA association analyses performed so far have often been too simplistic. A striking example is represented by haplogroup H, by far the most common haplogroup in Europe with a uniformly high frequency (30%–50%), which is formed by many sub-haplogroups whose frequencies vary considerably across Europe [20,21]. Such a degree of difference in frequency distribution of mtDNA sub-haplogroups alone could easily explain some of the inconsistent results obtained by association studies carried out in different European populations.

A second general area of investigation concerns the role of mtDNA variants or haplogroups in modulating susceptibility to develop diabetes complications, usually classified into macrovascular (cardiovascular disease, cerebrovascular accidents, and peripheral vascular disease) and microvascular complications (diabetic nephropathy, neuropathy, and retinopathy) [22,23], but the number of mtDNA studies that, in addition to the "whole" T2DM phenotype, have also evaluated diabetes complications is still limited [24–26].

In this study, to evaluate the role of mtDNA backgrounds, not only in T2DM as a whole but also in its associated complications, we have genotyped, at an extremely high level of phylogenetic resolution, the mitochondrial genome of a large number of subjects (466 T2DM patients and 438 controls) from the Marche region of central Italy.

Results

Before determining the extent and nature of mtDNA variation in control and diabetic subjects from the Marche region, we investigated the effects of a large number of phenotypical and clinical variables on the risk of T2DM. Some of the traits evaluated in the 904 subjects are shown in Table 1. No difference in the risk of T2DM was found only for fibrinogen and C-reactive protein. As expected, among the strongest predictors of diabetes were age, BMI (and consequently obesity), metabolic syndrome, insulin resistance evaluated by homeostasis model assessment (HOMA), glycated hemoglobin (HbA1c), high-density lipoprotein (HDL) cholesterol, triglycerides, and hypertension. All these parameters, except HDL cholesterol, were much higher in patients than in controls. However, there was also one unexpected finding, also in light of the randomly selected gender of participants: a significantly increased risk for males and smokers was noted (p-values of <0.0001 and 0.001, respectively). Assuming that BMI might be considered as a general indicator of health, we found that the BMI is just slightly lower among smokers (27.3 ± 4.2 vs 28.2 ± 4.7).

T2DM and mtDNA haplogroups

All 904 mtDNAs were genotyped and assigned to 57 different mtDNA haplogroups and sub-haplogroups (Table S1). This classification was based on the most updated phylogeny [27], thus reaching an unprecedented level of resolution. As summarized in Table 2, more than 97% of the mtDNAs belonged to typical Western Eurasian lineages, i.e. H*, H1, H3, H5, H6, H8, H9, HV*, HV0, V, R0a, J1, J2, T1, T2, U1, U2, U3, U4, U5, U6, U7, U8, U9, K1, K2, N1, I, W, X2. The only notable exceptions were represented by 24 mtDNAs: 8 attributed to the Eastern Asian clade D4 and 16 classified into three typical African haplogroups (M1, L1b and L3).

When we compared haplogroup distributions of T2DM cases and controls (Table 2), multiple logistic-regression analysis showed that subjects harboring haplogroup H1 (9.4% and 15.8% in patients and controls, respectively) might be characterized by a reduced risk of T2DM (OR = 0.5576, 95% CI: 0.3726–0.8344, p-value = 0.0045), and that H1 was indeed the only haplogroup included in the final step-wise model (p-value = 0.004). However, such a p-value does not reach the statistical significance established at $\alpha\leq0.003$, after the Bonferroni correction. We then examined whether the possible protective effect of haplogroup H1 towards T2DM was related to age, gender, obesity, smoking, and/or to some clinical traits such as BMI, metabolic syndrome, insulin resistance, fibrinogen, C-reactive protein, HbA1c, HDL, triglycerides and hypertension. None of the parameters showed significant differences between the subjects with haplogroup H1 and those without it (data not shown).

Table 2 illustrates a second interesting finding. Haplogroup R0a, which was not included in the logistic-regression analysis because of its low frequency (0.7%), was detected only in diabetic patients (six out of six R0a mtDNAs), thus raising the possibility of a potential effect by this rare haplogroup. The presence of three different R0a control-region haplotypes among the six subjects (Table S1) excludes the possibility of a founder event. Two possible scenarios can be envisioned to explain the detection of this haplogroup only in diabetic patients: (i) R0a might actually increase the risk of T2DM, consequently decreasing its detection rate in healthy subjects older than 40 years; (ii) the mtDNA background which may be modulating the appearance of diabetes is not the entire haplogroup R0a, but only one of its internal branches. To discriminate between the two alternative scenarios, we completely sequenced and included all six R0a mtDNAs in an updated R0a phylogeny (Figure 1). Data from the complete sequencing show that all six genomes from Marchigian diabetic patients belong to the same sub-clade named R0a2. This clade differs from the root of haplogroup R0a by three mutations. A T insertion in the control region at nucleotide position (np) 60 and

Table 1. Clinical characteristics of diabetic patients and controls.

Variables	All samples[a]			Males[a]			Females[a]			N analyzed (Males;Females)
	Patients (N = 466)	Controls (N = 438)	p-value	Patients (N = 257)	Controls (N = 176)	p-value	Patients (N = 209)	Controls (N = 262)	p-value	
Traits:										
Age [years]	65.84±8.19	59.96±9.97	<0.0001	65.09±8.55	59.34±9.40	<0.0001	66.76±7.64	60.38±10.32	<0.0001	904 (433;471)
Sex [M/F (%)]	257/209 (55.15%/44.85%)	176/262 (40.18%/59.82%)	<0.0001							
BMI [Kg/m2]	28.76±4.62	27.14±4.46	<0.0001	28.24±4.15	27.29±3.51	0.0107	29.40±5.07	27.04±5.00	<0.0001	902 (432;470)
Obesity[b] (%)	152 (32.69%)	96 (21.97%)	0.0003	71 (27.73%)	35 (19.89%)	0.0696	81 (38.76%)	61 (23.37%)	0.0004	902 (432;470)
Smokers (%)	124 (28.64%)	76 (16.14%)	0.0010	92 (35.80%)	32 (18.18%)	<0.0001	36 (17.22%)	40 (15.27%)	0.6147	904 (433;471)
Metabolic Syndrome[c] (%)	267 (57.42%)	56 (12.90%)	<0.0001	114 (44.53%)	16 (9.25%)	<0.0001	153 (73.21%)	40 (15.33%)	<0.0001	899 (429;470)
Insulin Resistance[d] (%)	190 (40.77%)	54 (12.47%)	<0.0001	97 (37.74%)	26 (15.12%)	<0.0001	93 (44.50%)	28 (10.73%)	<0.0001	899 (429;470)
Fibrinogen [mg/dL]	303.50±79.49	295.29±71.76	0.1590	294.04±77.85	281.95±78.17	0.2012	315.36±80.11	302.89±66.90	0.1064	706 (342;364)
C-reactive protein [mg/L]	4.55±7.01	3.43±7.37	0.0200	4.20±6.74	3.62±10.45	0.5179	4.97±7.31	3.30±4.17	0.0035	901 (431;470)
HbA1c [%]	7.43±1.25	5.67±0.40	<0.0001	7.37±1.28	5.59±0.36	<0.0001	7.51±1.20	5.72±0.42	<0.0001	904 (433;471)
HDL [mg/dL]	52.75±14.85	58.32±15.17	<0.0001	49.44±12.10	51.77±13.50	0.0682	56.82±16.80	62.64±14.68	<0.0001	901 (430;471)
Triglycerides	138.38±93.16	103.28±68.45	<0.0001	136.12±101.92	119.09±88.70	0.0674	141.16±81.26	92.85±48.34	<0.0001	899 (429;470)
Hypertension (%)	293 (62.88%)	137 (31.35%)	<0.0001	155 (60.31%)	40 (22.86%)	<0.0001	138 (66.03%)	97 (37.02%)	<0.0001	903 (432;471)
Complications:										
Retinopathy (%)	132 (28.33%)	...	...	69 (26.85%)	...	...	63 (30.14%)	...	...	904 (433;471)
Somatic Neuropathy (%)	94 (20.17%)	...	...	64 (24.90%)	...	...	30 (14.35%)	...	...	904 (433;471)
Cardiac Ischemia (%)	81 (8.96%)	...	...	50 (19.46%)	...	...	31 (14.83%)	...	...	904 (433;471)
Nephropathy (%)	64 (13.73%)	...	...	45 (17.51%)	...	–	19 (9.09%)	...	...	904 (433;471)
Peripheral Artery Occlusive Disease (PAOD)(%)	30 (3.2%)	...	...	17 (6.61%)	...	...	13 (6.22%)	...	...	904 (433;471)
Renal Failure (%)	20 (2.21%)	...	...	15 (5.84%)	...	...	5 (2.39%)	...	...	904 (433;471)
Index:										
HOMA-IR	2.99±3.52	1.59±1.55	<0.0001	3.14±4.22	1.74±1.78	<0.0001	2.81±2.39	1.49±1.36	<0.0001	904 (433;471)

[a]Values are means ± standard deviation (or absolute number and percentages).
[b]BMI ≥30.
[c]Diagnosed according to the criteria proposed by the National Cholesterol Education Program (NCEP) Adult Treatment Panel III (ATP III).
[d]HOMA-IR >2.5.

Table 2. Frequencies of the major mitochondrial DNA haplogroups and sub-haplogroups in diabetic patients and controls.

Haplogroup[a]		All samples		Males		Females		Total (%)
		Patients (%)	Controls (%)	Patients (%)	Controls (%)	Patients (%)	Controls (%)	
		N = 466	N = 438	N = 257	N = 176	N = 209	N = 262	N = 904
H:		161 (34.55%)	181 (41.34%)	90 (35.01%)	66 (37.50%)	71 (33.96%)	115 (43.89%)	342 (37.83%)
	H*	77 (16.52%)	72 (16.44%)	43 (16.73%)	29 (16.48%)	34 (16.27%)	43 (16.41%)	149 (16.48%)
	H1	44 (9.44%)	69 (15.75%)	23 (8.95%)	23 (13.07%)	21 (10.05%)	46 (17.56%)	113 (12.50%)
	H3	10 (2.15%)	13 (2.97%)	6 (2.33%)	8 (4.55%)	4 (1.91%)	5 (1.91%)	23 (2.54%)
	H5	16 (3.43%)	17 (3.88%)	11 (4.28%)	3 (1.70%)	5 (2.39%)	14 (5.34%)	33 (3.65%)
	H6	10 (2.15%)	7 (1.60%)	5 (1.95%)	2 (1.14%)	5 (2.39%)	5 (1.91%)	17 (1.88%)
	H8	...	2 (0.46%)	...	1 (0.57%)	...	1 (0.38%)	2 (0.22%)
	H9	4 (0.86%)	1 (0.23%)	2 (0.78%)	...	2 (0.96%)	1 (0.38%)	5 (0.55%)
HV[b]:		37 (7.94%)	29 (6.62%)	25 (9.73%)	13 (7.39%)	12 (5.74%)	16 (6.11%)	66 (7.30%)
	HV*	15 (3.22%)	17 (3.88%)	8 (3.11%)	9 (5.11%)	7 (3.35%)	8 (3.05%)	32 (3.54%)
	HV0	4 (0.86%)	1 (0.23%)	3 (1.17%)	...	1 (0.48%)	1 (0.38%)	5 (0.55%)
	V	18 (3.86%)	11 (2.51%)	14 (5.45%)	4 (2.27%)	4 (1.91%)	7 (2.67%)	29 (3.21%)
R0:		6 (1.29%)	...	3 (1.17%)	...	3 (1.44%)	...	6 (0.66%)
	R0a	6 (1.29%)	...	3 (1.17%)	...	3 (1.44%)	...	6 (0.66%)
J:		33 (7.08%)	37 (8.45%)	21 (8.17%)	19 (10.80%)	12 (5.74%)	18 (6.87%)	70 (7.75%)
	J1	27 (5.79%)	31 (7.08%)	18 (7.00%)	16 (9.09%)	9 (4.31%)	15 (5.73%)	58 (6.42%)
	J2	6 (1.29%)	6 (1.37%)	3 (1.17%)	3 (1.70%)	3 (1.44%)	3 (1.15%)	12 (1.33%)
T:		71 (15.24%)	57 (13.01%)	37 (14.39%)	23 (13.07%)	34 (16.27%)	34 (12.98%)	128 (14.16%)
	T1	12 (2.58%)	11 (2.51%)	7 (2.72%)	3 (1.70%)	5 (2.39%)	8 (3.05%)	23 (2.54%)
	T2	59 (12.66%)	46 (10.50%)	30 (11.67%)	20 (11.36%)	29 (13.88%)	26 (9.92%)	105 (11.62%)
UK:								
	U	80 (17.17%)	65 (14.84%)	48 (18.68%)	25 (14.20%)	32 (15.31%)	40 (15.26%)	145 (16.04%)
	U1	3 (0.64%)	4 (0.91%)	3 (1.17%)	2 (1.14%)	...	2 (0.76%)	7 (0.77%)
	U2	1 (0.21%)	1 (0.23%)	1 (0.39%)	...	...	1 (0.38%)	2 (0.22%)
	U3	13 (2.79%)	11 (2.51%)	10 (3.89%)	4 (2.27%)	3 (1.44%)	7 (2.67%)	24 (2.65%)
	U4	12 (2.58%)	8 (1.83%)	6 (2.33%)	5 (2.84%)	6 (2.87%)	3 (1.15%)	20 (2.21%)
	U5	39 (8.37%)	34 (7.76%)	21 (8.17%)	10 (5.68%)	18 (8.61%)	24 (9.16%)	73 (8.08%)
	U6	2 (0.43%)	1 (0.23%)	...	1 (0.57%)	2 (0.96%)	...	3 (0.33%)
	U7	4 (0.86%)	2 (0.46%)	2 (0.78%)	1 (0.57%)	2 (0.96%)	1 (0.38%)	6 (0.66%)
	U8	5 (1.07%)	4 (0.91%)	4 (1.56%)	2 (1.14%)	1 (0.48%)	2 (0.76%)	9 (1.00%)
	U9	1 (0.21%)	...	1 (0.39%)	...	...	...	1 (0.11%)
	K	31 (6.65%)	24 (5.48%)	12 (4.67%)	15 (8.52%)	19 (9.09%)	9 (3.44%)	55 (6.08%)
	K1	30 (6.44%)	22 (5.02%)	12 (4.67%)	13 (7.39%)	18 (8.61%)	9 (3.44%)	52 (5.75%)
	K2	1 (0.21%)	2 (0.46%)	...	2 (1.14%)	1 (0.48%)	...	3 (0.33%)
N1:		17 (3.65%)	9 (2.05%)	9 (3.50%)	1 (0.57%)	8 (3.83%)	8 (3.05%)	26 (2.88%)
	N1	9 (1.93%)	6 (1.37%)	6 (2.33%)	1 (0.57%)	3 (1.44%)	5 (1.91%)	15 (1.66%)
	I	8 (1.72%)	3 (0.68%)	3 (1.17%)	...	5 (2.39%)	3 (1.15%)	11 (1.22%)
N2:		6 (1.29%)	8 (1.83%)	3 (1.17%)	4 (2.27%)	3 (1.44%)	4 (1.53%)	14 (1.55%)
	W	6 (1.29%)	8 (1.83%)	3 (1.17%)	4 (2.27%)	3 (1.44%)	4 (1.53%)	14 (1.55%)
X:		13 (2.79%)	15 (3.42%)	4 (1.56%)	5 (2.84%)	9 (4.31%)	10 (3.82%)	28 (3.10%)
	X2	13 (2.79%)	15 (3.42%)	4 (1.56%)	5 (2.84%)	9 (4.31%)	10 (3.82%)	28 (3.10%)
M:		10 (2.15%)	8 (1.82%)	5 (1.95%)	3 (1.70%)	5 (2.39%)	5 (1.91%)	18 (1.99%)
	D4	5 (1.07%)	3 (0.68%)	4 (1.56%)	2 (1.14%)	1 (0.48%)	1 (0.38%)	8 (0.88%)
	M1	5 (1.07%)	5 (1.14%)	1 (0.39%)	1 (0.57%)	4 (1.91%)	4 (1.53%)	10 (1.11%)
L:		1 (0.21%)	5 (1.14%)	...	2 (1.14%)	1 (0.48%)	3 (1.15%)	6 (0.66%)
	L1b	...	1 (0.23%)	...	...	...	1 (0.38%)	1 (0.11%)
	L3	1 (0.21%)	4 (0.91%)	...	2 (1.14%)	1 (0.48%)	2 (0.76%)	5 (0.55%)

Table 2. Cont.

[a]H* is a paragroup that encompasses all H mtDNAs that did not belong to any of the tested subclades of H.
[b]Without H.

the non-synonymous transition MTCYB-T15674C/S310P are shared with the sister branch R0a3, whereas the third mutation, the transition A2355G in the 16S rRNA gene, is distinctive of R0a2 (Figure 1).

T2DM complications and mitochondrial haplogroups

Many studies have evaluated mtDNA variation in T2DM patients. However, only a few studies have tested mtDNA haplogroups for association with diabetes complications. In an attempt to investigate a potential role of mtDNA backgrounds in complications rather than in T2DM as a whole, we evaluated this issue in our population sample. Table 3 reports the haplogroup distributions observed in patients with only the diabetic phenotype and no complications and in T2DM patients characterized by the

development of at least one (or at least two) of six common T2DM complications. These complications include the following: retinopathy, somatic neuropathy, nephropathy, renal failure, cardiac ischemia, and peripheral artery occlusive disease (see Tables S2, S3, S4, S5, S6, and S7 for details concerning each complication). Even if T2DM complications were determined by different molecular mechanisms, the concomitant analysis of grouped complications provides some initial clues concerning the role of mitochondrial haplogroups in modulating the pathology course. Then, this is further investigated by analyzing each candidate haplogroup in relation to patients' traits and complications. Evidence of association was observed only for haplogroup H3 that seemed to increase the probability of developing at least one complication by almost 8.5 fold (Table 4). In particular, when we

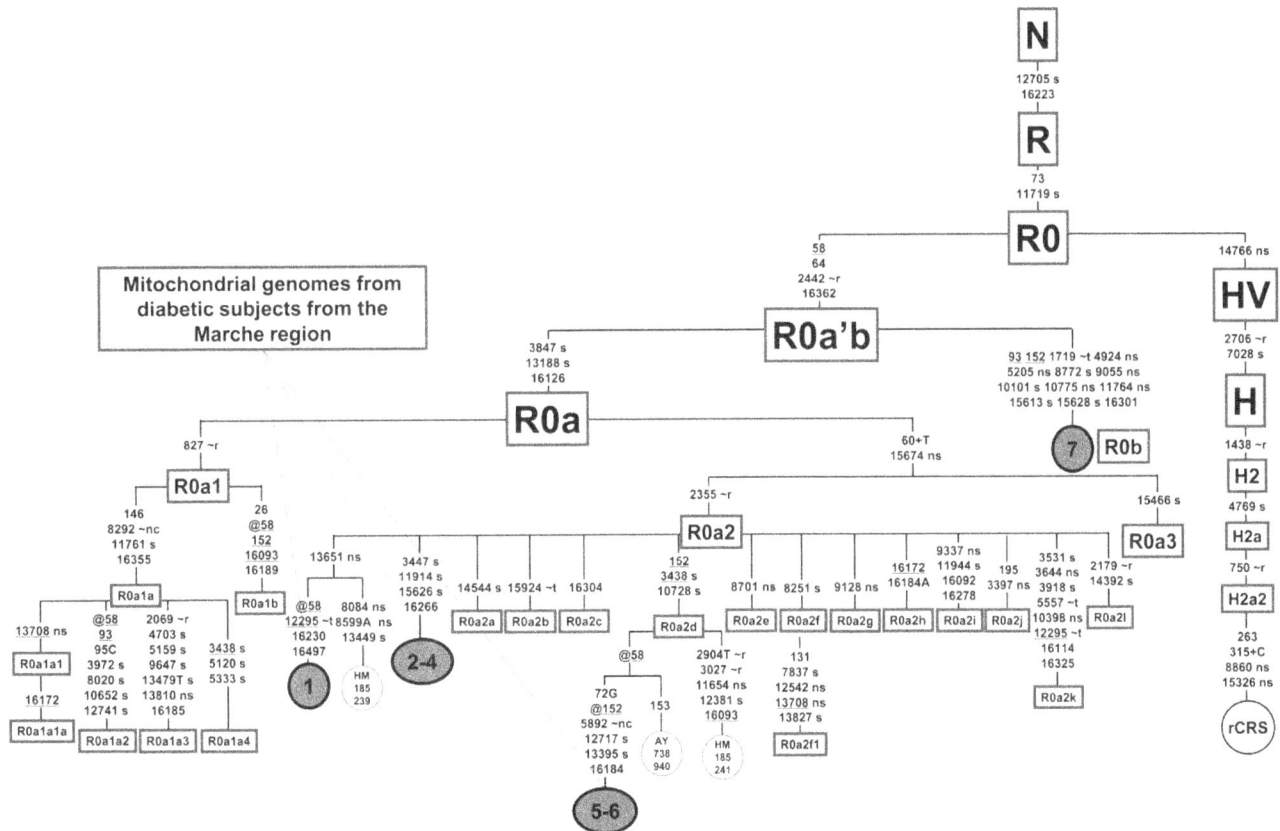

Figure 1. Schematic phylogeny of haplogroup R0a encompassing seven complete mtDNA sequences from diabetic patients. The schematic classification of the R0a sub-clades is based on Černý et al. [42], while the R0a'b node is newly defined on the basis of the complete genome #7. Sequences #1–7 were obtained in the course of this study and are from Italian diabetic patients: sequences #1–6 (GenBank accession numbers JF717355-JF717360) are from subjects of the Marche region sample, while sequence #7 (GenBank accession number JF717361) is from a diabetic patient not included in the current study because the maternal ancestry was from a different region (Campania, Southern Italy). Three control mtDNA sequences from the literature (GenBank accession numbers HM185239, HM185241 [42] and AY738940 [20]), which clustered in the same sub-branches of the sequences obtained from the diabetic subjects, were also included in the tree. The position of the revised Cambridge Reference Sequence (rCRS) [43] – a member of haplogroup H2a2 – is indicated for reading off sequence motifs. Mutations are shown on the branches; they are transitions unless a base is explicitly indicated. The prefix @ designates reversions, while suffixes indicate transversions (to A, G, C, or T), insertions (+), gene locus (~t, tRNA; ~r, rRNA; nc, non coding region outside of the control region) and synonymous or non synonymous changes (s or ns). Recurrent mutations within the phylogeny are underlined.

Table 3. Frequencies of mtDNA haplogroups and sub-haplogroups in patients with only the diabetic phenotype and diabetic patients also affected by at least one or two of six common complications [retinopathy, somatic neuropathy, cardiac ischemia, nephropathy, peripheral artery occlusive disease (PAOD), and/or renal failure].

	All Samples[a]			Males			Females		
	No complications	At least one complication	At least two complications	No complications	At least one complication	At least two complications	No complications	At least one complication	At least two complications
	N = 223	N = 243	N = 109	N = 111	N = 146	N = 69	N = 112	N = 97	N = 40
H:	68 (30.49%)	93 (38.27%)	49 (44.95%)	34 (30.64%)	56 (38.38%)	29 (42.03%)	34 (30.36%)	37 (38.16%)	20 (50.00%)
H*	34 (15.25%)	43 (17.70%)	26 (23.85%)	18 (16.22%)	25 (17.12%)	14 (20.29%)	16 (14.29%)	18 (18.56%)	12 (30.00%)
H1	19 (8.52%)	25 (10.29%)	12 (11.01%)	9 (8.11%)	14 (9.59%)	8 (11.59%)	10 (8.93%)	11 (11.34%)	4 (10.00%)
H3	1 (0.45%)	9 (3.70%)	6 (5.50%)	⋯	6 (4.11%)	3 (4.35%)	1 (0.89%)	3 (3.09%)	3 (7.50%)
H5	8 (3.59%)	8 (3.29%)	3 (2.75%)	6 (5.41%)	5 (3.42%)	3 (4.35%)	2 (1.79%)	3 (3.09%)	⋯
H6	4 (1.79%)	6 (2.47%)	2 (1.83%)	1 (0.90%)	4 (2.74%)	1 (1.45%)	3 (2.68%)	2 (2.06%)	1 (2.50%)
H9	2 (0.90%)	2 (0.82%)	⋯	⋯	2 (1.37%)	⋯	2 (1.79%)	⋯	⋯
HV:	20 (8.97%)	17 (7.00%)	8 (7.34%)	11 (9.91%)	14 (9.59%)	8 (11.59%)	9 (8.04%)	3 (3.09%)	⋯
HV*	10 (4.48%)	5 (2.06%)	⋯	5 (4.50%)	3 (2.05%)	⋯	5 (4.46%)	2 (2.06%)	⋯
HV0	2 (0.90%)	2 (0.82%)	1 (0.92%)	2 (1.80%)	1 (0.68%)	1 (1.45%)	⋯	1 (1.03%)	⋯
V	8 (3.59%)	10 (4.12%)	7 (6.42%)	4 (3.60%)	10 (6.85%)	7 (10.14%)	4 (3.57%)	⋯	⋯
R0:	2 (0.90%)	4 (1.65%)	1 (0.92%)	⋯	3 (2.05%)	1 (1.45%)	2 (1.79%)	1 (1.03%)	⋯
R0a	2 (0.90%)	4 (1.65%)	1 (0.92%)	⋯	3 (2.05%)	1 (1.45%)	2 (1.79%)	1 (1.03%)	⋯
J:	17 (7.62%)	16 (6.58%)	5 (4.59%)	10 (9.01%)	11 (7.53%)	4 (5.80%)	7 (6.25%)	5 (5.15%)	1 (2.50%)
J1	13 (5.83%)	14 (5.76%)	5 (4.59%)	7 (6.31%)	11 (7.53%)	4 (5.80%)	6 (5.36%)	3 (3.09%)	1 (2.50%)
J2	4 (1.79%)	2 (0.82%)	⋯	3 (2.70%)	⋯	⋯	1 (0.89%)	2 (2.06%)	⋯
T:	41 (18.39%)	30 (12.35%)	13 (11.93%)	22 (19.82%)	15 (10.27%)	7 (10.14%)	19 (16.96%)	15 (15.46%)	6 (15.00%)
T1	6 (2.69%)	6 (2.47%)	3 (2.75%)	2 (1.80%)	5 (3.42%)	2 (2.90%)	4 (3.57%)	1 (1.03%)	1 (2.50%)
T2	35 (15.70%)	24 (9.88%)	10 (9.17%)	20 (18.02%)	10 (6.85%)	5 (7.25%)	15 (13.39%)	14 (14.43%)	5 (12.50%)
UK:									
U	36 (16.14%)	44 (18.10%)	19 (17.43%)	18 (16.22%)	30 (20.55%)	12 (17.39%)	18 (16.06%)	14 (14.43%)	7 (17.50%)
U1	1 (0.45%)	2 (0.82%)	1 (0.92%)	1 (0.90%)	2 (1.37%)	1 (1.45%)	⋯	⋯	⋯
U2	⋯	1 (0.41%)	⋯	⋯	1 (0.68%)	⋯	⋯	⋯	⋯
U3	6 (2.69%)	7 (2.88%)	6 (5.50%)	5 (4.50%)	5 (3.42%)	4 (5.80%)	1 (0.89%)	2 (2.06%)	2 (5.00%)
U4	7 (3.14%)	5 (2.06%)	1 (0.92%)	2 (1.80%)	4 (2.74%)	⋯	5 (4.46%)	1 (1.03%)	1 (2.50%)
U5	19 (8.52%)	20 (8.23%)	8 (7.34%)	8 (7.21%)	13 (8.90%)	5 (7.25%)	11 (9.82%)	7 (7.22%)	3 (7.50%)
U6	⋯	2 (0.82%)	⋯	⋯	⋯	⋯	⋯	2 (2.06%)	⋯
U7	2 (0.90%)	2 (0.82%)	⋯	1 (0.90%)	1 (0.68%)	⋯	1 (0.89%)	1 (1.03%)	⋯
U8	1 (0.45%)	4 (1.65%)	2 (1.83%)	1 (0.90%)	3 (2.05%)	1 (1.45%)	⋯	1 (1.03%)	1 (2.50%)
U9	⋯	1 (0.41%)	1 (0.92%)	⋯	1 (0.68%)	1 (1.45%)	⋯	⋯	⋯
K	12 (5.38%)	19 (7.82%)	4 (3.67%)	2 (1.80%)	10 (6.85%)	4 (5.80%)	10 (8.93%)	9 (9.28%)	⋯
K1	12 (5.38%)	18 (7.41%)	4 (3.67%)	2 (1.80%)	10 (6.85%)	4 (5.80%)	10 (8.93%)	8 (8.25%)	⋯
K2		1 (0.41%)	⋯	⋯	⋯	⋯	⋯	1 (1.03%)	⋯
N1:	7 (3.14%)	10 (4.12%)	5 (4.59%)	5 (4.50%)	4 (2.74%)	1 (1.45%)	2 (1.79%)	6 (6.19%)	4 (10.00%)
I	4 (1.79%)	5 (2.06%)	2 (1.83%)	4 (3.60%)	2 (1.37%)	⋯	⋯	3 (3.09%)	2 (5.00%)
N1	3 (1.35%)	5 (2.06%)	3 (2.75%)	1 (0.90%)	2 (1.37%)	1 (1.45%)	2 (1.79%)	3 (3.09%)	2 (5.00%)
N2:	4 (1.79%)	2 (0.82%)	1 (0.92%)	2 (1.80%)	1 (0.68%)	1 (1.45%)	2 (1.79%)	1 (1.03%)	⋯
W	4 (1.79%)	2 (0.82%)	1 (0.92%)	2 (1.80%)	1 (0.68%)	1 (1.45%)	2 (1.79%)	1 (1.03%)	⋯
X:	8 (3.59%)	5 (2.06%)	2 (1.83%)	3 (2.70%)	1 (0.68%)	1 (1.45%)	5 (4.46%)	4 (4.12%)	1 (2.50%)
X2	8 (3.59%)	5 (2.06%)	2 (1.83%)	3 (2.70%)	1 (0.68%)	1 (1.45%)	5 (4.46%)	4 (4.12%)	1 (2.50%)
M:	7 (3.14%)	3 (1.23%)	2 (1.83%)	4 (3.60%)	1 (0.68%)	1 (1.45%)	3 (2.68%)	2 (2.06%)	1 (2.50%)
D4	4 (1.79%)	1 (0.41%)	1 (0.92%)	3 (2.70%)	1 (0.68%)	1 (1.45%)	1 (0.89%)	⋯	⋯
M1	3 (1.35%)	2 (0.82%)	1 (0.92%)	1 (0.90%)	⋯	⋯	2 (1.79%)	2 (2.06%)	1 (2.50%)
L:	1 (0.45%)	⋯	⋯	⋯	⋯	⋯	1 (0.89%)	⋯	⋯

Table 3. Cont.

	All Samples[a]			Males			Females		
No complications	At least one complication	At least two complications	No complications	At least one complication	At least two complications	No complications	At least one complication	At least two complications
N = 223	N = 243	N = 109	N = 111	N = 146	N = 69	N = 112	N = 97	N = 40
L1b	...	...	...	...	...	...	...	...	...
L3	1 (0.45%)	...	...	...	...	...	1 (0.89%)	...	...

[a]Haplogroup frequencies in males and females are reported for congruency with previous tables. However, gender was not considered in statistical analyses dealing with complications.

inverted the analysis, only neuropathy turned out to be related to H3 (*p-value* = 0.0007) (Table 5). The significance of the association with H3 was confirmed in the logistic regression with two or more complications, but also other groupings – the paragroup H* and the haplogroups U3 and V – turned out to be risk factors (Table 4). Considering the combined effect of H* and H3, it is conceivable that the entire haplogroup H (and its basal mutational motif) might play an important role in the development of T2DM-related complications. This scenario is supported by the finding that the incidence of retinopathy (Table S2) was significantly increased (*p-value* = 0.0007) in subjects harboring H mtDNAs (OR = 2.0075, 95% CI: 1.3080-3.0812, *p-value* 0.0014), who also showed a slight decrease in HDL cholesterol (50.73±12.22 mg/dL *vs.* 53.82± 15.98 mg/dL, t-test *p-value* = 0.0202).

Finally, U3 and V subjects showed an increased occurrence of nephropathy (OR = 4.1518, 95% CI: 1.3118–13.1401, *p-value* 0.0154) and renal failure (OR = 5.8429, 95% CI: 1.5159–22.5206, *p-value* 0.0103), respectively (Table 5).

In order to compute confidence bounds around the predictions, we tested the significant haplogroups trough a decision tree analysis. Actually, all the reported associations were supported (Figure S1): H3 entered in the final decision tree when analyzing one T2DM complication, more than one complication and neuropathy (*p-values* 0.027, 0.034 and <0.001, respectively); while H, U3 and V were significant predictors for retinopathy (*p-value* 0.036), nephropathy (*p-value* 0.011) and renal failure (*p-value* 0.019), respectively.

Discussion

As a first step in this study, we examined the relationships between T2DM and a wide range of mtDNA haplogroups and sub-haplogroups in a large-scale association study carried out on an Italian regional population. A reduced susceptibility to diabetes was possibly detected only for the H1 mtDNA background (9.4% and 15.8% in patients and controls, respectively). This H sub-branch is common in Western Europe (~22% in the Iberian Peninsula, ~13.7% in France and ~15.3% in Scandinavia) and North Africa (average frequency of ~16%) [28] and probably marks the expansions from the Franco-Cantabrian refuge zone when climatic conditions improved after the Last Glacial Maximum [29]. As shown in the schematic tree of figure 2, which illustrates the basal mutational motifs of all haplogroups associated with T2DM and/or its complications until now, H1 differs from the root of H only for the G3010A transition in the MTRNR2 gene. It is important to note that the same nucleotide change, due to an independent mutational event, characterizes also haplogroup J1 (Figure 2), whose protective role in diabetes has been previously postulated [13]. It is also worth mentioning that polymorphic variations in the mtDNA rRNA genes have been proposed as

Table 4. Logistic-regression analyses of haplogroups associated with T2DM complications.

Modeled Outcome	Haplogroup	*p-value*	O.R.[b]	95% C.I.[c]
One complication (*Sig.* [a] = 0.0090)				
	H3	0.0427	8.5385	1.0730–67.9460
Two complications (*Sig.* = 0.0007)[§]				
	H*	0.0083	2.0682	1.2055–3.5481
	H3	0.0044	6.5625	1.7993–23.9349
	U3	0.0211	3.7500	1.2190–11.5361
	V	0.0418	2.7841	1.0389–7.4610

[a]*Significance (p-value)* relative to the final model considering all slopes = zero (no effect of the included I.V., taken together, on the outcome), obtained by the likelihood ratio test. The symbol § highlights significant values (α≤0.003).
[b]*Odd ratio.*
[c]*Confidence interval.*

Table 5. "Inverted" logistic-regression analyses employed to evaluate characteristics associated with candidate haplogroups.

Modeled Outcome [a]	Characteristics	*p-value*	O.R.	95% C.I.
H3 subjects (*Sig.* [b] = 0.0007)[§]				
	Neuropathy	0.0012	9.6389	2.4411–38.0594
H [c] subjects (*Sig.* = 0.0007)[§]				
	Retinopathy	0.0014	2.0075	1.3080–3.0812
	HDL	0.0259	0.9836	0.9694–0.9980
U3 subjects (*Sig.* = 0.0247)				
	Nephropathy	0.0154	4.1518	1.3118–13.1401
V subjects (*Sig.* = 0.0276)				
	Renal Failure	0.0103	5.8429	1.5159–22.5206

[a]The candidate haplogroup was analyzed in relation to the patients' traits and complications reported in Table 1.
[b]*Significance (p-value)* relative to the final model considering all slopes = zero (no effect of the included I.V., taken together, on the outcome), obtained by the likelihood ratio test. The symbol § highlights significant values (α≤0.003).
[c]H here represents the entire clade, thus including H*, H1, H3, H5, H6 and H9.

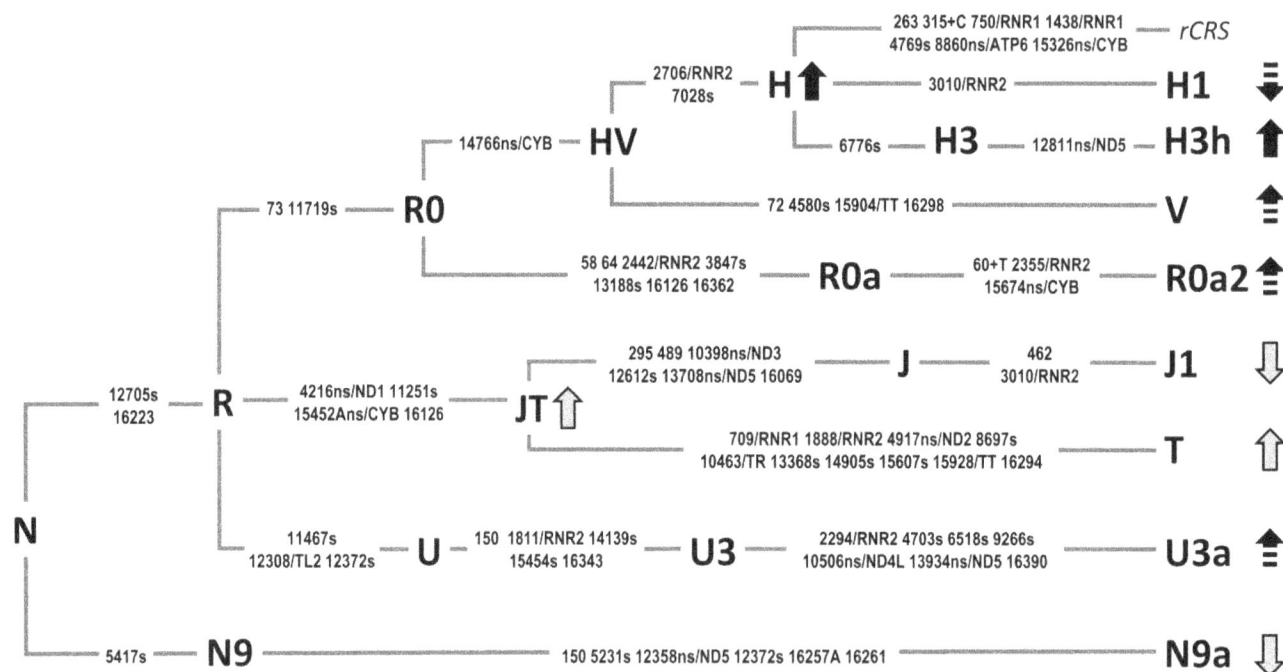

Figure 2. MtDNA tree encompassing the roots of haplogroups associated with T2DM and/or its complications. The distinguishing mutational motifs for the haplogroups shown in the tree are reported on the branches and they are transitions unless a base is explicitly indicated. The position of the rCRS [43] is indicated for reading off sequence motifs. Suffixes indicate transversions (to A), insertions (+), synonymous or non-synonymous changes (s or ns), gene locus (for tRNA, rRNA and non-synonymous mutations – following the nomenclature proposed by MITOMAP). A role for haplogroups R0a/R0a2, H, H1, H3/H3 h, V, and U3/U3a has been proposed in this study. The protective or pejorative haplogroup effect is indicated by down or up arrows. Continuous arrow lines mean highly significant values. Previous analyses found associations (gray arrows) with J1 [13], JT and T [14], and N9a [11,12].

modulators affecting the penetrance of some specific pathogenic mutations causing non-syndromic deafness and LHON [30,31]. Taking into account that the entire haplogroup H is characterized by another base substitution in MTRNR2 (G2706A), it is conceivable that such a combination of polymorphisms in the same gene might modulate susceptibility to diabetes.

Similar to haplogroup H1, the rare R0a2 branch (Figure 2), which was found only among diabetic patients in our sample (Table 2 and Figure 1), is also characterized by a mutation (A2355G) in the MTRNR2 gene (Figures 2). This subclade of the rare R0a haplogroup – 0.9% in Italy [32] – harbors also the non-synonymous transition MTCYB-T15674C/S310P affecting an amino acid position with a very high conservation index (C.I. = 92.31, calculated using the mtPhyl program http://eltsov. org/mtphyl.aspx). Thus, such a molecular change might affect the biochemical efficiency of the respiratory chain complex III. Moreover, it should be also considered that all R02a mtDNAs harbor a T insertion at np 60 in the H-strand replication origin, a sequence stretch whose variation has been recently associated to an increase of mtDNA content in T2DM patients [33].

Unfortunately, neither the association with haplogroup H1 nor that with haplogroup R0a was statistically supported. In fact, the R0a mtDNAs were too few to be included in the logistic regression, and H1 did not reach the established level of significance after the Bonferroni correction (p-value>0.003). Thus, European mtDNA haplogroups, even when analyzed at a very high level of molecular and phylogenetic resolution, do not appear to play a major role in T2DM as a whole, at least in the context of a well defined population of central Italy, as that of the Marche region.

In contrast, when we evaluated the potential role of mtDNA backgrounds in complications rather than in T2DM as a whole, we were able to build a very significant logistic model (p-value

<0.001). We observed that four mtDNA haplogroups (H, H3, U3 and V) were associated with an increased risk of complications, in particular with the risk of developing at least two common T2DM complications (Table 4). Intriguingly, we found that each haplogroup was related to a different pathology: U3 to nephropathy, V to renal failure, H to retinopathy, and H3 to neuropathy (Table 5).

The excess of U3 mtDNAs among nephropathic subjects (7.8% vs. 2.0% in T2DM controls, Table S5) is difficult to explain since this branch is characterized only by control-region mutations and synonymous coding-region transitions (Figure 2). A plausible explanation might dwell in the incidence of its subclade U3a that is almost 4-fold more represented in nephropathic cases (4.7% vs. 1.2%). The U3a mtDNAs share at least two non-synonymous mutations in two different subunits of the NADH dehydrogenase complex (MTND4L-A10506G/T13A, C.I. = 46.15; MTND5-T13934C/T533M, C.I. = 15.38).

As for haplogroup V, it was found to be associated with renal failure (15.0% in cases vs. 3.4% in T2DM controls, Table S7), which is a pejorative condition of nephropathy. Actually, the nephrological problems of the three identified V patients (Table S5) always ended with renal failure (Table S7). Their mtDNAs harbor the transition C15904T in the tRNA threonine gene that might accentuate the possible effect of the amino-acid change isoleucine to threonine (MTCYB-C14766T/I7L, C.I. = 48.72) distinctive of the entire superhaplogroup HV. The latter mutation, together with the MTRNR2-G2706A transition, could be also involved in the 2-fold increased risk of retinopathy for diabetic patients (44.7% in patients vs. 30.5% in T2DM controls, Table S2) belonging to H, the most common European haplogroup (Table 5). Within haplogroup H, it is difficult to provide an explanation for the pejorative role of H3 with regard to neuropathy. Indeed haplogroup H3 is defined only by the synonymous mutation MTCOI-T6776C (Figure 2). However, through a complete sequence analysis of H3 mtDNAs (data not shown), we were able to identify a new internal branch of H3 (named H3h in Figure 2) defined by the amino acid change MTND5-T12811C/Y53H (C.I. = 53.85). The incidence of this subgroup within H3 is much higher among the neuropathic patients (57%) than in controls (37%).

Overall, we observed that most of the candidate branches in the mtDNA tree are characterized by mutations in the MTRNR2 gene and amino acid changes affecting cytochrome b and subunits of the respiratory enzyme complex I (Figure 2). Actually, recent evidence of a stable mitochondrial supercomplex (I–III) [34–36] raises the possibility that amino acid changes in the two complexes might directly interact with each other, eventually increasing ROS production and in this way influencing the onset of diabetic complications involving neuronal tissues (neuropathy and retinopathy) [37] and nephronal structures (nephropathy and renal failure) [38], tissues that are highly susceptible to oxidative damage.

In conclusion, our data appear to indicate that mitochondrial backgrounds do not play a significant role in causing the onset of type 2 diabetes, despite indications of a protective effect for haplogroup H1 – possibly due to the G3010A transition in the MTRNR2 gene. As H1 is common in Western Europe, such a possibility might be further evaluated by assaying diabetic cohorts (and matched controls) of other European populations (see below). In contrast, we found significant associations between some European mtDNA haplogroups and typical diabetes complications. We cannot exclude that these associations might be influenced by nuclear genomic backgrounds and genetic substructure of the analyzed population, or biased by the reduced statistical power due to the decreased sample size of subgroups (patients with T2DM complications ascribed to different haplogroups) [39]. When we evaluated the latter scenario by calculating the power values for each haplogroup (Table 6) according to a previously described method [40], we observed, as would be expected due to the high haplogroup resolution of this study, rather low power values ranging from 4.4% to 42.8%. Taking into account the size of our samples (about 450 cases and 450 controls), even for haplogroup H - the most common in our study - we would be able to reach a 90% power value only if there was a frequency difference ≥40% in the T2DM group relative to the control group (41%). On the other hand, the finding that the highest power values were generally observed for the same haplogroups for which we found an association with T2DM (H1 and possibly R0a) and T2DM complications (H, H3, U3 and V) tends to support the scenario that these haplogroups do indeed play a role in T2DM complications. It should also be pointed out that our power analysis results raise the possibility that additional associations between mtDNA haplogroups and diabetes complications might exist and that they were not detected in our study simply because the analyzed cohorts were not large enough to have the power to identify small effects.

In brief, our study provides important clues indicating that certain mtDNA haplogroups might modulate diabetes complications. Obviously to definitively link mtDNA backgrounds with T2DM complications additional studies at the same level of phylogenetic resolution in other populations with similar haplogroup/subhaplogroup profiles are required. It is also likely that

Table 6. Power values calculated for each haplogroup in different comparisons.

Haplogroup[a]	Power (%)[b]		
	T2DM Patients/Controls	At least one complication/ No complications	At least two complications/ One or no complications
H1	42.81	6.12	5.28
H3	6.60	31.46	18.30
H5	4.99	4.49	4.79
H6	6.07	5.43	4.53
H[c]	4.42	5.07	14.59
HV[d]	4.37	11.98	17.81
V	10.15	4.67	9.51
R0a	31.50	n.d.	n.d.
J	6.78	5.06	8.08
T1	4.40	4.44	4.44
T2	8.62	19.82	8.60
U3	4.67	20.66	11.77
U5	4.79	4.42	4.91
U4/U9	8.37	4.97	5.82
U8b/K	6.65	13.91	7.08
N1	12.86	5.69	5.13
X2	5.42	8.18	5.82

[a]These haplogroups (excluding R0a) correspond to those tested in the logistic regression models.
[b]Power percentages were calculated as reported in [40]. The number of cases (N_C) was assumed different in each comparison, while the number of haplogroups (N_H) was always set at 16. The underlined power values refer to haplogroups H1, R0a and the other haplogroups that were statistically significant in the logistic models (see Table 4).
[c]H here includes H*, H8 and H9 of Tables 2 and 3.
[d]HV here includes HV* and HV0 of Tables 2 and 3.

for many uncommon subhaplogroups only meta-analyses encompassing data from multiple studies will be able to reach power values that are adequate to provide definitive answers on the issue.

Materials and Methods

Ethics Statement

All experimental procedures and written informed consent, obtained from all donors, were reviewed and approved by the Ethics Committee of the National Institute on Health and Science on Aging (INRCA), Ancona, Italy, in accordance with the European Union Directive 86/609.

Samples

A sample of 904 unrelated subjects (433 males and 471 females) age 40 years and older was collected by the Diabetology Unit, INRCA (National Institute on Health and Science on Aging) in Ancona (Italy). This included 466 patients affected with T2DM – whose diagnosis was made according to the American Diabetes Association Criteria (http://www.diabetes.org/) – and 438 control cases. The mean age for each group was 65.84 ± 8.19 and 59.96 ± 9.97, respectively. To avoid population stratification effects, only patients and controls with at least two generations of maternal ancestry from the Marche region (Central Italy) were included in this study. All five provinces of the region are represented: 794 from Ancona; 42 from Macerata; 15 from Ascoli Piceno; 3 from Pesaro and Urbino; 1 from Fermo; 49 of unspecified Marchigian descent.

The basic phenotypical and clinical characteristics (including data on vital signs, anthropometric factors, medical history, behavior and lifestyle, etc.) of the sample are summarized in Table 1. A predominantly Mediterranean diet was reported by all subjects. Controls did not show signs of illness and did not take any prescription drugs. The presence/absence of microvascular and macrovascular diabetic complications was evidenced as follows: microvascular: (1) diabetic retinopathy by fundoscopy through dilated pupils and/or fluorescence angiography, (2) incipient nephropathy, defined by an excessive urinary albumin excretion (>30 mg/24 h) and a normal creatinine clearance, (3) renal failure, detected as an estimated glomerular filtration rate >60 mL/min per 1.73 m^2, and (4) neuropathy established by electromyography; macrovascular: (1) ischemic heart disease diagnosed by clinical history, and/or ischemic electrocardiographic alterations, and (2) peripheral artery occlusive diseases (PAOD) including atherosclerosis obliterans and cerebrovascular disease, established on the basis of history, physical examinations and Doppler velocimetry.

Hypertension was defined as a systolic blood pressure >140 mmHg and/or a diastolic blood pressure >90 mmHg. The values were measured while the subjects were sitting and confirmed at least three times. Overnight fasting venous blood samples from all subjects were collected from 8:00 to 9:00 a.m. The biological samples were either analyzed immediately or stored at -80°C for no more than ten days. Blood concentrations for HDL cholesterol, triglycerides, HbA1c, fasting insulin, fibrinogen, high-sensitivity C reactive protein (hsCRP), creatinine, urea nitrogen, and white blood cells count were measured by standard procedures.

MtDNA analysis

Total DNA was extracted from peripheral blood using standard commercial kits (Qiamp DNA Blood Maxi Kit, Qiagen) and stored at -20°C. The mtDNA from the 904 subjects was first analyzed by sequencing ~800 bp from the control region for each subject (at least from nucleotide position [np] 16024 to np 220),

thus including the entire hypervariable segment [HVS]-I [nps 16024–16383] and part of the HVS-II [nps 57–372]. The GenBank accession numbers for the 904 mtDNA control-region sequences are JF716451-JF717354. This analysis was followed by a hierarchical survey of haplogroup and sub-haplogroup diagnostic markers in the coding region, which allowed the classification of mtDNAs into different haplogroups and sub-haplogroups [32]. Also some paragroups were evaluated, for example paragroups H* and HV* (Tables 2–3). A paragroup is a term used to indicate lineages within a haplogroup that are not defined by additional marker mutations either because the marker mutation(s) are absent, or as yet undiscovered, or simply because they were not evaluated in the molecular screening. They are generally represented by an asterisk placed after the name of the haplogroup. For instance, our paragroup H* contains all (rather numerous) H mtDNAs that did not cluster within any of the subclades of H defined in the course of this study (H1, H3, H5, H6, H8 and H9). Therefore, there is no specific marker(s) for H* in addition to those that define the entire haplogroup H but, when statistically evaluating H*, the potential role of the unknown markers within H* can be assayed, eliminating the possible confounding effects of H1, H3, H5, H6, H8 and H9.

Sequencing of entire mtDNA genomes (belonging to haplogroups R0a and H3) and phylogenetic analysis were performed as previously described [5].

Statistics

Statistical analyses were performed using the SPSS statistical package. Quantitative clinical data were compared between patients with diabetes and control individuals by the unpaired Student's t test. Qualitative data were compared using the Fisher's exact test. Because multiple comparisons were made, the established statistical significance ($\alpha\leq0.050$) was Bonferroni corrected to $\alpha\leq0.004$.

Binary logistic regressions were used to determine, simultaneously across the whole sample, whether the susceptibility to develop T2DM or T2DM complications – represented by binary dependent variables (or outcomes) taking on values 0 and 1 – differed among haplogroups. This approach reduces the chance of type 1 error (false-positive result) and controls for differences in the frequency of key variables among the different groups. MtDNA haplogroups are phylogenetically related, but they are also defined by different clusters of haplotype-specific polymorphisms. Thus, the categorical variable "haplogroup" is converted into different dummy variables (or predictors, one for each haplogroup) and introduced separately into the regression equation. To avoid small sample sizes, some of the haplogroups were grouped following phylogenetic considerations, whenever possible. The threshold was established at >10 subjects across the whole patients' group, in keeping with the "rule of thumb" whereby logistic regression should be performed only when the number of studied subjects is one order of magnitude greater than each parameter. Thus, the uncommon haplogroups H8 and H9 went into H (together with H*); HV0 was grouped with the sister paragroup HV*; U4 and U9 were clustered together; U8b, K1 and K2 were considered as U8b/K; R0a, W, the remaining U subclades (namely U1, U2, U6 and U7), and the African/Asian haplogroups were not included in the logistic computation. After this correction, 16 (haplogroup) classes were obtained. To find out how these combined predictors affect the outcome variable (T2DM or T2DM complications) we used a stepwise forward method with the likelihood ratio (LR) test employed for entering the terms (probability thresholds: entry 0.05, since we have modeled two outcomes i.e. T2DM and T2DM complications; removal 0.100): the initial model contained only the constant (B0); then the program searched for the predictor which has the highest simple correlation with the outcome variable; if this significantly improved the model, it was retained; then the program searched for the predictor which has the second highest semi-partial correlation with the outcome; if this significantly improved the model, it was retained, and so on. The chi-squared significance of the obtained model was computed by calculating the difference between log-likelihood statistic (-2LL) of the final block and that of the first step. Since we have modeled 16 haplogroups only the model *p-values* less than 0.003 were considered statistically significant.

In order to verify the relationship between mitochondrial haplogroups and T2DM complications we applied a decision tree analysis. In particular, the significant groupings in the logistic analyses (i.e. H3, H, U3 and V) were tested as predictors by Chi-squared Automatic Interaction Detection (CHAID) [41]. The CHAID tree was built by splitting subsets of the space into two or more child nodes repeatedly. To determine the best split at any node the CHAID algorithm merges each pair of categories of the predictor variable until a non-significant pair is found with regard to target variables. The process is repeated recursively until one of the stopping rules is triggered. The CHAID algorithm incorporates a sequential merge and split procedure based on Chi-square test statistics. In growing the tree the convergence criteria for CHAID were: epsilon = 0.001 and 100 maximum iterations. For each node chi square tests are computed.

Power values for each haplogroup were calculated by following the procedure previously described by Samuels et al. [40].

Supporting Information

Figure S1 CHAID diagrams assessing the association between T2DM complications and candidate haplogroups. Chi-squared Automatic Interaction Detector (CHAID) was used to develop decision-tree analyses for the evaluation of T2DM complications, using those haplogroups that were significant in logistic analyses (H3, H, U3 and V) as predictors. As shown on panels "a-c", only H3 haplogroup entered in the decision tree when predicting the presence of one or more complications and specifically neuropathy. Panel "d" confirms that H haplogroup was the predictor of retinopathy, while panels "e–f" confirm U3 and V as predictors of nephropathy and renal failure, respectively.

Table S1 Control-region haplotypes and haplogroup/sub-haplogroup classification of the 904 mtDNAs from the Marche region.

Table S2 Frequencies of mtDNA haplogroups and sub-haplogroups in diabetic patients also affected by retinopathy.

Table S3 Frequencies of mtDNA haplogroups and sub-haplogroups in diabetic patients also affected by somatic neuropathy.

Table S4 Frequencies of mtDNA haplogroups and sub-haplogroups in diabetic patients also affected by cardiac ischemia.

Table S5 Frequencies of mtDNA haplogroups and sub-haplogroups in diabetic patients also affected by nephropathy.

Table S6 Frequencies of mtDNA haplogroups and sub-haplogroups in diabetic patients also affected by Peripheral Artery Occlusive Disease (PAOD).

Table S7 Frequencies of mtDNA haplogroups and sub-haplogroups in diabetic patients also affected by renal failure.

Acknowledgments

The authors thank Norman Angerhofer (Sorenson Molecular Genealogy Foundation, Utah, USA) for providing bioinformatics support and Alessia Grinzato (University of Pavia) for helping with experimental work.

Author Contributions

Conceived and designed the experiments: AT CF RT MNG. Performed the experiments: AA AO MP BHK HL ACormio VC FG VG. Analyzed the data: AA AO VB CS LS. Contributed reagents/materials/analysis tools: AT CF RT. Wrote the paper: AA AO UAP ACeriello OS AT. Performed the collection of clinical/biometric data, blood and DNA samples: RT AS MM ARB MB IT.

References

1. De Silva NM, Frayling TM (2010) Novel biological insights emerging from genetic studies of type 2 diabetes and related metabolic traits. Curr Opin Lipidol 21: 44–50.

2. Prokopenko I, McCarthy MI, Lindgren CM (2008) Type 2 diabetes: new genes, new understanding. Trends Genet 24: 613–621.

3. Sladek R, Rocheleau G, Rung J, Dina C, Shen L, et al. (2007) A genome-wide association study identifies novel risk loci for type 2 diabetes. Nature 445: 881–885.

4. Shriner D, Vaughan LK, Padilla MA, Tiwari HK (2007) Problems with genome-wide association studies. Science 316: 1840–1842.

5. Torroni A, Achilli A, Macaulay V, Richards M, Bandelt H-J (2006) Harvesting the fruit of the human mtDNA tree. Trends Genet 22: 339–345.

6. Underhill PA, Kivisild T (2007) Use of Y chromosome and mitochondrial DNA population structure in tracing human migrations. Annu Rev Genet 41: 539–564.

7. Lowell BB, Shulman GI (2005) Mitochondrial dysfunction and type 2 diabetes. Science 307: 384–387.

8. Maechler P, Wollheim CB (2001) Mitochondrial function in normal and diabetic beta-cells. Nature 414: 807–812.

9. Petersen KF, Dufour S, Befroy D, Garcia R, Shulman GI (2004) Impaired mitochondrial activity in the insulin-resistant offspring of patients with type 2 diabetes. N Engl J Med 350: 664–671.

10. Wallace DC (2010) Mitochondrial DNA mutations in disease and aging. Environ Mol Mutagen 51: 440–450.

11. Fuku N, Park KS, Yamada Y, Nishigaki Y, Cho YM, et al. (2007) Mitochondrial haplogroup N9a confers resistance against type 2 diabetes in Asians. Am J Hum Genet 80: 407–415.

12. Tanaka M, Fuku N, Nishigaki Y, Matsuo H, Segawa T, et al. (2007) Women with mitochondrial haplogroup N9a are protected against metabolic syndrome. Diabetes 56: 518–521. Erratum in: Diabetes (2007) 56: 1486.

13. Feder J, Ovadia O, Blech I, Cohen J, Wainstein J, et al. (2009) Parental diabetes status reveals association of mitochondrial DNA haplogroup J1 with type 2 diabetes. BMC Med Genet 10: 60.

14. Crispim D, Canani LH, Gross JL, Tschiedel B, Souto KE, et al. (2006) The European-specific mitochondrial cluster J/T could confer an increased risk of insulin-resistance and type 2 diabetes: an analysis of the m.4216T > C and m.4917A > G variants. Ann Hum Genet 70: 488–495.

15. Chinnery PF, Mowbray C, Patel SK, Elson JL, Sampson M, et al. (2007) Mitochondrial DNA haplogroups and type 2 diabetes: a study of 897 cases and 1010 controls. J Med Genet 44: e80.

16. Mohlke KL, Jackson AU, Scott LJ, Peck EC, Suh YD, et al. (2005) Mitochondrial polymorphisms and susceptibility to type 2 diabetes-related traits in Finns. Hum Genet 118: 245–254.

17. Saxena R, de Bakker PI, Singer K, Mootha V, Burtt N, et al. (2006) Comprehensive association testing of common mitochondrial DNA variation in metabolic disease. Am J Hum Genet 79: 54–61.

18. Carelli V, Achilli A, Valentino ML, Rengo C, Semino O, et al. (2006) Haplogroup effects and recombination of mitochondrial DNA: novel clues from the analysis of Leber hereditary optic neuropathy pedigrees. Am J Hum Genet 78: 564–574.

19. Ji Y, Zhang AM, Jia X, Zhang YP, Xiao X, et al. (2008) Mitochondrial DNA haplogroups M7b1'2 and M8a affect clinical expression of leber hereditary optic neuropathy in Chinese families with the m.11778G–>a mutation. Am J Hum Genet 83: 760–768.

20. Achilli A, Rengo C, Magri C, Battaglia V, Olivieri A, et al. (2004) The molecular dissection of mtDNA haplogroup H confirms that the Franco-Cantabrian glacial refuge was a major source for the European gene pool. Am J Hum Genet 75: 910–918.

21. Roostalu U, Kutuev I, Loogväli EL, Metspalu E, Tambets K, et al. (2007) Origin and expansion of haplogroup H, the dominant human mitochondrial DNA lineage in West Eurasia: the Near Eastern and Caucasian perspective. Mol Biol Evol 24: 436–448.

22. Fowler MJ (2008) Microvascular and macrovascular complications of diabetes. Clin. Diabetes 26: 77–82.

23. Melendez-Ramirez LY, Richards RJ, Cefalu WT (2010) Complications of type 1 diabetes. Endocrinol Metab Clin North Am 39: 625–640.

24. Brownlee M (2001) Biochemistry and molecular cell biology of diabetic complications. Nature 414: 813–820.

25. Feder J, Blech I, Ovadia O, Amar S, Wainstein J, et al. (2008) Differences in mtDNA haplogroup distribution among 3 Jewish populations alter susceptibility to T2DM complications. BMC Genomics 9: 198.

26. Kofler B, Mueller EE, Eder W, Stanger O, Maier R, et al. (2009) Mitochondrial DNA haplogroup T is associated with coronary artery disease and diabetic retinopathy: a case control study. BMC Med Genet 10: 35.

27. Van Oven M, Kayser M (2009) Updated comprehensive phylogenetic tree of global human mitochondrial DNA variation. Hum Mutat 30: E386–E394.

28. Ottoni C, Primativo G, Hooshiar Kashani B, Achilli A, Martinez-Labarga C, et al. (2010) Mitochondrial haplogroup H1 in North Africa: an early Holocene arrival from Iberia. PLoS ONE 5: e13378.

29. Soares P, Achilli A, Semino O, Davies W, Macaulay V, et al. (2010) The archaeogenetics of Europe. Curr Biol 70: R174–R183.

30. Hudson G, Carelli V, Spruijt L, Gerards M, Mowbray C, et al. (2007) Clinical expression of Leber hereditary optic neuropathy is affected by the mitochondrial DNA-haplogroup background. Am J Hum Genet 81: 228–233.

31. Prezant TR, Agapian JV, Bohlman MC, Bu X, Oztas S, et al. (1993) Mitochondrial ribosomal RNA mutation associated with both antibiotic-induced and non-syndromic deafness. Nat Genet 4: 289–294.

32. Achilli A, Olivieri A, Pala M, Metspalu E, Fornarino S, et al. (2007) Mitochondrial DNA variation of modern Tuscans supports the Near Eastern origin of Etruscans. Am J Hum Genet 80: 759–768.

33. Cormio A, Milella F, Marra M, Pala M, Lezza AM, et al. (2009) Variations at the H-strand replication origins of mitochondrial DNA and mitochondrial DNA content in the blood of type 2 diabetes patients. Biochim Biophys Acta 1787: 547–552.

34. Dudkina NV, Eubel H, Keegstra W, Boekema EJ, Braun HP (2005) Structure of a mitochondrial supercomplex formed by respiratory-chain complexes I and III. Proc Natl Acad Sci U S A 102: 3225–3229.

35. Lenaz G, Genova ML (2009) Structural and functional organization of the mitochondrial respiratory chain: a dynamic super-assembly. Int J Biochem Cell Biol 41: 1750–1772.

36. Lenaz G, Genova ML (2010) Structure and organization of mitochondrial respiratory complexes: a new understanding of an old subject. Antioxid Redox Signal 12: 961–1008.

37. Abramov AY, Smulders-Srinivasan TK, Kirby DM, Acin-Perez R, Enriquez JA, et al. (2010) Mechanism of neurodegeneration of neurons with mitochondrial DNA mutations. Brain 133: 797–807.

38. Ha H, Hwang IA, Park JH, Lee HB (2008) Role of reactive oxygen species in the pathogenesis of diabetic nephropathy. Diabetes Res Clin Pract 82: Suppl 1: S42–45.

39. Cai XY, Wang XF, Li SL, Qian J, Qian DG, et al. (2009) Association of mitochondrial DNA haplogroups with exceptional longevity in a Chinese population. PLoS One 4: e6423.

40. Samuels DC, Carothers AD, Horton R, Chinnery PF (2006) The power to detect disease associations with mitochondrial DNA haplogroups. Am J Hum Genet 78: 713–720.

41. Kass GV (1980) An exploratory technique for investigating large quantities of categorical data. Appl Stat 29: 119–127.

42. Černý V, Mulligan CJ, Fernandes V, Silva NM, Alshamali F, et al. (2011) Internal diversification of mitochondrial haplogroup R0a reveals post-Last Glacial Maximum demographic expansions in South Arabia. Mol Biol Evol 28: 71–78.

43. Andrews RM, Kubacka I, Chinnery PF, Lightowlers RN, Turnbull DM, et al. (1999) Reanalysis and revision of the Cambridge reference sequence for human mitochondrial DNA. Nat Genet 23: 147.

Indicators of Acute and Persistent Renal Damage in Adult Thrombotic Microangiopathy

Firuseh Dierkes[1]❦, **Nikolaos Andriopoulos**[2]❦, **Christoph Sucker**[3], **Kathrin Kuhr**[4], **Markus Hollenbeck**[5], **Gerd R. Hetzel**[1], **Volker Burst**[2], **Sven Teschner**[2], **Lars C. Rump**[1], **Thomas Benzing**[2,6], **Bernd Grabensee**[1], **Christine E. Kurschat**[2,6]*

1 Department of Nephrology, Medical Faculty, Heinrich-Heine-University, Düsseldorf, Germany, 2 Renal Division, Department of Medicine and Center for Molecular Medicine, University of Cologne, Cologne, Germany, 3 Department of Hemostasis and Transfusion Medicine, Heinrich-Heine-University Medical Center, Düsseldorf, Germany, 4 Institute of Medical Statistics, Informatics and Epidemiology, University of Cologne, Cologne, Germany, 5 Department of Nephrology and Rheumatology, Knappschaftskrankenhaus, Bottrop, Germany, 6 Cologne Excellence Cluster on Cellular Stress Responses in Aging-Associated Diseases, University of Cologne, Cologne, Germany

Abstract

Background: Thrombotic microangiopathies (TMA) in adults such as thrombotic thrombocytopenic purpura (TTP) and hemolytic uremic syndrome (HUS) are life-threatening disorders if untreated. Clinical presentation is highly variable and prognostic factors for clinical course and outcome are not well established.

Methods: We performed a retrospective observational study of 62 patients with TMA, 22 males and 40 females aged 16 to 76 years, treated with plasma exchange at one center to identify clinical risk factors for the development of renal insufficiency.

Results: On admission, 39 of 62 patients (63%) had acute renal failure (ARF) with 32 patients (52%) requiring dialysis treatment. High systolic arterial pressure (SAP, p = 0.009) or mean arterial pressure (MAP, p = 0.027) on admission was associated with acute renal failure. Patients with SAP>140 mmHg on admission had a sevenfold increased risk of severe kidney disease (OR 7.464, CI 2.097–26.565). MAP>100 mmHg indicated a fourfold increased risk for acute renal failure (OR 4.261, CI 1.400–12.972). High SAP, diastolic arterial pressure (DAP), and MAP on admission were also independent risk factors for persistent renal insufficiency with the strongest correlation for high MAP. Moreover, a high C-reactive protein (CRP) level on admission correlated with renal failure in the course of the disease (p = 0.003). At discharge, renal function in 11 of 39 patients (28%) had fully recovered, 14 patients (23%) remained on dialysis, and 14 patients (23%) had non-dialysis-dependent chronic kidney disease. Seven patients (11%) died. We identified an older age as risk factor for death.

Conclusions: High blood pressure as well as high CRP serum levels on admission are associated with renal insufficiency in TMA. High blood pressure on admission is also a strong predictor of sustained renal insufficiency. Thus, adult TMA patients with high blood pressure may require special attention to prevent persistent renal failure.

Editor: Shree Ram Singh, National Cancer Institute, United States of America

Funding: The authors have no support or funding to report.

Competing Interests: The authors have declared that no competing interests exist.

* E-mail: christine.kurschat@uk-koeln.de

❦ These authors contributed equally to this work.

Introduction

Thrombotic microangiopathies (TMA) such as HUS or TTP are rare microangiopathic thrombotic disorders characterized by hyaline thrombi in the arterial microvasculature, Coombs-negative hemolytic anemia, and thrombocytopenia. Prior to the introduction of plasma infusion and plasma exchange therapy, TMA was associated with a mortality rate of more than 90% in adults [1,2]. In recent years, with the advent of plasma exchange in TMA mortality rate could be drastically decreased, but TMA can still be viewed as a life-threatening disorder with the outcome depending on the underlying disease, the age of the patient, severity of organ damage (e.g. kidney, heart, brain), and on the time lapse between the onset of symptoms and initiation of plasma therapy.

A variety of possible triggers such as gastrointestinal infection with *E.coli O157:H7*, *E.coli O104:H4* or *Shigella* for typical HUS and genitourinary or respiratory infections, human immunodeficiency virus infection, hormonal dysbalance, drugs, tumours, inherited and acquired defects in complement components and autoimmune diseases for TTP and adult atypical HUS have been identified [3,4,5]. However, in up to 30% of cases the underlying cause remains unclear. Recently, a large outbreak of *E.coli O104:H4* in Germany demonstrated the clinical severity of this disease [6]. New pathophysiological approaches identified a low activity of ADAMTS13, a metalloprotease responsible for cleavage of unusually large *von Willebrand factor* (ULvWF) multimers, to be responsible for TTP development [3,7,8]. However, according to epidemiologic studies ADAMTS13 activity was reduced below 5% in only 15% of patients with TMA [9], suggesting the presence of additional unrecognized risk factors predisposing for the onset and clinical course of TMA. Patients with atypical HUS may have a deficiency of complement factor H or auto-antibodies directed against this protein. Furthermore, mutations in the membrane cofactor protein gene (MCP/CD46), in the complement factor I gene, in the complement factor B gene or in the thrombomodulin gene may also be present [10,11,12]. In atypical HUS and selected Shiga-toxin-induced HUS cases the humanized monoclonal anti-C5 antibody eculizumab was reported to be beneficial [13,14,15]. In contrast to HUS patients, classic TTP patients usually present with predominant neurological symptoms. Since there is considerable clinical overlap between these two entities the disease is often referred to as HUS/TTP [16].

Presently, there is a need for risk stratification to guide therapy and follow-up. Therefore, we analysed 62 consecutive adult patients with TMA admitted to our hospital between 1989 and 2006.

Methods

Study design

The aim of this study was to identify clinical risk factors for acute renal failure, persistent renal insufficiency and for mortality in adult TMA patients. Data of 62 patients (22 males, 40 females) consecutively admitted to our hospital between June 1989 and June 2006 at the age of 16 to 76 years with their first episode of acute TMA were analyzed. This study was reviewed and approved by the Institutional Review Board of Düsseldorf University as exempt research without requirement for informed consent as this was review of existing data. TMA was diagnosed on the basis of clinical criteria: thrombocytopenia of less than 100,000/µl, Coombs-negative hemolytic anemia (Hb<12 g/dl, LDH>240 U/l), and the presence of more than two schistocytes per visual field in the peripheral blood smear. Other causes of severe thrombocytopenia, in particular disseminated intravascular coagulation or idiopathic thrombocytopenic purpura, were excluded. Almost all patients in this study were treated with plasmapheresis. 57 of the patients underwent plasma exchange therapy within 12 hours after admission; three patients received plasma infusion due to less severe disease. Two patients died from severe cerebral hemorrhage before initiation of plasma therapy. Medical records of all patients were examined for clinical signs of TMA and potential risk factors for the disease. In this study, we did not classify patients into TTP, HUS, or overlap syndromes by determining ADAMTS13 levels, factor H, B, I, MCP or thrombomodulin gene mutations [11,12,17] because these data were only available in a subset of patients. Furthermore, although the concept of ADAMTS13 deficiency or mutations in complement factors being responsible for the development of TMA is important, TMA patients still represent a very heterogenous group. Thus, the known pathophysiologic approaches are applicable to some, but not all TMA patients [9,12,18,19,20].

Clinical parameters (age, sex, SAP, DAP, MAP, white blood cell count, hemoglobin concentration, platelet count, LDH, serum creatinine, blood urea nitrogen (BUN), CRP) were analysed on admission and at discharge. For plasmapheresis, we routinely administered 250 mg methylprednisolone i.v. per day initially for the first three days followed by 1–4 mg/kg body weight of prednisone orally per day, usually at the same time as plasma therapy.

Acute renal failure (ARF) in patients with no prior history of kidney disease was defined by an increase of serum creatinine

levels of >0.5 mg/dl in 48 hours. In patients with renal insufficiency (baseline creatinine ≥1.5 mg/dl) ARF was defined by a rise in serum creatinine of ≥1 mg/dl from baseline over a period of 48 hours. Patients with elevated serum creatinine ≥1.5 mg/dl at discharge were categorized to have persistent renal insufficiency. All patients were treated on the intensive care unit (ICU) until platelet levels rose to more than 50 000/µl. Symptomatic treatment consisted of blood pressure control, electrolyte and water balance control, and whole blood transfusions if necessary.

"Remission" was defined as normalization of serum creatinine ≤1.2 mg/dl and reversal of neurological symptoms. All patients categorized as remission did not exhibit proteinuria at the time of discharge. Systolic blood pressure was normalized in 9 of 11 patients with renal insufficiency on admission and remission at discharge. Diastolic blood pressure was normalized in all these patients.

Statistical Analysis

The objective of this study was (1) to analyse potential differences between patients with renal impairment and patients with normal renal function on admission, (2) to find potential risk factors for persistent renal insufficiency and (3) to find potential risk factors for mortality. For this purpose we used the non-parametric Mann-Whitney test and performed pairwise comparisons for the baseline factors CRP, blood pressure, platelets, LDH and white blood cell count (WBC). Additionally, SAP and MAP were defined with 140 and 100 mmHg as cut-off, and odds ratios (OR) and their 95% confidence intervals (CI) were assessed to describe the strength of association between these factors and the renal status on admission (situation 1).

For persistent renal insufficiency, the prognostic impacts of the baseline factors were first explored one at a time by logistic regression analyses, adjusted for renal status on admission. Factors associated with a p value of the Wald type <20% were examined more closely in a multivariate logistic regression model, using forward selection. Results are expressed as OR with their 95% CI. The variables CRP, WBC, platelets and LDH were natural logarithm transformed for inclusion in regression analyses (situation 2).

In situation 3, we analysed additionally to the parameters from situation 1 and 2 the factors age, haemoglobin, schistocytes and creatinine. Due to small sample sizes, a logistic regression analysis was not feasible, thus we used a non-parametric Mann Whitney test and performed pairwise comparisons for surviving and deceased patients.

If not stated otherwise, continuous variables were presented as median (interquartile range (IQR)), categorical variables were presented as proportions (%). Because of the explorative character of this study we did not adjust the significance level α = 0.05 to account for multiple testing. Therefore, all p-values are of an explorative nature and p values<0.05 were considered to be statistically significant. All reported p-values are two-sided. The analyses were performed using PASW Statistics 18.0.3 for Windows (SPSS 2010, Chicago, Il., USA).

Results

Clinical characteristics of patients on initial presentation

62 consecutive patients diagnosed with adult TMA were analysed in this study (table 1). Median age at presentation was 35 years with a wide range of 16 to 76 years (interquartile range (IQR): 27–49). Two thirds of our patients were female. 82% of patients only had a single episode of TMA whereas 18% relapsed

Table 1. Clinical characteristics of patients on admission.

	n (%)	Median (IQR)	Associated risk factors for the development of TMA	n (%)
Total number of patients	62		Infection	18 (29.0)
Age at first event (yr)		35 (27–49)	Pulmonary infection	5 (8.1)
Female gender	40 (64.5)		Diarrhea	7 (11.3)
Male gender	22 (35.5)		Pregnancy / oral contraceptives	8 (12.9)/2 (3.2)
Patients with single event	51 (82.3)		Renal transplantation	4 (6.5)
Patients with relapsing TMA	11 (17.7)		Malignancy	4 (6.5)
Neurological symptoms	32 (51.6)		SLE	3 (4.8)
Renal impairment	39 (62.9)		Systemic sclerosis	2 (3.2)
Dialysis treatment	32 (51.6)		Drugs	2 (3.2)
			Unknown	19 (30.6)

IQR: Interquartile range.

at least once during the study period. Half of our patients exhibited neurological impairment varying from less severe symptoms such as headache and dizziness to severe seizures and coma. Renal insufficiency at presentation was very common (table 1). Most of our patients had no history of renal insufficiency prior to their first TMA episode. In patients with history of chronic renal failure, 3 patients had received a renal transplant, 2 patients had SLE, and one patient had scleroderma.

The different underlying causes of TMA in our patients are summarized in table 1. 31% of all patients had no obvious clinical trigger for the development of TMA.

19% of our patients were known to suffer from hypertension prior to the onset of TMA, whereas 81% did not show any medical history of hypertension.

Clinical outcome

At discharge, remission (no renal insufficiency, no proteinuria, no neurological symptoms) was achieved in 42% of patients (table 2). Renal failure had resolved in 11 of 39 patients. The number of dialysis-dependent patients decreased from 52% to 23% (table 2). Only two patients, one with renal insufficiency on admission and one without, still had a neurological deficit at discharge. Among those patients with no previous hypertension, 32% required antihypertensive treatment at the time of discharge. 7 patients with TMA died (table 2), one of sepsis, three of severe cerebral hemorrhage, and three of TMA-associated acute myocardial infarction where immediate lysis therapy was unsuccessful.

Clinical markers for renal insufficiency on admission

C-reactive protein (CRP) levels on admission were significantly higher in patients with renal insufficiency compared to patients with normal renal function (table 3, figure 1). Taking the median of CRP values (2.7 mg/dl) to divide patients into two subgroups, 10 patients with CRP≥2.7 mg/dl had infections whereas 20 patients did not have signs of infection (6 patients with unknown trigger of TMA, 5 patients post-partum, 3 patients with tumour, 3 patients with drug-induced TMA, 2 patients with SLE).

Blood pressure levels, MAP and SAP, were also significantly higher in patients with renal impairment on admission (table 3, figure 1). Patients with SAP>140 mmHg on admission had a sevenfold increased probability of renal insufficiency on admission (odds ratio (OR) 7.464, CI 2.097–26.565). Patients with MAP>100 mmHg on admission had a fourfold increased probability (OR 4.261, CI 1.400–12.972) of acute renal insufficiency. There was a tendency for lower DAP in patients with normal renal function. Platelet count was significantly lower in patients with normal renal function (Table 3). This finding reflects the high proportion of patients with a clinical diagnosis of TTP in this group who often present with very low thrombocyte counts but with normal renal function. No significant difference was observed for LDH levels or white blood cell count (WBC), as described previously [21].

In our study, schistocytes remained elevated in some patients although LDH levels and platelet count were already normalized (data not shown). Therefore, as published earlier [22], schistocytes were unreliable markers for the detection of disease activity.

Table 2. Clinical outcome.

	All patients n (%)	Renal impairment on admission n (%)	Normal renal function on admission (n = 23) n (%)
Remission	26 (41.9)	8 (20.5)	18 (78.3)
Renal insufficiency without dialysis	14 (22.6)	10 (25.6)	2 (8.7)
Dialysis	14 (22.6)	11 (28.2)	0 (0)
Neurological deficit	2 (3.2)	1 (2.6)	1 (4.3)
Death	7 (11.3)	5 (12.8)	2 (8.7)

Table 3. Characteristic factors for acute renal failure on admission.

	All patients (*n*=62) Median (IQR)	Renal impairment (*n*=39) Median (IQR)	Normal renal function (*n*=23) Median (IQR)	p-value (Mann-Whitney-U test)
MAP (mmHg)	106 (90–117)	110 (95–120)	97 (87–110)	**0.027***
SAP (mmHg)	140 (120–150)	150 (130–160)	130 (120–140)	**0.009***
DAP (mmHg)	85 (70–100)	89 (80–100)	80 (70–90)	0.067
CRP (mg/dl)	2.7 (0.9–5.4)	2.9 (1.4–8.7)	0.95 (0.3–2.8)	**0.003***
Platelets (/µl)	25 000 (9 000–56 000)	40 000 (18 000–85 000)	9 000 (8 000–26 000)	**0.001***
LDH (U/l)	1 259 (714–2 001)	1 430 (765–2 799)	1 002 (630–1 650)	0.147
WBC (/µl)	10 800 (7 000–13 500)	11 900 (7 100–15 600)	9 400 (6 200–12 000)	0.062

*values significantly higher in patients with impaired renal function compared to patients with normal renal function on admission (p<0.05). IQR: Interquartile range.

Risk factors for persistent renal insufficiency

Our objective of this study was to identify clinical markers to detect patients at risk for TMA-induced sustained renal insufficiency. We performed logistic regression analyses, adjusted for renal status on admission (table 4), comparing patients on admission and at discharge. Potential risk factors influencing renal status at discharge were high MAP, SAP, DAP, and LDH levels on admission (table 4). We observed a strong association of elevated MAP on admission with renal insufficiency at discharge in multivariate analysis (table 5). An increase in MAP by 10 mmHg was associated with a twofold increased chance for renal insufficiency at discharge. This finding indicates that patients with renal dysfunction on admission as well as at discharge have higher blood pressure levels compared to patients with normal renal function.

In our logistic regression analysis (table 4), LDH levels were higher in patients with renal impairment on admission and at discharge compared to patients with normal renal function.

Risk factors for death from TMA

The only associated risk factor for death in our study population was older age (table 6). MAP, SAP, DAP, LDH levels, CRP levels, WBC, haemoglobin levels, thrombocyte counts, schistocyte levels or creatinine levels were not significantly different in patients who died from TMA compared to surviving patients. Multivariate analysis was not performed due to the small number of deceased patients.

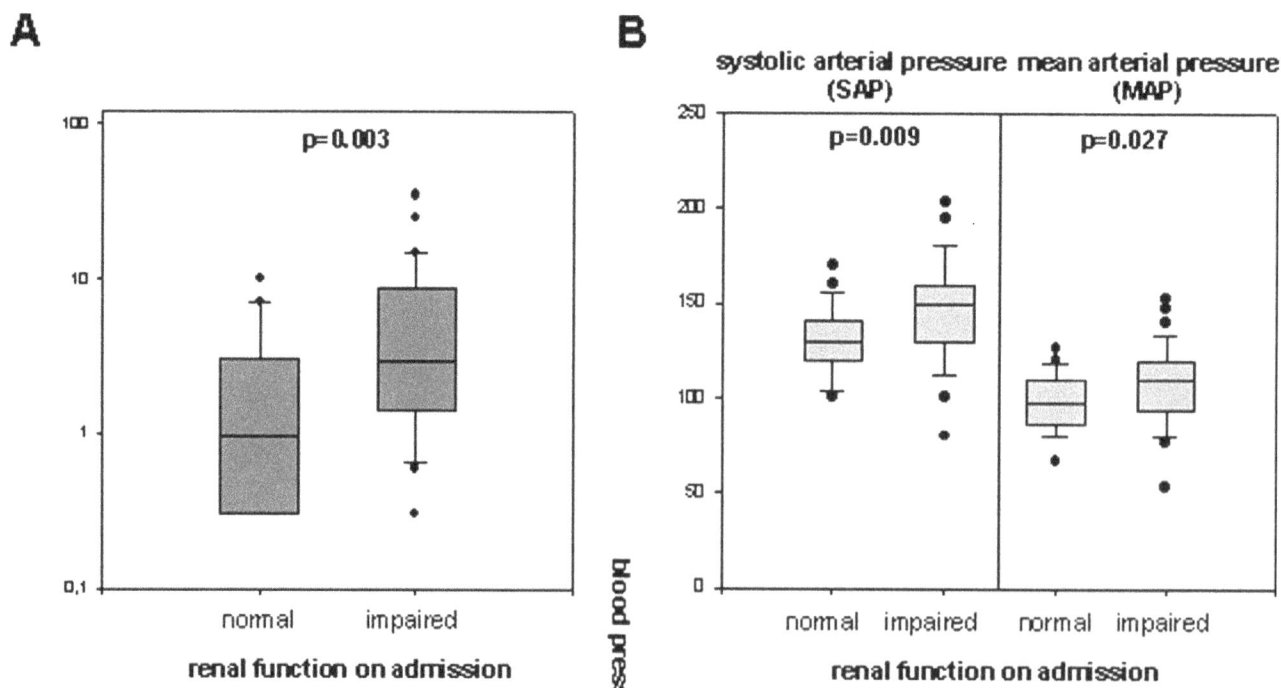

Figure 1. Risk factors for renal insufficiency in TMA. A: CRP serum levels on admission are significantly higher in patients with renal insufficiency compared to patients with normal renal function. B: Systolic arterial pressure (SAP) and mean arterial pressure (MAP) on admission are significantly higher in TMA patients with renal insufficiency.

Table 4. Risk factors for renal insufficiency at discharge. Logistic regression analyses, adjusted for renal status on admission.

	Renal impairment on admission only ($n=8$) Median (IQR)	Renal impairment on admission and at discharge ($n=26$) Median (IQR)	Normal renal function on admission and at discharge ($n=19$) Median (IQR)	p-value (Wald-Test)
MAP (mmHg)	96 (88–111)	113 (105–124)	93 (83–107)	**0.011***
SAP (mmHg)	133 (120–148)	150 (139–173)	120 (110–140)	**0.025***
DAP (mmHg)	80 (70–93)	90 (80–100)	80 (70–90)	**0.023***
CRP (mg/dl)	2.75 (1.1–4.9)	2.9 (1.5–9.5)	1.1 (0.3–3.9)	0.816
LDH (U/l)	1 835 (1 038–3 655)	1 346 (670–2 001)	1 002 (630–1 650)	**0.082***
WBC (/µl)	11 900 (6 600–13 900)	11 050 (7 000–16 300)	9 400 (6 100–12 000)	0.894

*values higher in patients with impaired renal function compared to patients with normal renal function at discharge (p<0.20). IQR: Interquartile range.

Discussion

TMA is a life-threatening disease that was previously associated with a high mortality of more than 90% before plasmapheresis was introduced as therapy for TMA patients. Nowadays, survival rates have significantly improved, but sporadic non-Shiga-toxin-induced HUS still has a mortality rate of up to 50% in some patient subgroups [17]. The 2011 outbreak of *E.coli O104:H4* in Germany demonstrated the severity of this disease very clearly, where at least 27 patients died from diarrhea-associated HUS [6].

This study was designed to evaluate clinical risk factors predisposing TMA patients to renal insufficiency. The clinical course of a single patient presenting with TMA is often difficult to predict. Therefore, we analyzed data of 62 consecutively treated TMA patients to identify markers for the development of renal insufficiency and for the lack of renal recovery after successful TMA treatment.

Attempts to clinically define prognostic factors for the development of renal insufficiency in TMA have already been made earlier [21,23,24,25]. Hollenbeck and co-workers demonstrated the importance of plasmapheresis to prevent the development of end-stage renal disease compared to plasma infusion alone [21]. In three studies pre-existing nephropathy or severe renal involvement were identified as risk factors for chronic renal failure [23,24,25]. Four studies correlated chronic renal failure to the severity of arterial and glomerular damage on renal biopsy [23,24,25], whereas one study did not find any correlation between renal histology and renal prognosis [21]. Compared to the present analysis patient subgroups were different. In the study by Hollenbeck et al. only 71% of patients were treated with plasmapheresis. Tostivint and colleagues reported exclusively on HUS patients, not on TTP patients,

mostly treated with plasma infusion [23], with a large cohort of HIV positive cases. In our study patients were treated almost exclusively with plasmapheresis.

Acute renal failure (ARF) in TMA patients is frequently seen. In our study, more than 60% of patients showed renal impairment at presentation confirming results that have been published earlier (for review, see [17],[26],[27]). We identified high CRP and high blood pressure as clinical markers associated with ARF in TMA patients. CRP serum levels on admission were significantly increased in patients with ARF compared to patients with normal renal function. Therefore, high CRP may serve as a risk factor for ARF in TMA. CRP is a non-specific acute phase protein synthesized and degraded in the liver. It is markedly elevated in septic states in which ARF develops with a prevalence of 9–40% [28]. In our study, sepsis only played a minor role as a potential cause of ARF. The reason for high CRP levels in our patient subgroup with ARF is unclear. They usually occur in response to infection and inflammation. In the renal insufficiency group they may reflect additional, clinically undetected infection, possibly facilitating the development of ARF. Since WBC was not elevated in patients with higher CRP levels it is unlikely that severe infections were the reason for CRP elevation. Therefore, high CRP levels should rather be interpreted as an indicator for the severity of TMA-induced organ damage, including the kidney. Going along the same line with our observation, a Japanese study on diarrhea-associated typical HUS in children (D+ HUS) identified high CRP serum levels as a risk factor for the development of severe CNS disorders [29]. High CRP has also been recognized as a prognostic indicator in chronic renal disease. [30,31]. Serum CRP levels predict death in dialysis patients [32,33]. In severe renal insufficiency, elevation of CRP is associated with a higher

Table 5. Risk factors for renal insufficiency at discharge, multivariate logistic regression analysis.

	β[a]	SE[b]	p-value (Wald Test)	Odds Ratio (95% CI)
Renal impairment on admission[c]	3.290	0.927	<0.001	26.84 (4.36–165.11)
MAP (mmHg)	0.070	0.028	0.011	1.07 (1.02–1.13)
Constant	−12.869	3.630	<0.001	

[a] β, estimated regression coefficient,
[b] standard error of β,
[c] "yes" coded 1.

Table 6. Risk factors for TMA-associated death.

	Surviving patients (n=55) Median (IQR)	Deceased patients (n=7) Median (IQR)	p-value
Age (yrs)	34 (26–45)	48 (41–65)	**0.009 ***
MAP (mmHg)	106 (93.33–116.67)	95 (90–106.67)	0.346
SAP (mmHg)	140 (120–150)	130 (120–150)	0.512
DAP (mmHg)	87 (70–100)	80 (70–85)	0.280
LDH (U/l)	1 241 (694–1 935)	1 430 (1 086–3 570)	0.171
CRP (mg/dl)	2.5 (0.9–4.4)	3.6 (2.2–8.7)	0.386
WBC (/μl)	10 600 (6 400–13 800)	12 600 (10 000–13 500)	0.182
Hemoglobin (g/dl)	8.2 (7.1–9.8)	7.7 (5.7–11.3)	0.730
Platelets (/μl)	26 000 (9 000–58 000)	12 000 (5 000–56 000)	0.344
Schistocytes per field of view	6 (3–9)	7 (7–8)	0.528
Creatinine (mg/dl)	2.5 (1–5.2)	1.5 (1–4.3)	0.815

IQR: Interquartile range.

cardiovascular mortality due to the contribution of CRP in endothelial damage and atherogenesis [34,35]. CRP might therefore play an active role in endothelial damage also in TMA patients, independently of its elevation in septic states. Thus, high CRP levels may reflect TMA activity itself, leading to more severe end-organ damage and ARF.

In our cohort, high blood pressure (MAP) in patients with renal insufficiency on admission was a risk factor for acute and persistent renal insufficiency. Tostivint and co-workers already indicated that high DAP was associated with chronic renal failure but they did not identify high DAP as independent risk factor in multivariate analysis [23]. Higher blood pressure is either due to pre-existing hypertension or due to secondary hypertension caused by TMA-related renal involvement. Interestingly, only a minority of patients was known to be hypertensive prior to their episode of TMA. Most of our patients also did not have any previous history of kidney disease. Our data suggest that adequate treatment of hypertension in TMA patients may be essential to prevent additional renal damage. By lowering blood pressure into the normal range renal function might be preserved and may lead to a better renal outcome.

LDH serum levels at the time of admission were higher in patients with sustained renal insufficiency at discharge compared to patients with normal renal function. This finding is not surprising since LDH levels indicate the severity of hemolysis and of end-organ damage. Higher LDH levels in patients with persisting renal insufficiency suggest a more severe course of TMA and presumably also more severe kidney damage.

Several risk factors for the development of TMA, such as infection, pregnancy, autoimmune disease or drugs, have been published. We found these to be present in 69% of our patients. One third of patients did not show any apparent trigger. Genetic testing of genes encoding complement factors and determination of ADAMTS13 activity have been demonstrated to be useful to clarify the etiology of TMA [12]. Recent studies show that 20% of HUS patients have a familiar form of HUS [26], and 80% of TTP is triggered by deficient activity of ADAMTS13 [12]. Unfortunately, these data were only available in a minority of our patients.

11% of patients in our study died due to sepsis, hemorrhage, and acute myocardial infarction. This mortality rate is comparable to mortality rates previously published for this disorder [17,25,36]. We identified older age as a risk factor for death confirming results of Shiepatti and co-workers [24]. We did not observe any association between risk of death and blood pressure, CRP serum levels, LDH serum levels, Hb, WBC, thrombocytes, schistocytes, or creatinine serum levels on admission. Data published earlier suggested that low hemoglobin levels as well as high WBC were also associated with a higher risk of death [21]. In our study, we were not able to confirm these findings. This may reflect differences between patient subgroups in both studies.

For interpretation of this study some limitations should be taken into account. The study took place in a single hospital with a particular clientele of patients that might be different compared to hospitals in other regions or other countries. For example, we did not observe any HIV infections in our patient cohort. Furthermore, a single site investigation often presents data on only a limited number of cases.

In summary, we were able to identify parameters significantly correlated with unfavorable outcomes in TMA patients. High CRP serum levels and high blood pressure indicate a predisposition for ARF and persistent renal insufficiency. These parameters could help to detect TMA patients at risk for sustained kidney function impairment. Therapy of the underlying cause of CRP elevation as well as immediate and sufficient lowering of blood pressure may improve renal prognosis.

Acknowledgments

Michael Menges and Ivonne Theobald are gratefully acknowledged for valuable help on data transfer.

Author Contributions

Conceived and designed the experiments: CEK. Performed the experiments: FD. Analyzed the data: CEK KK NA. Wrote the paper: CEK. Critical revision of the manuscript and important intellectual contribution: CS MH GRH VB ST LCR TB BG.

References

1. Bell WR, Braine HG, Ness PM, Kickler TS (1991) Improved survival in thrombotic thrombocytopenic purpura-hemolytic uremic syndrome. Clinical experience in 108 patients. N Engl J Med 325: 398–403.
2. Remuzzi G, Ruggenenti P (1998) The hemolytic uremic syndrome. Kidney Int Suppl 66: S54–57.
3. Tsai HM (2003) Advances in the pathogenesis, diagnosis, and treatment of thrombotic thrombocytopenic purpura. J Am Soc Nephrol 14: 1072–1081.
4. Ruggenenti P, Remuzzi G (1998) Pathophysiology and management of thrombotic microangiopathies. J Nephrol 11: 300–310.
5. Mayer SA, Aledort LM (2005) Thrombotic microangiopathy: differential diagnosis, pathophysiology and therapeutic strategies. Mt Sinai J Med 72: 166–175.
6. Frank C, Werber D, Cramer JP, Askar M, Faber M, et al. (2011) Epidemic Profile of Shiga-Toxin-Producing Escherichia coli O104:H4 Outbreak in Germany - Preliminary Report. N Engl J Med.
7. Moake JL (2002) Thrombotic microangiopathies. N Engl J Med 347: 589–600.
8. Moake JL (2004) von Willebrand factor, ADAMTS-13, and thrombotic thrombocytopenic purpura. Semin Hematol 41: 4–14.
9. Terrell DR, Williams LA, Vesely SK, Lammle B, Hovinga JA, et al. (2005) The incidence of thrombotic thrombocytopenic purpura-hemolytic uremic syndrome: all patients, idiopathic patients, and patients with severe ADAMTS-13 deficiency. J Thromb Haemost 3: 1432–1436.
10. Zipfel PF, Misselwitz J, Licht C, Skerka C (2006) The role of defective complement control in hemolytic uremic syndrome. Semin Thromb Hemost 32: 146–154.
11. Kavanagh D, Goodship T (2011) Haemolytic uraemic syndrome. Nephron Clin Pract 118: c37–42.
12. Noris M, Bresin E, Mele C, Remuzzi G, Caprioli J (2007) Atypical Hemolytic-Uremic Syndrome. in: Pragon RA, Bird TC, Dolan CR, Stephens K, eds. GeneReviews. Seattle (WA): University of Washington, Seattle.
13. Noris M, Remuzzi G (2009) Atypical hemolytic-uremic syndrome. N Engl J Med 361: 1676–1687.
14. Nurnberger J, Philipp T, Witzke O, Opazo Saez A, Vester U, et al. (2009) Eculizumab for atypical hemolytic-uremic syndrome. N Engl J Med 360: 542–544.
15. Lapeyraque AL, Malina M, Fremeaux-Bacchi V, Boppel T, Kirschfink M, et al. (2011) Eculizumab in severe Shiga-toxin-associated HUS. N Engl J Med 364: 2561–2563.
16. Sadler JE, Moake JL, Miyata T, George JN (2004) Recent advances in thrombotic thrombocytopenic purpura. Hematology Am Soc Hematol Educ Program. pp 407–423.
17. Noris M, Remuzzi G (2005) Hemolytic uremic syndrome. J Am Soc Nephrol 16: 1035–1050.
18. Veyradier A, Obert B, Houllier A, Meyer D, Girma JP (2001) Specific von Willebrand factor-cleaving protease in thrombotic microangiopathies: a study of 111 cases. Blood 98: 1765–1772.
19. Wolf G (2004) Not known from ADAM(TS-13)-novel insights into the pathophysiology of thrombotic microangiopathies. Nephrol Dial Transplant 19: 1687–1693.
20. Coppo P, Bengoufa D, Veyradier A, Wolf M, Bussel A, et al. (2004) Severe ADAMTS13 deficiency in adult idiopathic thrombotic microangiopathies defines a subset of patients characterized by various autoimmune manifestations, lower platelet count, and mild renal involvement. Medicine (Baltimore) 83: 233–244.
21. Hollenbeck M, Kutkuhn B, Aul C, Leschke M, Willers R, et al. (1998) Haemolytic-uraemic syndrome and thrombotic-thrombocytopenic purpura in adults: clinical findings and prognostic factors for death and end-stage renal disease. Nephrol Dial Transplant 13: 76–81.
22. Egan JA, Hay SN, Brecher ME (2004) Frequency and significance of schistocytes in TTP/HUS patients at the discontinuation of plasma exchange therapy. J Clin Apher 19: 165–167.
23. Tostivint I, Mougenot B, Flahault A, Vigneau C, Costa MA, et al. (2002) Adult haemolytic and uraemic syndrome: causes and prognostic factors in the last decade. Nephrol Dial Transplant 17: 1228–1234.
24. Schieppati A, Ruggenenti P, Cornejo RP, Ferrario F, Gregorini G, et al. (1992) Renal function at hospital admission as a prognostic factor in adult hemolytic uremic syndrome. The Italian Registry of Haemolytic Uremic Syndrome. J Am Soc Nephrol 2: 1640–1644.
25. Matsumae T, Takebayashi S, Naito S (1996) The clinico-pathological characteristics and outcome in hemolytic-uremic syndrome of adults. Clin Nephrol 45: 153–162.
26. Zipfel PF, Wolf G, John U, Kentouche K, Skerka C (2011) Novel developments in thrombotic microangiopathies: is there a common link between hemolytic uremic syndrome and thrombotic thrombocytic purpura? Pediatr Nephrol.
27. Zipfel PF, Heinen S, Skerka C. Thrombotic microangiopathies: new insights and new challenges. Curr Opin Nephrol Hypertens 19: 372–378.
28. Neveu H, Kleinknecht D, Brivet F, Loirat P, Landais P (1996) Prognostic factors in acute renal failure due to sepsis. Results of a prospective multicentre study. The French Study Group on Acute Renal Failure. Nephrol Dial Transplant 11: 293–299.
29. Kamioka I, Yoshiya K, Satomura K, Kaito H, Fujita T, et al. (2008) Risk factors for developing severe clinical course in HUS patients: a national survey in Japan. Pediatr Int 50: 441–446.
30. Hashimoto K, Ikeda Y, Korenaga D, Tanoue K, Hamatake M, et al. (2005) The impact of preoperative serum C-reactive protein on the prognosis of patients with hepatocellular carcinoma. Cancer 103: 1856–1864.
31. Nakanishi H, Araki N, Kudawara I, Kuratsu S, Matsumine A, et al. (2002) Clinical implications of serum C-reactive protein levels in malignant fibrous histiocytoma. Int J Cancer 99: 167–170.
32. Iseki K, Tozawa M, Yoshi S, Fukiyama K (1999) Serum C-reactive protein (CRP) and risk of death in chronic dialysis patients. Nephrol Dial Transplant 14: 1956–1960.
33. Yeun JY, Levine RA, Mantadilok V, Kaysen GA (2000) C-Reactive protein predicts all-cause and cardiovascular mortality in hemodialysis patients. Am J Kidney Dis 35: 469–476.
34. Rao M, Jaber BL, Balakrishnan VS (2006) Inflammatory biomarkers and cardiovascular risk: association or cause and effect? Semin Dial 19: 129–135.
35. Mutluay R, Konca C, Erten Y, Pasaoglu H, Deger SM, et al. (2010) Predictive markers of asymptomatic atherosclerosis in end-stage renal disease patients. Ren Fail 32: 448–454.
36. Lara PN, Jr., Coe TL, Zhou H, Fernando L, Holland PV, et al. (1999) Improved survival with plasma exchange in patients with thrombotic thrombocytopenic purpura-hemolytic uremic syndrome. Am J Med 107: 573–579.

Inhibition of the Soluble Epoxide Hydrolase Promotes Albuminuria in Mice with Progressive Renal Disease

Oliver Jung[1,2], Felix Jansen[1], Anja Mieth[1], Eduardo Barbosa-Sicard[3], Rainer U. Pliquett[1,2], Andrea Babelova[1], Christophe Morisseau[4], Sung H. Hwang[4], Cindy Tsai[4], Bruce D. Hammock[4], Liliana Schaefer[5], Gerd Geisslinger[6], Kerstin Amann[7], Ralf P. Brandes[1]*

1 Institut für Kardiovaskuläre Physiologie, Fachbereich Medizin der Goethe-Universität, Frankfurt am Main, Germany, 2 Medizinische Klinik III, Klinikum der Goethe-Universität, Frankfurt am Main, Germany, 3 Institute for Vascular Signalling, Klinikum der Goethe-Universität, Frankfurt am Main, Germany, 4 Department of Entomology and Cancer Center, University of California Davis, Davis, California, United States of America, 5 Pharmazentrum Frankfurt/ZAFES/Institut für Allgemeine Pharmakologie, Klinikum der Goethe-Universität, Frankfurt am Main, Germany, 6 Pharmazentrum Frankfurt/ZAFES/Institut für Klinische Pharmakologie, Klinikum der Goethe-Universität, Frankfurt am Main, Germany, 7 Department of Pathology, Nephropathology, Friedrich-Alexander University, Erlangen-Nürnberg, Germany

Abstract

Epoxyeicotrienoic acids (EETs) are cytochrome P450-dependent anti-hypertensive and anti-inflammatory derivatives of arachidonic acid, which are highly abundant in the kidney and considered reno-protective. EETs are degraded by the enzyme soluble epoxide hydrolase (sEH) and sEH inhibitors are considered treatment for chronic renal failure (CRF). We determined whether sEH inhibition attenuates the progression of CRF in the 5/6-nephrectomy model (5/6-Nx) in mice. 5/6-Nx mice were treated with a placebo, an ACE-inhibitor (Ramipril, 40 mg/kg), the sEH-inhibitor cAUCB or the CYP-inhibitor fenbendazole for 8 weeks. 5/6-Nx induced hypertension, albuminuria, glomerulosclerosis and tubulo-interstitial damage and these effects were attenuated by Ramipril. In contrast, cAUCB failed to lower the blood pressure and albuminuria was more severe as compared to placebo. Plasma EET-levels were doubled in 5/6 Nx-mice as compared to sham mice receiving placebo. Renal sEH expression was attenuated in 5/6-Nx mice but cAUCB in these animals still further increased the EET-level. cAUCB also increased 5-HETE and 15-HETE, which derive from peroxidation or lipoxygenases. Similar to cAUCB, CYP450 inhibition increased HETEs and promoted albuminuria. Thus, sEH-inhibition failed to elicit protective effects in the 5/6-Nx model and showed a tendency to aggravate the disease. These effects might be consequence of a shift of arachidonic acid metabolism into the lipoxygenase pathway.

Editor: Carmine Zoccali, L' Istituto di Biomedicina ed Immunologia Molecolare, Consiglio Nazionale delle Ricerche, Italy

Funding: This study was supported by the Deutsche Forschungsgemeinschaft (BR1839/4-2 and SFB 423, Z2), the Exzellenzcluster 147 "Cardio-Pulmonary Systems", the Medical Faculty of the Goethe-University, the LOEWE Lipid Signaling Forschungszentrum Frankfurt (LiFF) and the National Institute of Environmental Health Sciences (grant R01 ER02710) and National Institutes of Health HL59699. The funders had no role in study design, data collection and analysis, decision to publish, or preparation of the manuscript.

Competing Interests: BDH is a George and Judy Marcus Senior Fellow of the American Asthma Foundation.

* E-mail: r.brandes@em.uni-frankfurt.de

Introduction

Epoxyeicosatrienoic acids (EETs) are anti-inflammatory derivatives of arachidonic acid (AA) which are generated by cytochrome P450 (CYP) epoxygenases [1]. EETs are antihypertensive, anti-inflammatory, anti-proliferative and pro-fibrinolytic. They act as an endothelium-derived hyperpolarizing factor (EDHF) in some vascular beds [1]. The CYP450 expression in the kidney is high and EETs promote renal sodium excretion [1,2]. EET levels are dependent on the activity and expression of the CYP epoxygenases, which generate them and the enzyme soluble epoxide hydrolase (sEH) which converts the EETs to their corresponding dihydroxyeicosatrienoic acids (DHETs) [3]. DHETs subsequently leave the cell, can be conjugated in the liver and be excreted by liver or kidney [2,4]. The activity of the sEH is therefore thought to be a major determinant of EET bioavailability [4]. Genetic deletion of the sEH as well as pharmacological inhibition increase plasma EET levels and potentiate their effects [5], and thus sEH inhibition elicits anti-hypertensive and anti-inflammatory effects [2,5,6]. Indeed, we have previously shown that sEH inhibition reduces angiotensin II-induced hypertension [7], neo-intima formation in hyperlipidemic mice [8] and vascular remodelling in the monocrotaline-model in rats [9].

Hypertension and inflammation are important progression factors for renal disease and thus it is logical to assume that sEH inhibition is a strategy to prevent progression of renal diseases [2,5]. Indeed, it has been demonstrated that sEH inhibition improves renal vascular function, decreased glomerular injury and renal inflammation in rat models of angiotensin-induced and DOCA-salt hypertension [10–12]. A main limitation of these models is however that their high inflammatory activity does not necessarily reflect the situation of chronic renal disease in man which is dominated by sclerotic and fibrotic processes and which is characterized by a progressive, self-perpetuating nature [13,14]. In animal experiments such a situation can be modelled by 5/6-nephrectomy (5/6-Nx). In this remnant kidney model, the substantial reduction in renal mass leads to compensatory renal hypertrophy, glomerula hyperfiltration and subsequently progressive chronic renal failure as consequence of glomerulo-sclerosis and interstitial fibrosis [15–17]. Although also in the remnant kidney model, the renin-angiotensin-system is involved in disease progression [18], it is only one of several factors contributing to a complex disease scenario.

Given the similarities between the remnant kidney model in rodents and the pathophysiology of progressive chronic renal failure in humans, we postulated that sEH inhibitors could be of therapeutic value. We tested this hypothesis in the rodent remnant kidney model. Unexpectedly and in contrast to previous data from inflammation driven renal failure models we observed that sEH inhibition had a tendency to accelerate the disease process in this model.

Methods

Animal preparations

SV129 which were purchased from Charles Rivers Laboratories (Sulzfeld, Germany) were used for this study, as other strains do not develop progressive renal failure mice [19]. Animals were housed in cages at constant temperature (22°C) and humidity (50%) and were exposed to a 12-hour dark/light cycle. Food and water were supplied ad libitum. The experiments were performed in accordance with the National Institutes of Health Guidelines on the Use of Laboratory Animals. Both, the University Animal Care Committee and the Federal Authorities for Animal Research of the Regierungspräsidium Darmstadt (Hessen, Germany) approved the study protocol (approval number V54-19c20/15-F28/05 and -F61/16). After 7 days of adaptation, the animals were randomly allocated to 5/6 nephrectomy (5/6-Nx) or sham operation. The surgery was performed under Isoflurane anaesthesia as previous described by others with modifications [19]. In brief: A left dorsal longitudinal incision was performed to expose the left kidney. The upper branch of the left renal artery was ligated by 6–0 prolene suture to produce about one third area with visible renal ischemia infarct; the lower pole of the left kidney (about one third kidney size) was removed by cautery. After 7 days of recovery, the right kidney was exposed in a similar preparation and removed after decapsulation and ligation of the vessels and the ureter to induce a total 5/6 nephrectomy (5/6-Nx). The control animals were sham operated in parallel by decapsulating the kidney. Early mortality within the first 3 days was approx. 20%. Subsequently, animals were randomized to the different treatment groups (n = 16 per group). The substances were administered as follows: The sEH inhibitor *cis*-4-[4-(3-adamantan-1-yl-ureido)-cyclohexyloxy]-benzoic acid (cAUCB, final concentration 8 mg/l), the ACE-inhibitor ramipril (final concentration 40 mg/l) were given with the drinking water, fenbendazole with the chow (100 mg/kg). Ramipril was kindly provided by Sanofi-Aventis, fenbendazole was from the university of Mainz (Zentrale Versuchstiereinheite - ZVTE) and cAUCB was synthesized by one of the coauthor as previously reported [20].

Blood pressure measurements

Systolic blood pressure was assessed at 4 and 8 weeks after initiation of treatment. By an automated tail-cuff Blood Pressure Monitor (Visitech) in conscious, trained mice at room temperature as reported previously [7]. In a subset of animals blood pressure measurements were confirmed by telemetry with the aid of the data science instruments (DSI) system with the catheter being placed in the right iliac artery.

Analysis of kidney function

Mice were placed in metabolic cages (Tecniplast) for 24-hour for urine collection. Urinary albumin was determined using the albumin-to-creatinine ratio (ACR). Urinary albumin and creati-

nine levels were measured by ELISA (Bethyl Laboratories, Montgomery, USA) and a creatinine assay kit (Labor+Technik, Berlin, Germany), respectively.

Histological analysis

After the induction of terminal anesthesia, the abdominal vessels were opened, the thoracic cavity was opened, a canula was inserted into the right ventricle and the animals were perfused with phosphate-buffered saline (PBS). After the perfusion, kidneys were removed and fixed with 4% paraformaldehyde/PBS solution. The samples were subsequently embedded in paraffin and 2-μm sections were cut and stained with haematoxylin/eosin (HE), periodic acid Schiff (PAS) and Sirius red (fibrous tissue stain). Thereafter, the stained kidney sections were analyzed by morphometry and stereology by investigations blinded to the study protocol. The following parameter were determined as reported previously [21]: To quantify mesangial matrix accumulation and sclerosis of the glomerular tuft, a score of 0 to 4 was determined on PAS and HE stained paraffin sections (GSI = Glomerulosclerosis index). A score of 0 was assigned for normal glomerulus, a score of 1 indicated mesangial expansion or sclerosis involving up to 25% of the glomerular tuft, a score of 2 indicated sclerosis of 25 to 50%, a score of 3 described sclerosis 50 to 75% and/or segmental extracapillary fibrosis or proliferation, and a score of 4 indicated global sclerosis >75%, global extracapillary fibrosis or complete collapse of the glomerular tuft.

The mesangiolysis score (MSI = Mesangiolysis index) was determined in PAS-stained paraffin sections and graded in 100 systematically subsampled glomeruli per animal using the following scoring system: score 0: no changes of capillaries, score 1: capillary dilatation <25% of the capillary convolute, score 2: capillary dilatation >25% of the capillary convolute or capillary aneurysms <50% of the capillary convolute, score 3: capillary aneurysms

Table 1. Primers for qRT-PCR.

ALOX5	forward	5'-CGGCTTCCCTTTGAGTATTGATGC-3'
	reverse	5'-CAGGAACTGGTAGCCAAACATGAG-3'
ALOX12	forward	5'-GGTTCTGCAACCTCATCACAGTTC -3'
	reverse	5'-CCAGCAGTAGGTCTGTTGTCTTTC -3'
ALOX15	forward	5'-GACACTTGGTGGCTGAGGTCTTTG-3'
	reverse	5'-GCTCCAGCTTGCTTGAGAAGATCC-3'
PLA2G4A	forward	5'-GTTCTACGTGCCACCAAAGTAACC-3'
	reverse	5'-TCCATGACGTAGTTGGCATCCATC-3'
Cyp2c38	forward	5'-CCCACTCCTTTCCCGATTAT-3'
	reverse	5'-CAGAAAACTCCTCCCCATGA-3'
	probe	5'-CY5-ATCAGAGCTTCCTTCACTGCTTCATCCCA-3'
Cyp2c40	forward	5'-AGGTCCAGCGGTACATTGAC-3'
	reverse	5'-CACAAATCCGTTTTCCTGCT-3'
	probe	5'-FAM-TTCATCCTCAAGGGAACACAGGTAA-3'
Cyp2c44	forward	5'-CAAAAAGGCTTGGTGGTGTT-3'
	reverse	5'-CCACAGATGGCCAAATTCTC-3'
	probe	5'-FAM-TTACATCGACTGTTTCCTCAGCAAGAT-3'
EEF2	forward	5'-GACATCACCAAGGGTGTGCAG-3'
	reverse	5'-GCGGTCAGCACACTGGCATA-3'
EPHX2	forward	5'-GAACATGAGTCGGACTTTCAAAAGCTTCTTC-3'
	reverse	5'-CCACAGTCCTCAATGTGTCCCCTTTTCAGG-3'

comprising 50–75% of the capillary convolute, score 4: capillary aneurysms comprising >75% of the capillary convolute [22].

Tubulointerstitial changes, i.e. tubular atrophy, dilatation, interstitial inflammation and interstitial fibrosis, and vascular damage, i.e. wall thickening and necrosis of the vessel wall, were assessed on HE stained paraffin sections as described at a magnification of 100× using a similar semi-quantitative scoring system from 0–4 [23]. In brief, for the determination of the tubulointerstitial damage, 10 fields per kidney were randomly sampled and graded as follows: grade 0 – normal tubulointerstitial structure; grade 1 – lesions involving less than 25% of the area; grade 2 – lesions affecting 25 to 50%; grade 3 – lesions involving more than 50% up to 75% and grade 4 with tubulointerstitial damage in almost the entire area (TSI = Tubulointerstitial damage index). Similarly, for the vascular damage score interlobular and smaller arteries were graded according to the following scheme: grade 0 – no wall thickening; grade 1, 2, 3 – mild, moderate and severe wall thickening, respectively; grade 4 – fibrinoid necrosis of the vascular wall.

Determination of Arachidonic acid metabolites by liquid chromatography/tandem mass spectrometry

Blood samples were collected at the end of the experiment. After coagulation and centrifugation, the serum was stored at −80°C.

At a later time point, samples were spiked with deuterated internal standards (5-HETE-d8, 12-HETE-d8, 15-HETE-d8, 20-HETE-d6, 8,9-EET-d8, 11,12-EET-d8 and 14,15-EET-d8) and extracted twice with ethyl acetate (0.5 ml). The sEH assay was extracted similarly but here one-tenth of organic phase was used and spiked. After evaporation of the ethyl acetate in a vacuum block under a gentle stream of nitrogen, the residues were reconstituted with 50 μl of methanol/water (1:1, v/v) and analyzed with a Sciex API4000 mass spectrometer (AME Bioscience, Toroed, Norway) operating in multiple reaction monitoring (MRM) mode as described in detail elsewhere [24]. Chromatographic separation was performed on a Gemini C18 column (150×2 mm inner diameter, 5 μm particle size, Phenomenex, Aschaffenburg, Germany).

Immunoblotting

Kidney samples were mortared in liquid nitrogen. For western blot analysis, cytosolic kidney protein (100 000 g supernatant, 20 μg) was boiled in Laemmli buffer, separated on sodium dodecyl sulfate–polyacrylamide gel electrophoresis (SDS–PAGE; 8%) and transferred onto nitrocellulose membrane as described (102). Proteins were detected using antibodies against sEH (provided by one of the coauthors) and glyceraldehyde 3-phosphate dehydrogenase (GAPDH/Santa

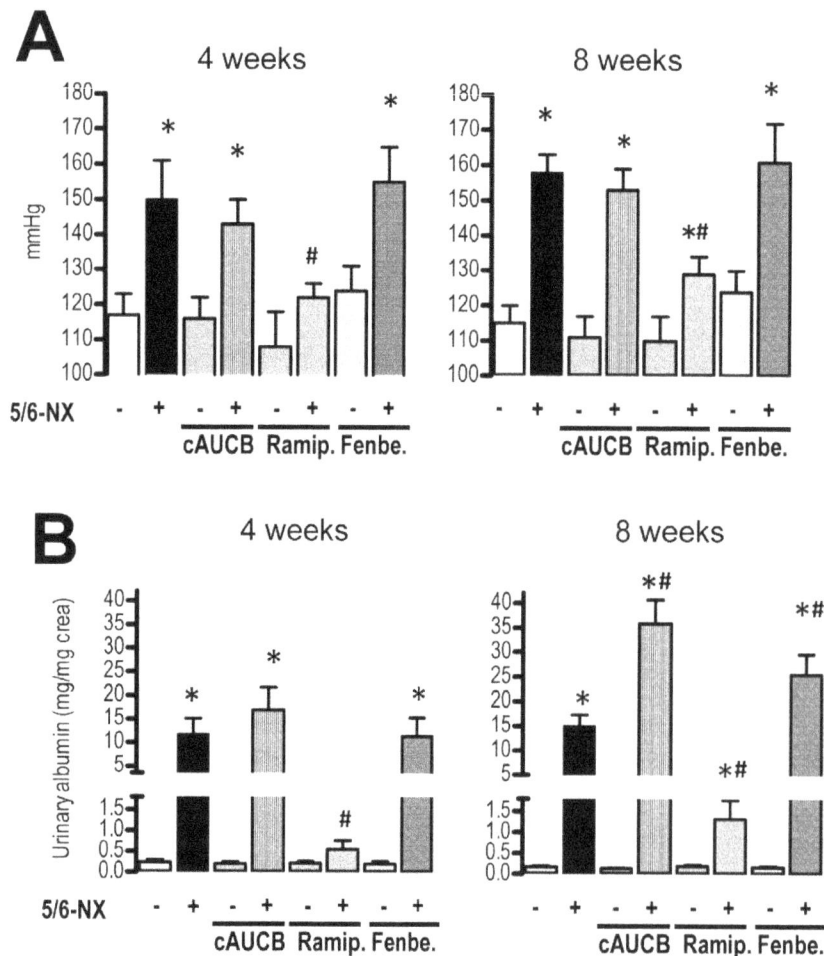

Figure 1. Blood pressure and albuminuria. Blood pressure measured by tail cuff technique (A) and albuminuria (B) were determined 4 and 8 weeks after initiation of treatment. Effects of placebo, sEH-inhibition by cAUCB, ACE-inhibition by ramipril (Ramip.) and CYP-inhibition by fenbendazole (Fenbe.) are shown on sham operated (−) and 5-6-Nx (+) animals. * p<0,05 vs. sham, # p<0,05 vs. placebo (n = 10–12/group).

Cruz Biotechnology, Santa Cruz, California, USA). Proteins were detected using appropriate secondary antibodies labeled with infrared dyes and visualized using the Odyssey infrared imaging system (Li-COR Biosciences, Bad Homburg, Germany) system. Densitometry was carried out using the integrated odyssey software.

Real-time quantitative reverse transcription PCR

Organs were removed, flash frozen in liquid nitrogen and disrupted by grounding with mortar and pestle. RNA isolation was done with Absolutely RNA Miniprep Kit (Stratagene), cDNA synthesis with SuperScript III Reverse Transcriptase (Invitrogen) and random hexamer primers, semiquantitative real-time PCR with ABsolute QPCR SYBR Green Mix and ROX as reference dye (Thermo Scientific) in Mx4000 (Stratagene) with appropriate primers. For primer sequences please see table 1. Relative expressions of target genes were normalized to eukaryotic translation elongation factor 2 (EEF2), analyzed by delta-delta-Ct method and given as percentage compared to control experiments. PCRs for Cyp2c genes were done without SYBR Green but with fluorescent labelled probes.

Data and statistical analysis

All values are mean ± SEM. Statistical analysis was performed using analysis of variance (ANOVA); ANOVA followed by Bonferroni-corrected Fisher's LSD test, respectively, or, wherever appropriate, using a paired or unpaired t-test. A P value less than 0.05 was considered statistically significant.

Results

sEH inhibition does not prevent hypertension development and augments proteinuria in the remnant kidney model

As compared to sham operated mice, 5/6-Nx induced systemic hypertension present 4 weeks after the operation ($p < 0.0.5$) that was maintained until the end of the observation period. Surprisingly, sEH-inhibition by cis-4-[4-(3-adamantan-1-yl-ur-cido)-cyclohexyloxy]-benzoic acid (cAUCB) had no effect on the development of hypertension, while ACE-inhibition by Ramipril significantly attenuated the process in 5/6-Nx mice at both time points (**Fig. 1A**). Tail-cuff measurements were verified by telemetry in a subset of animals (blood pressure in placebo treated animals: systolic blood pressure in sham-operated mice was 114 ± 9 mmHg after 4 weeks and 112 ± 4 mmHg after 8 weeks as compared to 169 ± 11 mmHg after 4 weeks and 168 ± 4 mmHg after 8 weeks in 5/6-Nx; diastolic blood pressure in sham-operated mice was 88 ± 8 mmHg after 4 weeks and 87 ± 5 mmHg after 8 weeks as compared to 128 ± 9 mmHg after 4 weeks and 125 ± 3 mmHg after 8 weeks in 5/6-Nx).

Albuminuria was determined after 4 and 8 weeks to assess renal damage (**Fig. 1B**). 5/6 nephrectomy induced marked albuminuria present at 4 weeks which was further increased 8 weeks after the operation. As expected, ACE-inhibition significantly attenuated the development of albuminuria. In contrast, sEH inhibition augmented albuminuria development in 5/6-Nx mice. While this effect was not statistically significant 4 weeks after operation,

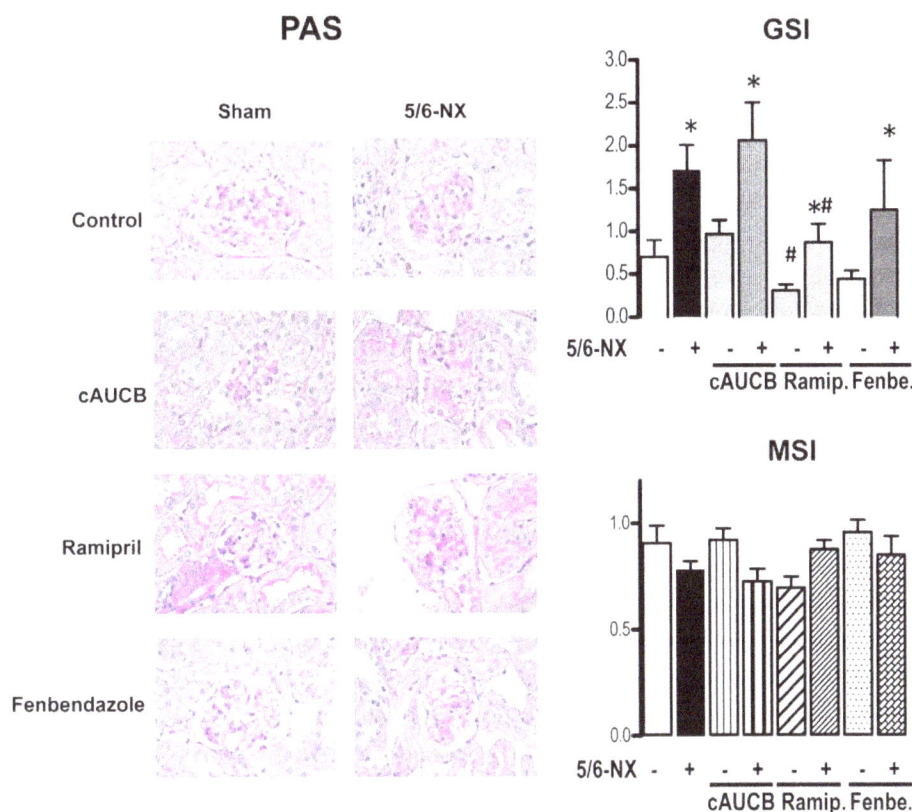

Figure 2. Histological glomerular changes. Representative kidney sections (magnification ×400) stained by periodide acid - Schiff (PAS) scoring glomerulosclerosis index (GSI) and mesangiolysis score (MSI) after 8 weeks of treatment. Effects of placebo, sEH-inhibition by cAUCB, ACE-inhibition by ramipril (Ramip.) and CYP-inhibition by fenbendazole (Fenbe.) are shown on sham operated (−) and 5-6-Nx (+) animals. * p<0,05 vs. sham, # p<0,05 vs. placebo (n = 5–8/group).

urinary albumin excretion after 8 weeks was 2-fold higher in the sEH inhibitor treated group as compared to placebo-treated animals ($p < 0.05$).

sEH inhibition does not prevent progression of renal damage

To determine the extent of renal damage, semi-quantitative analyses of renal damage scores were performed on histological sections of the whole kidney. 5/6 nephrectomy lead to a significant increase in glomerulosclerosis index (**Fig. 2**) and tubulo-interstitial damage index compared to sham operated animals (**Fig. 3**), while mesangiolysis index was comparable (**Fig. 2 und 3**). cAUCB

treatment had no effect on the development of glomerulosclerosis and tubulo-interstitial damage compared to the placebo treated group. In contrast, histological damage score was significantly lower in 5/6-Nx-mice receiving ramipril ($p < 0.05$). Accordingly, late mortality in mice subjected to ACE inhibition but not to the sEH inhibitor was significantly reduced as compared to placebo-treated animals (**Fig. 4**).

EET plasma level are elevated in the 5/6-Nx model

In order to determine whether or not a possible shortage of basal EET formation after 5/6-Nx underlies the failure of sEH inhibitors to interfere with disease progression, plasma levels were

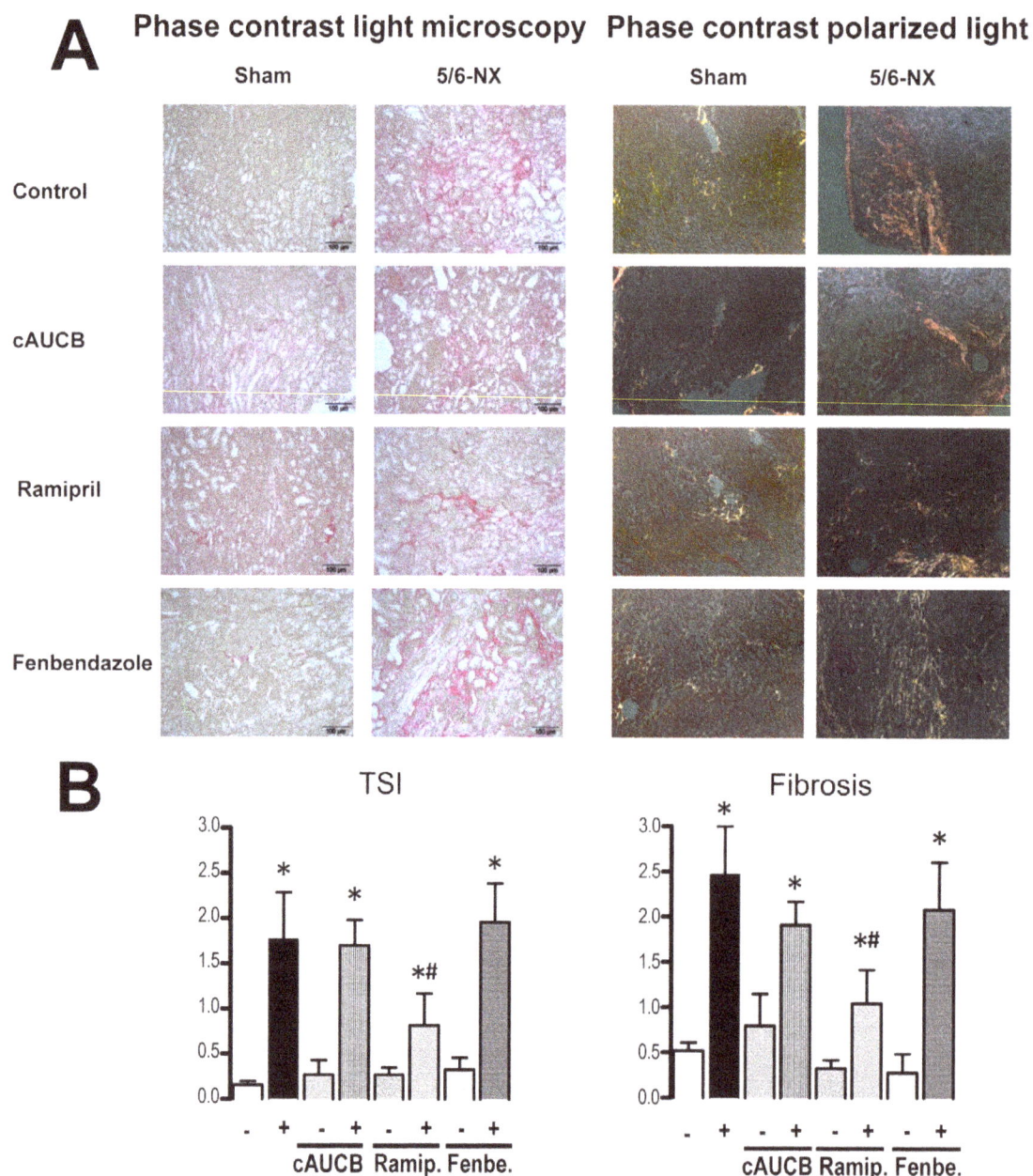

Figure 3. Histological tubulointerstitial changes. Representative kidney sections (magnification ×100) stained by Sirius Red in phase contrast light microscopy and polarized light microscopy scoring tubulointerstitial damage index (TSI) and interstitial fibrosis after 8 weeks of treatment. Effects of placebo, sEH-inhibition by cAUCB, ACE-inhibition by ramipril (Ramip.) and CYP-inhibition by fenbendazole (Fenbe.) are shown on sham operated (−) and 5-6-Nx (+) animals. * $p < 0,05$ vs. sham, # $p < 0,05$ vs. placebo (n = 5–8/group). The scale bar denotes 100 μmeter.

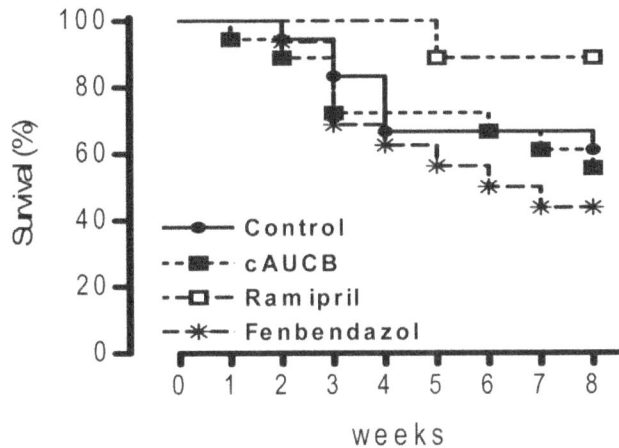

Figure 4. Survival data. Kaplan-Meier survival curves after 5/6-Nx in mice receiving the treatment indicated. n = 16, Survial was significantly better only in mice receiving ramipril.

measured. Animals subjected to 5/6-Nx presented with significantly increased EET plasma levels as shown for 11,12-EET (**Fig. 5**). This effect was equally strong as the increase of EETs in response to sEH inhibition by cAUCB in sham animals. Although EET levels were already elevated in 5/6-Nx mice, sEH-inhibition by cAUCB in 5/6-Nx- animals further increased the EET-levels (**Fig. 5**). ACE-inhibitor therapy had no effect on EET plasma levels (data not shown). Similar effects were seen for 5,6-EET, 8,9-EET and 14,15-EET (data not shown). No significant effects were seen on DHET plasma levels excluding product inhibition of sEH as a possible mechanism for EET accumulation in chronic renal failure. The latter observation suggest that renal function is not a limiting factor for DHET excretion and my suggest that these lipids are, potentially after conjugation in the liver, excreted via the bile.

In order to determine whether changes in EET production underlie the effects observed, the renal expression of sPLA2, sEH and CYP450 enzymes was determined. Whereas the expression of Cyp2c40 and 2c38 was unaffected by 5/6-Nx, sPLA$_2$-mRNA expression was increased, suggesting a possible enhanced supply of

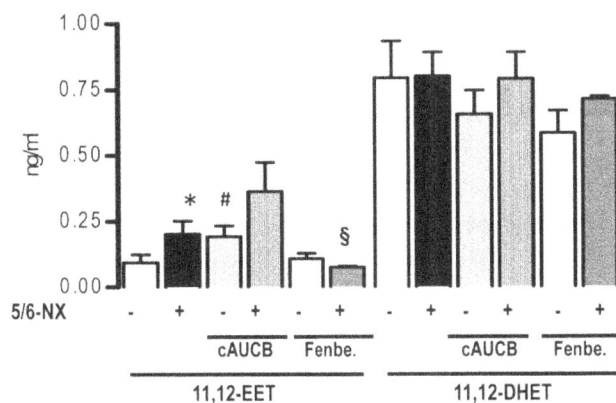

Figure 5. EET plasma level. 11,12-EET and 11,12-DHET plasma levels 8 weeks after initiation of treatment. Effects of placebo, sEH-inhibition by cAUCB, and CYP-inhibition by fenbendazole (Fenbe.) are shown on sham operated (−) and 5-6-Nx (+) animals. * p<0,05 vs. sham, # p<0,05 vs. placebo, § p<0.05 vs. placebo and cAUCB (n = 5–8/group).

CYP450-enzymes with arachidonic acid (**Fig. 6A**). Interestingly, 5/6-Nx also resulted in a marked decrease in the renal expression of the sEH on the protein, as well as on the mRNA level (**Fig. 6B**). This observation may suggest that in the diseased kidney local effects of sEH inhibitors are less pronounced than it could be assumed from the changes in plasma EET level. It also indicates that the renal sEH, although highly expressed in the kidney, only has a minor contribution to the systemic turnover of EETs.

Inhibition of sEH and 5/6-Nx results in increased plasma level of lipoxygenase products

To further elucidate the lack of beneficial effects of sEH inhibition on the progression of chronic renal failure, we investigated the pro-inflammatory lipoxygenase system. 5/6-Nx had no significant effect on the renal expression of 5-Lox and 12-Lox, whereas a trend towards increased expression of 15-Lox was observed. (**Fig. 6C**) Although this did not reach statistical significance, 15-HETE plasma levels were the only lipoxygenase products which were significantly higher in the plasma of mice after 5/6-Nx receiving placebo treatment (**Fig. 7**). Interestingly, this lipoxygenase product was also increased in mice receiving sEH-inhibitor treatment and this effect was additive leading to more than 4-fold higher plasma levels in 5/6-Nx under sEH inhibitor treatment as compared to control animals not receiving treatment. Also 5-HETE was increased in 5/6-Nx mice on sEH-inhibitor treatment. In contrast, 12-HETE and the Cyp450a4-product 20-HETE were unaffected in this scenario, excluding that unspecific accumulation of lipid peroxides are responsible for the effects observed. 5-HETE and 12-HETE levels were decreased under ACE inhibitor treatment, but ACE inhibition had no effect on 15-HETE and 20 HETE levels.

Inhibition of the CYP450 pathway in 5/6-Nx results in accumulation of lipoxygenase products

A possible explanation for the effects on the pro-inflammatory hydroxylipids is that high levels of EETs shift arachidonic acid into the LOX pathways. In order to test this hypothesis, we treated a subgroup of mice with the unspecific CYP450 inhibitor fenbendazole. Fenbendazole was effective in inhibiting CYP as demonstrated by decreased 11,12-EET (**Fig. 5**) and 20-HETE plasma levels (**Fig. 7**). Importantly, the compound had a similar effect on the progression of renal failure in 5/6-Nx mice as the sEH inhibitor: It did not affect blood pressure (**Fig. 1A**) or histological lesion scores (**Fig. 2 and 3**) but significantly increased albuminuria after 8 weeks of treatment in 5/6-Nx mice (**Fig. 1B**). Moreover, fenbendazole basically increased all lipoxygenase products measured in this study, demonstrating that under CYP-inhibition substantial amounts of AA are shifted into the lipoxygenase pathway (**Fig. 7**).

Discussion

In this study, we determined the impact of sEH inhibition on the progression of renal failure in mice subjected to the 5/6-Nx model. In contrast to our expectations, sEH inhibition did not delay disease progression but rather resulted in an increase in albuminuria. sEH inhibition increased some lipoxygenase products and resulted in similar changes as observed with the broad-spectrum CYP450 inhibitor fenbendazole. These findings may suggest that EETs are less important in protecting the kidney than initially anticipated but that increased formation of lipoxygenase products by shifting of arachidonic acid from the CYP450 pathway into the LOX pathway might be important for the progression of the disease.

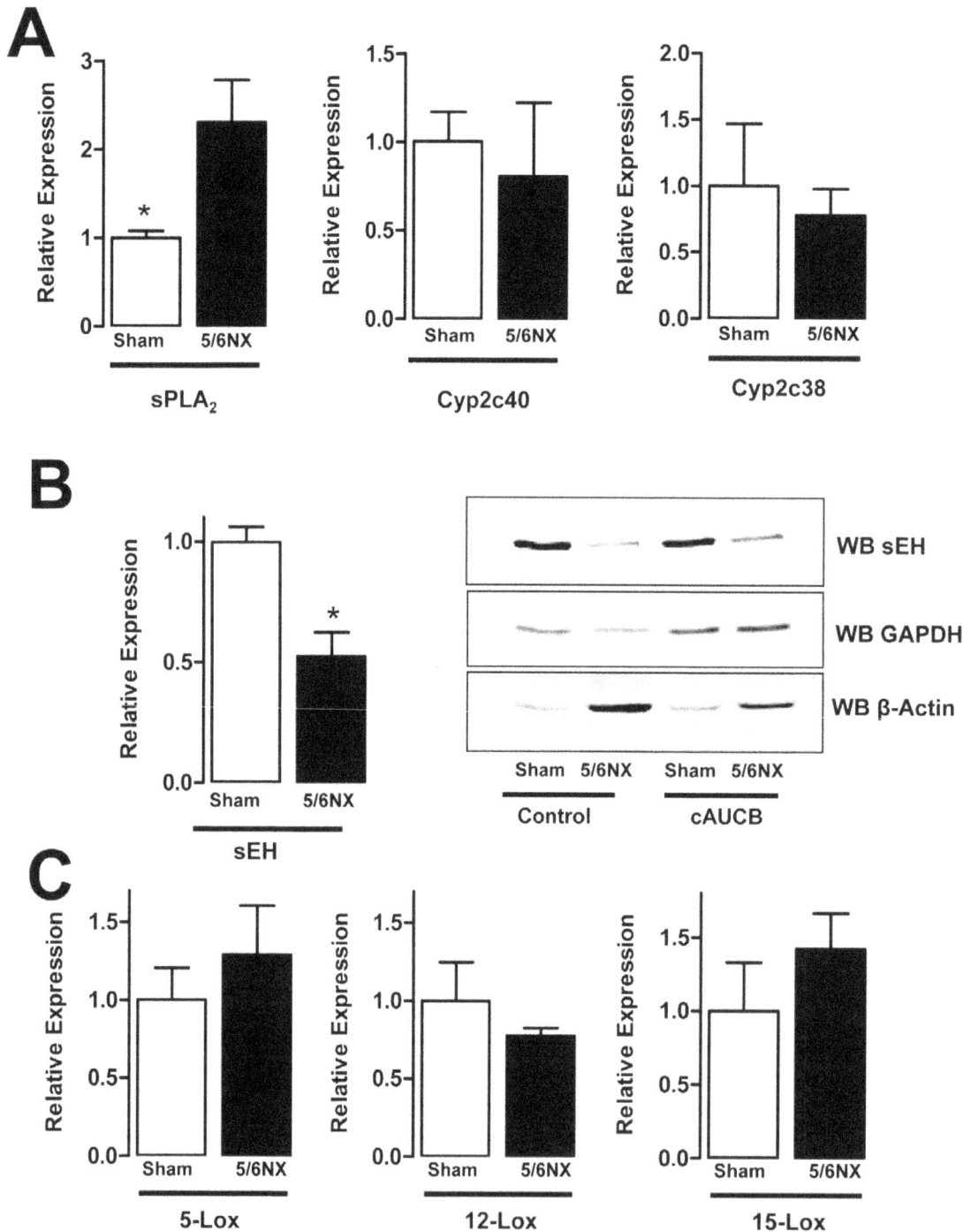

Figure 6. mRNA expression of arachidonic acid metabolizing enzymes. Relative mRNA expression (2^-ΔΔCT) determined by realtime RT-PCR for the factors indicate and representative sEH Western blot (WB sEH) from the kidney of sham operated and 5/6-Nx mice at the end of the study. A: Determination of EET-producing systems, B: qRT-PCR and Western blot for sEH. GAPDH and β-actin were used as loading control for the Western blots. C: Expression of Lox enzymes on the RNA level. n = 6, *p<0.05.

One important progression factor of chronic renal disease is hypertension. The antihypertensive effect of sEH inhibition has been demonstrated in numerous rat and mouse models, like spontaneously hypertensive rats, angiotensin II-induced hypertension and DOCA and salt-induced and salt-sensitive hypertension [7,11,25,26]. The antihypertensive effect was mediated by a decrease in vascular resistance and enhanced renal Na⁺ excretion

[2,7,10,11], and all these resemble biological effects of EETs [25,27,28].

In contrast to these observations, in the present study, sEH inhibition had no effect on blood pressure in 5/6-Nx mice. The pathogenesis of hypertension in chronic renal failure is however complex: In addition to an activation of the renin angiotensin system (RAS), sodium and water retention and thus increased

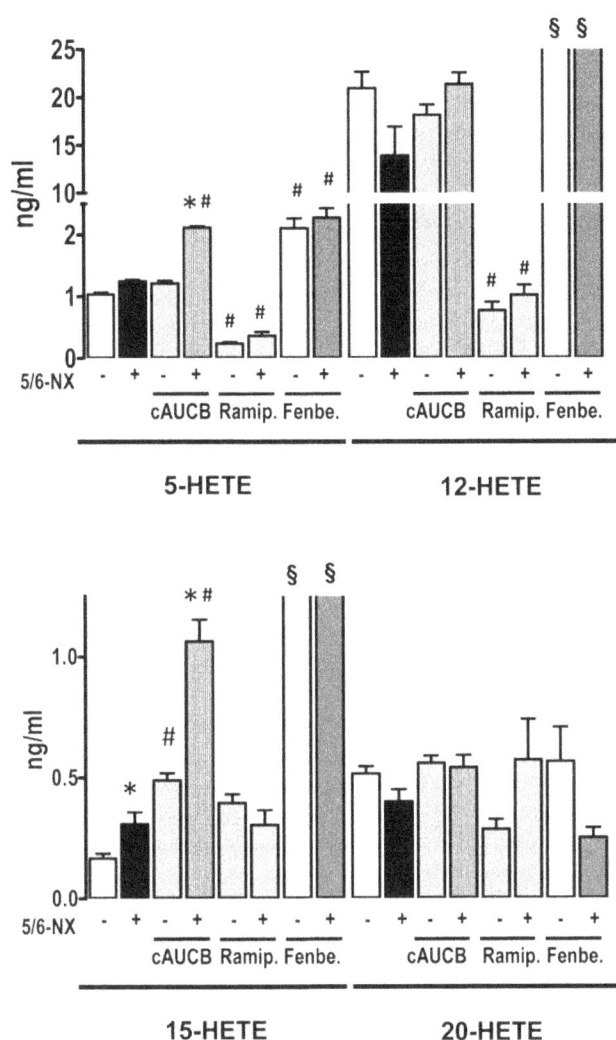

Figure 7. Plasma levels of hydroxyeicosatetraenoic (HETE) acids. Plasma level of 5-HETE, 12-HETE, 15-HETE and 20-HETE as determined by LC-MS/MS 8 weeks after initiation of treatment. Effects of placebo, sEH-inhibition by cAUCB, ACE-inhibition by ramipril (Ramip.) and CYP-inhibition by fenbendazole (Fenbe.) are shown on sham operated (−) and 5-6-Nx (+) animals. * $p < 0.05$ vs. sham, # $p < 0.05$ vs. placebo, § $p < 0.05$ vs. placebo all groups (n = 5–8/group).

As one would expect, sEH inhibition-mediated lowering in blood pressure exerts reno-protective effects in models of hypertensive kidney injury [10–12]. In hypertensive models in which sEH inhibitors failed to lower the blood pressure this reno-protective effect was observed, too [32,35]. Also the acute renal injury by the tubulotoxic chemotheraptic agent cisplatin was attenuated by sEH inhibitors [36]. The latter three studies had in common that sEH inhibition lowered several markers of inflammation, another progression factor for renal disease.

The data of the present study demonstrated that sEH inhibition in 5/6-Nx rather increased than decreased disease progression. In keeping with a possible role of inflammation, we could demonstrate that lipoxygenase products, particularly of the 15-LOX pathway, but also of the 5-LOX pathway accumulated in 5/6-Nx mice treated with sEH inhibitors. The biological effects of the two LOX enzymes differ to some extent. 5-LOX is considered pro-inflammatory in general [37] and 5-LOX inhibitors exerted reno-protective effects [38]. 15-LOX in contrast, not only generates pro-inflammatory lipids but 15-HETE is further metabolized to lipoxins, which have strong anti-inflammatory properties [39]. On the other hand, inhibition of 15-LOX had beneficial effects on diabetic models [40] or renal injury and mesangial cells of 12/15-LOX knockout mice had a reduced level of activation after stimulation, which was associated with reduced matrix production [41]. Indeed, it is important to remember that chronic progressive renal failure is a complex disease with a strong fibrotic contribution. Interestingly, a strong positive interplay exists between 15-LOX-products and the pro-fibrotic transforming growth factor β (TGF β)-pathway [42]. One limitation of all these studies, however, is that they are predominantly performed in glomerular cells or culture and that therefore the role of LOX for tubulo-interstitial fibrosis has to remain unclear. Thus, also a limitation of the present study is that we did not determine the effect of sEH inhibition in animals lacking LOX activity and therefore we cannot provide definite proof for an involvement of LOX in the progression of renal failure after sEH inhibitor treatment.

A potential explanation for the observations of the present study is that sEH inhibition shifted arachidonic acid from the CYP450 pathway into the LOX pathway. That such shifting occurs is well known for COX inhibitors and the basis of NSAIDS-induced asthma [43]. Direct inhibition of CYP450 with the compound fenbendazole [44] also increased the products of the LOX pathway, demonstrating that shifting of arachidonic acid also from the CYP450 pathway can occur. Given the low plasma concentrations of EETs, it is however difficult to imagine that the somewhat modest increase in response to sEH inhibition or renal failure is sufficient to induce a significant product inhibition of the CYP enzymes, although other observations supporting the complex crosstalk have been published for inflammatory models [45]. An alternative explanation could therefore be that the increase in sPLA₂ mRNA observed in this study results to in overall increase in all arachidonic acid pathways. Unfortunately, the amount of plasma samples obtained in the course of this study did not allow us to analyze the lipidom in more detail to further clarify this point. We therefore also did not measure the different enantiomers of the HETEs to definitely prove that the increase of this hydroxylipids is a consequence of the action of LOX and not of lipid peroxidation.

In this study we observed that the sEH expression decreases during progressive renal failure. As this effect occurred on the message as well as on the protein level, it is unlikely that changes in the matrix composition which occur during the fibrotic remodeling of the kidney could account for this observation. Interest-

cardiac output contribute to the situation [13,14,29]. The contribution of RAS to the hypertension thereby is not easy to estimate. Although the ACE inhibitor ramipril prevented the development of hypertension in the present study, it also interfered with disease progression, making it highly probable that also sodium and water retention were reduced by ramipril [30]. Moreover, the compound had a natriuretic effect on its own and promotes sodium excretion by multiple ways.

It should also be mentioned that the antihypertensive effect of sEH inhibitors is model dependent and not observed in stroke prone SHR [31] and Goto-Kakizaki rats [32] and of a variable degree in the different strains of SHR [31,33,34]. Also conflicting results have been published in sEH $^{-/-}$ mice, in which the antihypertensive effect was lost after backcrossing on the C57/BL6 background [12,30,35]. Although blood pressure lowering effects of sEH inhibition depend on their vasodilative and natriuretic effects, it is also possible that the renal dysfunction after 5/6-Nx [29] attenuates the efficacy of sEH inhibition on blood pressure.

ingly, also in the lung we previously observed that fibrosis occurring during pulmonary hypertension reduced the sEH expression [9] suggesting that this effect is more important than the previously reported induction of sEH by angiotensin II [46]. The fact that the relative increase in plasma EET level were similar between normal mice and those in renal failure suggest that the renal sEH contributes little to the EET plasma level. The increase in EET plasma level in response to 5/6-Nx is either a consequence of a reduced renal excretion or of a greater formation of EET under this condition.

Independently of the mechanism of increased EET plasma level, the present study demonstrates that lowering sEH activity is not necessarily beneficial. Importantly, this notion is also supported by data on human polymorphisms: In kidney transplanted patients a gene polymorphism leading to reduced sEH activity was linked to allograft dysfunction and decreased graft survival [47].

In conclusion, in the present study we demonstrate that sEH inhibition rather promotes than delays the progression of chronic renal failure in mice. As a possible mechanism we suggest the accumulation of inflammatory lipoxygenase products. Thus, chronic renal failure as a possible drug target for sEH inhibitors should be reconsidered.

Acknowledgments

We are grateful for the excellent technical assistance of Susanne Schütz, Sina Bätz and Miriam Reutelshöfer.

Author Contributions

Conceived and designed the experiments: OJ CM BH RPB. Performed the experiments: OJ FJ AM EBS RUP AB CT LS KA. Analyzed the data: FJ AM EBS RUP CT LS KA RPB. Contributed reagents/materials/analysis tools: CM SHH BH GG. Wrote the paper: OJ BH RPB.

References

1. Fleming I (2008) Vascular cytochrome p450 enzymes: physiology and pathophysiology. Trends Cardiovasc Med 18: 20–25.
2. Imig JD, Navar LG, Roman RJ, Reddy KK, Falck JR (1996) Actions of epoxygenase metabolites on the preglomerular vasculature. J Am Soc Nephrol 7: 2364–2370.
3. Arand M, Cronin A, Adamska M, Oesch F (2005) Epoxide hydrolases: structure, function, mechanism, and assay. Methods Enzymol 400: 569–588.
4. Yu Z, Xu F, Huse LM, Morisseau C, Draper AJ, et al. (2000) Soluble epoxide hydrolase regulates hydrolysis of vasoactive epoxyeicosatrienoic acids. Circ Res 87: 992–998.
5. Chiamvimonvat N, Ho CM, Tsai HJ, Hammock BD (2007) The soluble epoxide hydrolase as a pharmaceutical target for hypertension. J Cardiovasc Pharmacol 50: 225–237.
6. Revermann M (2010) Pharmacological inhibition of the soluble epoxide hydrolase-from mouse to man. Curr Opin Pharmacol 10: 173–178.
7. Jung O, Brandes RP, Kim IH, Schweda F, Schmidt R, et al. (2005) Soluble epoxide hydrolase is a main effector of angiotensin II-induced hypertension. Hypertension 45: 759–765.
8. Revermann M, Schloss M, Barbosa-Sicard E, Mieth A, Liebner S, et al. (2010) Soluble Epoxide Hydrolase Deficiency Attenuates Neointima Formation in the Femoral Cuff Model of Hyperlipidemic Mice. Arterioscler Thromb Vasc Biol 30: 909–914.
9. Revermann M, Barbosa-Sicard E, Dony E, Schermuly RT, Morisseau C, et al. (2009) Inhibition of the soluble epoxide hydrolase attenuates monocrotaline-induced pulmonary hypertension in rats. J Hypertens 27: 322–331.
10. Zhao X, Yamamoto T, Newman JW, Kim IH, Watanabe T, et al. (2004) Soluble epoxide hydrolase inhibition protects the kidney from hypertension-induced damage. J Am Soc Nephrol 15: 1244–1253.
11. Imig JD, Zhao X, Zaharis CZ, Olearczyk JJ, Pollock DM, et al. (2005) An orally active epoxide hydrolase inhibitor lowers blood pressure and provides renal protection in salt-sensitive hypertension. Hypertension 46: 975–981.
12. Manhiani M, Quigley JE, Knight SF, Tasoobshirazi S, Moore T, et al. (2009) Soluble epoxide hydrolase gene deletion attenuates renal injury and inflammation with DOCA-salt hypertension. Am J Physiol Renal Physiol 297: F740–F748.
13. Klahr S, Morrissey J (2003) Progression of chronic renal disease. Am J Kidney Dis 41: S3–S7.
14. Yu HT (2003) Progression of chronic renal failure. Arch Intern Med 163: 1417–1429.
15. Shimamura T, Morrison AB (1975) A progressive glomerulosclerosis occurring in partial five-sixths nephrectomized rats. Am J Pathol 79: 95–106.
16. Anderson S, Meyer TW, Rennke HG, Brenner BM (1985) Control of glomerular hypertension limits glomerular injury in rats with reduced renal mass. J Clin Invest 76: 612–619.
17. Griffin KA, Picken M, Bidani AK (1994) Method of renal mass reduction is a critical modulator of subsequent hypertension and glomerular injury. J Am Soc Nephrol 4: 2023–2031.
18. Ibrahim HN, Hostetter TH (1998) The renin-aldosterone axis in two models of reduced renal mass in the rat. J Am Soc Nephrol 9: 72–76.
19. Ma LJ, Fogo AB (2003) Model of robust induction of glomerulosclerosis in mice: importance of genetic background. Kidney Int 64: 350–355.
20. Hwang SH, Tsai HJ, Liu JY, Morisseau C, Hammock BD (2007) Orally bioavailable potent soluble epoxide hydrolase inhibitors. J Med Chem 50: 3825–3840.
21. Haas CS, Amann K, Schittny J, Blaser B, Muller U, et al. (2003) Glomerular and renal vascular structural changes in alpha8 integrin-deficient mice. J Am Soc Nephrol 14: 2288–2296.

22. Dimmler A, Haas CS, Cho S, Hattler M, Forster C, et al. (2003) Laser capture microdissection and real-time PCR for analysis of glomerular endothelin-1 gene expression in mesangiolysis of rat anti-Thy 1.1 and murine Habu Snake Venom glomerulonephritis. Diagn Mol Pathol 12: 108–117.
23. Veniant M, Heudes D, Clozel JP, Bruneval P, Menard J (1994) Calcium blockade versus ACE inhibition in clipped and unclipped kidneys of 2K-1C rats. Kidney Int 46: 421–429.
24. Michaelis UR, Fisslthaler B, Barbosa-Sicard E, Falck JR, Fleming I, et al. (2005) Cytochrome P450 epoxygenases 2C8 and 2C9 are implicated in hypoxia-induced endothelial cell migration and angiogenesis. J Cell Sci 118: 5489–5498.
25. Imig JD (2005) Epoxide hydrolase and epoxygenase metabolites as therapeutic targets for renal diseases. Am J Physiol Renal Physiol 289: F496–F503.
26. Loch D, Hoey A, Morisseau C, Hammock BO, Brown L (2007) Prevention of hypertension in DOCA-salt rats by an inhibitor of soluble epoxide hydrolase. Cell Biochem Biophys 47: 87–98.
27. Capdevila JH, Falck JR (2001) The CYP P450 arachidonic acid monooxygen-ases: from cell signaling to blood pressure regulation. Biochem Biophys Res Commun 285: 571–576.
28. Moreno C, Maier KG, Hoagland KM, Yu M, Roman RJ (2001) Abnormal pressure-natriuresis in hypertension: role of cytochrome P450 metabolites of arachidonic acid. Am J Hypertens 14: 90S–97S.
29. Chamberlain RM, Shirley DG (2007) Time course of the renal functional response to partial nephrectomy: measurements in conscious rats. Exp Physiol 92: 251–262.
30. Chiurchiu C, Remuzzi G, Ruggenenti P (2005) Angiotensin-converting enzyme inhibition and renal protection in nondiabetic patients: the data of the meta-analyses. J Am Soc Nephrol 16 Suppl 1: S58–S63.
31. Dorrance AM, Rupp N, Pollock DM, Newman JW, Hammock BD, et al. (2005) An epoxide hydrolase inhibitor, 12-(3-adamantan-1-yl-ureido)dodecanoic acid (AUDA), reduces ischemic cerebral infarct size in stroke-prone spontaneously hypertensive rats. J Cardiovasc Pharmacol 46: 842–848.
32. Olearczyk JJ, Quigley JE, Mitchell BC, Yamamoto T, Kim IH, et al. (2009) Administration of a substituted adamantyl urea inhibitor of soluble epoxide hydrolase protects the kidney from damage in hypertensive Goto-Kakizaki rats. Clin Sci (Lond) 116: 61–70.
33. Fornage M, Hinojos CA, Nurowska BW, Boerwinkle E, Hammock BD, et al. (2002) Polymorphism in soluble epoxide hydrolase and blood pressure in spontaneously hypertensive rats. Hypertension 40: 485–490.
34. Simpkins AN, Rudic RD, Schreihofer DA, Roy S, Manhiani M, et al. (2009) Soluble epoxide inhibition is protective against cerebral ischemia via vascular and neural protection. Am J Pathol 174: 2086–2095.
35. Sinal CJ, Miyata M, Tohkin M, Nagata K, Bend JR, et al. (2000) Targeted disruption of soluble epoxide hydrolase reveals a role in blood pressure regulation. J Biol Chem 275: 40504–40510.
36. Parrish AR, Chen G, Burghardt RC, Watanabe T, Morisseau C, et al. (2009) Attenuation of cisplatin nephrotoxicity by inhibition of soluble epoxide hydrolase. Cell Biol Toxicol 25: 217–225.
37. Hao CM, Breyer MD (2007) Physiological and pathophysiologic roles of lipid mediators in the kidney. Kidney Int 71: 1105–1115.
38. Guasch A, Zayas CF, Badr KF (1999) MK-591 acutely restores glomerular size selectivity and reduces proteinuria in human glomerulonephritis. Kidney Int 56: 261–267.
39. Ryan A, Godson C (2010) Lipoxins: regulators of resolution. Curr Opin Pharmacol 10: 166–172.
40. Ma J, Natarajan R, LaPage J, Lanting L, Kim N, et al. (2005) 12/15-lipoxygenase inhibitors in diabetic nephropathy in the rat. Prostaglandins Leukot Essent Fatty Acids 72: 13–20.

41. Kim YS, Reddy MA, Lanting L, Adler SG, Natarajan R (2003) Differential behavior of mesangial cells derived from 12/15-lipoxygenase knockout mice relative to control mice. Kidney Int 64: 1702–1714.

42. Kim YS, Xu ZG, Reddy MA, Li SL, Lanting L, et al. (2005) Novel interactions between TGF-{beta}1 actions and the 12/15-lipoxygenase pathway in mesangial cells. J Am Soc Nephrol 16: 352–362.

43. Hamad AM, Sutcliffe AM, Knox AJ (2004) Aspirin-induced asthma: clinical aspects, pathogenesis and management. Drugs 64: 2417–2432.

44. Keseru B, Barbosa-Sicard E, Popp R, Fisslthaler B, Dietrich A, et al. (2008) Epoxyeicosatrienoic acids and the soluble epoxide hydrolase are determinants of pulmonary artery pressure and the acute hypoxic pulmonary vasoconstrictor response. FASEB J 22: 4306–4315.

45. Liu JY, Yang J, Inceoglu B, Qiu H, Ulu A, et al. (2010) Inhibition of soluble epoxide hydrolase enhances the anti-inflammatory effects of aspirin and 5-lipoxygenase activation protein inhibitor in a murine model. Biochem Pharmacol 79: 880–887.

46. Ai D, Fu Y, Guo D, Tanaka H, Wang N, et al. (2007) Angiotensin II up-regulates soluble epoxide hydrolase in vascular endothelium in vitro and in vivo. Proc Natl Acad Sci U S A 104: 9018–9023.

47. Lee SH, Lee J, Cha R, Park MH, Ha JW, et al. (2008) Genetic variations in soluble epoxide hydrolase and graft function in kidney transplantation. Transplant Proc 40: 1353–1356.

11

Potassium and the Excitability Properties of Normal Human Motor Axons *In Vivo*

Delphine Boërio[1], Hugh Bostock[1,2]*, Romana Spescha[1], Werner J. Z'Graggen[1,3]

1 Department of Neurology, Inselspital, Bern University Hospital and University of Bern, Bern, Switzerland, **2** Sobell Department of Motor Neuroscience and Movement Disorders, Institute of Neurology, University College London, London, United Kingdom, **3** Department of Neurosurgery, Inselspital, Bern University Hospital and University of Bern, Bern, Switzerland

Abstract

Hyperkalemia is an important cause of membrane depolarization in renal failure. A recent theoretical model of axonal excitability explains the effects of potassium on threshold electrotonus, but predicts changes in superexcitability in the opposite direction to those observed. To resolve this contradiction we assessed the relationship between serum potassium and motor axon excitability properties in 38 volunteers with normal potassium levels. Most threshold electrotonus measures were strongly correlated with potassium, and superexcitability decreased at higher potassium levels ($P = 0.016$), contrary to the existing model. Improved modelling of potassium effects was achieved by making the potassium currents obey the constant-field theory, and by making the potassium permeabilities proportional to external potassium, as has been observed *in vitro*. This new model also accounted well for the changes in superexcitability and other excitability measures previously reported in renal failure. These results demonstrate the importance of taking potassium levels into account when assessing axonal membrane dysfunction by excitability testing, and provide evidence that potassium currents are activated by external potassium *in vivo*.

Editor: Steven Barnes, Dalhousie University, Canada

Funding: This study was supported by a grant of the Swiss National Science Foundation (320030_125160/1) (http://www.snf.ch) to W.J.Z. The funders had no role in study design, data collection and analysis, decision to publish, or preparation of the manuscript.

* E-mail: H.Bostock@ucl.ac.uk

Introduction

Nerve excitability tests [1,2] have been increasingly applied in clinical neurophysiology to assess the excitability properties of motor axons, and to infer likely underlying changes in membrane properties (*e.g.* membrane potential and ion channel functions)[3–6]. Recent clinical applications include prediction of survival in amyotrophic lateral sclerosis [7] and early warning of chemotherapy-induced neurotoxicity [8], but an early and continuing contribution has been towards the understanding and possible prevention of uraemic neuropathy. The pathophysiological basis of uraemic neuropathy is not well understood, and unidentified neurotoxic factors have been blamed, but nerve excitability studies have provided evidence that peripheral nerves are chronically depolarized in renal failure, due to hyperkalemia which is only temporarily relieved by dialysis [9–13]. This has led to the hypothesis that hyperkalemic depolarization may be an underestimated cause of neuropathy in chronic renal failure [14] and to attempts to prevent the development of neuropathy by maintaining normokalemia.

Despite the importance of potassium effects on peripheral nerve and nerve excitability, the biophysical basis of these effects is only partly understood. Since the resting potential depends primarily on the selective permeability of the axolemma to potassium ions, it is expected that hyperkalemia will cause membrane depolarization with a consequent increase in potassium permeability and

membrane conductance, and thereby a 'fanning-in' of threshold electrotonus. This behaviour is well accounted for by a model of nerve excitability, in which myelinated axons are represented by two linked compartments (node and internode), with different assortments of ion channels following Hodgkin-Huxley equations [3,15–17]. However this model, which predicts quite well the effects of altering membrane potential by applied currents and the effects of reducing different ion currents, does not account for the effects of hyperkalemia on nerve excitability in end-stage kidney disease (ESKD)[13]. Arnold *et al.* found that the excitability abnormalities in ESKD patients were 'profoundly worse than that expected for normal axons exposed to similarly high potassium concentrations'. Moreover, whereas superexcitability in the ESKD patients falls steeply with increasing potassium, the model predicts a slight increase [13], because of the reduction in the post-spike hyperpolarization by slow potassium currents. Since their modelling suggested that nodal fast potassium conductance was increased in the patients, Arnold *et al.* proposed that the hyperkalaemia may have disrupted the paranodal myelin, thereby exposing juxtaparanodal potassium channels. However, an alternative interpretation is that their results exposed a deficiency in the modelling of the potassium channels.

There has only been one previous study exploring the relationship between superexcitability and serum potassium in normal subjects ($n = 12$), which found a significant relationship ($p = 0.02$), again contradicting the model [18]. The present study was undertaken on a larger group of normal subjects, to define more clearly the potassium dependence of superexcitability and other excitability measures, to clarify any difference from the relationship in uraemic patients, and to improve the model as necessary to account for potassium effects. The results confirm that superexcitability decreases as serum potassium increases, and indicate that potassium currents are more sensitive to external potassium than the present model predicts. A new model is proposed in which the potassium currents in human motor axons depend on extracellular potassium as if 1:1 binding of potassium ions to the outside of the channel were necessary for their function, a suggestion earlier made to account for the effects of altered potassium concentrations on single myelinated axons of the frog [19].

Methods

Ethics statement

All procedures were approved by the local ethical committee: Kantonale Ethikkommission, Bern, Switzerland (KEK-Nr. 180/10), and conformed to the Declaration of Helsinki. Experimental procedures were fully explained and all subjects gave their written informed consent to participate.

Subjects

Forty healthy volunteers were enrolled to participate in this study. There were 23 women and 17 men, aged between 21 and 79 years. None of the subjects suffered from carpal tunnel syndrome or had any history of a neuromuscular disorder or any risk factor for peripheral neuropathy (including diabetes, neurotoxic medication and alcohol abuse). Finally, subjects with abnormal potassium serum or creatinine were not included. Normal ranges were defined as follows: serum potassium [3.5–4.7 mmol/l] and creatinine [women: 45–84 µmol/l; men: 59–104 µmol/l].

Laboratory examination

Subjects were comfortably rested on a bed in a warm room. A 5 ml blood sample was taken from one arm and the rest of the examination was performed on the other side. Serum levels of potassium and creatinine were measured. Serum creatinine was used as marker of normal renal function [20].

Peripheral nerve excitability

Excitability properties of the peripheral nerve were assessed by means of Qtrac software (copyright Institute of Neurology, London, UK), as previously reported [2]. Since temperature affects some excitability parameters [21], cutaneous temperature was carefully monitored and maintained above 32°C through the entire session.

Multiple measures of nerve excitability were performed on the median motor nerve at the wrist, using surface electrodes, as previously described [2,22,23]. Electrical stimuli were applied via non-polarizable electrodes (Red Dot, 3 M Health Care, Borken, Germany), the cathode being placed on the median nerve at the wrist and the anode being placed about 10 cm proximal, over the muscle. Stimulus waveforms generated by a computer were converted to current with a purpose-built isolated linear bipolar constant current stimulator (DS5, Digitmer Ltd., Welwyn Garden City, UK) (maximum output 50 mA).

Compound muscle action potentials (CMAP) were recorded from abductor pollicis brevis (APB), using adhesive disposable surface electrodes (REF 9013L0203, Alpine BioMed, Skovlunde, Denmark) with the active electrode at the motor point and the

reference electrode on the proximal phalanx. The ground electrode (Red Dot surface electrode) was taped on the top of the hand. The signal was amplified (gain: 1000, bandwidth: 1.6–2 kHz) and digitized with a data acquisition unit (National Instruments NI DAQCARD-6062E, National Instruments Europe Corp., Debrecen, Hungary) using a sampling rate of 10 kHz.

Nerve excitability measurements were made using the TRONDNF protocol. Initially the 1 ms stimulus was set manually to a supramaximal level, and then the computer generated a stimulus-response relationship by progressively decreasing the strength of the stimulus in 2% steps. Next, computer feedback was used to track the stimulus that excited a CMAP equal to 40% of maximal amplitude and threshold comparisons were used to evaluate strength-duration curve, threshold electrotonus, current-threshold (I/V) relationship and recovery cycle. For the strength-duration relationship, the threshold current required to generate the target CMAP was tracked as the pulse duration was reduced from 1 ms to 0.2 ms. During threshold electrotonus, excitability was tested at 26 intervals during and after 100 ms polarizing currents set to ±20% and ±40% of the control threshold current. For the I/V relationship, excitability was tested after 200 ms current pulses that were varied from 50% to −100% of control threshold, in 10% steps. Finally, for the recovery cycle, excitability was tested at 18 inter-stimulus intervals (ISI) from 200 ms to 2 ms after a supra-maximal conditioning stimulus.

Data analysis

The nerve excitability data were analyzed by means of the QtracP program, as previously described [2]. Multiple excitability measure files were generated for each recording. These files contained all the threshold estimates (e.g. for 26 time points on the threshold electrotonus), and also a set of derived excitability measurements that was retained for analysis:

i) from the strength-duration relationship: strength-duration time constant and rheobase

ii) from the threshold electrotonus: mean threshold reductions between the specified times after the start of polarization, for the 40% depolarizing current (TEd40[10–20 ms], TEd40[90–100 ms]), the 20% depolarizing current (TEd20[10–20 ms], TEd20[90–100 ms]), the 20% hyperpolarizing current (TEh20[10–20 ms], TEh20[90–100 ms]), and for the 40% hyperpolarizing current (TEh40[10–20 ms], TEh40[90–100 ms]). Also, the maximal threshold reductions were measured for the 40% and 20% depolarizing currents (TEd40[peak], TEd20[peak]).

iii) from the I/V relationship: resting and minimum I/V slope (an analogue of conductance)

iv) from the recovery cycle: refractoriness, superexcitability and late subexcitability.

Statistical analysis

All data are reported as mean ±SD. Correlations were assessed by the Pearson product moment correlation coefficient R. The level of significance was set at $P<0.05$.

Nerve models

The dependence of nerve excitability properties on extracellular potassium was modelled in 3 different ways:

Model 1. The first model was the human motor axon model described in detail by Howells et al.[17]. In this model, potassium and leakage channels are modelled as conductances, as in the original Hodgkin-Huxley model of the squid giant axon, and the first model of human nodal membrane currents [24], e.g.

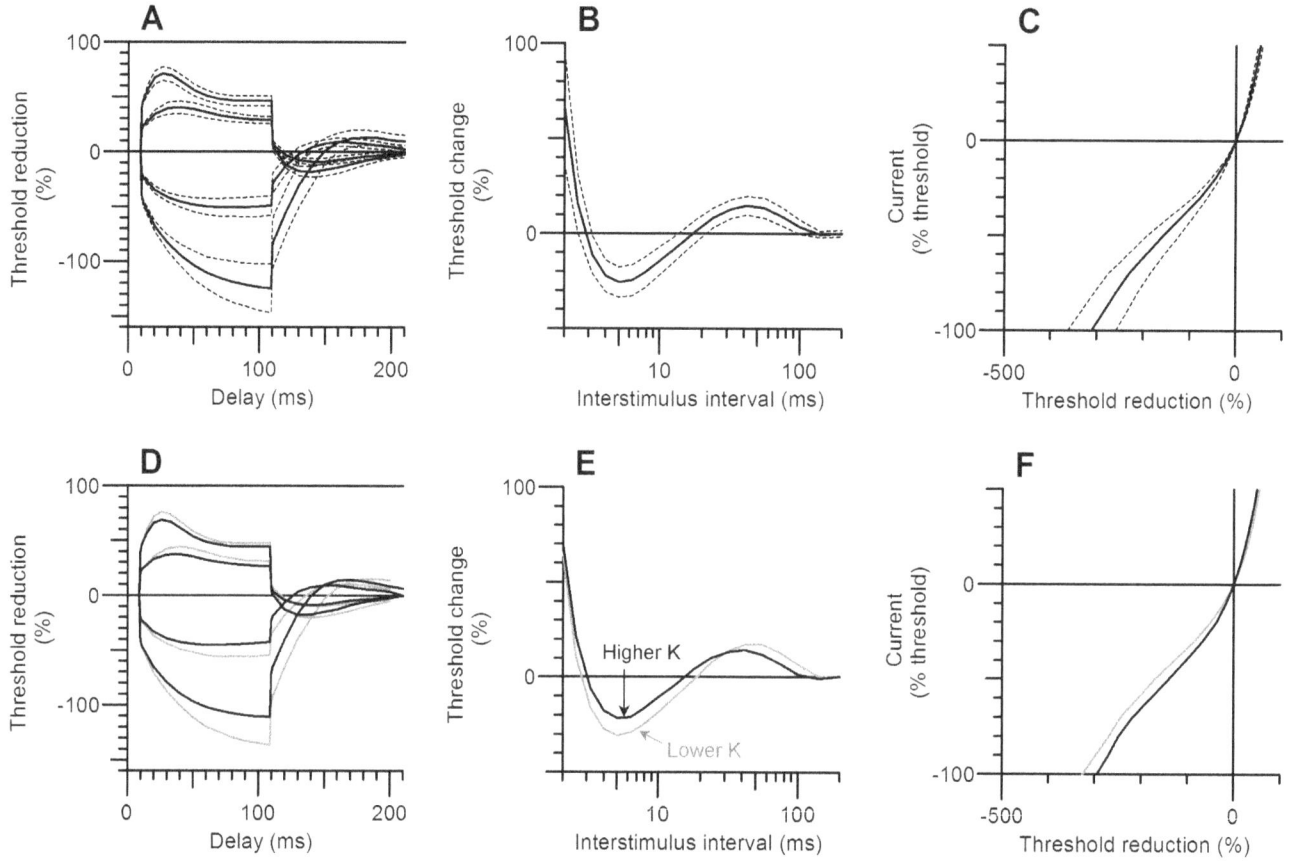

Figure 1. Multiple excitability measurements recorded from normal subjects: motor axons in the median nerve were tested at the wrist and compound muscle action potentials recorded from the abductor pollicis brevis muscle. A–C: Mean +/− SD for all 38 subjects. D–F: Comparisons between means of Lower K (grey) and Higher K (black) groups. A, D: Threshold electrotonus, *i.e.*, threshold changes during and after polarizing currents set to +40 (top), +20, −20 and −40% (bottom) of threshold. B, E: Recovery cycle showing successive phases of refractoriness, superexcitability, and late subexcitability. C,F: Current-threshold (I/V) relationship.

$$I_{Kf} = G_{Kf} \cdot n^4 (E - E_K) \tag{1}$$

where I_{Kf} is the fast potassium current, G_{Kf} is the maximum fast potassium conductance (a constant), n is the fraction of activated gates, E is the membrane potential, and E_K is the reversal potential for potassium currents, given by the Nernst equation: $E_K = RT/F \times \ln([K]_o/[K]_i)$. Similarly,

$$I_{Ks} = G_{Ks} \cdot s (E - E_K) \tag{2}$$

where I_{Ks} is the slow potassium current and s is the fraction of activated channels, and

$$I_{Lk} = G_{Lk}(E - E_r) \tag{3}$$

where I_{Lk} is the leakage current, G_{Lk} the leak conductance, and E_r is the resting potiential. Equations (1)–(3) are written separately for the nodal and internodal axon membrane. In this model, changes in extracellular potassium only affect potassium currents through their effects on the potassium reversal potential E_K.

Model 2. To allow for the fact that potassium ions more readily diffuse from a region of high concentration to one of low concentration than *vice versa*, the potassium currents can alterna-

tively be modelled by the constant field equation, as used by Frankenhaeuser and Huxley to account for the potential dependence of the nodal potassium currents of *Xenopus laevis* [25]. In this formulation, potassium conductances (G_K) are replaced by potassium permeabilities (P_K), and equations (1) and (2) are replaced by equations (4) and (5) respectively:

$$I_{Kf} = P_{Kf} \cdot n^4 \cdot \frac{EF^2}{RT}[K]_x \tag{4}$$

$$I_{Ks} = P_{Ks} \cdot s \cdot \frac{EF^2}{RT}[K]_x \tag{5}$$

where F, R and T are Avogadro's number, the gas constant and absolute temperature, respectively, and

$$[K]_x = \frac{\left([K]_o - [K]_i e^{EF/RT}\right)}{1 - e^{EF/RT}} \tag{6}$$

Model 3. Dubois [26] found that for both fast and slow potassium currents at voltage-clamped frog nodes there was a linear relationship between $1/G_K$ and $1/[K]_o$ at low values of $[K]_o$, consistent with channel opening being dependent on a 1:1

binding with extracellular K^+ ions [19]. When $[K]_o$ is small, as it is *in vivo*, potassium currents therefore become almost directly proportional to $[K]_o$, and this relationship was represented in Model 3 by multiplying $[K]_x$ in equations (4) and (5) of Model 2 by the factor $[K]_o/(\text{average } [K]_o)$.

Model fitting procedure. The fitting of the models to the nerve excitability data was performed with the MEMFIT facility in QtracP, which minimizes the 'discrepancy' (D), scored as the weighted mean of the error terms: $([x_m - x_n]/s_n)^2$, where x_m is the threshold of the model, x_n is the mean, and s_n is the standard deviation of the thresholds for the real nerves. To keep the D values consistent in this study, the s_n values were always based on the 14 medium K subjects (see below). The weights were the same for all thresholds of the same type (*e.g.* recovery cycle) and were chosen to give total weights to the four different types of threshold measurement: threshold electrotonus, current–threshold relation, recovery cycle, and strength–duration properties in the ratio 2:1:1:0.5. Parameter values for Model 1 were obtained from the recently described model [17] by minimizing the discrepancy between the model and the average of the data from the 38 subjects with an iterative least squares procedure, until alteration of any of the membrane parameters would make the discrepancy worse. For Model 2, starting values of the potassium permeabilities were estimated by making each channel contribution to the resting current the same as in model 1, then the iterative procedure was

repeated until the discrepancy was again minimized. Parameter values for Model 3 were the same as for model 2.

Results

All subjects participated in the study without any adverse effects and none of them requested an early termination of the recording session. However, two subjects had potassium levels outside the normal range (3.1 and 3.4 mmol/l) and were therefore excluded from analysis. Potassium serum levels in the remaining 38 subjects varied from 3.5 to 4.5 mmol/l (average concentration: 4.11 ± 0.25 mmol/l). The subjects were divided into 3 groups on the basis of these potassium levels: Lower K (3.5–3.9, mean 3.82 mmol/l, n = 11); Medium K (4.0–4.2, mean 4.06 mmol/l, n = 14) and Higher K (4.3–4.5, mean 4.39 mmol/l, n = 13). (It should be emphasized that the 3 groups were all within the normal range of 3.5 to 4.7 mmol/l.). Creatinine values were also all within the normal ranges, and varied from 57 to 80 µmol/l (average: 69.4 µmol/l) in women and from 62 to 100 µmol/l (average: 83.2 µmol/l) in men. Average cutaneous temperature at the stimulation site was $32.92\pm0.73°C$. The potassium levels in the subjects were not correlated with age (Pearson $R=0.141$, $P=0.40$), temperature ($R=0.247$, $P=0.$ 14) or sex ($R=0.018$, $P=0.88$). However, comparing the younger subjects (14 under 30) with the older ones (24 over 30), although the mean potassium levels were similar in the two age groups (younger 4.09 ± 0.18,

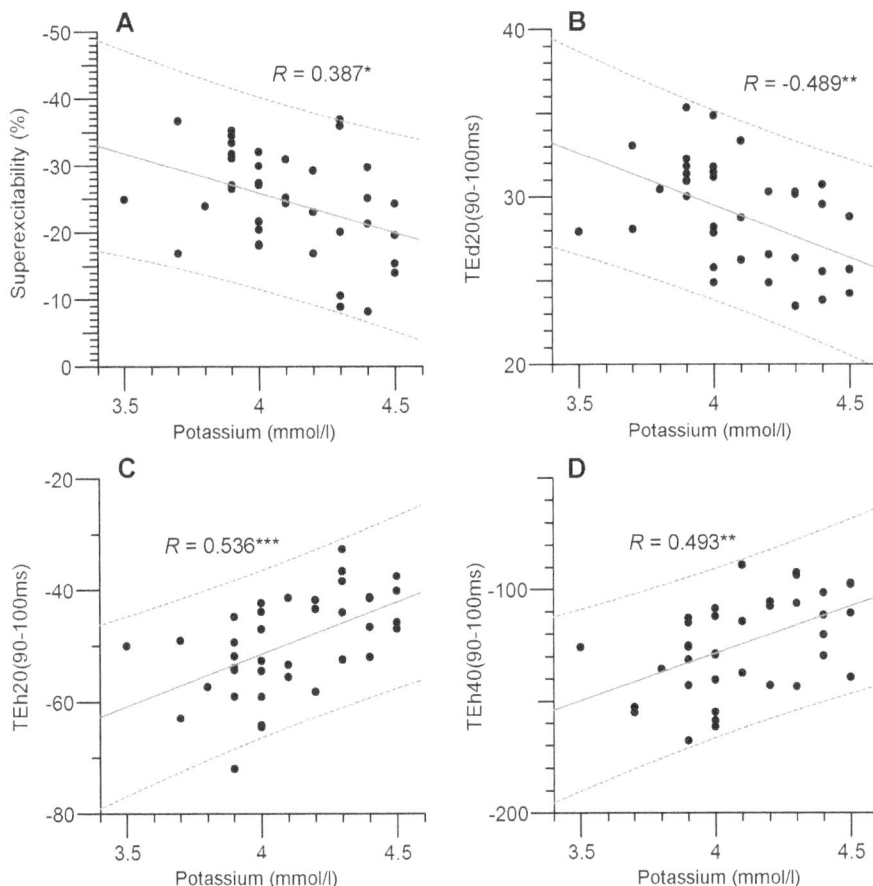

Figure 2. Examples of nerve excitability measures showing significant relationship to serum potassium levels. A: Superexcitability, **B**: TEd20(90–100 ms) threshold decrease at end of 20% depolarizing current, **C,D**: TEh20(90–100 ms) and TEh40(90–100 ms) threshold decrease at end of 20% and 40% hyperpolarizing current (NB Negative threshold decrease indicates threshold were increased by hyperpolarization).

Table 1. Mean values of excitability parameters derived from the multiple measures of nerve excitability performed on the median nerve in 38 normal subjects.

	Mean ±SD	R v. [K]$_o$	P
Strength-duration relationship			
SDTC (ms)	0.47±0.14	0.187	0.27
Rheobase (mA)	3.84±2.05	0.079	0.65
Depolarizing threshold electrotonus			
TEd40[10–20 ms] (%)	69.5±5.8	−0.364	0.024*
TEd40[peak](%)	68.7±5.7	−0.348	0.030*
TEd40[90–100 ms] (%)	46.2±4.5	−0.254	0.12
TEd20[10–20 ms](%)	36.7±4.5	−0.318	0.049*
TEd20[peak] (%)	39.5±3.4	−0.341	0.035*
TEd20[90–100 ms]	28.8±3.2	−0.489	0.0019**
Hyperpolarizing threshold electrotonus			
TEh20[10–20 ms] (%)	−38.3±3.6	0.429	0.0070**
TEh20[90–100 ms] (%)	−49.5±8.8	0.536	0.00061***
TEh40[10–20 ms] (%)	−75.8±5.9	0.480	0.0024**
TEh40[90–100 ms] (%)	−124.1±21.6	0.493	0.0018**
Current-threshold relationship			
Resting I/V slope	0.597±0.105	0.529	0.00073***
Minimum I/V slope	0.246±0.050	0.097	0.57
Recovery cycle			
RRP (ms)	2.88±0.34	0.482	0.0023**
Superexcitability (%)	−24.7±7.7	0.387	0.016*
Late Subexcitability (%)	14.1±4.7	−0.145	0.39

First column shows mean ± standard deviation (SD). Second column shows Pearson product moment correlation coefficient between excitability measure and serum potassium. Third column shows p values (* = P<0.05, ** = P<0.01, *** = P<0.001). SDTC: strength-duration time constant. TEd20 and TEh20: threshold electrotonus changes due to depolarizing and hyperpolarizing currents respectively, set to 20% of control threshold; TEd40, TEh40 same, but for 40% polarizing currents; expressions in square brackets indicate times after start of 100 ms current, early [10–20 ms], late [90–100 ms] or around peak threshold change [peak]. I/V: current-threshold. RRP: relative refractory period.

older 4.11±0.29 mmol/l, Welch test $P = 0.79$), the variance of the potassium levels was higher in the older group (F test $P = 0.034$).

Nerve excitability and relation to serum potassium level

Nerve excitability waveforms recorded from the median motor nerve are illustrated in Figure 1 for the 38 subjects. In the top row are plotted the mean waveforms for the 38 subjects ±1 SD. These recordings are very similar to previously published normal median/APB recordings [2]. In the bottom row the mean recordings from the Lower K group are compared with those from the Higher K group. Conventional excitability measurements derived from the waveforms are listed in Table 1, with their correlation to the serum potassium values. As previously reported by Kuwabara and colleagues [18], there was a significant tendency for axons to become less superexcitable at higher potassium levels ($R = 0.39$, $P = 0.016$). There was a clear tendency for electrotonus to 'fan in' at higher potassium levels (*i.e.* TEd values to decrease, TEh values to increase, Table 1 and Figure 2). Over this limited potassium range, there was no significant dependence of rheobase or strength-duration time constant on potassium.

Comparison with Models 1–3

Figure 3 shows electrotonus and recovery cycle waveforms generated by the three models for potassium concentrations equal to the Lower K (3.82 mmol/l) and Higher K (4.39 mmol/l)

groups, which can be compared with the recordings in Figures 1D and 1E. Only Model 3 shows an increase in superexcitability at lower potassium levels and fanning-out of depolarising as well as hyperpolarising threshold electrotonus as seen in the recordings.

To further explore the potassium dependence of nerve excitability according to the 3 models, and how they predict extrapolation to hyperkalaemic levels, Figure 4 shows 2 excitability measures plotted as a function of potassium concentration, and compares the 3 models with the 3 groups of normal subjects, and also with the previously published data for patients with chronic renal failure, who had varying degrees of hyperkalemia prior to dialysis [9]. In Figure 4A it can be seen that only Model 3 predicts a marked reduction in superexcitability with increasing potassium, and when model 3 is extrapolated to abnormally high potassium levels, it predicts quite accurately the relationship previously found in patients with renal failure prior to dialysis, as indicated by the ellipse. The changes in electrotonus with potassium were too small to distinguish between the models as far as the normal subjects are concerned, but Fig 4B indicates that the changes in depolarizing electrotonus (TEd40[90–100 ms]) in the renal failure patients with hyperkalemia are also best explained by model 3.

Model 3 also provided the best fits taking into account all the excitability measurements (i.e. current-voltage and charge-duration relationships as well as threshold electrotonus and recovery cycle) as judged by the discrepancy scores D (see Methods for

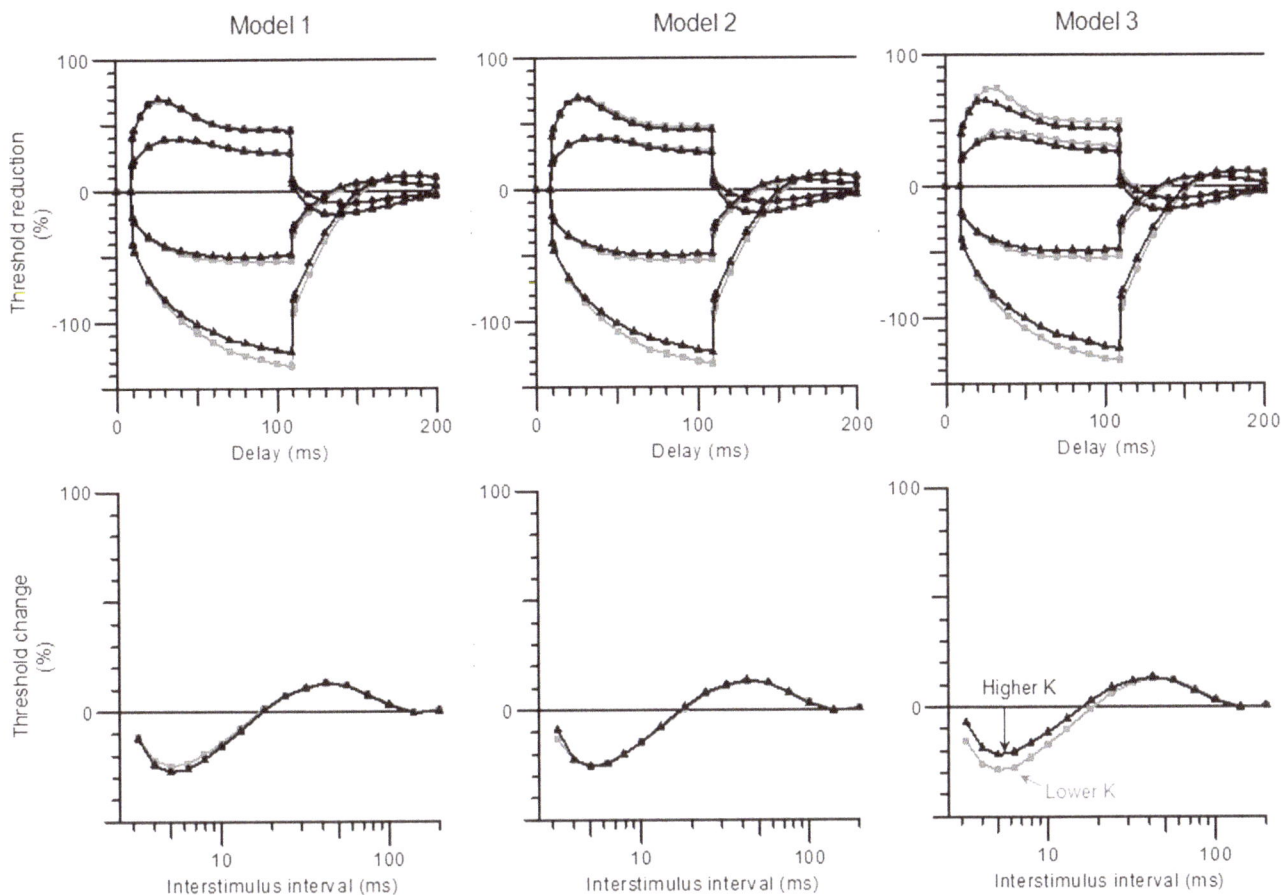

Figure 3. Threshold electrotonus (top row) and recovery cycle (bottom row) waveforms generated by Models 1–3 for values of extracellular potassium corresponding to the Lower K (grey) and Higher K (black) groups.

definition). The mean data for the Medium K group could be fitted well by either the constant conductance or constant permeability models (D = 0.094 and 0.104 respectively). Without allowance for the differences in potassium, the fits to the Lower K and Higher K group recordings were, not surprisingly, worse (D = 0.412, 0.419 respectively, Table 2). When allowance for the differences in potassium were made according to Model 1, the fits were improved by 14.1% for the Higher K group, but actually made 1.5% worse for the lower K group. Model 2 produced better fits, and Model 3 the best fits, with a reduction in discrepancy of 63.2% for the Higher K group, just by changing the $[K^+]_o$ value from 4.06 to 4.39. Although the discrepancy scores were

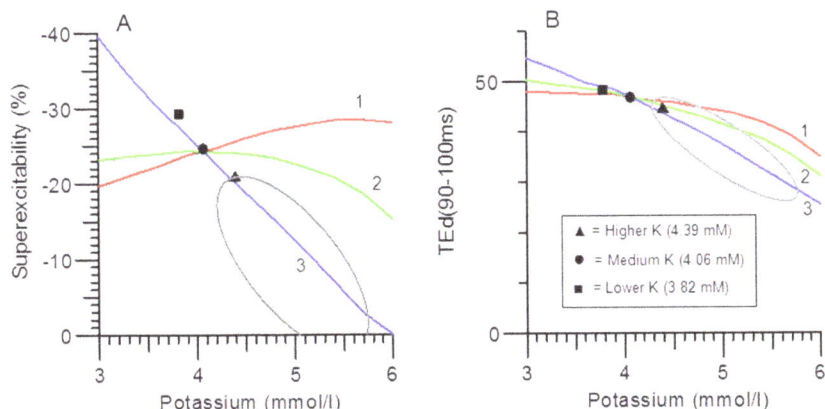

Figure 4. Potassium dependence of 2 nerve excitability measurements predicted by Models 1 (red line), 2 (green line) and 3 (blue line) compared with mean measurements for Higher K (▲), Medium K (●) and Lower K (■) groups, and ellipse representing 1 SD limits for 9 patients with chronic renal failure (reproduced from Kiernan et al.).[9] Only Model 3 predicts an appropriate drop in superexcitability with increasing potassium level.

Table 2. Comparison between the three models in their ability to account for the effects of changes in serum potassium levels on multiple measures of nerve excitability.

	Lower K$^+$ normal subjects (n = 11)	Higher K$^+$ normal subjects (n = 13)	High K$^+$ CRF patients * (n = 9)
Medium [K$^+$]$_o$ (mmol/l)	3.82	4.39	5.02
Discrepancy from Medium K data (n = 14)	0.412	0.419	3.85
Discrepancy from Model 1 (% reduction)	0.418 (−1.5%)	0.360 (14.1%)	3.503 (9.0%)
Discrepancy from Model 2 (% reduction)	0.368 (10.7%)	0.259 (38.2%)	2.545 (33.9%)
Discrepancy from Model 3 (% reduction)	**0.243 (41.0%)**	**0.154 (63.2%)**	**1.218 (68.4%)**

Data from Medium K data was fitted to nerve model, and then adjusted for different potassium levels according to Models 1, 2 and 3. Discrepancies score difference between model and recorded data and discrepancy reductions score improvement over no allowance for potassium. For each data set Model 3 provides lowest discrepancy (figures in bold).

appreciably higher for the patients with chronic renal failure (who had serum potassium values ranging from 4.3 to 6.1 mmol/l), the discrepancy reductions obtained by the different ways of modelling the effects of the hyperkalemia were similar to those obtained for the Higher K normal subjects (Table 2).

In addition to the Models 1, 2 and 3, we have also explored the consequences of other assumptions about the effects of changes in [K]$_o$, for example a constant conductance model with conductances proportional to [K]$_o$, and permeability models with only fast potassium channel permeability or slow potassium channel permeability proportional to [K]$_o$. These alternative models produced results intermediate between Model 2 and Model 3. Thus Model 3 provided the best simulation of the potassium dependence of both the normal nerves recorded in this study and also the earlier recordings from patients with chronic renal failure.

Discussion

This study has shown that even within a narrow range of normal serum potassium levels (3.5–4.5 mmol/l), potassium has a significant effect on nerve excitability properties, including superexcitability and the responses to depolarizing and hyperpolarizing currents as measured by threshold electrotonus. In this we have confirmed a previous study by Kuwabara and colleagues [18], using a somewhat different protocol in which 12 normal subjects were each tested on 3 occasions, and in which there was a wider range of potassium levels (3.5–5.0 mmol/l). The principle new finding of this study is that the current model of human nerve excitability cannot account for these relationships. To overcome this deficiency we have presented a new model, in which potassium currents are not only dependent on membrane potential, but also proportional to extracellular potassium concentration. Here we first relate these findings to previous evidence about the potassium dependence of axonal potassium currents, and then consider the implications for future nerve excitability studies.

Potassium dependence of potassium currents

The dependence on external potassium concentration of potassium currents in frog nodes was studied in detail by Dubois and Bergman [19]. They concluded that the potassium conductance (g_K) behaved as if proportional to 1:1 binding of external K$^+$ ions to membrane sites, i.e. $g_K = G_K.[K]_o/(K_{app} + [K]_o)$, where G_K is the maximum conductance when all sites are occupied, and K_{app} is the apparent dissociation constant. K_{app} depended on membrane potential and external calcium concentration, but was

sufficiently high in the physiological region of excitability studies that g_K was effectively directly proportional to [K]$_o$. The notion of an external binding site was strengthened by the finding that external caesium ions could replace potassium ions in enabling outward potassium currents, so long as their concentration was kept low [19]. That study was re-evaluated by Dubois [26] in the light of his evidence for 3 different types of potassium channel. He concluded that the apparent voltage dependence of K_{app} in the earlier study was attributable to the existence of different potassium channels with different voltage dependence, and that potassium conductance increased with [K]$_o$ for both fast and slow potassium channels.

The question of the potassium dependence of potassium currents has received little attention in mammalian myelinated axons. The first nodal voltage clamp studies of rabbit and rat fibers [27,28] found potassium currents to be almost non-existent, because the fast potassium channels are mainly restricted to the juxta-paranodal region, under the myelin sheath [29,30]. While later studies of mammalian, including human, nodal ion currents have recognized the importance of slow as well as fast potassium currents [24,31,32] the dependence of these currents on external potassium concentrations within the physiological range has never, so far as we are aware, been investigated. Single channel patch clamp studies have found higher unitary channel currents in the high [K]$_o$ solutions commonly used than in Ringer solution (e.g. 18 ps v. 10 ps for outward 'I channel' potassium currents) [33], but possible effects of [K]$_o$ on open channel probability have not been described. The present study provides evidence that the potassium channels in human myelinated axons are critically dependent on extracellular potassium, as in the frog.

Implications for nerve excitability studies

Nerve excitability studies can provide a considerable amount of information about altered nerve membrane properties in disease, but the evidence they provide is indirect and it has sometimes only been by modelling the excitability changes that interpretation has been possible (e.g. the effects of sodium channel block by tetrodotoxin) [3]. It is therefore important to ensure that the model can correctly take account of alterations in the nerve milieu, such as potassium concentration, with effects on excitability. In the case of patients with renal failure, the very high correlations found between excitability changes (including superexcitability) and serum potassium levels, provided good evidence of a strong causal connection [9,10]. Very recently, a causal connection has been proved more decisively by an elegant, two-stage dialysis procedure, in which the serum potassium level was kept constant for the first

3 hours [13]. However, the authors observed that the available model of human motor nerve excitability could not account well for the relationship between serum potassium concentration and excitability properties, especially superexcitability, and suggested that the hyperkalaemia might also be disrupting the myelin sheath. However, our new evidence clearly shows that that model is inadequate to account for the effects of potassium on nerve excitability, even in normal control subjects with potassium levels in the normal range. A better model is required, and the new model presented here provides a simple explanation of how hyperkalemia alone can be responsible for the superexcitability changes in uremia (as illustrated by the ellipse in Fig. 4A) as well as for the dependence of superexcitability on potassium in normal subjects.

The other important lesson of this study is to reinforce the conclusions of Kuwabara *et al.* [17] that excitability studies should be performed when serum potassium levels are stable (*e.g.* before a meal), and where possible a blood sample should be taken at the same time for electrolyte analysis. Model 3 (which is now incorporated in the Qtrac software) provides a means for predicting the likely contribution of serum potassium level to the nerve excitability measurements.

Author Contributions

Conceived and designed the experiments: WJZ DB RS HB. Performed the experiments: WJZ DB RS. Analyzed the data: WJZ DB HB. Contributed reagents/materials/analysis tools: HB. Wrote the paper: WJZ DB HB.

References

1. Bostock H, Cikurel K, Burke D (1998) Threshold tracking techniques in the study of human peripheral nerve. Muscle Nerve 21: 137–158.
2. Kiernan MC, Burke D, Andersen KV, Bostock H (2000) Multiple measures of axonal excitability: a new approach in clinical testing. Muscle Nerve 23: 399–409.
3. Kiernan MC, Isbister GK, Lin CS-Y, Burke D, Bostock H (2005) Acute tetrodotoxin-induced neurotoxicity following ingestion of puffer fish. Ann Neurol 57: 339–348.
4. Nodera H, Kaji R (2006) Nerve excitability testing and its clinical application to neuromuscular diseases. Clin Neurophysiol 117: 1902–1916.
5. Krarup C, Moldovan M (2009) Nerve conduction and excitability studies in peripheral nerve disorders. Curr Opin Neurol 22: 460–466.
6. Krishnan AV, Lin CS, Park SB, Kiernan MC (2009) Axonal ion channels from bench to bedside: A translational neuroscience perspective. Prog Neurobiol 89: 288–313.
7. Kanai K, Shibuya K, Sato Y, Misawa S, Nasu S, et al. (2012) Motor axonal excitability properties are strong predictors for survival in amyotrophic lateral sclerosis. J Neurol Neurosurg Psychiatry 83: 734–738.
8. Park SB, Lin CS, Kiernan MC (2012) Nerve excitability assessment in chemotherapy-induced neurotoxicity. J Vis Exp 62: e3439.
9. Kiernan MC, Walters RJ, Andersen KV, Taube D, Murray NM, et al. (2002) Nerve excitability changes in chronic renal failure indicate membrane depolarization due to hyperkalaemia. Brain 125: 1366–1378.
10. Krishnan AV, Phoon RK, Pussell BA, Charlesworth JA, Bostock H, et al. (2005) Altered motor nerve excitability in end-stage kidney disease. Brain 128: 2164–2174.
11. Krishnan AV, Phoon RK, Pussell BA, Charlesworth JA, Bostock H, et al. (2006a) Neuropathy, axonal Na+/K+ pump function and activity-dependent excitability changes in end-stage kidney disease. Clin Neurophysiol 117: 992–999.
12. Krishnan AV, Phoon RK, Pussell BA, Charlesworth JA, Kiernan MC (2006b) Sensory nerve excitability and neuropathy in end stage kidney disease. J Neurol Neurosurg Psychiatry 77: 548–551.
13. Arnold R, Pussel BA, Howells J, Grinius V, Kiernan MC, et al. (2014) Evidence for a causal relationship between hyperkalaemia and axonal dysfunction in end-stage kidney disease. Clin Neurophysiol 125: 179–85.
14. Bostock H, Walters RJ, Andersen KV, Murray NM, Taube D, et al. (2004) Has potassium been prematurely discarded as a contributing factor to the development of uraemic neuropathy? Nephrol Dial Transplant 19: 1054–1057.
15. Bostock H, Baker M, Reid G (1991) Changes in excitability of human motor axons underlying post-ischaemic fasciculations: evidence for two stable states. J Physiol 441: 537–557.
16. Lin CS-Y, Krishnan AV, Lee M-J, Zagami AS, You H-L, et al. (2008) Nerve function and dysfunction in acute intermittent porphyria. Brain 131: 2510–2519.
17. Howells J, Trevillion L, Bostock H, Burke D (2012) The voltage dependence of Ih in human myelinated axons. J Physiol 500: 1625–1640.
18. Kuwabara S, Misawa S, Kanai K, Tamura N, Nakata M, et al. (2007) The effects of physiological fluctuation of serum potassium levels on excitability properties in healthy human motor axons. Clin Neurophysiol 118: 278–282.
19. Dubois JM, Bergman C (1977) The steady-state potassium conductance of the Ranvier node at various external K-concentrations. Pflugers Arch 370: 185–194.
20. Rutherford WE, Blondin J, Miller JP, Greenwalt AS, Vavra JD (1977) Chronic progressive renal disease: rate of change of serum creatinine concentration. Kidney Int 11: 62–70.
21. Kiernan MC, Cikurel K, Bostock H (2001) Effects of temperature on the excitability properties of human motor axons. Brain 124: 816–825.
22. Kuwabara S, Kanai K, Sung JY, Ogawara K, Hattori T, et al. (2002) Axonal hyperpolarization associated with acute hypokalemia: multiple excitability measurements as indicators of the membrane potential of human axons. Muscle Nerve 26: 283–287.
23. Z'Graggen WJ, Lin CS, Howard RS, Beale RJ, Bostock H (2006) Nerve excitability changes in critical illness polyneuropathy. Brain 129: 2461–2470.
24. Schwarz JR, Reid G, Bostock H (1995) Action potentials and membrane currents in the human node of Ranvier. Pflugers Arch 430: 283–292.
25. Frankenhaeuser B, Huxley AF (1964) The action potential in the myelinated nerve fibre of *Xenopus Laevis* as computed on the basis of voltage clamp data. J Physiol 171: 302–315.
26. Dubois JM (1981) Evidence for the existence of three types of potassium channels in the frog Ranvier node membrane. J Physiol 318: 297–316.
27. Chiu SY, Ritchie JM, Rogart RB, Stagg D (1979) A quantitative description of membrane currents in rabbit myelinated nerve. J Physiol 292: 149–166.
28. Brismar T (1980) Potential clamp analysis of membrane currents in rat myelinated nerve fibres. J Physiol 298: 171–184.
29. Chiu SY, Ritchie JM (1981) Evidence for the presence of potassium channels in the paranodal region of acutely demyelinated mammalian single nerve fibres. J Physiol 313: 415–437.
30. Arroyo EJ, Scherer SS (2000) On the molecular architecture of myelinated fibers. Histochem Cell Biol 113: 1–18.
31. Röper J, Schwarz JR (1989) Heterogeneous distribution of fast and slow potassium channels in myelinated rat nerve fibres. J Physiol 416: 93–110.
32. Scholz A, Reid G, Vogel W, Bostock H (1993) Ion channels in human axons. J Neurophysiol 70: 1274–1279.
33. Safronov BV, Kampe K, Vogel W (1993) Single voltage-dependent potassium channels in rat peripheral nerve membrane. J Physiol 460: 675–691.

12

Geldanamycin Derivative Ameliorates High Fat Diet-Induced Renal Failure in Diabetes

Hong-Mei Zhang[1,2], Howard Dang[3], Amrita Kamat[2,4], Chih-Ko Yeh[3,4], Bin-Xian Zhang[2,3,4]*

1 Department of Clinical Oncology, Xijing Hospital, The Fourth Military Medical University, Xi'an, China, **2** Department of Medicine, Health Science Center, University of Texas, San Antonio, Texas, United States of America, **3** Department of Comprehensive Dentistry, Health Science Center, University of Texas, San Antonio, Texas, United States of America, **4** Audie L. Murphy Division, Geriatric Research, Education and Clinical Center, South Texas Veterans Health Care System, San Antonio, Texas, United States of America

Abstract

Diabetic nephropathy is a serious complication of longstanding diabetes and its pathogenesis remains unclear. Oxidative stress may play a critical role in the pathogenesis and progression of diabetic nephropathy. Our previous studies have demonstrated that polyunsaturated fatty acids (PUFA) induce peroxynitrite generation in primary human kidney mesangial cells and heat shock protein 90β1 (hsp90β1) is indispensable for the PUFA action. Here we investigated the effects of high fat diet (HFD) on kidney function and structure of db/db mice, a widely used rodent model of type 2 diabetes. Our results indicated that HFD dramatically increased the 24 h-urine output and worsened albuminuria in db/db mice. Discontinuation of HFD reversed the exacerbated albuminuria but not the increased urine output. Prolonged HFD feeding resulted in early death of db/db mice, which was associated with oliguria and anuria. Treatment with the geldanamycin derivative, 17-(dimethylaminoehtylamino)-17-demethoxygeldanamycin (17-DMAG), an hsp90 inhibitor, preserved kidney function, and ameliorated glomerular and tubular damage by HFD. 17-DMAG also significantly extended survival of the animals and protected them from the high mortality associated with renal failure. The benefit effect of 17-DMAG on renal function and structure was associated with a decreased level of kidney nitrotyrosine and a diminished kidney mitochondrial Ca^{2+} efflux in HFD-fed db/db mice. These results suggest that hsp90β1 is a potential target for the treatment of nephropathy and renal failure in diabetes.

Editor: Shree Ram Singh, National Cancer Institute, United States of America

Funding: This work was supported by the Mike Hogg Fund, National Institutes of Health (NIH), The Department of Veterans Health Care, the National Natural Science Foundation of China (No. 30900673), and Natural Science Foundation of Shaanxi Province(SJ08-ZT10). The funders had no role in study design, data collection and analysis, decision to publish, or preparation of the manuscript.

Competing Interests: The authors have declared that no competing interests exist.

* E-mail: zhangb2@uthscsa.edu

Introduction

Diabetic nephropathy is a progressive disorder in diabetic patients and worsens over time. Although hyperglycemia is known as the primary factor underlying the initiation and progression of diabetic nephropathy, the pathogenesis of diabetic nephropathy is complex and remains unclear [1]. Oxidative stress due to increased reactive oxygen species (ROS) production has been postulated to contribute to matrix accumulation, inflammation and tubulointerstitial fibrosis in the diabetic kidney [2–4]. Peroxynitrite, formed by the interaction of superoxide and nitric oxide, is a potent oxidant that attacks a variety of biomolecules including proteins, and causes structural and functional damage to tissues and cells. Increased level of nitrotyrosine in proximal tubules of diabetic patients suggest that oxidative injury of the proximal tubules by peroxynitrite may play an important part in the pathogenesis and/or progression of diabetic nephropathy [5]. Improvement of glomerular filtration rate in type 2 diabetes patients with diminished kidney functions by bardoxolone methyl, an agonist of nuclear factor-erythroid 2-related factor 2 that regulates cytoprotective antioxidant pathways, demonstrated the efficacy of antioxidant in treating diabetic nephropathy [6,7].

Longstanding hyperglycemia, along with other factors, is associated with accelerated decline of kidney function in patients with type 2 diabetic nephropathy [8]. Despite the lack of benefits for all-cause mortality and cardiovascular mortality, intensive hyperglycemic control reduces the risk of diabetic nephropathy and other microvascular complications significantly [9]. In vitro studies also support the critical role of high glucose in regulating matrix protein levels in kidney cells including mesangial [10], endothelial and epithelial cells [11]. Hyperglycemia exposure, albuminuria and other factors interact with the tubular system to cause oxidative stress and interstitial inflammation, which in turn contribute to tubulointerstitial fibrosis and progression of diabetic nephropathy [2,12]. Exposure of primary human renal proximal tubular cells to high glucose enhances cell proliferation and increases the level of collagen IV and fibronectin [13,14]. Increased collagen IV expression, mitochondrial dysfunction and excessive ROS generation were observed in murine proximal tubular cells exposed to high glucose [15–17].

Despite the critical role of hyperglycemia *per se* in vascular complications of type 2 diabetes, other metabolic factors, such as hyperlipidemia and elevated serum nonesterified fatty acids (NEFA), are clearly involved in the pathogenesis of diabetic nephropathy. Excessive NEFA not only contribute to insulin resistance by various mechanisms [18–22], but also cause mitochondrial defects [23]. Our previous studies indicate that polyunsaturated fatty acids (PUFA) induce peroxynitrite generation in various cell types including primary human mesangial cells [24,25]. The increasing peroxynitrite formation in response to PUFA requires heat shock protein 90β1 (HSP90β1) and is associated with Ca^{2+} efflux from the mitochondria [25,26]. In the current work, we investigated the role of hsp90 in high fat diet (HFD)-induced renal failure in db/db mice. Our results demonstrated that inhibition of hsp90 with 17-DMAG preserved kidney function, ameliorated glomerular and tubular damage, and improved animal survival in HFD- fed db/db mice. These beneficial effects of 17-DMAG in vivo may result from a reduction of peroxynitrite formation and oxidative damage in the kidney of db/db mice. Our findings provide new insights into molecular mechanisms underlying diabetic nephropathy.

Results

High fat diet (HFD) induces decline of kidney function in db/db mice

In these experiments, the challenge of db/db mice with HFD was divided into two phases with a four-week regular diet (RD) interval as illustrated in Figure 1A. This design allowed us to test the effect of HFD on kidney function in db/db mice and whether the HFD effects were reversible. Following the first phase of HFD feeding (on HFD for 2 weeks starting at 3 month old), all *db/db* mice showed dramatic increases in urinary albumin excretion and urine output (Figure 1 B and C), rapid bodyweight gain, and elevated blood glucose levels (Figure S1). The urinary albumin excretion (Figure 1 B) and bodyweight (Figure S1) were fully reversed to the pre-HFD treatment levels following discontinuation of HFD for four weeks. However, the increased urine output and blood glucose levels induced by HFD feeding persisted at four weeks following discontinuation of HFD. In parallel control experiments, two-week HFD challenge had no significant effects on urinary albumin excretion and urine output in the non-diabetic heterozygous littermate *db/+* mice (Figure 1 B and C).

The hsp90 inhibitor 17-DMAG antagonizes HFD-induced decline of kidney functions in db/db mice

Feeding db/db mice with HFD leads to rapid and reversible bodyweight gain because of the increase in fat tissues, which may further exacerbate circulating fatty acids, including PUFA. Linoleic acid (LA), a major component of PUFA in the plasma, interacts with hsp90β1 to cause mitochondrial Ca^{2+} ($[Ca^{2+}]_m$) efflux and peroxynitrite generation in cell cultures [25,26]. These pathways may contribute to HFD-induced decline of kidney functions in db/db mice by increasing oxidative stress. In the second phase of HFD challenge (Figure 1), db/db mice were treated with or without 17-DMAG (6.5 µg/kg bodyweight injected intraperitoneally once daily) to test the involvement of hsp90. The dose of 17-DMAG was chosen based on our previous studies showing 17-DMAG at that concentration exerting maximal inhibition on PUFA-induced $[Ca^{2+}]_m$ efflux but not producing apparent toxicity to cells [26]. In db/db mice without 17-DMAG treatment [injected with saline (vehicle) *db/db-HF-S* group, Figure 1 D], a dramatic increase in urine albumin excretion was observed following two weeks on HFD in the second phase of HFD challenge, mirroring the results in the first phase of HFD feeding (Figure 1B). Interestingly, treatment with 17-DMAG of the db/db mice during the second phase of HFD challenge significantly reduced albuminuria (*db/db-HF-G* group, Figure 1 D).

In contrast to the large increase of 24-h urine volume during two weeks of the first phase of HFD feeding, there was only a small and insignificant decrease of 24-h urine output following initial two weeks on HFD in the second phase (Figure 1E). Interestingly, starting from the 17th day of the second phase of HFD feeding, we observed a dramatic decrease of urine output or development of anuria in saline-injected db/db mice (*db/db-HF-S* group, Figure 1 E), indicating the loss of kidney function and the development of renal failure. Treatment with 17-DMAG resulted in significantly higher 24 h urine output (*db/db-HF-G* group, Figure 1 E), indicating preservation of renal function and prevent of renal failure by 17-DMAG. These beneficial effects of 17-DMAG on kidney functions were observed without measurable changes in blood glucose compared with that of saline-injected animals (*db/db-HF-S vs db/db-HF-G*, Figure 1 F).

The induction of renal failure by prolonged HFD feeding in db/db mice and the beneficial effect of 17-DMAG treatment were further supported by evidence based on serum creatinine measurement. Serum creatinine was determined in animals at the end of four weeks of the second phase HFD feeding. The results indicated that the serum creatinine was 283% higher in saline-injected db/db mice compared to *db/+* mice (*db/db-HF-S vs db/+*, Figure 1G). Interestingly, treatment with 17-DMAG significantly lowered the serum creatinine in HFD-fed db/db mice (*db/db-HF-G vs db/db-HF-S*, Figure 1G) and no significant difference was found between *db/db-HF-G* and *db/+* groups, indicating that 17-DMAG restored mice kidney function to normal creatinine clearance. These data provided evidence that HFD feeding resulted in renal failure in *db/db* mice and 17-DMAG treatment effectively preserved renal functions.

17-DMAG mitigates HFD-induced structural damage of glomeruli and tubules

The effect of HFD and treatment with 17-DMAG on kidney structure was examined with histopathology. The kidney samples were collected at the time of renal failure (as indicated by oliguria, anuria, and mortality) or at the end of the experiments (Day 33 of the second phase HFD feeding after total mortality was observed in saline-injected group of db/db mice) and analyzed by histopathological stains. Inspection of hematoxylin-eosin staining indicated segmental glomerulosclerosis, patches of tubular vacuolation, atrophy and degeneration in saline-injected db/db mice (*db/db-HF-S* group, Figure 2 C and E). These damages induced by HFD in the glomeruli and tubules were largely protected by 17-DMAG (*db/db-HF-G* group, Figure 2 D and F). In parallel experiments, HFD-fed *db/+* mice treated with saline (Figure 2 A) or 17-DMAG (Figure 2 B) did not exhibit any glomerular and tubular abnormalities. Structural damages in the db/db mice kidney was further confirmed by mesangial matrix expansion and tubulointerstitial fibrosis in PAS and Masson's trichrome stained sections (Figure 2 G and I). Interestingly, 17-DMAG treatment effectively ameliorated these abnormalities (Figure 2 H and J). Quantification with morphometric measurements confirmed significant alleviation of tubular damage (Figure 2 K), mesangial matrix expansion (Figure 2 L), and collagen accumulation (Figure 2 M) by 17-DMAG treatment.

High fat diet causes early death of db/db mice and 17-DMAG treatment improves animal survival

Renal failure is expected to cause mortality in the absence of additional treatments such as dialysis or kidney transplantation. Our results indicated that oliguria and anuria in HFD- fed db/db mice were associated with early mortality. As demonstrated in Figure 3, the earliest death among *db/db* mice injected with saline was

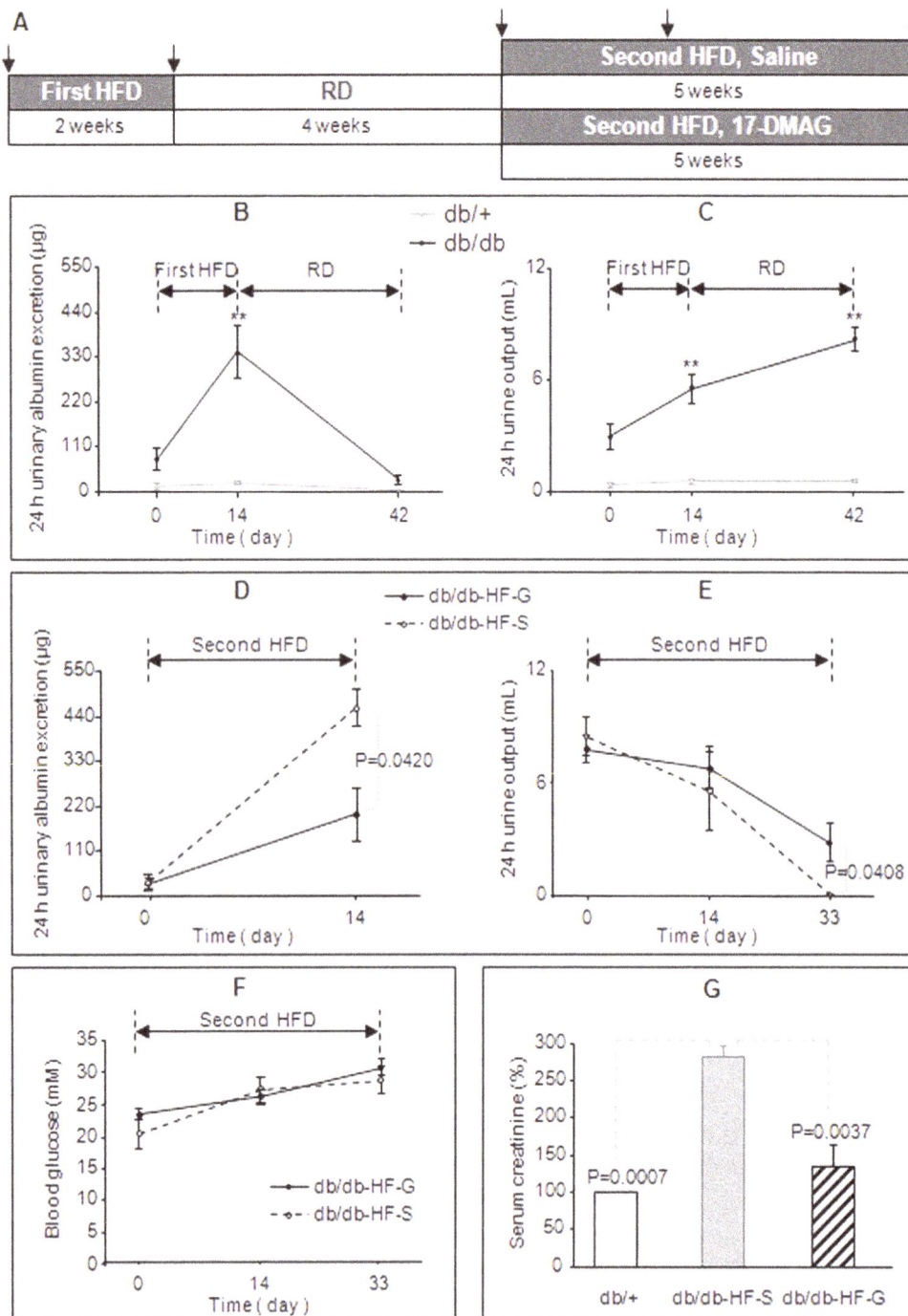

Figure 1. Effects of high fat diet (HFD) and 17-DMAG treatment on kidney function of *db/db* mice. (A) Schematic of two phases of HFD feeding and 17-DMAG treatment with the arrows indicating the scheduled kidney function assessments. During the first phase of HFD and the subsequent regular diet (RD) feeding, the 24 h urinary albumin excretion (B) and urine output (C) were measured to assess kidney functions in *db/db* and the non-diabetic control (*db/+*) mice. During the second phase of HFD feeding, the animals were either injected with saline (*HF-S*) or 17-DMAG (*HF-G*) and the kidney functions were initially assessed by the 24 h urinary albumin excretion (D) and urine output (E), and then by serum creatinine (G) when anuria or oliguria occurred. Blood glucose was measured as indicated in (F). **$P < 0.01$, compared with baseline assessed on day 0 with n = 6–12 per group.

observed on the 17th day of second phase HFD challenge and complete mortality was observed within 33 days. Treatment with 17-DMAG resulted in a significantly longer survival (*db/db-HF-S* vs *db/db-HF-G*, Figure 3). It is noteworthy that the second phase HFD feeding for 4–5 weeks did not cause renal failure or mortality in *db/+* mice regardless of saline or 17-DMAG treatments (Figure 3).

17-DMAG inhibits calcium efflux from the kidney mitochondrial of HFD-fed db/db mice

Elevated fatty acids, particularly LA and other PUFA, in diabetes may alter mitochondrial functions and ROS generation by $[Ca^{2+}]_m$ efflux. Treatment of cells with 17-DMAG downregulates hsp90β1 and inhibits LA-induced $[Ca^{2+}]_m$ efflux [25,26].

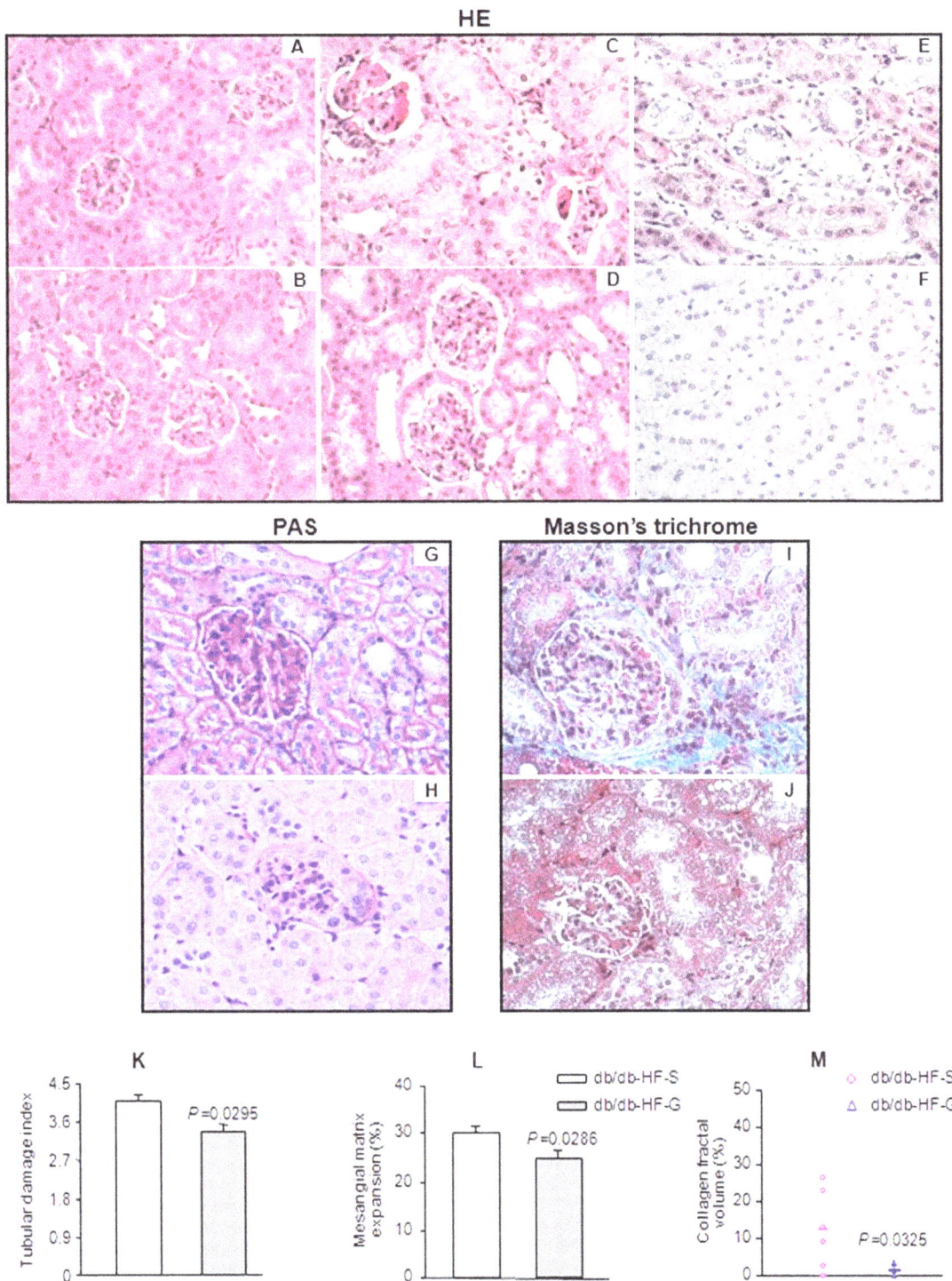

Figure 2. Kidney histopathology of HFD-fed *db/db* **mice.** Representative figures showing the photomicrographs of HE (*A–F*), PAS (*G, H*), and Masson's trichrome stained sections from *db/db-HF-S* group (*C, E, G, I*) and *db/db-HF-G* group (*D, F, H, J*) taken at 200× magnification. Image-based computer assisted analysis was performed to quantify tubular damage index (*K*), mesangial expansion (*L*), and interstitial collagen accumulation (*M*) from 6 animals per group. (A) and (B) showed parallel experiments with HFD-fed *db/+* mice injected with saline and 17-DMAG, respectively.

We thus determined whether the beneficial effect of 17-DMAG on HFD-fed db/db mice involved the regulation of the same pathways in the kidney. Hsp90β1 levels in the kidney of HFD-fed *db/db* mice was analyzed by immunoblotting and the results demonstrated similar hsp90β1 levels in the kidney homogenates and isolated mitochondria in animals treated with or without 17-

DMAG (*db/db-HF-S* vs *db/db-HF-G*, Figure 4 A and B). Interestingly, as shown in Figure 4 C–E, LA-induced $[Ca^{2+}]_m$ efflux was significantly diminished in the kidney mitochondria of *db/db* mice treated with 17-DMAG compared to saline. Both the rate and amplitude of LA-induced $[Ca^{2+}]_m$ efflux were significantly attenuated by 17-DMAG treatment (Figure 4 D and E).

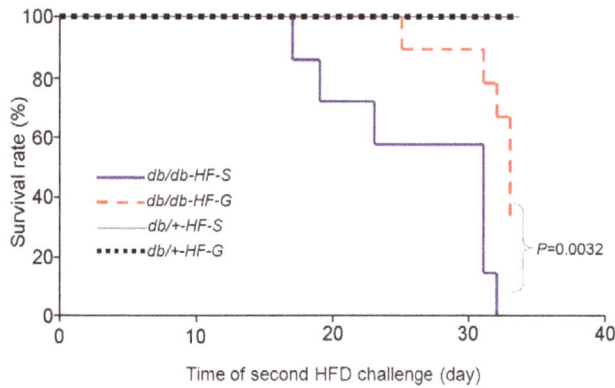

Figure 3. Effect of 17-DMAG on survival rate of HFD-fed *db/db* mice. Kaplan-Meyer survival analysis was performed using the log-rank statistics to measure the difference between the survival curves of d*b/db-HF-S* vs *db/db-HF-G* mice with n = 9 per group. Parallel experiments were performed with *db/+* mice (*db/+-HF-S* and *db/+-HF-G* groups) and no mortality was observed.

The peroxynitrite generation was also attenuated by 17-DMAG in the *db/db-HF-G* group even though the results did not reach statistical significance (Figure 4 F). These data demonstrate that in HFD-fed *db/db* mice, 17-DMAG reduces LA-induced $[Ca^{2+}]_m$ efflux, which may preserve Ca^{2+}-dependent mitochondrial functions and reduce oxidative stress in the kidney.

17-DMAG reduces nitrotyrosine level in HFD-fed db/db mice kidney

Since LA-induced $[Ca^{2+}]_m$ efflux is coupled to peroxynitrite generation [25] and nitrotyrosine level indicates oxidative damage by peroxynitrite, we measured nitrotyrosine levels in kidney tissues by immunoblotting and immunohistochemistry (Figure 5). As demonstrated in Figure 5 A, nitrotyrosine level in proteins with molecular weight ≤50 kDa was significantly higher in HFD-fed db/db mice injected with saline than in *db/+* mice. Interestingly, 17-DMAG treatment significantly lowered renal tissue nitrotyrosine levels in HFD-fed db/db mice (Figure 5A), indicating a protective effect against nitrosative injury by HFD. The results of immunohistochemistry also indicated high nitrotyrosine levels in HFD-fed db/db mice, particularly in the glomerular region, and

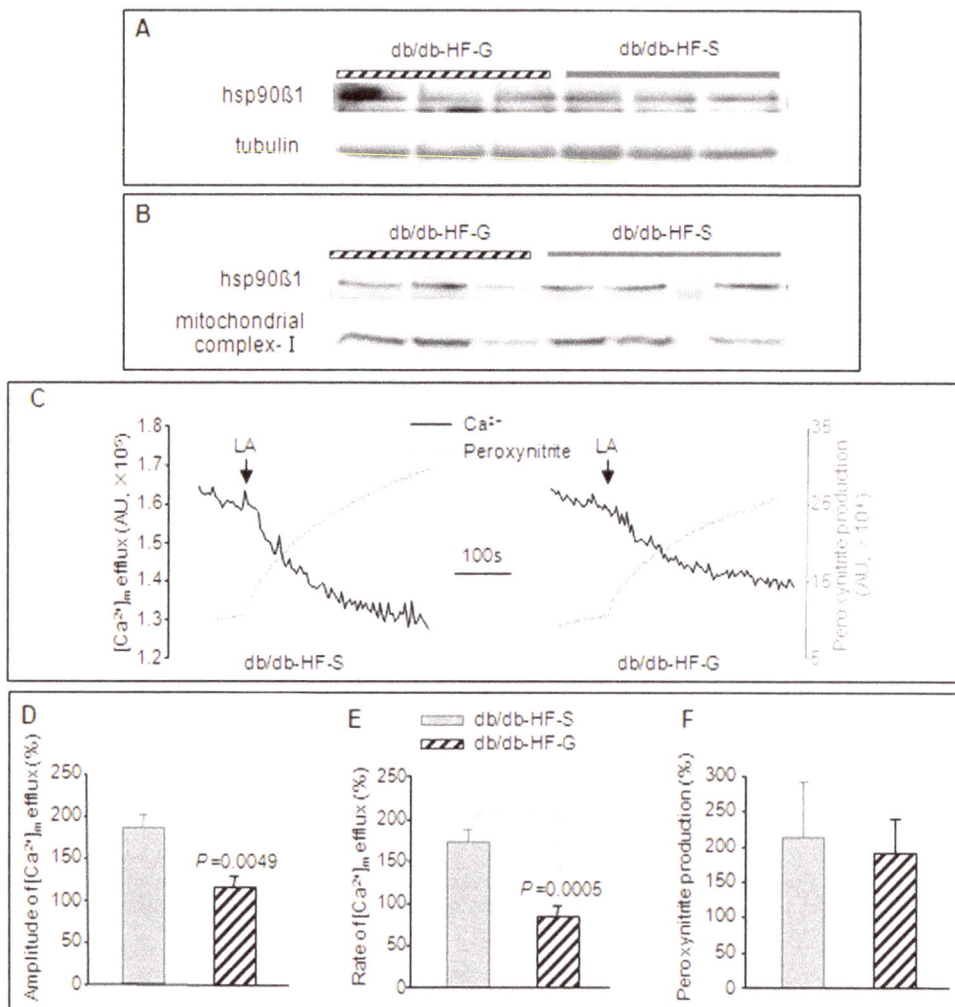

Figure 4. Impact of 17-DMAG on hsp90β1, $[Ca^{2+}]_m$, and peroxynitrite generation in the kidney. Western blot analysis was performed to assess hsp90β1 in kidney homogenate (*A*) and isolated mitochondria (*B*) of HFD-fed *db/db* mice with 6 animals per group. Linoleic acid (LA)-induced $[Ca^{2+}]_m$ efflux and peroxynitrite generation (*C–F*) in kidney mitochondria were measured.

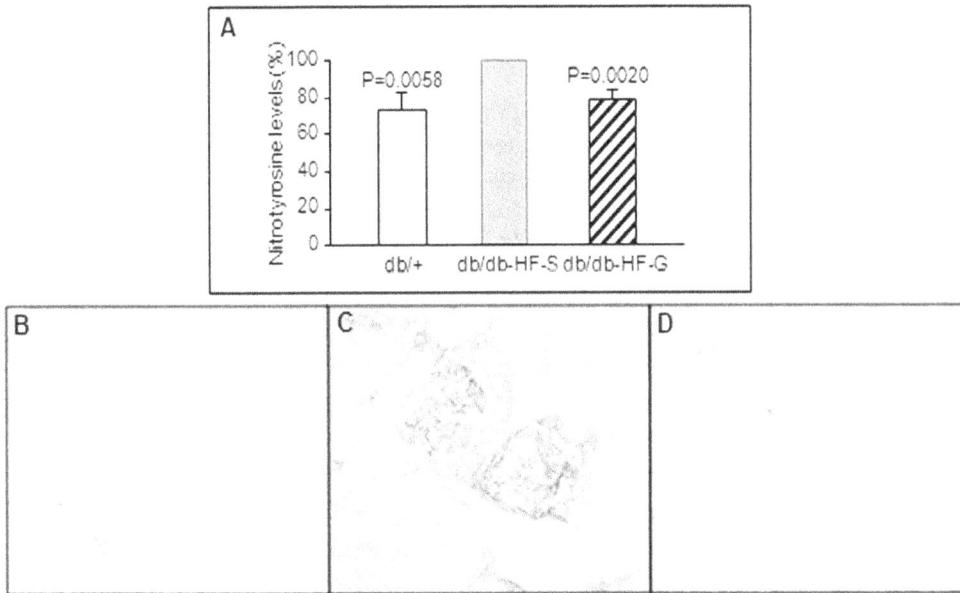

Figure 5. Effect of 17-DMAG on nitrotyrosine levels in the kidney. (A) Western blot analysis of nitrotyrosine was performed with monoclonal antibodies in kidney homogenates. The bar graphs were mean±SE density values from proteins ≤50 kDa normalized to the *db/db-HF-S* group from 6 animals per group. The nitrotyrosine level in kidney sections of *db/+* (C), *db/db-HF-S* (D) and *db/db-HF-G* (E) groups was assessed by immunohistochemistry with same monoclonal antibodies.

17-DMAG treatment effectively reduced renal tissue nitrotyrosine levels (Figure 5 B–D).

Discussion

Diabetic renal disease is a complication that develops in a subpopulation of patients with longstanding diabetes [1]. The deterioration in kidney functions including albuminuria and reduction of glomerular filtration rate is associated with histopathological alterations characterized by mesangial matrix expansion, glomerulosclerosis and tubulointerstitial fibrosis [27]. All of these functional and histopathological changes are believed to be the result of an interaction between metabolic abnormality and genetic predisposition [28]. Our results provide evidence that HFD accelerates diabetic nephropathy and caused renal failure in db/db mice, a rodent model of type 2 diabetes (Figures 1, 2, 3). The exacerbated albuminuria but not the 24 h urine output caused by HFD was reversible following discontinuation of HFD (Figure 1). However, prolonged HFD feeding leads to oliguria and anuria, an indication of renal failure, associated with animal death in db/db mice. More severe damage to glomeruli and tubules was also observed in HFD-fed db/db mice (Figure 2). All these deleterious effects of HFD in db/db mice were significantly ameliorated by inhibition of hsp90 with 17-DMAG. Our results suggest that HFD may worsen diabetic nephropathy and cause renal failure by exacerbating the metabolic abnormality in db/db mice.

The levels of plasma glucose and nonesterified fatty acids (NEFA) are elevated in type 2 diabetes and are implicated in diabetic complications. Several clinical studies with large cohorts have shown the role of hyperglycemia as a causative factor in the development and progression of diabetic nephropathy [29–31]. Experimental evidence support that hyperglycemia alters the expression of a number of genes involved in matrix protein synthesis and degradation in the diabetic kidney [32]. Nevertheless, hyperglycemia alone is clearly not sufficient to account for the heterogeneity and variability of diabetic nephropathy. We thus used HFD-fed db/db mice to investigate the effect of high lipid ingestion on the progression of diabetic nephropathy. We found that following 2 weeks of HFD feeding, both db/+ and db/db mice exerted excessive accumulation of adipose tissues as indicated by the rapid extra bodyweight gains (11.5% in db/+ and 22% in db/db on HFD, $P<0.05$, n = 5), which were coupled with significantly increased albuminuria in the kidney of db/db mice. Both dietary lipid ingestion and deregulated lipolysis due to insulin resistance may lead to higher circulated NEFA in HFD-fed db/db mice. These observations suggest that the deleterious effect of HFD on the kidney of db/db mice may be due to the exacerbating metabolic abnormality associated with excessive fat accumulation and elevated NEFA.

Kidney mitochondria, the major site of catabolism and oxidation of carbohydrates and lipids, are readily exposed and vulnerable to damaging insults from the exacerbated hyperglycemia and hyperlipidemia in HFD-fed db/db mice and the damage to renal mitochondria may contribute to worsening of nephropathy and renal failure observed (Figures 1 and 2). Morphological and ultrastructural changes of the mitochondria in proximal tubules correlate with deterioration of renal function in diabetes [33,34]. Increased posttranslational modification of renal mitochondrial proteins through glycation [35], nitration and oxidation [36] is associated with the development of diabetic nephropathy in animal models. Moreover, glycation of mitochondrial proteins is associated with excess superoxide generation [35]. It has been reported that repetitive intraperitoneal injection of NEFA-bond bovine serum albumin leads to functional and structural alterations in mouse kidney with characteristics similar to those of diabetic nephropathy [37]. These renal abnormalities were associated with a decrease in catalase, superoxide dismutase, enzymes involved in NEFA oxidation, and antiapoptotic proteins, and an increase of proinflammatory factors and macrophage infiltration. We noted an imbalance in mitochondrial complex I and III in the renal mitochondria in db/db mice [38,39]. In cultured cells, linoleic acid and other NEFA has been shown to cause loss of mitochondrial membrane potential, activation of caspase 3, 7, and 9, cytochrome c release and apoptosis, $[Ca^{2+}]_m$ efflux and peroxynitrite generation [25,40]. We provided evidence that the last action of NEFA is mediated by hsp90β1 [26]. It is possible that all these NEFA actions upon mitochondria may contribute to the deterioration of diabetic kidney and development of renal failure in HFD-fed db/db mice. The beneficial effect of 17-DMAG on renal function and structure and the counteraction of 17-DMAG upon linoleic acid induced $[Ca^{2+}]_m$ efflux in renal mitochondria in HFD-fed db/db mice suggest the involvement of these pathways.

As a highly water soluble derivative of geldanamycin, 17-DMAG is an hsp90 inhibitor with potent anticancer activities against a wide range of malignancies. Its application has been expanded to treat a mouse model of spinal and bulbar muscular atrophy [41]. In this study, treatment of db/db mice with 17-DMAG during HFD challenge preserves renal function and ameliorates damages to glomeruli and tubules, indicating involvement of hsp90β1 in the pathology of diabetic nephropathy and renal failure. As a chaperone protein, hsp90β1 is abundantly expressed in cells and tissues and is widely distributed in most subcellular organelles, such as plasma membrane, cytosol, endoplasmic reticulum, mitochondrion, and nucleus [26,42–44]. Hsp90 were detected in outer medulla and glomeruli of rat kidney, but no significant alterations were observed in type 1 diabetic rats [45]. Increased hsp90β levels have been observed in muscles of type 2 diabetes patients [46]. Our previous in vitro studies have indicated that mitochondrial hsp90β1 is involved in regulating cytosolic Ca^{2+} and $[Ca^{2+}]_m$ homeostasis [24–26]. A major role of $[Ca^{2+}]_m$ is to stimulate oxidative phosphorylation by activation of multiple dehydrogenases [47] and ATP synthesis [48]. $[Ca^{2+}]_m$ inhibits the generation of ROS from complexes I and III under normal conditions whereas its overload promotes ROS generation and apoptosis [49]. The enhanced $[Ca^{2+}]_m$ efflux in renal mitochondria of HFD-fed db/db mice may diminish the inhibitory effect of $[Ca^{2+}]_m$ on ROS production and thus leads to overproduction of superoxide and peroxynitrite. Furthermore, elevated NEFA, particularly linoleic acid, may augment the interaction with hsp90β1 and $[Ca^{2+}]_m$ efflux to deplete $[Ca^{2+}]_m$ and overproduce peroxynitrite, which exaggerates kidney oxidative/nitrosative injuries and eventuates renal failure. This paradigm is supported by the facts that enhanced $[Ca^{2+}]_m$ efflux and nitrotyrosine levels were found in the kidney of HFD-fed db/db mice and inhibition of hsp90 with 17-DMAG ameliorated these HFD effects (Figures 4 and 5). The significant elevation of plasma linoleic acids and arachidonic acids [50,51] and kidney nitrotyrosine levels [5,52,53] in type 2 diabetes patients indicate that a similar scenario may also occur in human beings.

Although 17-DMAG effectively reduced $[Ca^{2+}]_m$ efflux and nitrotyrosine levels in the kidney of HFD-fed db/db mice, we did not observe a significant reduction in the peroxynitrite generation coupled to linoleic acid-induced $[Ca^{2+}]_m$ efflux (Figures 4 and 5). The reason for the different responses to hsp90 inhibition with 17-DMAG on peroxynitrite generation in mitochondria from db/db mice and cultured human mesangial cells [25] is currently unclear. Whether mitochondria in different cell types of kidney (predominantly epithelial cells with few other cell types including mesangial cells) respond to 17-DMAG distinctly requires further investigations.

In summary, our results indicate that HFD aggravates nephropathy and causes renal failure in diabetes and these effects of HFD are antagonized by 17-DMAG. Decreased $[Ca^{2+}]_m$ efflux and lowered nitrotyrosine levels may account for the beneficial effect of 17-DMAG in diminishing nitrosative injury, preserving kidney function and structure, and improving animal survival. These results suggest that hsp90β1 is a potential target for prevention or treatment of nephropathy and renal failure in diabetes. 17-DMAG or other hsp90 inhibitors might represent new and promising therapeutic candidates for diabetic nephropathy and renal failure.

Materials and Methods

Animals

The animal protocols were approved by the Institutional Animal Care and Use Committee, South Texas Veterans Health Care System. Male db/db (BKS.Cg-m+/+Lepr^{db}/J), age and sex matched db/+ mice were acquired from Jackson Laboratories at age of 10 weeks and housed 4/cage or less. Animals were habitat for 2 weeks in a temperature- and humidity-controlled facility with a 12:12-h light-dark cycle, fed ad libitum with regular diet (7012 Teklad LM-485, Harlan Laboratories) and had free access to water. The mice were challenged with high fat diet (HFD) (TD.06414, Harlan Laboratories, 60.3% calories from fat) starting at 12 weeks of age as depicted in Figure 1A. The HFD challenge was divided into two phases: in the first phase the mice were fed with HFD for 2 weeks followed by a 4-week regular diet period. The second phase of HFD feeding was started after the 4-week regular diet interval and continued for 5 weeks because of a total mortality in HFD-fed db/db mice. At the beginning of the second HFD feeding, db/db mice were randomly assigned to 2 groups and intraperitoneally injected with either saline (vehicle, db/db-HF-S) or 17-DMAG (6.5 μg/kg bodyweight, db/db-HF-G; InvivoGen). Bodyweight of the animals was followed weekly and the dose of 17-DMAG was adjusted according to bodyweight gains.

Assessment of renal function by 24-h urine output and urinary albumin or serum creatinine

Urine collection and other physical parameters were measured following the schedule in Figure 1A. The animals were fasted for 6 h (9:00 AM-3:00 PM) prior to blood glucose measurement with a glucometer (Accu-Chek, Roche). 24 h urine samples were collected from individual mice housed in metabolic cages and the total urine volume was measured to index urine output. Urinary albumin concentrations were determined using a murine albumin ELISA kit (Albuwell M Kit; Exocell, Philadelphia, PA). In mice with oliguria or anuria, serum creatinine concentrations were determined by the Creatinine Companion kit (Exocell) to indicate renal functions.

Histopathology

Formalin-fixed, paraffin-embedded kidney sections were stained with haematoxylin and eosin (HE), periodic acid-Schiff (PAS), or Masson's trichrome and analyzed to evaluate kidney damages in a blinded manner. The area of glomerular PAS staining was measured by image analysis using Image-Pro Plus 4.5 (Media Cybernetics, Silverspring, MD) as described [54]. A semi-quantitative assessment was performed [55] in HE-stained slides to evaluate the extent of tubular damage and graded from 1 to 5 as follows: 1: vacuolation of cytoplasm in <20% of tubules; 2: vacuoles in 20% to 40% of tubules; 3: vacuoles in 40% to 60% tubules with minimal distortion of tubular structures; 4: vacuoles in 60% to 80% of tubules with large and marked distortion of tubular profiles, pyknotic nuclei, patches of tubular atrophy and tubular degeneration; and 5: >80% of tubules with severe vacuolation, or tubular atrophy and degeneration. The fractal collagen volume was assessed by point counter grid using ImageJ (NIH) program to quantify the blue stain in the trichrome-stained sections [56].

Measurement of $[Ca^{2+}]_m$ and peroxynitrite in mitochondria

Kidney mitochondria were prepared from mice and LA-induced $[Ca^{2+}]_m$ efflux and peroxynitrite generation were assessed as previously described [25,26]. Briefly, fresh kidney tissues (0.1–0.2 g) were homogenized in 5–10 ml MB1 solution containing 250 mM mannitol, 75 mM succinic acid, 0.1 mM EDTA, 0.5 mM EGTA, 10 mM HEPES, pH 7.4 at 4°C. The homogenates were centrifuged at 329 g for 15 min and mitochondria in the supernatant were collected by further centrifugation at 10000 g for 30 min. Mitochondria were double labeled with X-rhod-1 AM (2 μM) and 2′,7′-dichlorodihydrofluorescein diacetate (1 μM) at 37°C for 60 min and LA-induced $[Ca^{2+}]_m$ efflux and peroxynitrite generation were measured by changes in X-rhod-1 and 2′,7′-dichlorodihydrofluorescein fluorescence, respectively [25].

Assessment of hsp90β1 and nitrotyrosine

Immunoblotting and immunochemistry were performed to detect hsp90β1 and nitrotyrosine levels. In immunoblotting experiments, total and mitochondrial protein were isolated from mice kidney as previously described [25]. The primary antibodies used were as follows: mAb anti-mouse nitrotyrosine (1:1000, clone 1A6, Millipore); pAb anti-mouse GRP94 (1:1000, Santa Cruz Biotechnology), mAb anti-mitochondrial complex 1 NDUFS-3 subunit (1:2000, Invitrogen) and mAb anti-α-tubulin (1:1000, Invitrogen). The secondary antibodies were HRP-linked anti-rabbit or anti-mouse IgG (1:5000, GE Healthcare UK Limited). For the immunochemistry staining with mouse mAb, a specific procedure was performed as previously described [57] to eliminate the direct interaction between antigen and secondary antibody. Prior to application to the specimen, the primary mAb was incubated with secondary biotinylated anti-mouse immunoglobulin, resulting in the binding of biotinylated secondary antibody to the primary mAb. Normal mouse serum was added to the mixture to bind the residual biotinylated anti-mouse immunoglobulin,

preventing the potential interaction with endogenous immunoglobulin in the specimen. The nitrotyrosine levels were detected by streptavidine-peroxidase (Dako ARK Kit) and peroxidase substrate solution (DAB Substrate Kit, Vector Laboratories).

Statistical analysis

Results presented as mean±S.E and Student's t-test was used to evaluate the differences between two groups. Kaplan-Meyer survival analysis was performed using the log-rank statistic to test for a significant difference among the survival curves. Differences were considered statistically significant at $P<0.05$.

Supporting Information

Figure S1   Effects of HFD and 17-DMAG treatment on bodyweight and blood glucose levels of db/db mice. HFD caused rapid gains in bodyweight that was reversed to the baseline values measured prior to HFD feeding following four weeks discontinuation of HFD. The elevation of blood glucose after first HF seemed irreversible even after four weeks on RD feeding. The bodyweight gain was significantly potentiated in db/db-HF-D group compared to db/db-HF-S group (Figure S1). The persistently elevated blood glucose level that were not reversed during the four week interval of RD did not show further significant increases in the second HFD challenge (Figure S1, right panels). *$P<0.05$, **$P<0.001$, compared to baseline values assessed on day 0 from 6–12 animals per group.

Acknowledgments

We thank Dr. JL Barnes for help with mesangial expansion analysis and critical review of the manuscript and Dr. MA Hanes for help with inspection and interpretation of histopathology slides.

Author Contributions

Conceived and designed the experiments: HMZ BXZ. Performed the experiments: HMZ HD AK CKY BXZ. Analyzed the data: HMZ BXZ. Contributed reagents/materials/analysis tools: AK HD BXZ. Wrote the paper: HMZ BXZ.

References

1. Ismail-Beigi F, Moghissi E, Tiktin M, Hirsch IB, Inzucchi SE, et al. (2011) Individualizing glycemic targets in type 2 diabetes mellitus: implications of recent clinical trials. Ann Intern Med 154: 554–559.
2. Vallon V (2011) The proximal tubule in the pathophysiology of the diabetic kidney. Am J Physiol Regul Integr Comp Physiol 300: R1009–R1022.
3. Giacco F, Brownlee M (2010) Oxidative stress and diabetic complications. Circ Res 107: 1058–1070.
4. Sivitz WI, Yorek MA (2010) Mitochondrial dysfunction in diabetes: from molecular mechanisms to functional significance and therapeutic opportunities. Antioxid Redox Signal 12: 537–577.
5. Thuraisingham RC, Nott CA, Dodd SM, Yaqoob MM (2000) Increased nitrotyrosine staining in kidneys from patients with diabetic nephropathy. Kidney Int 57: 1968–1972.
6. Pergola PE, Raskin P, Toto RD, Meyer CJ, Huff JW, et al. (2011) Bardoxolone methyl and kidney function in CKD with type 2 diabetes. N Engl J Med 365: 327–336.
7. Pergola PE, Krauth M, Huff JW, Ferguson DA, Ruiz S, et al. (2011) Effect of bardoxolone methyl on kidney function in patients with T2D and Stage 3b-4 CKD. Am J Nephrol 33: 469–476.
8. Rossing K, Christensen PK, Hovind P, Tarnow L, Rossing P, et al. (2004) Progression of nephropathy in type 2 diabetic patients. Kidney Int 66: 1596–1605.
9. Hemmingsen B, Lund SS, Gluud C, Vaag A, Almdal T, et al. (2011) Targeting intensive glycaemic control versus targeting conventional glycaemic control for type 2 diabetes mellitus. Cochrane Database Syst Rev 6: CD008143.
10. Liu W, Tang F, Deng Y, Li X, Lan T, et al. (2009) Berberine reduces fibronectin and collagen accumulation in rat glomerular mesangial cells cultured under high glucose condition. Mol Cell Biochem 325: 99–105.

11. Danne T, Spiro MJ, Spiro RG (1993) Effect of high glucose on type IV collagen production by cultured glomerular epithelial, endothelial, and mesangial cells. Diabetes 42: 170–177.
12. Gilbert RE, Cooper ME (1999) The tubulointerstitium in progressive diabetic kidney disease: more than an aftermath of glomerular injury? Kidney Int 56: 1627–1637.
13. Jones SC, Saunders HJ, Pollock CA (1999) High glucose increases growth and collagen synthesis in cultured human tubulointerstitial cells. Diabet Med 16: 932–938.
14. Phillips AO, Steadman R, Morrisey K, Martin J, Eynstone L, et al. (1997) Exposure of human renal proximal tubular cells to glucose leads to accumulation of type IV collagen and fibronectin by decreased degradation. Kidney Int 52: 973–984.
15. Ziyadeh FN, Snipes ER, Watanabe M, Alvarez RJ, Goldfarb S, et al. (1990) High glucose induces cell hypertrophy and stimulates collagen gene transcription in proximal tubule. Am J Physiol 259: F704–F714.
16. Sun L, Xiao L, Nie J, Liu FY, Ling GH, et al. (2010) p66Shc mediates high-glucose and angiotensin II-induced oxidative stress renal tubular injury via mitochondrial-dependent apoptotic pathway. Am J Physiol Renal Physiol 299: F1014–F1025.
17. Munusamy S, MacMillan-Crow LA (2009) Mitochondrial superoxide plays a crucial role in the development of mitochondrial dysfunction during high glucose exposure in rat renal proximal tubular cells. Free Radic Biol Med 46: 1149–1157.
18. Adams JM, 2nd, Pratipanawatr T, Berria R, Wang E, DeFronzo RA, et al. (2004) Ceramide content is increased in skeletal muscle from obese insulin-resistant humans. Diabetes 53: 25–31.
19. Itani SI, Ruderman NB, Schmieder F, Boden G (2002) Lipid-induced insulin resistance in human muscle is associated with changes in diacylglycerol, protein kinase C, and IkappaB-alpha. Diabetes 51: 2005–2011.

20. Groop LC, Saloranta C, Shank M, Bonadonna RC, Ferrannini E, et al. (1991) The role of free fatty acid metabolism in the pathogenesis of insulin resistance in obesity and noninsulin-dependent diabetes mellitus. J Clin Endocrinol Metab 72: 96–107.

21. Golay A, Swislocki AL, Chen YD, Reaven GM (1987) Relationships between plasma-free fatty acid concentration, endogenous glucose production, and fasting hyperglycemia in normal and non–insulin-dependent diabetic individuals. Metabolism 36: 692–696.

22. Saloranta C, Groop L (1996) Interactions between glucose and FFA metabolism in man. Diabetes Metab Rev 12: 15–36.

23. Krebs M, Roden M (2005) Molecular mechanisms of lipid-induced insulin resistance in muscle, liver and vasculature. Diabetes Obes Metab 7: 621–632.

24. Zhang BX, Ma X, Zhang W, Yeh CK, Lin A, et al. (2006) Polyunsaturated fatty acids mobilize intracellular Ca2+ in NT2 human teratocarcinoma cells by causing release of Ca2+ from mitochondria. Am J Physiol Cell Physiol 290: C1321–C1333.

25. Zhang H-M, Dang H, Yeh C-K, Zhang B-X (2009) Linoleic acid-induced mitochondrial Ca(2+) efflux causes peroxynitrite generation and protein nitrotyrosylation. PLoS ONE 4: e6048.

26. Zhang H, Li ZH, Zhang MQ, Katz MS, Zhang BX (2008) Heat shock protein 90beta 1 is essential for polyunsaturated fatty acid-induced mitochondrial Ca2+ efflux. J Biol Chem 283: 7580–7589.

27. Sharma K, McCue P, Dunn SR (2003) Diabetic kidney disease in the db/db mouse. Am J Physiol Renal Physiol 284: F1138–F1144.

28. Dronavalli S, Duka I, Bakris GL (2008) The pathogenesis of diabetic nephropathy. Nat Clin Pract Endocrinol Metab 4: 444–452.

29. The Diabetes Control and Complications Trial Research Group (1993) The effect of intensive treatment of diabetes on the development and progression of long-term complications in insulin-dependent diabetes mellitus. N Engl J Med 329: 977–986.

30. UK Prospective Diabetes Study (UKPDS) Group (1998) Intensive blood-glucose control with sulphonylureas or insulin compared with conventional treatment and risk of complications in patients with type 2 diabetes (UKPDS 33). Lancet 352: 837–853.

31. Members of the ADVANCE collaborative group (2008) Intensive blood glucose control and vascular outcomes in patients with type 2 diabetes. N Engl J Med 358: 2560–2572.

32. Sanchez AP, Sharma K (2009) Transcription factors in the pathogenesis of diabetic nephropathy. Expert Rev Mol Med 11: e13.

33. Kaneda K, Iwao J, Sakata N, Takebayashi S (1992) Correlation between mitochondrial enlargement in renal proximal tubules and microalbuminuria in rats with early streptozotocin-induced diabetes. Acta Pathol Jpn 42: 855–860.

34. Nishi S, Ueno M, Hisaki S, Iino N, Iguchi S, et al. (2000) Ultrastructural characteristics of diabetic nephropathy. Med Electron Microsc 33: 65–73.

35. Rosca MG, Mustata TG, Kinter MT, Ozdemir AM, Kern TS, et al. (2005) Glycation of mitochondrial proteins from diabetic rat kidney is associated with excess superoxide formation. Am J Physiol Renal Physiol 289: F420–F430.

36. Ghosh S, Khazaei M, Moien-Afshari F, Ang LS, Granville DJ, et al. (2009) Moderate exercise attenuates caspase-3 activity, oxidative stress, and inhibits progression of diabetic renal disease in db/db mice. Am J Physiol Renal Physiol 296: F700–F708.

37. Takahashi K, Kamijo Y, Hora K, Hashimoto K, Higuchi M, et al. (2011) Pretreatment by low-dose fibrates protects against acute free fatty acid-induced renal tubule toxicity by counteracting PPARa deterioration. Toxicol Appl Pharmacol 252: 237–249.

38. Zhang H, Zhang H-M, Wu LP, Tan DX, Kamat A, et al. (2011) Impaired mitochondrial complex III and melatonin responsive reactive oxygen species generation in kidney mitochondria of db/db mice. J Pineal Res 51: 338–344.

39. Zhang H-M, Zhang Y, Zhang B-X (2011) The role of mitochondrial complex III in melatonin-induced ROS production in cultured mesangial cells. J Pineal Res 50: 78–82.

40. Tuo Y, Wang D, Li S, Chen C (2011) Long-term exposure of INS-1 rat insulinoma cells to linoleic acid and glucose in vitro affects cell viability and function through mitochondrial-mediated pathways. Endocrine 39: 128–138.

41. Tokui K, Adachi H, Waza M, Katsuno M, Minamiyama M, et al. (2009) 17-DMAG ameliorates polyglutamine-mediated motor neuron degeneration through well-preserved proteasome function in an SBMA model mouse. Hum Mol Genet 18: 898–910.

42. Kang BH, Plescia J, Dohi T, Rosa J, Doxsey SJ, et al. (2007) Regulation of tumor cell mitochondrial homeostasis by an organelle-specific hsp90 chaperone network. Cell 131: 257–270.

43. Kang BH, Plescia J, Song HY, Meli M, Colombo G, et al. (2009) Combinatorial drug design targeting multiple cancer signaling networks controlled by mitochondrial Hsp90. J Clin Invest 119: 454–464.

44. Sumanasekera WK, Tien ES, Davis JW, 2nd, Turpey R, Perdew GH, et al. (2003) Heat shock protein-90 (Hsp90) acts as a repressor of peroxisome proliferator-activated receptor-alpha (PPARalpha) and PPARbeta activity. Biochemistry 42: 10726–10735.

45. Barutta F, Pinach S, Giunti S, Vittone F, Forbes JM, et al. (2008) Heat shock protein expression in diabetic nephropathy. Am J Physiol Renal Physiol 295: F1817–F1824.

46. Hojlund K, Wrzesinski K, Larsen PM, Fey SJ, Roepstorff P, et al. (2003) Proteome Analysis Reveals Phosphorylation of ATP Synthase beta -Subunit in Human Skeletal Muscle and Proteins with Potential Roles in Type 2 Diabetes. J Biol Chem 278: 10436–10442.

47. Hansford R, Zorov D (1998) Role of mitochondrial calcium transport in the control of substrate oxidation. Mol Cell Biochem 184: 359–369.

48. Visch HJ, Koopman WJ, Zeegers D, van Emst-de Vries SE, van Kuppeveld FJ, et al. (2006) Ca2+-mobilizing agonists increase mitochondrial ATP production to accelerate cytosolic Ca2+ removal: aberrations in human complex I deficiency. Am J Physiol Cell Physiol 291: C308–C316.

49. Brookes PS, Yoon Y, Robotham JL, Anders MW, Sheu SS (2004) Calcium, ATP, and ROS: a mitochondrial love-hate triangle. Am J Physiol Cell Physiol 287: C817–C833.

50. Kamijo A, Kimura K, Sugaya T, Yamanouchi M, Hase H, et al. (2002) Urinary free fatty acids bound to albumin aggravate tubulointerstitial damage. Kidney Int 62: 1628–1637.

51. Yi L, He J, Liang Y, Yuan D, Gao H, et al. (2007) Simultaneously quantitative measurement of comprehensive profiles of esterified and non-esterified fatty acid in plasma of type 2 diabetic patients. Chem Phys Lipids 150: 204–216.

52. Shishehbor MH, Aviles RJ, Brennan ML, Fu X, Goormastic M, et al. (2003) Association of nitrotyrosine levels with cardiovascular disease and modulation by statin therapy. JAMA 289: 1675–1680.

53. Ceriello A, Mercuri F, Quagliaro L, Assaloni R, Motz E, et al. (2001) Detection of nitrotyrosine in the diabetic plasma: evidence of oxidative stress. Diabetologia 44: 834–838.

54. Danda RS, Habiba NM, Rincon-Choles H, Bhandari BK, Barnes JL, et al. (2005) Kidney involvement in a nongenetic rat model of type 2 diabetes. Kidney Int 68: 2562–2571.

55. Lauronen J, Häyry P, Paavonen T (2006) An image analysis-based method for quantification of chronic allograft damage index parameters. APMIS 114: 440–448.

56. Serón D, Moreso F (2007) Protocol biopsies in renal transplantation: prognostic value of structural monitoring. Kidney Int 72: 690–697.

57. van der Loos CM, Göbel H (2000) The animal research kit (ARK) can be used in a multistep double staining method for human tissue specimens. J Histochem Cytochem 48: 1431–1438.

13

High-Dose Enalapril Treatment Reverses Myocardial Fibrosis in Experimental Uremic Cardiomyopathy

Karin Tyralla[1], Marcin Adamczak[2,3], Kerstin Benz[1], Valentina Campean[1], Marie-Luise Gross[2], Karl F. Hilgers[4], Eberhard Ritz[5], Kerstin Amann[1]*

1 Department of Pathology, University of Erlangen-Nürnberg, Erlangen, Germany, 2 Department of Pathology, University of Heidelberg, Heidelberg, Germany, 3 Department of Nephrology, Endocrinology and Metabolic Diseases, Silesian University School of Medicine, Katowice, Poland, 4 Department of Internal Medicine-Nephrology, University of Erlangen-Nürnberg, Erlangen, Germany, 5 Department of Internal Medicine, University of Heidelberg, Heidelberg, Germany

Abstract

Aims: Patients with renal failure develop cardiovascular alterations which contribute to the higher rate of cardiac death. Blockade of the renin angiotensin system ameliorates the development of such changes. It is unclear, however, to what extent ACE-inhibitors can also reverse existing cardiovascular alterations. Therefore, we investigated the effect of high dose enalapril treatment on these alterations.

Methods: Male Sprague Dawley rats underwent subtotal nephrectomy (SNX, n = 34) or sham operation (sham, n = 39). Eight weeks after surgery, rats were sacrificed or allocated to treatment with either high-dose enalapril, combination of furosemide/dihydralazine or solvent for 4 weeks. Heart and aorta were evaluated using morphometry, stereological techniques and TaqMan PCR.

Results: After 8 and 12 weeks systolic blood pressure, albumin excretion, and left ventricular weight were significantly higher in untreated SNX compared to sham. Twelve weeks after SNX a significantly higher volume density of cardiac interstitial tissue ($2.57 \pm 0.43\%$ in SNX vs $1.50 \pm 0.43\%$ in sham, $p < 0.05$) and a significantly lower capillary length density (4532 ± 355 mm/mm^3 in SNX vs 5023 ± 624 mm/mm^3 in sham, $p < 0.05$) were found. Treatment of SNX with enalapril from week 8–12 significantly improved myocardial fibrosis ($1.63 \pm 0.25\%$, $p < 0.05$), but not capillary reduction (3908 ± 486 mm/mm^3) or increased intercapillary distance. In contrast, alternative antihypertensive treatment showed no such effect. Significantly increased media thickness together with decreased vascular smooth muscles cell number and a disarray of elastic fibres were found in the aorta of SNX animals compared to sham. Both antihypertensive treatments failed to cause complete regression of these alterations.

Conclusions: The study indicates that high dose ACE-I treatment causes partial, but not complete, reversal of cardiovascular changes in SNX.

Editor: Costanza Emanueli, University of Bristol, United Kingdom

Funding: Parts of the study were sponsored by a grant from the IZKF Erlangen (project A11). The funders had no role in study design, data collection and analysis, decision to publish, or preparation of the manuscript.

Competing Interests: The authors have declared that no competing interests exist.

* E-mail: kerstin.amann@uk-erlangen.de

Introduction

The development of left ventricular hypertrophy (LVH) and structural abnormalities of the heart and vessels is a key abnormality in chronic kidney disease (CKD) that potentially contributes to the high rate of cardiac death in this population [1]. Among the myocardial changes that accompany LVH in experimental renal failure as well as in patients with CKD the following play major roles: myocardial fibrosis [2,3], loss of cardiomyocytes [4], thickening of intramyocardial arterioles [5–6] and finally marked capillary deficit causing a mismatch between cardiomyocyte hypertrophy and capillary density [7–8].

Recent clinical and experimental studies document that the pathogenesis of these cardiovascular abnormalities is complex. Certainly, these abnormalities are not fully explained by increased pre- or afterload or by anemia [9–12]. Amongst others, the local renin aldosteron angiotensin system (RAS) seems to play a decisive role [1,13]. Other studies documented elevated angiotensin II and renin mRNA expression in the myocardium of subtotally nephrectomized animals (SNX) with moderate chronic renal failure [14,15]. In experimental renal failure blocking the RAS with an angiotensin converting enzyme (ACE) inhibitor (ACE-I) prevented development and progression of LVH and associated structural alterations such as myocardial fibrosis and loss of cardiomyocytes [16]. In patients with CKD evidence of regression of LVH after long-term treatment with either ACE-I or combination treatment was found [17,18]. Regression of LVH was also seen in hemodialysed patients with a policy of negative sodium balance, thus lowering blood pressure in the absence of any medication [19,20]. These studies in human beings could not address the issue how structural alterations of the heart in CKD were affected by either ACE-I or blood pressure lowering, respectively.

Whether in experimental renal failure ACE-I can also regress prevalent cardiac abnormalities and how these were affected in detail has not been investigated so far.

These considerations prompted the present study in subtotally nephrectomized rats which had developed major cardiovascular pathology. It was particularly designed to investigate the hypothesis that high-dose treatment with the ACE-I enalapril, but not treatment with alternative blood pressure lowering drugs reversed such existing cardiovascular pathology, i.e. LVH, interstitial myocardial fibrosis, reduced myocardial capillary supply, intramyocardial arteriolar and aortic wall thickening. In a standard model of moderate experimental renal failure [21] we assessed structural changes of the heart and the aorta in untreated SNX animals at 8 weeks and in addition compared at 12 weeks untreated SNX with SNX that had been treated for 4 weeks (week 8–12) with high-dose enalapril. To exclude confounding by lowering of blood pressure we studied in parallel SNX and sham operated animals treated with the non-specific antihypertensive combination furosemide and dihydralazine.

Materials and Methods

1. Animals and study design (fig. 1A)

Three months old male Sprague Dawley rats (Charles River Co, Sulzfeld, Germany), mean body weight 379 ± 27 g, were housed at constant room temperature ($21°C$) and humidity (75%) and exposed to a 12 h light on, 12 h light off cycle. The animals had free access to water and were fed pellets (23.4% protein, 4.5% fat, 6% fiber, 0.4% sodium; Altromin GmbH, Lage, Germany). After a 7 days adaptation period, rats were randomly allotted to subtotal nephrectomy (SNX, n = 34) or sham operation (sham, n = 39). As described before [16] rats were subtotally nephrectomized in two steps: first, the right kidney was surgically removed and kidney weight was carefully protocolled, then, one week later weight controlled removal of cortical tissue of the hypertrophied left kidney corresponding to 2/3 of the weight of the right kidney. This standardized procedure of two-step, weight controlled surgical resection of renal cortex resulted in a very moderate and stable degree of renal failure with a minor increase in systolic blood pressure, if any. Using the above procedure of moderate two-step subtotal nephrectomy the total nephron number is reduced from approximately 60,000 to 15,000.

Eight weeks after the second operation, one group of sham and SNX animals was sacrificed in order to clearly demonstrate the findings before the onset of therapy (sham 8 wks, SNX 8 wks). The remaining sham and SNX rats were randomly allotted to 2 treatment arms for another 4 weeks (fig. 1A): (i) enalapril treatment (E, 48 mg/kg bw per day, sham+E, SNX+E), (ii) furosemide (F) + dihydralazine (D) treatment (F/D, 15+20 mg/kg bw, sham+F/D, SNXF/D). One group of sham and SNX animals was left untreated (sham 12 wks, SNX 12 wks). Treatment was given by adding the drugs to the drinking water at concentrations calculated to deliver the above mentioned dose. Daily food and water consumption were monitored and the doses were adjusted. The enalapril dose used in the current study exceeds the antihypertensive dose used in previous prevention studies by a factor of 4. In previous studies our group had shown that treatment with the ACE-I ramipril prevented the development of LVH and myocardial fibrosis in SNX rats [4,16]. When designing the present study we reasoned that in contrast to prevention [16], regression of already altered heart morphology might require a higher dose of E, e.g. 48 mg/kg body weight [22] similar to the high doses necessary to cause regression of glomerular sclerosis [23]. In the absence of studies on regression of cardiovascular alterations we chose the dose used by Ikoma et al. [22] who

showed that in SNX a dose of 48 mg/kg bw enalapril, but not lower doses caused regression of glomerular lesions. The doses of F and D were chosen according to a previous study[5] and adjusted to induce a comparable blood pressure lowering.

Ethics statement. All animal work has been conducted according to relevant national and international guidelines. Formal approval was given by the local authorities (Regierungspräsidium Karlsruhe, AZ 35-9185.81/69/98).

2. Blood pressure (bp) and urinary albumin measurements

Systolic bp and heart rate were measured at weeks 2, 5, 7, 9 and 11 using tail plethysmography in conscious rats that were acquainted to the measuring conditions. In each animal 6 consecutive measurements per session were performed.

Seven and 11 weeks after SNX animals were placed in metabolic cages and 24 h urine was collected to measure urine volume, electrolyte and albumin excretion [24].

3. Tissue preparation, morphometry and stereology

After the above mentioned recordings and blood sampling the experiment was terminated by retrograde perfusion fixation via the abdominal aorta Perfusion pressure was adapted according to the in vivo blood pressure of the animals, i.e. 120–140 mmHg. Perfusion was started with rheomacrodex/procainhydrochloride in order to prevent interstitial edema and artifacts due to various states of vasodilation, followed by either glutaraldehyde for morphometric and stereological investigations or icecold NaCl for molecular studies [5]. After the perfusion, the heart of each animal was taken out and the total heart weight aswell as the left ventricular weight were determined. From glutaraldehyde fixed hearts tissue samples and sections were obtained and stained according to the orientator method (for details see [16,25]). Thus, semithin sections of 8 random samples of the left ventricular muscle including the septum were cut and examined by light microscopy with oil immersion and phase contrast at a magnification of 1:1000. All investigations were performed in a blinded manner, i.e. the observer was unaware of the study group the animal belonged to. Volume density (V_V) of capillaries, interstitial tissue and myocytes was obtained using the point counting method according to the equation $P_P = V_V$ (with P_P is point density). Reference volume was the total myocardial tissue (exclusive of non-capillary vessels, i.e. arterioles and veins, and tissue clefts). Vascular geometry of intramyocardial arterioles, i.e. vessels with lumen diameters between 20 and 120 μm and at least one muscular layer, was analysed using planimetry and a semiautomatic image analysis system (Analysis, SIS, Münster, Germany) as described in detail [5,6]. Thereby, mean wall thickness, lumen diameter, media and lumen area were determined in every arteriole that was present in all semithin sections per animal.

A 3 mm thick slice of the descending aorta was also embedded in Epon Araldite and semithin sections were prepared for quantitative and qualitative evaluation of the aortic wall. The remaining cardiac and aortic tissue was embedded in paraffin and 3 μm thick sections were prepared and stained with HE and Sirius red (for visualization and quantification of fibrous tissue).

4. TaqMan PCR for cardiac TGF-β, TIMP-1 and TMP-2 gene expression

Total RNA was extracted with the Qiagen MiniKit (Qiagen GmbH, Hilden, Germany). First-strand cDNA was synthesized with TaqMan reverse transcription reagents (Applied Biosystems, Darmstadt, Germany) using random hexamers as primers. Reactions without Multiscribe reverse transcriptase were used as

A

73 Sprague Dawley rats, 8 groups:

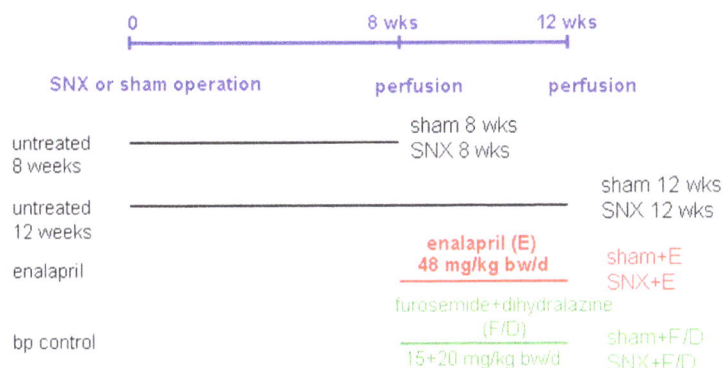

B

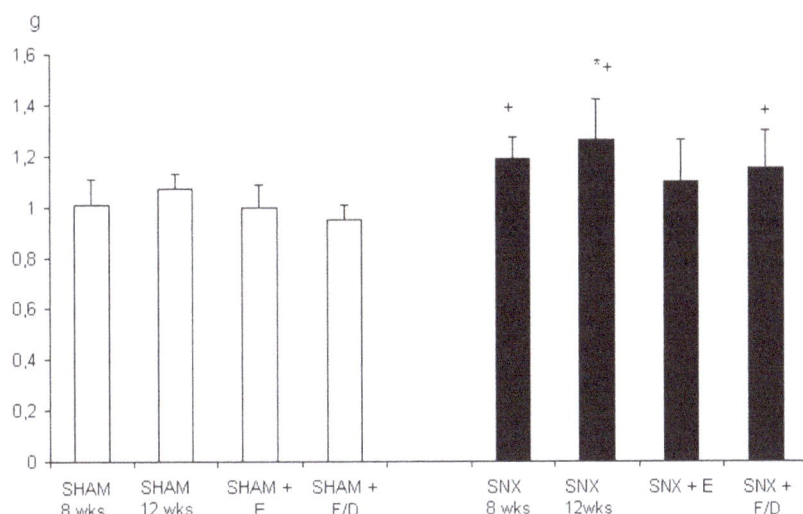

Figure 1. Experimental protocol (A) and left ventricular weight (B). A. Experimental protocol. B. Effect of treatment with the ACE-I enalapril or furosemide/dihydralazine on left ventricular weight (g). The increase in left ventricular weight (g) in untreated SNX at week 12 is completely prevented by enalapril, not by furosemide/dihydralazine treatment.

negative controls for genomic DNA contamination. PCR was performed with a Step One Plus Sequence Detector System FastSYBR Green Universal PCR Master Mix (Applied Biosystems), as described previously [26]. All samples were run in triplicate. Specific mRNA levels in hypertensive animals relative to UNX controls were calculated and normalized to a housekeeping gene with the Δ-Δ-C_T method as specified by the manufacturer (http://www3.appliedbiosystems.com/cms/groups/mcb_support/documents/generaldocuments/cms_040980.pdf).

Primer pairs and probes for transforming growth factor- β (TGF-β) [27] and tissue inhibitor of metalloproteases-1 and -2 (TIMP-1) were designed using Primer Express software (Perkin Elmer, Foster City, CA, USA) [28]. The relative amount of the specific mRNA was normalized with respect to 18S rRNA. All samples were run in triplicate.

5. Statistics

All statistical analysis was performed with SPSS 13. Data are given as mean $\pm$ standard deviation apart from the results of the TaqMan PCR which are provided as box plots. ANOVA was used for comparison of means followed by appropriate post-hoc tests. If distributional assumptions were in doubt the nonparametric Kruskal-Wallis-test was chosen. The zero-hypothesis was rejected at $p < 0.05$.

Results

1. Animal data

Enalapril (E) had no effect on body weight, but reversed left ventricular hypertrophy (LVH) in SNX animals (table 1, fig. 1B). At the end of the present experiment body weight was not significantly different between the groups. Eight and 12 weeks after SNX the weight of the left ventricle (LVW) was significantly higher in untreated SNX and SNX+F/D compared to sham indicating left ventricular hypertrophy (LVH). After 12 weeks LVW was significantly lower in SNX+E compared to untreated SNX documenting regression of LVH in SNX animals (fig. 1B). S-creatinine and urea as well as albuminuria were significantly higher in all SNX groups compared to sham (table 1). Of note, neither enalapril (E) nor furosemide/dihydralazine (F/D) treatment significantly lowered these parameters.

Comparable effects of enalapril (E) and furosemide/dihydralazine (F/D) on systolic blood pressure (bp) (fig. 2A). Two weeks after SNX systolic bp was not significantly different between the groups. From week 5 onward bp was moderately, but significantly higher in untreated SNX than in untreated sham. Treatment with E and F/D significantly and comparably lowered bp in SNX and sham compared to untreated animals. Of note, at week 7, i.e. 1 week before the initiation of antihypertensive treatment bp was highest in the SNX+F/D group and this might have some potential effect on any of the readout parameters although this remains speculative.

2. Effect of RAS blockade and alternative antihypertensive treatment on interstitial myocardial fibrosis and capillarisation in SNX (table 2, *figs. 2B,3,4*)

Enalapril (E), but not furosemide/dihydralazine (F/D) treatment caused regression of myocardial fibrosis in SNX animals (fig. 2B,3). At weeks 8 and 12 volume density of interstitial tissue (Vv int in %) as an index of myocardial fibrosis was significantly higher in untreated SNX than in sham operated rats (fig. 2B,3). Whereas RAS blockade with E significantly lowered the percentage of myocardial fibrous tissue compared to the values of untreated SNX at weeks 8 and 12, alternative antihypertensive treatment with F/D did not show such an effect.

The effect of Enalapril (E) on cardiac fibrosis in SNX animals was only partly dependent on lowering of TGF-β and TIMP expression (fig. 4). In the hearts of untreated SNX at 12 weeks markedly increased TGF-β, TIMP-1 and TIMP-2 mRNA expression compared to control animals was found by TaqMan PCR (fig. 4). Due to the high standard deviation of cardiac gene expression the difference was only statistically significant for TIMP-1 (fig. 4B). Expression of all 3 profibrotic genes was again markedly lowered by both antihypertensive treatments, but the differences were not statistically significant (fig. 4).

Enalapril (E) and furosemide/dihydralazine (F/D) treatment had no beneficial effect on reduced myocardial capillary density in SNX (table 2). At 8 weeks after SNX capillary length density (Lv), i.e. the total length of capillaries per unit myocardial volume, as a three-dimensional parameter of myocardial capillary supply was comparable in untreated SNX and sham animals. After 12 weeks myocardial capillary length density was markedly lower in untreated SNX compared to sham. Because of the high standard deviation this marked difference failed to be statistically significant. Antihypertensive treatment with either E or F/D did not improve myocardial capillary density in either SNX or sham animals. In SNX+E animals Lv was even lower compared to untreated SNX and F/D treatment. Changes in intercapillary distance, an important parameter of myocardial blood supply, went in parallel. In addition, myocardial intercapillary distance was significant higher in SNX 8 weeks than in sham (table 2).

3. Effect of RAS blockade and alternative antihypertensive treatment on changes of intramyocardial arterioles

Treatment with furosemide/dihydralazine (F/D), but not with Enalapril reversed wall thickening of intramyocardial

Table 1. Animal data: Effect of treatment with enalapril (E) or furosemide/dihydralazine (F/D) from week 8–12 in sham-op and SNX rats, respectively.

group	body weight [g]	S-creatinine [mg/dl]	S-urea [mg/dl]	albuminuria [mg/day]
SHAM 8 wks n = 10	500±20	0.48±0.08	40.8±2.9	2.76±2.65
SHAM 12 wks n = 10	552±24	0.49±0.06	44.2±3.3	4.38±4.90
SHAM +E n = 11	538±28	0.53±0.08	56.1±11.8	0.81±0.63
SHAM + F/D n = 8	586±39	0.4±0.05	42.4±5.26	1.31±1.34
SNX 8 wks n = 8	486±31	0.85±0.19 **a**	86.5±13.9 **a**	115±116 **a**
SNX 12 wks n = 8	531±52	0.88±0.23 **a**	97.9±32.1 **a**	277±148 **a**
SNX +E n = 11	491±25	0.92±0.08 **a**	107±19 **a**	258±220 **a**
SNX + F/D n = 7	544±19	1.01±0.57 **a**	118.1±67 **a**	192±195 **a**
analysis of variance	ns	p<0.001	p<0.05	p<0.001

mean ± standard deviation, [1] weight after perfusion fixation.
a) p<0.05 vs. corresponding SHAM.
b) p<0.05 vs. SNX 8 wks.
c) p<0.05 vs. SNX 12 wks.
d) p<0.05 vs. SNX+E.

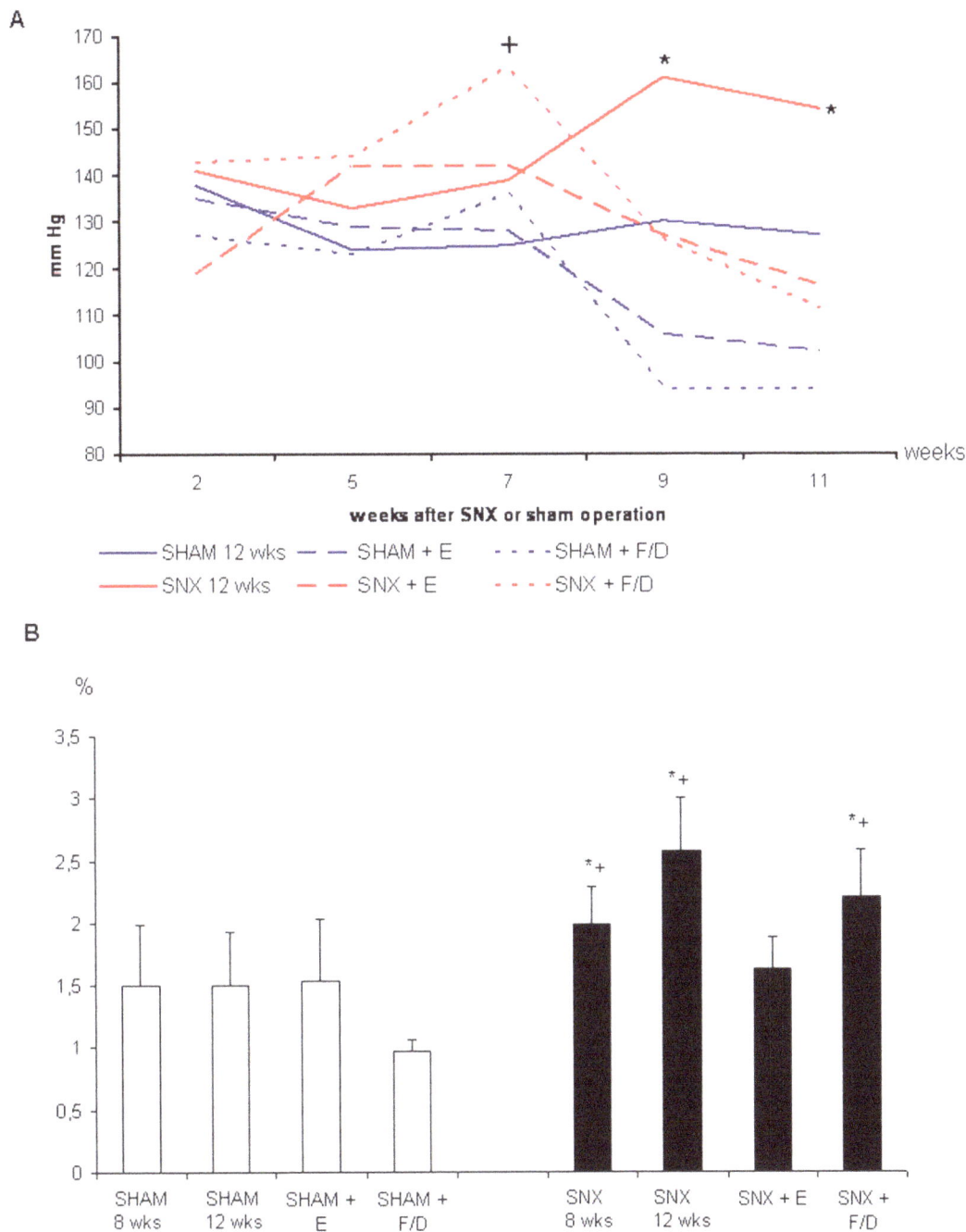

Figure 2. Effect of treatment with the ACE-I enalapril or furosemide/dihydralazine on systolic blood pressure (A) and myocardial interstitial fibrosis (B). A. Enalapril (E) and furosemide/dihydralazine (F/D) treatment lowered systolic blood pressure (bp) in sham and SNX to the same extent. Two weeks after SNX systolic bp was not significantly different between the groups. From week 5 onward bp was significantly higher ($p<0.01$) in untreated SNX than in untreated sham. At week 7 bp was highest in the SNX+F/D group. Treatment with E and F/D significantly and comparably lowered bp in SNX and sham compared to untreated animals. Mean of systolic blood pressure measurements at weeks 2, 5, 7, 9 and 11 using tail plethysmography in conscious rats that were acquainted to the measuring conditions. *: $p<0.01$ compared to all other groups. +: $p<0.05$ compared to all other groups. **B.** The increase in myocardial interstitial tissue (%) in untreated SNX at week 12 is completely prevented by enalapril, but not by furosemide/dihydralazine treatment. *: $p<0.05$ vs SNX 12 weeks. +: $p<0.05$ vs corresponding sham.

arterioles in SNX (table 2). All intramyocardial arterioles with lumen diameters between 15 and 50 μm were measured. The mean number of intramyocardial arterioles assessed per animal ranged from 6 to 32. The cumulative frequencies of arteries were not different between the groups excluding a sampling error. This conclusion is further supported by the fact that the mean lumen diameter was not significantly different between untreated sham and SNX 8 weeks (table 2). Lumen diameter in SNX 12 weeks and SNX+E was significantly lower than in SNX 8 weeks. In addition, it was significantly higher in SNX+F/D than in SNX+E. Wall thickness, wall:lumen ratio and media area (not shown) of intramyocardial arterioles were significantly higher in SNX 12

Table 2. Effect of enalapril (E) or furosemide/dihydralazine (F/D) treatment from week 8–12 in sham-op and SNX on intramyocardial arterioles and capillaries.

group	lumen diameter [μm]	wall thickness [μm]	wall:lumen ratio [μm/μm*10^{-2}]	Lv [mm/mm^3]	Intercapillary distance [μm]
SHAM 8 wks n = 10	30.0±4.9	3.3±0.5	12.4±2.7	4139±486	16.8±1.1
SHAM 12 wks n = 10	25.9±2.7	4.3±1.0	17.7±4.7	5023±624	15.3±1.0 **b**
SHAM +E n = 11	27.9±6.9	4.8±2.0	18.8±10.4	5339±915	14.9±1.2 **b**
SHAM + F/D n = 8	33.5±4.8	2.9±0.4	10.7±4.4	4641±429	15.7±0.7
SNX 8 wks n = 8	32.3±5.4 **c,d**	4.1±0.6 **c,d**	13.9±4.1 **c,d**	4086±517	16.9±1.1
SNX 12 wks n = 8	26.9±2.7 **b**	5.4±0.7 **b**	21.8±3.2 **b**	4532±355 **d**	16.0±0.7 **d**
SNX +E n = 11	25.2±4.3 **b**	5.9±1.7 **a,b**	24.7±8.8 **a,b**	3908±486 **a,c**	17.3±1.2 **a,c**
SNX + F/D n = 7	32.1±4.4 **d**	3.7±0.6 **c,d**	12.9±3.2 **c,d**	4610±553 **d**	15.9±1.0 **d**
analysis of variance	p<0.05	p<0.05	p<0.05	p<0.05	p<0.05

Mean ± standard deviation.
a) p<0.05 vs. corresponding SHAM.
b) p<0.05 vs. SNX 8 wks.
c) p<0.05 vs. SNX 12 wks.
d) p<0.05 vs. SNX+E.

weeks and SNX+E than in SNX 8 weeks. Interestingly, values were significantly lower in the SNX+F/D group.

4. Effect of RAS blockade and alternative antihypertensive treatment on changes of the aortic wall

Enalapril (E), but not furosemide/dihydralazine (F/D) lowered increased aortic wall thickness in SNX (table 3, fig. 5). Aortic lumen diameter and lumen area were not

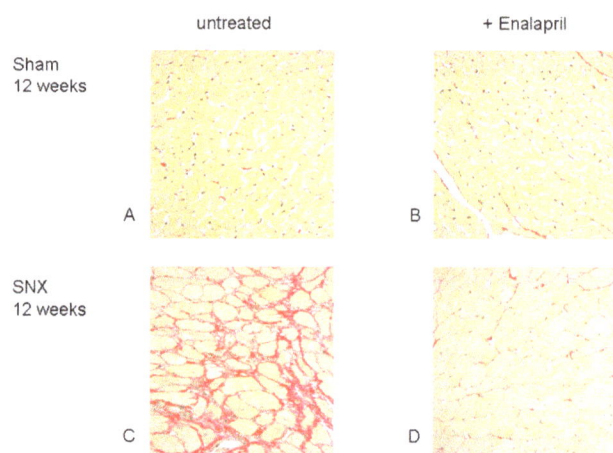

Figure 3. Myocardial fibrosis in untreated sham operated animals (A), sham+enalapril (B), untreated SNX 12 weeks (C) and SNX + enalapril (D). Note increased myocardial fibrous tissue content (depicted in red) in untreated SNX at 12 weeks (C) compared to untreated and treated sham (A,B). Complete regression of interstitial fibrosis is seen at 12 weeks after 4 weeks treatment with enalapril (D).Sirius red stain, magnification x 400.

significantly different between untreated sham and untreated SNX at 8 and 12 weeks. Lumen diameter was significantly lower in SNX+E compared to sham+E and significantly higher in SNX+F/D than in SNX 8 weeks presumably indicating vessel dilatation. In contrast, aortic media thickness at week 8 was significantly higher in SNX than in sham, whereas at week 12 due to the somewhat higher standard deviation there was only a tendency to higher values in SNX. Treatment of SNX with E, but not with F/D lowered aortic media thickness (table 3).

Enalapril (E) and furosemide/dihydralazine (F/D) improved aortic VSMC/matrix ratio in SNX animals (table 3, fig. 5). At weeks 8 and 12 the number of aortic VSMC per unit media area was significantly lower in untreated SNX compared to sham (table 3). In parallel, aortic extracellular matrix content as seen in fibrous tissue stains and semithin sections (fig. 5) was higher in untreated SNX (fig. 5C) than in sham (fig. 5A) indicating structural remodelling of the aortic wall. Of note, in both treated SNX groups (SNX+E, SNX+F/D) the number of VSMC per aortic media area was significantly increased compared to untreated SNX (tab. 3), but there was no effect on elastic fibre content (data not shown).

Discussion

In the present study the effect of 4 weeks of ACE inhibition (ACE-I) with high-dose enalapril (E) treatment on the regression of LVH and accompanying abnormalities of myocardium and aorta were investigated in an experimental model of chronic renal failure, i.e. the subtotally nephrectomized rats (SNX). Potential effects of blood pressure (bp) lowering by E were controlled for by a treatment arm with comparable bp lowering, i.e. a combination of furosemide and dihydralazine (F/D). Treatment with E, but not with F/D led to regression of LVH and myocardial interstitial fibrosis. In contrast, no beneficial effect of E was seen on reduction

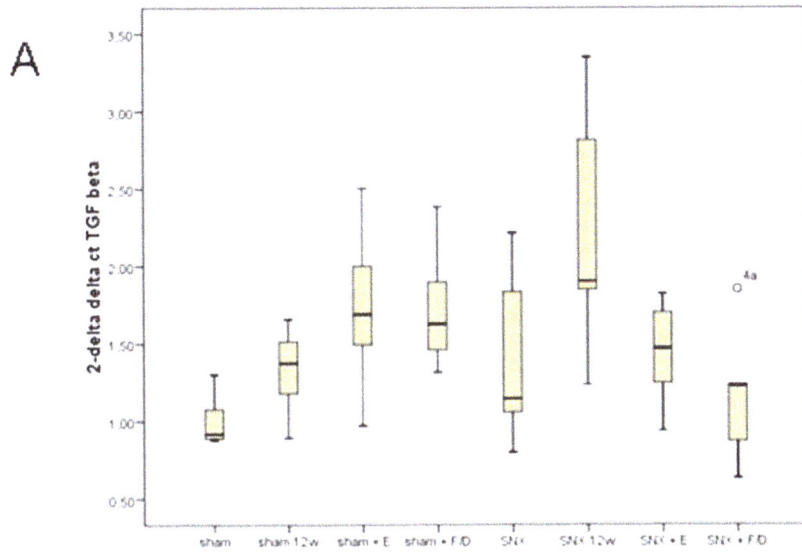

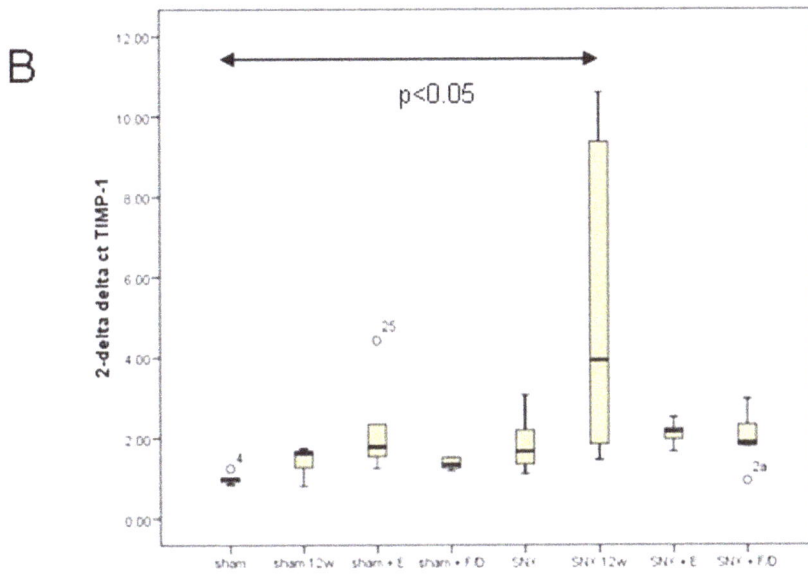

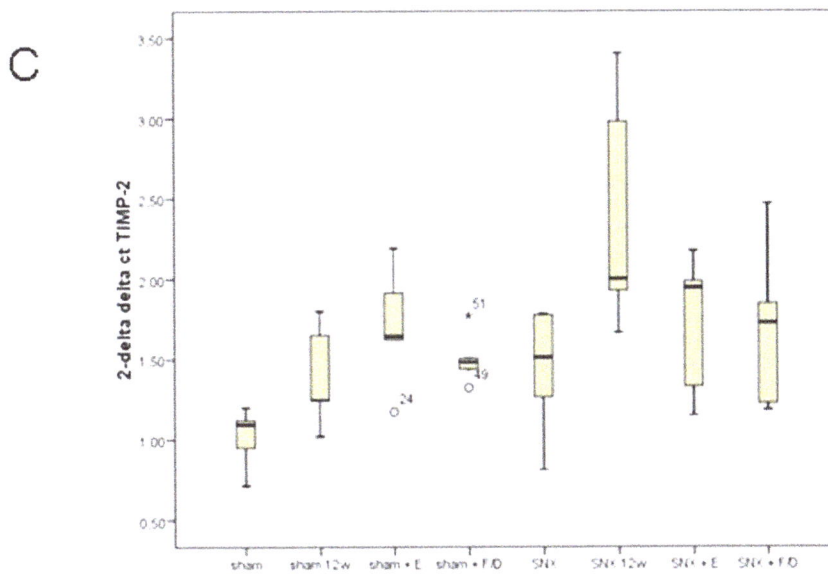

Figure 4. Effect of treatment with the ACE-I enalapril or furosemide/dihydralazine on cardiac mRNA expression of TGF-β (A), TIMP-1 (B) and TIMP-2 (B). Increased TGF-β mRNA expression in untreated SNX was lowered by both antihypertensive treatments. Cardiac TIMP-1 gene expression was also significantly higher in untreated SNX 12 weeks than in sham and SNX 8 weeks; RAS blockade by ACE-I and alternative antihypertensive treatment both lowered cardiac TIMP-1 gene expression in SNX animals. The same tendency was seen for TIMP-2 mRNA expression. The data are provided as box plots of the ΔCT analysis. ° indicate outlyers.

of myocardial capillary density, increased intercapillary distance or thickening of intramyocardial arteries in SNX, respectively.

Thickening of the aortic media in SNX was only partly, but not completely regressed by E treatment. The structural alterations of aortic media in SNX, i.e. decreased ratio VSMC:extracellular matrix were positively affected by both antihypertensive treatments.

Some methodological aspects of the present study deserve further comments:

In our hands the standard model of SNX induces reproducibly stable moderate chronic renal failure that is accompanied by only moderately increased systolic bp [5,16]. This is in contrast to findings in alternative models of renal insufficiency, i.e. the renal artery ligation model where bp is markedly increased [29]. In the SNX model by surgical ablation plasma Ang II is decreased, presumably due to volume overload, while increased local formation of Ang II has been reported in extrarenal resistance vessels [30]. The mechanisms contributing to higher local Ang II levels may include higher levels of the precursor protein angiotensinogen, and a decreased degradation of Ang II [30]. We are not aware of studies directly addressing such mechanisms in the heart. However, an upregulation of Ang II AT1 receptors and increased local renin mRNA in the myocardium has been reported after subtotal nephrectomy [7,13,31]. Higher AT1 receptor density may lead to a more pronounced local cardiac effect of Ang II. Of note, in a recent study [32] renal AT1 receptors were found to be required for the development of Ang II-dependent hypertension and cardiac hypertrophy suggesting

that the major mechanism of action of RAS inhibitors in hypertension is attenuation of Ang II effects in the kidney.

In previous studies our group had shown that treatment with the ACE-I ramipril prevented the development of LVH and myocardial fibrosis in SNX rats [4,16]. When designing the present study we reasoned that in contrast to prevention [33], regression of already altered heart morphology might require a higher dose of E, e.g. 48 mg/kg body weight [22] similar to the high doses necessary to cause regression of glomerular sclerosis [23]. In addition, there is accumulating data in the proteinuric nephropathy setting that using super-high doses of AT1 blockers can indeed be of added clinical benefit [34]. The combination of furosemide and dihydralazine was used to achieve comparable bp control; previous studies in this laboratory had documented that this combination did not affect morphological changes of the heart in SNX [5]. This is also in line with our past observation that the development of LVH in SNX is bp independent [4,10,11] since it cannot be prevented by bp lowering with either calcium channel blockers or other bp lowering agents, but only with ACE-I, endothelin receptor blockade or sympatholytic agents. These observations point so some pathogenetic involvement of these and other systems like for example increased PTH [1–3].

As already mentioned [32] Ang II was shown to affect hypertension and subsequent heart hypertrophy through its AT1 receptors in the kidney. In the absence of hypertension (due to the renal knockout of AT1), cardial AT1 receptors were not sufficient to cause hypertrophy. At first glance, these findings appear to conflict with the notion that the effects of RAS blockade were

Table 3. Effect of enalapril (E) or furosemide/dihydralazine (F/D) treatment from week 8–12 in sham-op and SNX on the aortic wall.

group	lumen diameter [μm]	lumen area [mm²]	media thickness [μm]	media area [mm²]	number of VSMC per media area [1/mm²]
SHAM 8 wks n = 10	1177±375	1.19±0.71	88.9±8.9	0.422±0.17	19.2±7.07
SHAM 12 wks n = 10	1487±464	1.89±0.85	97.6±11.7	0.658±0.25	18.4±2.60
SHAM +E n = 11	1109±395	1.08±0.78	83.2±7.32	0.431±0.12	18.3±2.27
SHAM + F/D n = 8	1809±294	2.63±0.77	100±11.9	0.705±0.21	20.4±2.94
SNX 8 wks n = 8	1312±383	1.45±0.82	105±6.47 **a**	0.582±0.20	14.4±2.53 **a**
SNX 12 wks n = 8	1676±298	2.27±0.81	109±21.9	0.792±0.30	10.8±2.36 **a.d**
SNX + E n = 11	1471±270 **a**	1.75±0.59	98.6±18.4 **a**	0.634±0.21 **a**	14.8±2.00 **a.c**
SNX + F/D n = 7	1854±530 **b**	2.89±1.26 **b.d**	109±19.7	0.859±0.25 **b.d**	15.4±2.22 **a.c**
analysis of variance	p<0.05	p<0.05	p<0.05	p<0.05	p<0.05

Mean ± standard deviation.
a) p<0.05 vs. corresponding SHAM.
b) p<0.05 vs. SNX 8 wks.
c) p<0.05 vs. SNX 12 wks.
d) p<0.05 vs. SNX+E.

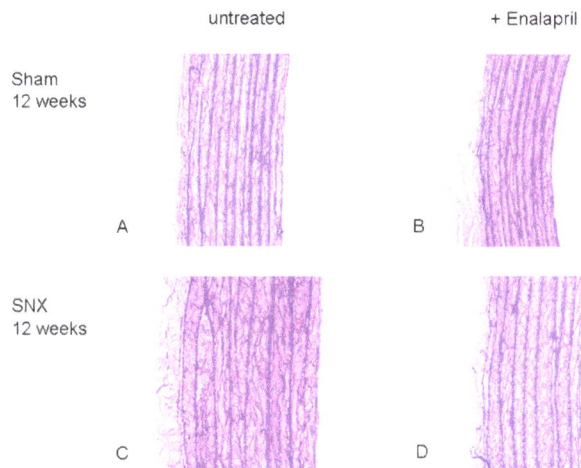

Figure 5. Effect of treatment with the ACE-I enalapril (E) on aortic wall thickness and aortic remodelling in sham (A,B) and SNX rats (C,D). The increase in aortic wall thickness in untreated SNX (C) compared to untreated and E-treated sham (A,B) reversed by antihypertensive treatment with enalapril (D).

independent from bp in our model. However, several aspects of the experimental setup were different. Apart from species differences and different strategies to interfere with the RAS, kidney AT1 receptors were not knocked out in our model but some degree of Ang II signaling through AT1 was certainly present in the kidney. Further, the effects of local RAS activation on the heart may be more pronounced in the presence of volume overload which could occur in subtotal nephrectomy. We have to acknowledge, however, that some of the effects of F/D treatment can be presumably explained by differences in bp before the start of treatment and particulary by increased natriuresis which has been shown to help to prevent and regress LVH [19,20].

There is good evidence for a role of the local cardiac RAS (and possibly bradykinin) in the pathogenesis of myocardial fibrosis [35]. Gonzalez et al. [36] showed that AngII signalling via the AT-1 receptor, MAPK/ERK and SMAD stimulates procollagen I formation and inhibits the activity of collagenases resulting in increased collagen I accumulation. This cascade is further modulated by TGF-β, PDGF, aldosterone, integrins and PAI-1 [36]. Of note, in the present experimental study TGF-β, TIMP-1 and TIMP-2 mRNA expression was not specifically altered by E treatment (and this was also confirmed for TGF-β on the protein level using immunohistochemistry, data not shown). In experimental renal failure as well, ACE-I therapy attenuated the development of myocardial fibrosis and cardiomyocyte hypertrophy as a result of activating lysosomal proteinases [37]. In past experiments we treated SNX animals with a combination of ACE-I and bradykinin antagonist; thereby the bradykinin antagonist abrogated the beneficial effect of ACE-I [35]. In addition to inhibiting cardiac fibrosis, ACE-I also reduced the loss of cardiomyocytes by apoptosis in SNX rats [4].

Apart from activation of the local RAS in the heart, changed elasticity of central arteries, mainly the aorta, also contribute to the development of LVH in CKD. This was documented by London et al in CKD patients [38]. Reduced aortic elasticity increases the pressure load imposed upon the left ventricle thus aggravating LVH. It is therefore of note that in the present study we confirmed reduced elastic fibre content and disturbed architecture of elastic fibres in the aorta of SNX animals [5,16]. This will increase aortic stiffness together with the observed reduced VSMC numbers and

increased extracellular matrix. Of note, on a qualitative base these structural alterations were positively affected by high-dose ACE-I. This is in line with data on a protective effect of ramipril in animal models of hypertension without renal dysfunction [39].

Our previous studies had documented a selective and marked increase of myocardial interstitial non-vascular tissue in SNX rats [3] and in uremic patients [40]. In uremic patients myocardial fibrosis was shown to be independent of potential confounders such as hypertension, diabetes or duration of dialysis [41]. In SNX animals treatment with the ACE-I ramipril, but not with the sympatholytic agent moxonidine or the calcium channel blocker nifedipine prevented the development of myocardial fibrosis [4]. This finding is confirmed and extended by the results of the present study: Enalapril, but not alternative antihypertensive treatment with furosemide/dihydralazine caused even regression of established myocardial fibrosis. Regression is proven by the observation that at week 12 the interstitial tissue area of SNX animals which had received high dose E for 4 weeks was even lower than the baseline value in untreated SNX at week 8. Apart from lowering of AngII by ACE-I a complementary explanation might be accumulation of bradykinin and we had already provided evidence for this in an earlier study using the SNX model [35]. Minshall et al. [42] documented bradykinin-2-receptors on neonatal and adult rat fibroblasts as well as cardiomyocytes. Stimulation of these receptors influences proliferation and protein synthesis directly and indirectly (via nitric oxide or prostacyclin) in various tissues [43]. It is therefore conceivable that bradykinin accumulation in the myocardium inhibits collagen synthesis by interstitial fibroblasts [44]. This idea is in line with increased PCNA positivity of interstitial cells indicating activation of fibroblasts and increased TGF-β expression in the heart of SNX animals compared to sham operated controls [10]. Of note, in renal failure PTH has a permissive role on the activation of interstitial fibroblasts in vitro and in vitro [3]. Ultrastructural analysis in SNX animals 14 days after subtotal nephrectomy documented early selective activation of cardiac interstitial fibroblasts, but not of endothelial cells [2]. Furthermore, Suzuki et al. documented that the increase in interstitial matrix is due to both increased production by activated fibroblasts and decreased matrix removal by MMPs [37].

The length density of intramyocardial capillaries as a three-dimensional parameter of myocardial capillary supply is significantly reduced in experimental renal failure[8] as well as in uremic patients [40]. Reduced myocardial capillary supply increases the intercapillary distance thus lowering pO2 midways between the capillaries thus rendering the myocardium more susceptible for ischemic injury [8,10]. Deficient capillary supply is a feature of LVH in renal failure. Its development is independent of bp [16]. In SNX reduced myocardial capillary supply is prevented by selective blockade of the sympathetic and endothelin systems [16,45] as well as by the antioxidant vitamin E [46] but not by ACE-I [16]. The present study extends the latter finding by documenting that low capillary density is not reversed by E either; we noted even a tendency to lower values after E treatment. This finding could be due to a blockade of the promitogenic effect of Ang II on endothelial cells [47] by ACE-I. An alternative explantation may be exhaustion of the endothelial cell pool after intense endothelial cell/mesenchymal transition [48]. As expected based on the findings of the various prevention studies treatment with F/D did not show any beneficial effect on reduced myocardial capillary density.

Thickening of intramyocardial arterioles as well as of extra-cardiac arteries and veins is found in SNX rats and in CKD patients [5,10,16]. In the present study we noted only a tendency to higher wall thickness in SNX at 8 weeks compared to sham animals which increased with the duration of renal failure and was significant at 12 weeks. This increase in wall thickness was not regressed or prevented by E which is in line with previous studies of our group [5,16], but contrasts to data of Kakinuma et al [49] who described a protective effect of ACE-I with respect to vascular thickening in experimental renal failure. The marked effect of F/D on intramyocardial arteriolar wall thickness and wall: lumen ratio was unexpected. F/D treatment had also an effect on the arteriolar diameter which is increased possibly indicating arteriolar dilatation.

In summary, in subtotally nephrectomized rats, high doses of the ACE-I enalapril cause regression of LVH and interstitial myocardial fibrosis. In addition, regression of abnormal aortic wall texture is observed. These results of this short term study extend previous experimental findings that lower doses of ACE-I prevent cardiac and aortic pathology and provide another argument for the clinical use of ACE-I in patients with CKD and established cardiovascular pathology. In remarkable contrast, myocardial capillary density and intercapillary distance, crucial determinants of tissue hypoxia tolerance, were not positively affected by ACE-I treatment. It remains to be investigated, however, whether longer treatment periods or addition of combination treatment with AT2 or aldosterone receptor blockers or renin inhibition, respectively, may increase the effects.

Acknowledgments

The authors thank Monika Klewer, Stefan Söllner, Miriam Reutelshöfer and Rainer Wachtveitl for expert technical assistance.

Author Contributions

Conceived and designed the experiments: MLG ER KA. Performed the experiments: KT MA. Analyzed the data: KT MA KB VC KFH KA. Contributed reagents/materials/analysis tools: KB VC KFH. Wrote the paper: KB KFH ER KA.

References

1. Amann K, Ritz E (1997) Cardiac disease in chronic uremia: Pathophysiology. Adv Ren Replace Ther 4: 212–224.
2. Mall G, Rambausek M, Neumeister A, Kollmar S, Vetterlein F, et al. (1988) Myocardial interstitial fibrosis in experimental uremia – implications for cardiac compliance. Kidney Int 33: 804–811.
3. Amann K, Ritz E, Wiest G, Klaus G, Mall G (1994) A role of parathyroid hormone for the activation of cardiac fibroblasts in uremia. J Am Soc Nephrol 4: 1814–1819.
4. Amann K, Tyralla K, Gross ML, Schwarz U, Törnig J, et al. (2003) Cardiomyocyte loss in experimental renal failure: Prevention by ramipril. Kidney Int 63: 1708–1713.
5. Amann K, Neusuess R, Ritz E, Irzyniec T, Wiest G, et al. (1995) Changes of vascular architecture independent of blood pressure in experimental renal failure. Am J Hypertens 8: 409–417.
6. Amann K, Törnig J, Flechtenmacher C, Nabokov A, Mall G, et al. (1995) Blood pressure independent wall thickening of intramyocardial arterioles in experimental uremia – evidence for a permissive action of PTH. Nephrol Dial Transplant 10: 2043–2048.
7. Amann K, Neimeier KA, Schwarz U, Törnig J, Matthias S, et al. (1997) Rats with moderate renal failure show capillary deficit in the heart but not in skeletal muscle. Am J Kidney Dis 30: 382–388.
8. Amann K, Wiest G, Zimmer G, Gretz N, Ritz E, et al. (1992) Reduced capillarydensity in the myocardium of uremic rats – a stereological study. Kidney Int 42: 1079–1085.
9. Rambausek M, Ritz E, Mall G, Mehls O, Katus H (1985) Myocardial hypertrophy in rats with renal insufficiency. Kidney Int 28: 775–787.
10. Amann K, Ritz E (2001) The heart in renal failure: Morphological changes of the myocardium – new insights. J Clin Basic Cardiol 4: 109–113.
11. Siedlecki AM, Jin X, Muslin AJ (2009) Uremic cardiac hypertrophy is reversed by rapamycin but not by lowering of blood pressure. Kidney Int 75: 800–8.
12. Eckardt KU, Scherhag A, Macdougall IC, Tsakiris D, Clyne N, et al. (2009) Left ventricular geometry predicts cardiovascular outcomes associated with anemia correction in CKD. J Am Soc Nephrol 20: 2651–60.
13. Ritz E (2009) Left ventricular hypertrophy in renal disease: beyond preload and afterload. Kidney Int 75: 771–3.
14. Kunczera M, Hilgers KF, Lisson C, Ganten D, Hilgenfeldt U, et al. (1991) Local angiotensin formation in hindlimbs of uremic hypertensive and renovascular hypertensive rats. J Hypertens 9: 41–48.
15. Ritz E, Amann K, Törnig J, Schwarz U, Stein G (1997) Some cardiac abnormalities in renal failure. Advances in Nephrology Vol. 27, Mosby, St. Louis, USA. pp 85–103.
16. Törnig J, Amann K, Ritz E, Nichols C, Zeier M, et al. (1996) Arteriolar wall thickening, capillary rarefaction and interstitial fibrosis in the heart of rats with renal failure: The effects of Ramipril, Nifedipin and Moxonidin. J Am Soc Nephrol 7: 667–675.
17. Cannella G, Paoletti E, Delfino R, Peloso G, Rolla D, et al. (1997) Prolonged therapy with ACE inhibitors induces a regression of left ventricular hypertrophy of dialyzed uremic patients independent from hypotensive effects. J Am Kidney Dis 30: 659–664.
18. Hampl H, Henning L, Rosenberger C, Amirkhalily M, Gogoll L, et al. (2005) Effects of optimized heart failure therapy and anemia correction with epoetin beta on left ventricular mass in hemodialysis patients. Am J Nephrol 25: 211–20.
19. Özkahya M, Ok E, Cirit M, Aydin S, Akçiçek F, et al. (1998) Regression of left ventricular hypertrophy in haemodialysis patients by ultrafiltration and reduced salt intake without antihypertensive drugs. Nephrol Dial Transplant 13: 1489–93.

20. Töz H, Ozkahya M, Dorhout Mees EJ (1999) Long-term evolution of cardiomyopathy in dialysis patients. Kidney Int 56: 350–1.
21. Gretz N, Meisinger E, Strauch M (1988) Partial nephrectomy and chronic renal failure: the "mature" rat model. Contrib Nephrol 60: 46–55.
22. Ikoma M, Kawamura T, Kakinuma J, Foga A, Ichikawa I (1991) Cause of variable therapeutic efficacy of angiotensin converting enzyme inhibitor on glomerular mesangial lesions. Kidney Int 40: 195–202.
23. Adamczak M, Gross ML, Krtil J, Koch A, Tyralla K, et al. (2009) Reversal of glomerulosclerosis after high-dose enalapril treatment in subtotally nephrectomised rats. J Am Soc Nephrol 14: 2833–42.
24. Schwarz U, Amann K, Orth SR, Simonaviciene A, Wessels S, et al. (1998) Effect of 1,25 (OH)2 vitamin D3 on glomerulosclerosis in subtotally nephrectomised rats. Kidney Int 53: 1696–705.
25. Mattfeldt T, Mall G, Gharehbaghi H, Möller P (1990) Estimation of surface area and length with the orientator. J Microsc 159: 301–317.
26. Hartner A, Veelken R, Wittmann M, Cordasic N, Hilgers KF (2005) Effects of diabetes and hypertension on macrophage infiltration and matrix expansion in the rat kidney. BMC Nephro 6: 6.
27. Ruiz V, Ordóñez RM, Berumen J, Ramirez R, Uhal B, et al. (2003) Unbalanced collagenases/TIMP-1 expression and epithelial apoptosis in experimental lung fibrosis. Am J Physiol Lung Cell Mol Physiol 285: L1026–36.
28. Hui AY, Leung WK, Chan HL, Chan FK, Go MY, et al. (2006) Effect of celecoxib on experimental liver fibrosis in rat. Liver Int 26: 125–36.
29. Griffin KA, Picken M, Bidani AK (1994) Method of renal mass reduction is a critical modulator of subsequent hypertension and glomerular injury. J Am Soc Nephrol 4: 2023–31.
30. Jackson B, Hodsman P, Johnston CI (1988) Changes in the renin-angiotensin system, exchangeable body sodium, and plasma and atrial content of atrial natriuretic factor during evolution of chronic renal failure in the rat. Am J Hypertens 1: 298–300.
31. Li Y, Takemura G, Okada H, Miyata S, Maruyama R, et al. (2007) Molecular signaling mediated by angiotensin II type 1A receptor blockade leading to attenuation of renal dysfunction-associated heart failure. J Card Fail 13: 155–62.
32. Crowley SD, Gurley SB, Herrera MJ, Ruiz P, Griffiths R, et al. (2006) Angiotensin II causes hypertension and cardiac hypertrophy through its receptors in the kidney. Proc Natl Acad Sci U S A 103: 17985–90.
33. Weiz MR (2007) Effects of renin-angiotensin system inhibition on end-organ protection: can we do better? Clin Ther 9: 1803–24.
34. Fernandez-Juárez G, Barrio V, de Vinuesa SG, Goicoechea M, Praga M, et al. (2006) Dual blockade of the renin-angiotensin system in the progression of renal disease: the need for more clinical trials. J Am Soc Nephrol 17: S250–4.
35. Amann K, Gassmann P, Buzello M, Orth SR, Törnig M, et al. (2000) Effects of ACE inhibition and bradykinin antagonism on cardiovascular changes in uremic rats. Kidney Int 58: 153–161.
36. González A, López B, Querejeta R, Diez J (2002) Regulation of myocardial fibrillar collagen by angiotensin II. A role in hypertensive heart disease? J Mol Cell Cardiol 34: 1585–93.
37. Suzuki H, Schaefer L, Ling H, Schaefer RM, Dammrich J, et al. (1995) Prevention of cardiac hypertrophy in experimental chronic renal failure by long-term ACE-inhibitior administration: Potential role of lysosomal proteinases. Am J Nephrol 15: 129–136.
38. London GM, Marchais SJ, Safar ME, Genest AF, Guerin AP, et al. (1990) Aortic and large artery compliance in end stage renal failure. Kidney Int 37: 137–142.
39. Gohlke P, Lamberty V, Kuwer I, Bartenbach S, Schnell A, et al. (1993) : Vascular remodelling in systemic hypertension. Am J Cardiol 72: 2E–7E.

40. Amann K, Breitenbach M, Ritz E, Mall G (1998) Myocyte/capillary mismatch in the heart of uremic patients. J Am Soc Nephrol 9: 1018–1022.

41. Mall G, Huther W, Schneider J, Lundin P, Ritz E (1990) Diffuse intermyocardiocytic fibrosis in uremic patients. Nephrol Dail Transplant 5: 39–44.

42. Minshall RD, Makamura F, Becker RP, Rabito SF (1995) Characterisation of bradykinin B2 receptors in adult myocardium and neonatal rat cardiomyocytes. Circ Res 76: 773–780.

43. Clerk A, Gillespie-Brown J, Fuller SJ, Sugden PH (1996) Stimulation of phosphatidylinositol hydrolysis, protein kinase C translocation, and mitogen-activated protein kinase activity by bradykinin in rat ventricular myocytes: Dissociaton from hypertrophic response. Biochem J 317: 109–118.

44. Imai C, Okamura A, Peng JF, Kitamura Y, Printz MB (2005) Interleukin-1beta enhanced action of kinins on extracellular matrix of spontaneous hypertensive rat cardiac fibroblasts. Clin Exp Hypertens 27: 59–69.

45. Amann K, Münter K, Wessels S, Wagner J, Balajew V, et al. (2000) Endothelin A receptor blockede prevents capillary/myocyte mismatch in he heart of uremic animals. J Am Soc Nephrol 11: 1702–1711.

46. Amann K, Törnig J, Buzello M, Kuhlmann A, Gross ML, et al. (2002) Effect of antoxidant therapy with dl-α-tocopherol on cardiovascular structure in experimental renal failure. Kidney Int 62: 877–884.

47. Wolf G, Ziyadeh FN, Zahner G, Stahl RAK (1996) Angiotensin II is mitogenic for cultured rat glomerular endothelial cells. Hypertension 27: 897–905.

48. Zeisberg EM, Tarnavski O, Zeisberg M, Dorfman AL, McMullen JR, et al. (2007) Endothelial-to-mesenchymal transition contributes to cardiac fibrosis. Nat Med 13: 952–61.

49. Kakinuma Y, Kawamura T, Bills T, Yoshioka T, Ichikawa I, et al. (1992) Blood pressure independent effect of angiotensin inhibitors on vascular lesions of chronic renal failure. Kidney Int 42: 46–55.

Treatment of Cryptococcal Meningitis in KwaZulu-Natal, South Africa

Josephine V. J. Lightowler[1,2], Graham S. Cooke[3,4]*, Portia Mutevedzi[3], Richard J. Lessells[3], Marie-Louise Newell[3,5], Martin Dedicoat[1,6]

1 Ngwelezane Hospital, Empangeni, KwaZulu-Natal, South Africa, 2 John Radcliffe Hospital, Oxford, United Kingdom, 3 Africa Centre for Health and Population Studies, University of KwaZulu-Natal, Mtubatuba, South Africa, 4 Department of Infectious Diseases, Imperial College London, London, United Kingdom, 5 UCL Institute of Child Health, London, United Kingdom, 6 University of Limpopo, Limpopo, South Africa

Abstract

Background: Cryptococcal meningitis (CM) remains a leading cause of death for HIV-infected individuals in sub-Saharan Africa. Improved treatment strategies are needed if individuals are to benefit from the increasing availability of antiretroviral therapy. We investigated the factors associated with mortality in routine care in KwaZulu-Natal, South Africa.

Methodology/Principal Findings: A prospective year long, single-center, consecutive case series of individuals diagnosed with cryptococcal meningitis 190 patients were diagnosed with culture positive cryptococcal meningitis, of whom 186 were included in the study. 52/186 (28.0%) patients died within 14 days of diagnosis and 60/186 (32.3%) had died by day 28. In multivariable cox regression analysis, focal neurology (aHR 11 95%C.I. 3.08–39.3, P<0.001), diastolic blood pressure <60 mmHg (aHR 2.37 95%C.I. 1.11–5.04, P = 0.025), concurrent treatment for tuberculosis (aHR 2.11 95%C.I. 1.02–4.35, P = 0.044) and use of fluconazole monotherapy (aHR 3.69 95% C.I. 1.74–7.85, P<0.001) were associated with increased mortality at 14 and 28 days.

Conclusions: Even in a setting where amphotericin B is available, mortality from cryptococcal meningitis in this setting is high, particularly in the immediate period after diagnosis. This highlights the still unmet need not only for earlier diagnosis of HIV and timely access to treatment of opportunistic infections, but for better treatment strategies of cryptococcal meningitis.

Editor: Dana Davis, University of Minnesota, United States of America

Funding: This work was funded in part by Wellcome Trust grant (GR085957). The funders had no role in study design, data collection and analysis, decision to publish, or preparation of manuscript.

Competing Interests: The authors have declared that no competing interests exist.

* E-mail: gcooke@africacentre.ac.za

Introduction

Despite the increasingly widespread availability of highly active antiretroviral therapy (HAART) throughout sub-Saharan Africa, HIV remains the leading cause of death amongst adults in many populations, particularly in rural Southern Africa [1] Prior to the availability of antiretrovirals, cryptococcal meningitis (CM) accounted for a significant proportion of deaths in HIV infected individuals [2–4] and even with increasing availability of HAART, recent data suggests that CM may account for more deaths amongst HIV positive individuals in sub-Saharan Africa than tuberculosis [5].

For many individuals with HIV, their first presentation to health services is with a major opportunistic infection such as CM and optimal management in these individuals is crucial if they are to benefit fully from antiretroviral therapy. Data from different healthcare settings is valuable for the identification of factors associated with treatment outcome and understanding which interventions are necessary to improve survival. The clinical diagnosis and management of CM differ between clinical settings depending on resources available [6]. Availability of diagnostics,

drugs and trained nursing and medical staff, as well as other broader health systems issues influencing timely access to healthcare are all likely to be relevant to outcomes.

We set out to understand the factors associated with outcome for patients with CM in a public sector hospital setting within northern KwaZulu-Natal, South Africa, where the prevalence of HIV infection reaches 20% or more among the general adult population.

Methods

This study was carried out at Ngwelezane hospital, a 550 bed regional government hospital in Northern KwaZulu-Natal, South Africa. KwaZulu-Natal is the South African province worst affected by HIV with an estimated 1.5 million infected individuals [7]. The hospital offers both district and regional services. 440,000 people fall under the hospital's district catchment area, only patients from this area were included in the study as for patients referred from other hospitals it was not possible to get baseline information.

All patients diagnosed with cerebrospinal fluid (CSF) culture positive CM during 2007 were included in the study. Verbal informed consent was obtained from the patient or relatives for the collection of relevant data from the patient's chart.

The decision to initiate CM treatment was based on a clinical diagnosis supported by positive Indian Ink microscopy. Patients were treated according to local hospital protocol with amphotericin B (AmB) 0.7 mg/kg daily for 14 days when supplies were available. Liposomal formulations were not available. 1 litre of normal saline was given before each dose of AmB, further intravenous fluids were given at the discretion of the treating doctor. Where possible lumbar puncture was repeated on days 7 and 14. Additional lumbar punctures were carried out if the patient developed severe headache believed by the clinician to be due to CM. CSF pressure measurement was not routinely performed as appropriate equipment was usually not available. Patients who had renal impairment on admission (define as serum creatinine >220 umol/l) were treated with fluconazole 400 mg daily rather than AmB in line with South African treatment guidelines at the time of the study. If a patient's renal function improved following hydration, AmB was started at standard dosage.

All patients had full blood counts, electrolytes (U&E) and liver function tests performed prior to initiating therapy with AmB. U&E was repeated every 48 hours. Electrolyte abnormalities were corrected where possible. Where possible, cannulation sites were rotated every 72 hours to prevent thrombophlebitis. Patients developing renal impairment were given increased intravenous fluids. If a patient's creatinine rose to >220 umol/l AmB was stopped and fluconazole 400 mg daily started. If the patients renal function improved AmB was restarted. If the patient's renal function deteriorated again AmB was terminated for good and substituted with fluconazole 400 mg daily. Flucytosine was not available during the study period.

As a regional centre, the hospital has both CT and MRI scans available. There is an on-site intensive care unit (ICU), but medical patients are not routinely admitted to the unit and none of the patients in this study were admitted to ICU. HAART has been available locally through public sector provision since 2004. All patients of unknown HIV status were offered VCT when clinically well enough to consent, no patients were tested anonymously or without consent. All patients not on HAART were offered treatment under South African guidelines that take any WHO stage IV illness (in this case CM) as an eligibility criterion for initiating HAART. HAART was started only after 14 days of AmB treatment, either as an inpatient, at a chronic care facility, or most usually, at an outpatient ART clinic following discharge.

Data were collected by a physician (MD) using a standardized data collection form. All patients were reviewed by the clinical team daily, and study data was updated every 48 hours. Data were entered into an excel spread sheet and verified on a separate occasion. For survival analysis, patients were right censored at date of discharge or date of later follow-up visit, with the outcome being mortality. Person time was calculated as days from date presenting at the hospital, as opposed to onset of disease, to date of death or date of discharge or review for those still alive. Kaplan-Meier analysis was used to determine the overall time to death and mortality rate as well as 14 and 28 day mortality rates. Cox regression analysis with Breslow method for ties was used to assess variables that were independently associated with 14 day and 28 days mortality. STATA 10 (College Station, Texas, USA) was used for analysis.

Results

Overall 92/186 (49.5%) individuals were male with a median age of 33.5 years (IQR 28–39.5). The median age for women

was 30.5 years (IQR 27–36), significantly lower than for men (P = 0.019). Baseline characteristics are shown in Table 1.

148/186 (79.6%) individuals received amphotericin B, 28/186 Fluconazole (15.1%) and one patient both treatments. In 25/28 (89.3%) patients receiving initial treatment with fluconazole, the treatment decision was based on the presence of renal failure. In 16 cases initially treated with amphotericin, patients were changed to fluconazole because of the development of renal failure. Other adverse events were uncommon, the most frequent side effect being hypokalaemia that developed in 7/186 (3.8%) Individuals.

Overall mortality rate was 2.13 deaths per 100 person days (95% CI 1.66–2.72). Mortality rates were higher in the first 14 days (2.54 per 100 person days, 95% C.I. 1.94–3.33) than the second 14 days (2.12 per 100 person years 95% C.I. 1.65–2.73). 52/186 (28.0%) patients died as in-patients within the first 14 days and 60/186 (32.3%) by 28 days (see Table 2). Data for overall outcomes are shown in Table 2.

Survival Analysis

Kaplan Meier plots are shown in figure 1. Risks factors for 14 day and 28 day mortality are shown in Table 3. The final model had 175 patients for 14 day mortality and 171 for 28 day mortality. For 14 day mortality, 11 individuals had data missing with respect to diastolic blood pressure. The presence of focal neurological abnormality, diastolic hypotension, concurrent treatment for TB and the use of fluconazole rather than amphotericin, were associated with increased mortality at 14 and 28 days (Table 3).

Discussion

Cryptococcal disease remains an important cause of mortality particularly in sub-Saharan Africa, despite the increasing availability of antiretrovirals. We describe a prospective series of individuals within a single health care setting operating within the public health sector of South Africa. The strengths of this data are that it is a large series, representative of outcomes in routine practice within South Africa.

A high proportion of the mortality observed in this unselected prospective case series was seen in the first 14 days. Unsurprisingly, the mortality rates observed are substantially higher than those in a western setting where mortality of 2.5–15% is more typical [8,9] and have improved since the advent of HAART[10]. A significant number of individuals left hospital prior to completion of CM treatment and thus the true mortality might be higher than observed, though even if it were pessimistically assumed that all patients discharged alive died within the first 14 days after starting treatment, mortality rate would rise to only 31%. By comparison to a recent study from a centre in central Kampala, Uganda [11] mortality rates observed here were higher than seen in the post-HAART era raising important questions as to what factors are predictive of a poor outcome to treatment, though such differences could be explained by exclusion of comatose patients and those on fluconazole in that study.

The association of focal neurology with poorer outcome is perhaps not surprising, suggesting as it does the presence of more severe disease. The association between diastolic hypotension and increased mortality has not been described previously. High blood pressure can reflect raised intracranial pressure and might be expected to be associated with a poorer outcome. However, in this study, headache (also a feature of raised intracranial pressure) was associated with better outcome. Diastolic hypotension might reflect other concurrent infections (for example, bacterial infection) or metabolic disturbance (for example, hypoadrenalism) that may

Table 1. Description of 186 patients diagnosed with Cryptococcal meningitis, presenting at Ngwelezana hospital.

Variable	n		n for group	%	
sex	186	Male	92	49.5	
		female	94	50.5	
			Over all	male	female
age	186	Mean	33.8	34.6	33.04
		Median	32	33.5	30.5
		IQR	27–38	28–39.5	27–36
			n for group	%	
Case type	186	New	154	82.8	
		Retreatment	32	17.2	
Headache	186	No	29	15.6	
		yes	157	84.4	
Fever	186	No	153	82.3	
		yes	33	17.7	
Fits	186	no	171	91.9	
		yes	15	8.1	
Confusion	186	No	144	77.4	
		yes	42	22.6	
Vomiting	186	No	101	54.3	
		yes	85	45.7	
Neck pain	186	No	43	23.1	
		yes	143	76.9	
Zoster	186	no	181	97.3	
		yes	5	2.7	
Focal Neurology	186	no	181	97.3	
		Yes	5	2.7	
CD4 cells/ul	119	Mean	90.8		
		Median	46		
		IQR	17–100		
Systolic BP	175	Mean	115		
		Median	113		
		IQR	101–125		
		<100	39	22.3	
		Normal (100–140)	114	65.1	
		>140	22	12.6	
Diastolic BP	175	Mean	74.1		
		Median	72		
		IQR	63–87		
		<60	30	17.1	
		Normal (60–90)	113	64.6	
		>90	32	18.3	
Glasgow Coma		Normal (15)	147	86	
Score		Abnormal (<15)	24	14	
Tuberculosis		Never	84	45.2	
		past	47	25.3	
		Current	38	20.4	
		Past and current	17	9.14	
HIV status	186	Positive on admission	112	60.2	
		Positive in hospital	26	14	

Table 1. Cont.

Variable	n		n for group	%
		unknown	48	25.8
On ART	186	No	159	85.5
		yes	27	14.5
Illness duration	174	Mean	13.1	
		Median	7	
		IQR	Apr-14	
Treatment given	186	Amphotericin	148	79.6
		Fluconazole	28	15.1
		Both	1	0.5
		none	9	4.8
Reason	164	None	139	84.8
		Renal failure	25	15.2

*P for differences in median age by sex = 0.019.

contribute to mortality. The association with concurrent tuberculosis treatment has not been described previously and is potentially specific to this population with very high rates of TB transmission. Assuming good adherence to medication, it is unlikely that these patients had active TB meningitis at the time of admission, although a small number of patients might have multi-drug resistant disease. Rifampicin can potentially reduce therapeutic levels of fluconazole but the effect on mortality was independent of treatment choice and most patients received amphotericin. Given the high burden of tuberculosis in local practice and limited diagnostics, there is a low threshold for initiation of empiric TB treatment in local practice and that it is possible that in some patients this delays the diagnosis of other conditions, including cryptococcal meningitis.

As results in table 3 demonstrate, there is clear evidence here for a poorer outcome in patients receiving fluconazole monotherapy rather than amphotericin. The majority of patients receiving fluconazole had co-existing renal failure which precluded the use of amphotericin (with liposomal formulations not available) and it is thus possible that the fluconazole-treated group over-represents individuals with severe disease. Given the co-linearity of The variables for choice of treatment and renal failure, it is not possible to separate these effects in analysis here, but a model including

Table 2. Period mortality rates in a cohort of 186 patients admitted in hospital due to cryptococcal meningitis.

Time		N	%	Exposure time in days	Mortality rate per 100 person days	95% C.I
Overall	Alive	123	66.13			
	Dead	63	33.87	2963	2.13	1.66–2.72
14 days	Alive	134	72.04			
	Dead	52	27.96	2047	2.54	1.94–3.33
28 days	Alive	126	67.74			
	Dead	60	32.26	2829	2.12	1.65–2.73

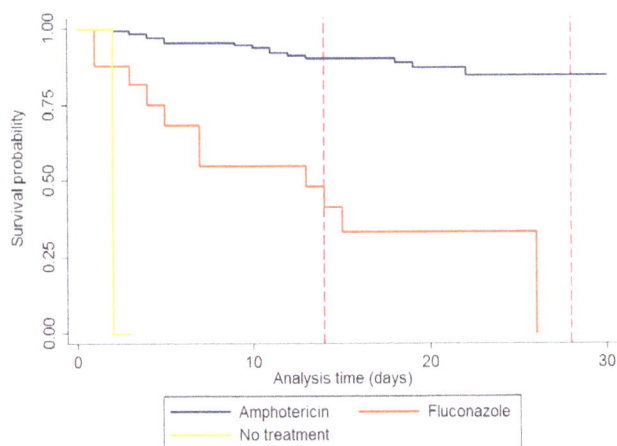

Figure 1. Kaplan-Meier time to death following diagnosis of cryptococcal meningitis and subsequent admission into hospital.

fluconazole monotherapy rather than renal failure provided a better fit to the data seen

Given the known superiority of AmB over fluconazole, a study of AmB in patients with renal failure could be justified from these data in resource-limited setting. In addition, studies using higher doses of fluconzaole will be helpful to improve the evidence base for non amphotericin based regimens[12]. Non-governmental guidelines issued during this study [13] recommend fluconazole at a higher dose of 800 mg/day and might offer additional benefit. Whether the addition of flucytosine to existing regimens would

substantially impact mortality is unknown and the drug remains expensive. There is good evidence that the addition of flucytosine to AmB treatment is more rapidly fungicidal than AmB alone [14] though in a large RCT in a western setting [9] of 408 patients, no difference in mortality could be seen at two weeks. However, it remains possible that improved drug treatment could have more impact in a setting with higher background mortality where the relative impact of drug choice on mortality might be higher. Recent work the relationship between rate of fungal CSF clearance over the first 14 days of treatment and clinical outcome suggests a method by which different treatment combinations could be tested [15].

Perhaps surprisingly, there was no positive effect on outcome for patients established on HAART prior to diagnosis of CM. However, the duration of follow-up was probably not long enough to see the benefits of HAART seen elsewhere [16]. However, other data has suggested a potential benefit for HAART as early as two weeks [17,18]. One of the limitations of this study was that it was not designed to study immune reconstitution inflammatory syndrome (IRIS). A proportion of those already on antiretrovirals might have experienced "unmasking IRIS" presenting early into treatment but data was not collected on duration of antiretroviral treatment to help understand this more. IRIS is undoubtedly a challenge for patients starting ART in the setting of CM [19]. Whilst ACTG 5164 [20], a strategic management trial largely recruiting in US centers with only a small number of CM patients, found no risk to early ART initiation, recent data from a larger study suggests a potential benefit to delaying the initiation of HAART in patients with CM [21]. However, early initiation of HAART following the diagnosis of CM was not common in this cohort and unlikely to have had a significant effect on mortality.

Table 3. Risk factors for in-hospital mortality within 14 days and 28 days in patients diagnosed with cryptococcal meningitis.

Variable		14 day mortality	95% C.I.	P	28 day mortality	95% C.I.	P
Sex	Female	0.63	0.32–1.27	0.2	0.95	0.52–1.73	0.862
Age		0.99	0.96–1.03	0.72	0.99	0.97–1.03	0.843
Headache	No	1			N/S		
	Yes	0.58	0.28–1.19	0.137			
Focal neurology	No	1			1		
	Yes	11	3.08–39.28	**<0.001**	8.14	2.58–25.7	**<0.001**
CD4	>50	1			1		
	<50	0.7	0.29–1.66	0.413	1.02	0.48–2.20	0.951
	Missing	1.49	0.68–3.26	0.322	2.06	1.00–4.31	**0.05**
Diastolic BP	Normal	1			1		
	<60	2.37	1.11–5.04	**0.025**	2.34	1.18–4.63	**0.015**
	>90	1.64	0.68–3.99	0.272	1.1	0.49–2.44	0.824
	Missing	0.86	0.21–3.52	0.837	0.61	0.17–2.21	0.454
GCS	Normal (15)	1			N/S		
	Abnormal (<15)	2.05	0.91–4.59	0.081			
	Missing	1.57	0.64–3.83	0.323			
TB	Never	1			1		
	Past	1.83	0.79–4.23	0.158	1.88	0.88–4.01	0.101
	Current	2.11	1.02–4.35	**0.044**	2.2	1.13–4.30	**0.02**
	Past and current	0.92	0.26–3.29	0.903	0.62	0.18–2.11	0.445
Treatment	Amphotericin	1			1		
	Fluconazole	3.69	1.74–7.85	**0.001**	5.16	2.71–9.83	**<0.001**

The context for our study was a regional referral hospital within the South African public sector. The facilities available lie between the extremes seen in developed countries and those in poorer (non-specialist) centres in sub-Saharan Africa. Drug treatment is available, with AmB the preferred first line option. Patients are usually managed by trained physicians but healthcare workers at all levels are in limited supply, drug and other medical supplies are inconsistent and supportive facilities (HDU,ICU), whilst theoretically available, are not routinely used for medically unwell patients. In well-resourced environments, it has become increasingly clear that the outcome for patients on ICU is not greatly different for those with HIV when compared to those without [22]. Data from this study can start to make an evidence based case for selecting those individuals who would benefit from more intensive support when it is available.

Detailed prevalence data from the nearby region [23] and experience of local antiretroviral programmes, suggests that the structure of the local population and relative prevalence of HIV between men and women, means more women both have HIV and access treatment. The similar proportions of men and women in this study therefore suggests that men within the local population are more likely than women to access care late and with WHO stage IV illness compared to what would be predicted. This cannot be fully substantiated with data from the wider immediate population, but is consistent with local experience. Late presentation is a key factor in improving outcome. With HAART widely available in many setting such as our own, all these deaths, and even disease presentations could be avoidable. The median duration of symptoms prior to presentation was 13 days in this study, very similar to that observed in Uganda [11]. Interventions that target earlier diagnosis and access to care are crucial if mortality is to be improved. In this regard, discussions within South Africa and elsewhere towards increasing the threshold at which individuals become eligible for antiretrovirals (in line with WHO recommendations) should be welcomed. In parallel to such efforts, studies looking to improve available treatments in resource poor settings should continue to be a priority.

Acknowledgments

The authors would like to thank Dr Tom Harrison, St George's Hospital, London for his helpful comments on the manuscript.

Author Contributions

Conceived and designed the experiments: JVL GC MD. Performed the experiments: MD. Analyzed the data: JVL GC PM RJL MLN MD. Wrote the paper: JVL GC PM RJL MLN MD.

References

1. Herbst AJ, Cooke GS, Barnighausen T, Kanykany A, Tanser F, et al. (2009) Adult mortality and antiretroviral treatment roll-out in rural KwaZulu-Natal, South Africa. Bull World Health Organ 87: 754–762.

2. Okongo M, Morgan D, Mayanja B, Ross A, Whitworth J (1998) Causes of death in a rural, population-based human immunodeficiency virus type 1 (HIV-1) natural history cohort in Uganda. Int J Epidemiol 27: 698–702.

3. French N, Gray K, Watera C, Nakiyingi J, Lugada E, et al. (2002) Cryptococcal infection in a cohort of HIV-1-infected Ugandan adults. Aids 16: 1031–1038.

4. Corbett EL, Churchyard GJ, Charalambos S, Samb B, Moloi V, et al. (2002) Morbidity and mortality in South African gold miners: impact of untreated disease due to human immunodeficiency virus. Clin Infect Dis 34: 1251–1258.

5. Park BJ, Wannemuehler KA, Marston BJ, Govender N, Pappas PG, et al. (2009) Estimation of the current global burden of cryptococcal meningitis among persons living with HIV/AIDS. Aids 23: 525–530.

6. Jarvis JN, Harrison TS (2007) HIV-associated cryptococcal meningitis. Aids 21: 2119–2129.

7. UNAIDS (2008) Report on the global AIDS epidemic. Geneva: UNAIDS.

8. Chuck SL, Sande MA (1989) Infections with Cryptococcus neoformans in the acquired immunodeficiency syndrome. N Engl J Med 321: 794–799.

9. van der Horst CM, Saag MS, Cloud GA, Hamill RJ, Graybill JR, et al. (1997) Treatment of cryptococcal meningitis associated with the acquired immunodeficiency syndrome. National Institute of Allergy and Infectious Diseases Mycoses Study Group and AIDS Clinical Trials Group. N Engl J Med 337: 15–21.

10. Antinori S, Ridolfo A, Fasan M, Magni C, Galimberti L, et al. (2009) AIDS-associated cryptococcosis: a comparison of epidemiology, clinical features and outcome in the pre- and post-HAART eras. Experience of a single centre in Italy. HIV Med 10: 6–11.

11. Kambugu A, Meya DB, Rhein J, O'Brien M, Janoff EN, et al. (2008) Outcomes of cryptococcal meningitis in Uganda before and after the availability of highly active antiretroviral therapy. Clin Infect Dis 46: 1694–1701.

12. Longley N, Muzoora C, Taseera K, Mwesigye J, Rwebembera J, et al. (2008) Dose response effect of high-dose fluconazole for HIV-associated cryptococcal meningitis in southwestern Uganda. Clin Infect Dis 47: 1556–1561.

13. McCarthy K, Meintjes G, Arthington-Skaggs B, Bicanic T, Cotton M, et al. (2007) Guidelines for the prevention, diagnosis and management of cryptococcal meningitis and disseminated cryptococcosis in HIV infected individuals. Southern African Journal of HIV Medicine 25–35.

14. Brouwer AE, Rajanuwong A, Chierakul W, Griffin GE, Larsen RA, et al. (2004) Combination antifungal therapies for HIV-associated cryptococcal meningitis: a randomised trial. Lancet 363: 1764–1767.

15. Bicanic T, Muzoora C, Brouwer AE, Meintjes G, Longley N, et al. (2009) Independent association between rate of clearance of infection and clinical outcome of HIV-associated cryptococcal meningitis: analysis of a combined cohort of 262 patients. Clin Infect Dis 49: 702–709.

16. Lortholary O, Poizat G, Zeller V, Neuville S, Boibieux A, et al. (2006) Long-term outcome of AIDS-associated cryptococcosis in the era of combination antiretroviral therapy. Aids 20: 2183–2191.

17. Bicanic T, Meintjes G, Wood R, Hayes M, Rebe K, et al. (2007) Fungal burden, early fungicidal activity, and outcome in cryptococcal meningitis in antiretroviral-naive or antiretroviral-experienced patients treated with amphotericin B or fluconazole. Clin Infect Dis 45: 76–80.

18. Bisson GP, Nthobatsong R, Thakur R, Lesetedi G, Vinekar K, et al. (2008) The use of HAART is associated with decreased risk of death during initial treatment of cryptococcal meningitis in adults in Botswana. J Acquir Immune Defic Syndr 49: 227–229.

19. Lawn SD, Bekker LG, Myer L, Orrell C, Wood R (2005) Cryptococcal immune reconstitution disease: a major cause of early mortality in a South African antiretroviral programme. Aids 19: 2050–2052.

20. Zolopa A, Andersen J, Powderly W, Sanchez A, Sanne I, et al. (2009) Early antiretroviral therapy reduces AIDS progression/death in individuals with acute opportunistic infections: a multicenter randomized strategy trial. PLoS One 4: e5575.

21. Makadzange A, Ndhlovu C, Takarinda K, Reid M, Kurangwa M, et al. (2009) Early vs Delayed ART in the Treatment of Cryptococcal Meningtis in Africa. CROI. Montreal.

22. Dickson SJ, Batson S, Copas AJ, Edwards SG, Singer M, et al. (2007) Survival of HIV-infected patients in the intensive care unit in the era of highly active antiretroviral therapy. Thorax 62: 964–968.

23. Barnighausen T, Tanser F, Gqwede Z, Mbizana C, Herbst K, et al. (2008) High HIV incidence in a community with high HIV prevalence in rural South Africa: findings from a prospective population-based study. Aids 22: 139–144.

15

Postoperative Adverse Outcomes in Intellectually Disabled Surgical Patients

Jui-An Lin[1,2,3], Chien-Chang Liao[1,2], Chuen-Chau Chang[1,2], Hang Chang[4,5,6], Ta-Liang Chen[1,2]*

1 Department of Anesthesiology, Taipei Medical University Hospital, Taipei, Taiwan, **2** School of Medicine, College of Medicine, Taipei Medical University, Taipei, Taiwan, **3** Graduate Institute of Clinical Medicine, College of Medicine, Taipei Medical University, Taipei, Taiwan, **4** Department of Emergency Medicine, Shin Kong Memorial Hospital, Taipei, Taiwan, **5** Graduate Institute of Injury Prevention and Control, College of Public Health and Nutrition, Taipei Medical University, Taipei, Taiwan, **6** Taiwan Joint Commission on Hospital Accreditation, New Taipei City, Taiwan

Abstract

Background: Intellectually disabled patients have various comorbidities, but their risks of adverse surgical outcomes have not been examined. This study assesses pre-existing comorbidities, adjusted risks of postoperative major morbidities and mortality in intellectually disabled surgical patients.

Methods: A nationwide population-based study was conducted in patients who underwent inpatient major surgery in Taiwan between 2004 and 2007. Four controls for each patient were randomly selected from the National Health Insurance Research Database. Preoperative major comorbidities, postoperative major complications and 30-day in-hospital mortality were compared between patients with and without intellectual disability. Use of medical services also was analyzed. Adjusted odds ratios using multivariate logistic regression analyses with 95% confidence intervals were applied to verify intellectual disability's impact.

Results: Controls were compared with 3983 surgical patients with intellectual disability. Risks for postoperative major complications were increased in patients with intellectual disability, including acute renal failure (odds ratio 3.81, 95% confidence interval 2.28 to 6.37), pneumonia (odds ratio 2.01, 1.61 to 2.49), postoperative bleeding (odds ratio 1.35, 1.09 to 1.68) and septicemia (odds ratio 2.43, 1.85 to 3.21) without significant differences in overall mortality. Disability severity was positively correlated with postoperative septicemia risk. Medical service use was also significantly higher in surgical patients with intellectual disability.

Conclusion: Intellectual disability significantly increases the risk of overall major complications after major surgery. Our findings show a need for integrated and revised protocols for postoperative management to improve care for intellectually disabled surgical patients.

Editor: Daniel Morgan, University of Maryland, School of Medicine, United States of America

Funding: The authors have no support or funding to report.

Competing Interests: The authors have declared that no competing interests exist.

* E-mail: tlc@tmu.edu.tw

Introduction

Intellectual disability (ID), defined as lower-than-normal intellectual function, is the most common developmental disorder [1]. It has a prevalence rate of 0.7–8.0% in various forms of severity [2] and is associated with a wide range of primary or secondary medical conditions complicating health management [2]. Earlier studies show severe ID as a negative predictor of life expectancy [3], and with more comorbidities compared with the general population [4]. Therefore intellectual disability's associated social services burden and related health care costs are high [5].

Patients with ID are susceptible to delayed diagnosis and adverse surgical outcomes due to associated anomalies, impaired communication and variable responses to pain and drugs [6]. A recent report found deaths of patients with ID are largely due to preventable causes and that these deaths result from poor medical practice [7].

A large-scale analysis of the global features of perioperative morbidity and mortality in surgical patients with ID is still lacking. Therefore we attempt to clarify whether ID is an independent risk factor for in-hospital major surgeries, and to validate the postoperative adverse outcomes in patients with ID.

Methods

Source of data and patient population

This study used reimbursement claims data from Taiwan's National Health Insurance Program, a universal insurance program that united 13 previous health insurance schemes starting from March 1995. More than 99% of the 22.6 million residents of Taiwan are enrolled in this system. The National Health Research Institutes established a National Health Insurance Research Database (NHIRD) that includes patient demographics and primary and secondary diagnoses of diseases, procedures, prescriptions and medical expenditures. It also records all reimbursements for inpatient and outpatient medical services. To protect personal privacy, the electronic database was decoded with patient identifications scrambled for further public access. The study was evaluated and approved by the NHIRD research committee.

We examined medical claims and identified 3983 surgical patients with preoperative diagnosis of ID from 2,010,412 persons who underwent inpatient major surgeries (defined as surgeries requiring general, epidural or spinal anesthesia, as well as hospitalization of more than one day) from 2004 to 2007 in Taiwan. For each surgical patient with ID, we randomly selected four non-ID subjects matched by sex, age and types of surgery from surgical patient populations as controls to increase statistical power.

Measures

We recorded preoperative major coexisting medical conditions from medical claims for the 24-month preoperative period. These illnesses included acute myocardial infarction, acute renal failure, chronic obstructive pulmonary disease, congestive heart failure, diabetes mellitus, hypertension, peripheral vascular disease, stroke and conditions requiring renal dialysis. We considered 30-day postoperative mortality as the study's primary outcome. The 30-day postoperative complications including acute renal failure, deep wound infection, pneumonia, postoperative bleeding, septicemia, stroke and any complications were considered as secondary outcomes in the present study [8]. Following the *International Classification of Diseases, 9th Revision, Clinical Modification* (ICD-9-CM), we defined ID (ICD-9-CM 317–319) and other comorbidities and postoperative complications in this study, including hypertension (ICD-9-CM 401–405), chronic obstructive pulmonary disease (ICD-9-CM 490–496), diabetes mellitus (ICD-9-CM 250), acute myocardial infarction (ICD-9-CM 410), stroke (ICD-9-CM 430–438), congestive heart failure (ICD-9-CM 428), peripheral vascular disease (ICD-9-CM 443), acute renal failure (ICD-9-CM 584), deep wound infection (ICD-9-CM 958), pneumonia (ICD-9-CM 480–486), postoperative bleeding (ICD-9-CM 998 and 999) and septicemia (ICD-9-CM 038, 998.0, and 778.52).

We calculated population density for each of Taiwan's 359 townships and city districts by dividing population by area (persons/km^2). The first, second, third and fourth quartiles of population density were considered as areas of low, moderate, high and very high urbanization, respectively [9]. We noted whether the surgery took place in a teaching hospital or not and examined use of medical services in terms of length of hospitalization, use of intensive care unit and in-hospital medical expenditures. To validate whether the severity of ID was associated with postoperative complications, we classified ID into unspecified, mild to moderate, and severe to profound groups according to ICD-9-CM codes; the correlation of these groups with postoperative adverse outcomes was analyzed.

Statistical analysis

Descriptive analyses concerning the distribution of demographic factors, coexisting medical conditions, intensive care unit stay and postoperative mortality and complication rates were compared between surgical patients with and without ID using chi-square tests. We used t-tests to compare the average of age, length of hospitalization and medical expenditure between surgical patients with and without ID.

Odds ratios (ORs) with 95% confidence intervals (CI) were analyzed for outcomes between patients with and without ID. Multivariate logistic regression with different models was used to

adjust covariates such as surgery in a teaching hospital, low income, urbanization and preoperative coexisting medical conditions. In order to verify the impact of ID severity on 30-day postoperative mortality, we calculated adjusted ORs and 95% CI of postoperative complications associated with unspecified, mild to moderate, and severe to profound ID using multivariate logistic regression analysis. In order to deal with possible multiplicity issues, we applied a Bonferroni correction testing at a significance level of α (0.05)/k (number of tests) to lower the chance of a type 1 error. Data were analyzed with SAS software version 9.1 (SAS Institute Inc., Carey, NC, USA), with two-sided probability value of <0.05 considered statistically significant.

Results

More ID patients were low-income (22.9% vs. 2.4%, p<0.001) and lived in less-urbanized areas (29.4% vs. 24.3%, p<0.001) compared with non-ID patients (Table S1). Compared with controls, ID patients were found to have higher prevalence of preoperative hypertension (12.9% vs. 9.1%, p<0.001), chronic obstructive pulmonary disease (26.8% vs. 15.3%, p<0.001), diabetes (9.5% vs. 5.4%, p<0.001), myocardial infarction (4.9% vs. 2.8%, p<0.001), stroke (9.3% vs. 2.3%, p<0.001), congestive heart failure (3.0% vs. 1.2%, p<0.001), peripheral vascular disease (1.0% vs. 0.5%, p = 0.001), dialysis (0.7% vs. 0.4%, p = 0.012) and acute renal failure (0.9% vs. 0.3%, p<0.001).

Surgical patients with ID had higher average length of hospitalization and use of intensive care, as well as higher rates of acute renal failure (1.0% vs. 0.3%, p<0.001), pneumonia (4.5% vs. 1.7%, p<0.001), postoperative bleeding (3.6% vs. 2.4%, p<0.001), septicemia (2.9% vs. 0.1%, p<0.001), stroke (3.5% vs. 2.2%, p<0.001) and any complications (13.7% vs. 7.6%, p<0.001) (Table 1). In-hospital medical expenditures differed significantly between patients with and without ID when categorizing participants into a quartet with equal numbers of patients (p<0.001). However, no significant difference was found in postoperative 30-day mortality of patients with and without ID.

After adjustment for confounding factors, surgical patients with ID had higher risks of postoperative acute renal failure (OR 3.81, 95% CI 2.28 to 6.37), pneumonia (OR 2.01, 1.61 to 2.49), bleeding (OR 1.35, 1.09 to 1.68), septicemia (OR 2.43, 1.85 to 3.21) and overall complications (OR 1.53, 1.35 to 1.73). Analyzed by multivariate logistic regression, postoperative 30-day mortality showed no significant difference between patients with or without ID after adjusting teaching hospital, low income, urbanization and coexisting disease (OR 1.52, 95% CI 0.91 to 2.54) (Table 2). The further analysis after Bonferroni correction on ID severity showed higher risk of postoperative septicemia in unspecified ID (OR 2.77, 95% CI 1.98 to 3.87), mild to moderate ID (OR 1.87, 1.29 to 2.71), and severe to profound ID (OR 4.12, 2.34 to 7.28) (Table 3). The corresponding ORs for overall postoperative complications associated with unspecified, mild to moderate, and severe to profound ID were 1.72 (95% CI 1.46 to 2.03), 1.26 (1.07 to 1.49) and 2.40 (1.74 to 3.31), respectively.

Discussion

This large-scale, population-based and cross-sectional study shows that compared with controls without intellectual disability, surgical patients with ID had significantly higher incidence of preoperative comorbidities and postoperative complications while consuming more medical resources. After adjustment for confounding variables, risks of overall postoperative 30-day complications increased in surgical patients with ID and highly correlated with ID severity, especially in septicemia.

Table 1. Outcome characteristics of surgical patients with intellectual disability and controls.

	Preoperative intellectual disability				
	No N = 15,932		Yes N = 3,983		p value
Postoperative complications					
Acute renal failure	40	(0.3)	41	(1.0)	<0.001
Deep wound infection	141	(0.9)	43	(1.1)	0.251
Pneumonia	275	(1.7)	181	(4.5)	<0.001
Postoperative bleeding	384	(2.4)	142	(3.6)	<0.001
Septicemia	157	(1.0)	117	(2.9)	<0.001
Stroke	350	(2.2)	139	(3.5)	<0.001
Any of the above	1,207	(7.6)	544	(13.7)	<0.001
Length of stay, days					<0.001
1–5	9,710	(60.9)	1,978	(49.7)	
6–10	3,266	(20.5)	908	(22.8)	
11–15	1,126	(7.1)	324	(8.1)	
>15	1,830	(11.5)	773	(19.4)	
Mean±SD	8.2±12.7		11.9±20.0		<0.001
ICU stay, %	1,619	(10.2)	609	(15.3)	<0.001
In-hospital expenditure, USD*					
Low	721	(132.5)	775	(149.3)	<0.001
Medium	1,054	(88.1)	1,204	(160.0)	<0.001
High	1,637	(270.8)	2,046	(383.2)	<0.001
Very high	7,265	(7,446.2)	9,001	(6,997.2)	<0.001
Postoperative 30-day mortality	69	(0.4)	25	(0.6)	0.109

Parenthesis indicates the percentage of patients in each group.
ICU, intensive care unit.
*Mean (standard deviation).

The prevalence of severe ID in low-income countries is at least double that in high-income countries [10]. Malnutrition, iodine deficiency, birth trauma and lead poisoning are all suspected factors in this difference in prevalence [5]. A previous study found

Table 2. Risk of postoperative 30-day mortality and complications associated with intellectual disability in multiple logistic regression models*.

	OR	(95% CI)
Postoperative 30-day complications		
Acute renal failure	3.81	(2.28–6.37)
Deep wound infection	1.32	(0.91–1.90)
Pneumonia	2.01	(1.61–2.49)
Postoperative bleeding	1.35	(1.09–1.68)
Septicemia	2.43	(1.85–3.21)
Stroke	1.18	(0.91–1.53)
Any of the above	1.53	(1.35–1.73)
Postoperative 30-day mortality	1.52	(0.91–2.54)

*Adjusted for age, sex, types of surgery, teaching hospital, low income, urbanization, and coexisting diseases.
OR, odds ratio; CI. Confidence interval.

61.3% of patients with ID belong to rural populations with low socioeconomic status [6]. Our result also showed that surgical patients with ID had lower incomes and lived in less-urbanized areas compared with the control group.

Respiratory diseases, followed by cardiovascular complications, are the leading causes of death in patients with ID [11], and pneumonia is the most common lethal illness [3]. Earlier reports showed ID is a risk factor of postoperative pulmonary complications [12,13], which is compatible with our data that surgical patients with ID were at higher risk of developing pneumonia than patients without ID. Risk of aspiration pneumonia in patients with ID is substantially high due to multiple factors, including ID-associated gastroesophageal reflux [14], dysfunctional pharyngo-esophageal sphincter [15], and anticonvulsants and/or tranquilizers that may cause hypersalivation when prescribed for ID-accompanying seizures [16]. Drugs for postoperative pain or agitation may also depress pharyngeal reflexes. In addition, significant physical impairment in ID patients further accentuates the risk of aspiration after surgery [17]. These studies confirm our results regarding intellectually disabled surgical patients' elevated risk of developing postoperative pneumonia.

Severe dental caries and periodontal disease were common handicaps associated with ID [18]. Poor oral hygiene is anticipated and leads to a higher rate of bacteremia after dental treatment in patients with ID than in others [19]; it is also reported as a risk factor for infective endocarditis [20]. As the most frequent genetic cause of ID [21], Down syndrome has been associated with

Table 3. Risk of postoperative 30-day mortality and complications by severity of intellectual disability in multiple logistic regression models[*].

Postoperative 30-day complications	Severity of intellectual disability							
	No disability N = 15,932		Unspecified N = 1,660		Mild to moderate N = 2,023		Severe to profound N = 300	
	OR	(95% CI)	OR	(95% CI)	OR	(95% CI)	OR	(95% CI)
Acute renal failure	1.00	(reference)	4.67	(2.61–8.36)[†]	3.04	(1.52–6.07)[†]	2.67	(0.71–10.0)
Deep wound infection	1.00	(reference)	1.56	(0.96–2.52)	1.18	(0.73–1.92)	0.86	(0.21–3.58)
Pneumonia	1.00	(reference)	2.51	(1.92–3.26)[†]	1.36	(1.00–1.84)	3.75	(2.36–5.97)[†]
Postoperative bleeding	1.00	(reference)	1.59	(1.20–2.10)[†]	1.13	(0.84–1.51)	1.65	(0.92–2.95)
Septicemia	1.00	(reference)	2.77	(1.98–3.87)[†]	1.87	(1.29–2.71)[†]	4.12	(2.34–7.28)[†]
Stroke	1.00	(reference)	1.30	(0.93–1.80)	1.09	(0.77–1.53)	0.98	(0.44–2.22)
Any of the above	1.00	(reference)	1.72	(1.46–2.03)[†]	1.26	(1.07–1.49)[†]	2.40	(1.74–3.31)[†]
Postoperative 30-day mortality	1.00	(reference)	1.99	(1.08–3.64)	0.91	(0.40–2.06)	2.53	(0.74–8.65)

[*]Adjusted for age, sex, types of surgery, teaching hospital, low income, urbanization, and coexisting diseases.
OR, odds ratio; CI, confidence interval.
[†]Statistically significant after Bonferroni correction (p<0.0125) ($\alpha = 0.05/4$ tests = 0.0125).

inherent immunodeficiency, and it may precipitate sepsis progression and increase mortality risk in children with sepsis [22]. Our results showed the severity of ID positively correlated with risk of septicemia following surgery, suggesting that poorer oral hygiene or immunity possibly correlates with disability severity.

Renal dysfunction has been reported in many ID-related syndromes, such as Williams-Beuren syndrome [23], Bardet-Biedl syndrome [24], oculocerebrorenal syndrome of Lowe [25] and Menkes disease [26]. Polycystic kidney can manifest as a ID-accompanying disorder, and all such patients progress to chronic renal failure early in their lives [27]. Our results showed the relative risk of acute renal failure was highest among major postoperative complications, which indicates that kidney function is most easily impaired by perioperative health care management in surgical patients with ID.

Several coexisting clotting defects have been reported in patients with ID, including factor V [28], factor VII (alone [29] or in combination with factor X [30]), and factor XI (alone [31] or in combination with factor XII [32]). Complicated bleeding diathesis (decreased factor XI, XII, von Willebrand's factor and platelet dysfunction) in some ID patients might be further exacerbated by physiological alterations in specific conditions (such as pregnancy) and result in postoperative bleeding [33]. The fragile X-ID syndrome, as one of the major causes of genetically determined ID, has a closely linked fragile mutated site with haemophilia B loci [34]. Bleeding resulting from therapy-related side effects is also a critical issue in these cases. Lorenzo's oil, as a choice of dietary management for ID patients with adrenoleukodystrophy, may cause thrombocytopenia [35]. Epilepsy was reported to be the most prevalent illness in patients with ID in Taiwan [36]; therefore valproate-associated coagulopathies should not be overlooked, even during short-term epileptic treatment [37], as risk of postoperative bleeding is increased.

Respiratory complications were the leading cause of death in patients with ID [11]. The incidence of postoperative pulmonary complications could be reduced significantly by routinely nursing patients in humidity tents for 24–48 h and by commencing vigorous chest physiotherapy immediately after surgery in patients with ID [14]. Moreover, perioperative antibiotic coverage and aggressive pulmonary hygiene are also crucial to prevent postoperative pulmonary complications in ID patients with high susceptibility,

including congenital central alveolar hypoventilation syndrome (Ondine's curse) [38], Langer-Giedion syndrome [39], mucopolysaccharide storage disorders [40] and cri du chat syndrome [41]. ID patients with congenital insensitivity to pain with anhidrosis should be managed as "full stomach" patients to prevent perioperative regurgitation and aspiration, because their gastric emptying is delayed due to autonomic nervous system dysfunction [42].

This study is limited to retrospective reimbursement claims without individual detailed biochemical data. A definite relationship between preoperative comorbidities and postoperative complications for each surgical patient with or without ID could not be verified. Information about physical activity, degree of family support and loading of caretakers was also unavailable in this study. Another limitation is that we investigated the global adverse outcome focusing on all ID patients receiving in-hospital surgeries. However, patients with definite diagnosis, such as Down syndrome, were not specified in our study due to patient collection in our study design as mental retardation (ICD-9-CM 317–319).

In conclusion, our results are the first to validate through a population-based study that risks for postoperative major complications were increased in patients with intellectual disability and correlated with ID severity. These findings confirmed the higher risks in surgical patients with ID for in-hospital major surgery and a corresponding need to provide integrated health care for both prevention and postoperative management. Efforts should be made to reallocate adequate resources for these purposes [5], and strategies are needed to reduce postoperative adverse outcomes in this population.

Author Contributions

Conceived and designed the experiments: TLC HC. Performed the experiments: CCL TLC. Analyzed the data: CCL TLC. Contributed reagents/materials/analysis tools: CCL TLC. Wrote the paper: JAL TLC CCL CCC.

References

1. Parmet S (2002) JAMA patient page. Mental retardation. JAMA 288: 1548.
2. Van Schrojenstein Lantman-de Valk HM, Walsh PN (2008) Managing health problems in people with intellectual disabilities. BMJ 337: a2507.
3. Eyman RK, Grossman HJ, Chaney RH, Call TL (1990) The life expectancy of profoundly handicapped people with mental retardation. N Engl J Med 323: 584–589.
4. Bittles AH, Petterson BA, Sullivan SG, Hussain R, Glasson EJ, et al. (2002) The influence of intellectual disability on life expectancy. J Gerontol A Biol Sci Med Sci 57: M470–M472.
5. Salvador-Carulla L, Saxena S (2009) Intellectual disability: between disability and clinical nosology. Lancet 374: 1798–1799.
6. Khalid K, Al-Salamah SM (2006) Surgery for acute abdominal conditions in intellectually-disabled adults. ANZ J Surg 76: 145–148.
7. Ali A, Hassiotis A (2008) Illness in people with intellectual disabilities. BMJ 336: 570–571.
8. Ghaferi AA, Birkmeyer JD, Dimick JB (2009) Variation in hospital mortality associated with inpatient surgery. N Engl J Med 361: 1368–1375.
9. Shih CC, Su YC, Liao CC, Lin JG (2010) Patterns of medical pluralism among adults: results from the 2001 National Health Interview Survey in Taiwan. BMC Health Serv Res 10: 191.
10. Durkin M (2002) The epidemiology of developmental disabilities in low-income countries. Ment Retard Dev Disabil Res Rev 8: 206–211.
11. Cooper SA, Melville C, Morrison J (2004) People with intellectual disabilities. BMJ 329: 414–415.
12. Anderson PR, Puno MR, Lovell SL, Swayze CR (1985) Postoperative respiratory complications in non-idiopathic scoliosis. Acta Anaesthesiol Scand 29: 186–192.
13. Spitz L, Kirtane J (1985) Results and complications of surgery for gastro-oesophageal reflux. Arch Dis Child 60: 743–747.
14. Spitz L (1982) Surgical treatment of gastrooesophageal reflux in severely mentally retarded children. J R Soc Med 75: 525–529.
15. Ekedahl C, Mansson I, Sandberg N (1974) Swallowing dysfunction in the brain-damaged with drooling. Acta Otolaryngol 78: 141–149.
16. Frederick FJ, Stewart IF (1982) Effectiveness of transtympanic neurectomy in management of sialorrhea occurring in mentally retarded patients. J Otolaryngol 11: 289–292.
17. McNeeley SG, Elkins TE (1989) Gynecologic surgery and surgical morbidity in mentally handicapped women. Obstet Gynecol 74: 155–158.
18. Smith DC, Decker HA, Herberg EN, Rupke LK (1969) Medical needs of children in institutions for the mentally retarded. Am J Public Health Nations Health 59: 1376–1384.
19. Messini M, Skourti I, Markopulos E, Koutsia-Carouzou C, Kyriakopoulou E, et al. (1999) Bacteremia after dental treatment in mentally handicapped people. J Clin Periodontol 26: 469–473.
20. Lockhart PB, Brennan MT, Thornhill M, Michalowicz BS, Noll J, et al. (2009) Poor oral hygiene as a risk factor for infective endocarditis-related bacteremia. J Am Dent Assoc 140: 1238–1244.
21. Hassold TJ, Jacobs PA (1984) Trisomy in man. Annu Rev Genet 18: 69–97.
22. Garrison MM, Jeffries H, Christakis DA (2005) Risk of death for children with down syndrome and sepsis. J Pediatr 147: 748–752.
23. Biesecker LG, Laxova R, Friedman A (1987) Renal insufficiency in Williams syndrome. Am J Med Genet 28: 131–135.
24. Green JS, Parfrey PS, Harnett JD, Farid NR, Cramer BC, et al. (1989) The cardinal manifestations of Bardet-Biedl syndrome, a form of Laurence-Moon-Biedl syndrome. N Engl J Med 321: 1002–1009.
25. Charnas LR, Bernardini I, Rader D, Hoeg JM, Gahl WA (1991) Clinical and laboratory findings in the oculocerebrorenal syndrome of Lowe, with special reference to growth and renal function. N Engl J Med 324: 1318–1325.
26. Ozawa H, Kodama H, Kawaguchi H, Mochizuki T, Kobayashi M, et al. (2003) Renal function in patients with Menkes disease. Eur J Pediatr 162: 51–52.
27. Seeman T, Malikova M, Blahova K, Seemanova E (2009) Polycystic kidney and hepatic disease with mental retardation and hand anomalies in three siblings. Pediatr Nephrol 24: 1409–1412.
28. Tsuda H, Mizuno Y, Hara T, Ohtsuki T, Ueda K, et al. (1990) A case of congenital factor V deficiency combined with multiple congenital anomalies: successful management of palatoplasty. Acta Haematol 83: 49–52.
29. Girolami A, Ruzzon E, Tezza F, Allemand E, Vettore S (2007) Congenital combined defects of factor VII: a critical review. Acta Haematol 117: 51–56.
30. Girolami A, Ruzzon E, Tezza F, Scandellari R, Scapin M, et al. (2008) Congenital FX deficiency combined with other clotting defects or with other abnormalities: a critical evaluation of the literature. Haemophilia 14: 323–328.
31. Futterweit W, Ritch R, Teekhasaenee C, Nelson ES (1986) Coexistence of Prader-Willi syndrome, congenital ectropion uveae with glaucoma, and factor XI deficiency. JAMA 255: 3280–3282.
32. Singer G, Schalamon J, Ainoedhofer H, Petek E, Kroisel PM, et al. (2005) Williams-Beuren syndrome associated with caudal regression syndrome and coagulopathy: a case report. J Pediatr Surg 40: e47–e50.
33. Grange CS, Heid R, Lucas SB, Ross PL, Douglas MJ (1998) Anaesthesia in a parturient with Noonan's syndrome. Can J Anaesth 45: 332–336.
34. Camerino G, Mattei MG, Mattei JF, Jaye M, Mandel JL (1983) Close linkage of fragile X-mental retardation syndrome to haemophilia B and transmission through a normal male. Nature 306: 701–704.
35. Zinkham WH, Kickler T, Borel J, Moser HW (1993) Lorenzo's oil and thrombocytopenia in patients with adrenoleukodystrophy. N Engl J Med 328: 1126–1127.
36. Lin JD, Wu JL, Lee PN (2003) Healthcare needs of people with intellectual disability in institutions in Taiwan: outpatient care utilization and implications. J Intellect Disabil Res 47: 169–180.
37. Kose G, Arhan E, Unal B, Ozaydin E, Guven A, et al. (2009) Valproate-associated coagulopathies in children during short-term treatment. J Child Neurol 24: 1493–1498.
38. Strauser LM, Helikson MA, Tobias JD (1999) Anesthetic care for the child with congenital central alveolar hypoventilation syndrome (Ondine's curse). J Clin Anesth 11: 431–437.
39. Michalek P, Doherty JT, Vesela MM (2009) Anesthetic management of a child with Langer-Giedion (TRPS II) syndrome. J Anesth 23: 456–459.
40. Semenza GL, Pyeritz RE (1988) Respiratory complications of mucopolysaccha-ride storage disorders. Medicine (Baltimore) 67: 209–219.
41. Yamashita M, Tanioka F, Taniguchi K, Matsuki A, Oyama T (1985) Anesthetic considerations in cri du chat syndrome: a report of three cases. Anesthesiology 63: 201–202.
42. Zlotnik A, Gruenbaum SE, Rozet I, Zhumadilov A, Shapira Y (2010) Risk of aspiration during anesthesia in patients with congenital insensitivity to pain with anhidrosis: case reports and review of the literature. J Anesth 24: 778–782.

16

Vitamin C: Intravenous Use by Complementary and Alternative Medicine Practitioners and Adverse Effects

Sebastian J. Padayatty[1][9], Andrew Y. Sun[1][9], Qi Chen[2], Michael Graham Espey[1], Jeanne Drisko[2], Mark Levine[1]*

1 Molecular and Clinical Nutrition Section, National Institute of Diabetes and Digestive and Kidney Diseases, National Institutes of Health, Bethesda, Maryland, United States of America, 2 Program in Integrative Medicine, University of Kansas Medical Center, Kansas City, Kansas, United States of America

Abstract

Background: Anecdotal information and case reports suggest that intravenously administered vitamin C is used by Complementary and Alternate Medicine (CAM) practitioners. The scale of such use in the U.S. and associated side effects are unknown.

Methods and Findings: We surveyed attendees at annual CAM Conferences in 2006 and 2008, and determined sales of intravenous vitamin C by major U.S. manufacturers/distributors. We also queried practitioners for side effects, compiled published cases, and analyzed FDA's Adverse Events Database. Of 199 survey respondents (out of 550), 172 practitioners administered IV vitamin C to 11,233 patients in 2006 and 8876 patients in 2008. Average dose was 28 grams every 4 days, with 22 total treatments per patient. Estimated yearly doses used (as 25g/50ml vials) were 318,539 in 2006 and 354,647 in 2008. Manufacturers' yearly sales were 750,000 and 855,000 vials, respectively. Common reasons for treatment included infection, cancer, and fatigue. Of 9,328 patients for whom data is available, 101 had side effects, mostly minor, including lethargy/fatigue in 59 patients, change in mental status in 21 patients and vein irritation/phlebitis in 6 patients. Publications documented serious adverse events, including 2 deaths in patients known to be at risk for IV vitamin C. Due to confounding causes, the FDA Adverse Events Database was uninformative. Total numbers of patients treated in the US with high dose vitamin C cannot be accurately estimated from this study.

Conclusions: High dose IV vitamin C is in unexpectedly wide use by CAM practitioners. Other than the known complications of IV vitamin C in those with renal impairment or glucose 6 phosphate dehydrogenase deficiency, high dose intravenous vitamin C appears to be remarkably safe. Physicians should inquire about IV vitamin C use in patients with cancer, chronic, untreatable, or intractable conditions and be observant of unexpected harm, drug interactions, or benefit.

Editor: Joel Joseph Gagnier, University of Michigan, Canada

Funding: This work was supported in part by the Intramural Research Program, National Institute of Diabetes and Digestive and Kidney Diseases, National Institutes of Health. The funders had no role in study design, data collection and analysis, decision to publish, or preparation of the manuscript.

Competing Interests: The authors have declared that no competing interests exist.

* E-mail: MarkL@intra.niddk.nih.gov

9 These authors contributed equally to this work.

Introduction

Among the most enduring of alternative medical treatments, vitamin C (ascorbic acid, ascorbate) is also one of the most popular. In 2007, it was the most widely sold single vitamin, with sales of 884 million dollars in the US1 [1]. Independent of its use to treat the deficiency disease scurvy, vitamin C has been used by non-mainstream physicians orally and parenterally for more than 60 years as a therapeutic agent [2–7]. Oral vitamin C is widely used by the public to prevent or treat infections, especially the common cold [8]. In one of its more controversial applications, gram doses of vitamin C were promoted by the two-time Nobel Laureate Linus Pauling as a cancer treatment agent [9,10]. Anecdotal evidence led us to posit that intravenous (IV) vitamin C is still used by Complementary and Alternative Medicine (CAM) practitioners to treat diverse conditions including infections, autoimmune diseases, cancer and illnesses of uncertain origin [11–13].

Despite its purported popularity, the extent of use of IV vitamin C is unknown. Its use in CAM has not been well publicized by practitioners and their patients, and is likely to be unrecognized by mainstream physicians. Benefits if any and especially side effects of such use may be unreported or under-reported. It is useful to know if high dose IV vitamin C therapy is widely used, and if so how and for what, so that conventional physicians can improve patient care by identifying any ill effects or drug interactions, and reporting benefit if any.

New knowledge has elucidated possible mechanisms of action of IV vitamin C and for the first time made therapeutic effects biologically plausible [14]. It is now known that IV but not oral administration of vitamin C produces pharmacologic plasma concentrations of the vitamin [15,16]. Past studies used oral and/ or IV routes inconsistently, making such studies, in retrospect, flawed and difficult to interpret [17]. Recent *in vitro* experiments indicated that vitamin C only in pharmacologic concentrations killed cancer cells but not normal cells, and that the mechanism was via hydrogen peroxide formation [18]. *In vivo* animal data indicated that hydrogen peroxide was produced selectively in extracellular fluid around normal and tumor tissues by pharmacologic vitamin C concentrations [19,20]. At these concentrations, vitamin C slowed tumor growth [20,21]. Pharmacologic vitamin C concentrations produced in animals by parenteral administration were reproduced in patients in a recent phase I clinical trial [16].

Because of the new interest in IV vitamin C, coupled to need to characterize use and uncover side effects, we surveyed CAM practitioners anonymously. We also searched for side effects of IV vitamin C administration in the published medical literature and in the Food and Drug Administration (FDA) adverse events database, and estimated sales volumes of IV vitamin C preparations.

Our study obtained quantitative information that substantiated previous anecdotal reports. Despite unexpected wide use, we found side effects of vitamin C were surprisingly few when patients were properly screened. The findings in this paper will alert conventional practitioners about unrecognized wide use of IV vitamin C, will remind them to query patients about such use, and may help to uncover either unexpected adverse events or benefit and spur further research in this area.

Methods

Survey Methods

The study was reviewed by the Human Subjects Committee/Institutional Review Board at the University of Kansas Medical Center. The survey was categorized as an exempt study. It contained no personal identifiers; therefore informed consent was not necessary under exempt status and was not obtained. Survey forms were distributed to practitioners attending a conference on CAM in 2006 and 2008. Participants were requested to return completed survey forms before the end of each conference. Participants were asked whether they used high dose IV vitamin C during the preceding 12 months, and if so, to detail its use by answering specific questions in the survey form (see Survey S1 for the survey form used). It was not possible to identify the respondent from the survey form or survey data. The same form was used in both years, with an additional line on the 2008 form inquiring whether the respondent had also responded in 2006 (See Survey S1).

Vitamin C doses sold

The major manufacturers/importers in the US of vitamin C preparations that can be administered IV were contacted by telephone. Data on annual sales of vitamin C in the US were obtained with the understanding that the names and sales figures of individual companies would not be linked nor made public.

Side effects of high dose IV vitamin C

We searched the Adverse Events Reporting System, a database of drug side effects maintained by the Food and Drug Administration (FDA). Data from 20 consecutive quarters available from 2004–2008 were queried. We also searched for side effects in publications on therapeutic use of high dose IV vitamin C. We searched Medline, Web of Science (ISI Thompson) and Scopus databases for papers in English that reported IV vitamin C administration in humans. Several different search terms and possible variants of each search term were used to capture the maximum number of papers. Papers reporting oral vitamin C treatment only, or those using IV doses of 1g or less, were excluded. Because vitamin C is sometimes administered IV

in patients undergoing hemodialysis, there are many published studies in this area. A separate search was conducted for papers reporting these to ensure that these were excluded from our analysis. IV administered vitamin C is also used to study the acute effects of antioxidants or of vitamin C itself on metabolism and physiology, particularly on cardiovascular and endothelial reactivity. This does not constitute a therapeutic use of vitamin C. Hence publications reporting these were identified and removed from the search results. Separately, we searched the same databases for specific reports of side effects of IV administered vitamin C and followed up references and cited papers. From papers so collected, we manually eliminated duplicate citations and those that did not meet the above criteria. From the remaining reports, adverse reactions attributable to IV administered vitamin C were noted.

Results

Survey response

We distributed 300 survey forms in 2006 to attendees at their annual CAM conference. 106 forms were returned, a response rate of 35%. In 2008, 250 survey forms were distributed and 93 completed forms were returned, a response rate of 37%. Of the 2008 respondents, 22 (24%) had previously responded in 2006. An unknown number of conference attendees were not practitioners but spouses, researchers or industry representatives who did not return survey forms, reducing response rates.

Vitamin C usage

Of 199 total respondents for 2006 and 2008: 172 practitioners administered vitamin C; 27 did not use IV Vitamin C; 48 practitioners treated more than 100 patients each per year; and 5 treated more than 1000 patients each per year (Figure 1A, B). 11,233 patients received IV vitamin C in 2006 and 8876 in 2008 (figure 1A, B). On average, each patient received 22 treatments (Table 1). Treatments occurred at a mean of once every 4 days, each at a mean dose of 28 grams (Table 1). Doses used were as low as 1gram or as high as 200grams, with a similar wide range for each of the parameters queried. Based on dosing vials of 25g/50ml, estimated total yearly dosing vials administered were 318,539 in 2006 and 354,647 in 2008. Estimated total number of dosing vials sold was independently obtained from the major manufacturers of vitamin C in the U.S. Total dosing vials of IV vitamin C sold in the United States were approximately 750,000 in 2006 and 855,000 in 2008 (Table 1).

Seventy seven percent of respondents reported the numbers of patients treated for broad indications, labeled as infection (44%), cancer (19%) or other conditions (37%) (Table 2). Numbers of practitioners who listed specific indications for treatment are shown in figure 2. Practitioners listed fatigue as the most common specific single indication for treatment in 2006, and breast cancer in 2008. There were a large number of indications for which less than four practitioners used high dose IV vitamin C (Table S1).

Adverse effects

Adverse events reported by survey respondents were minor (Table 3). No side effects were reported for 9227 patients while 59 were reported to have lethargy or fatigue. A single practitioner listed change in mental status in 10% of his patients (20 patients) but provided no details. One patient with pre existing renal impairment and cancer metastases to kidneys was reported to have developed unconfirmed renal failure. Some practitioners reported side effects without reporting patient numbers. The most common of these side effects were lethargy or fatigue (reported by 27

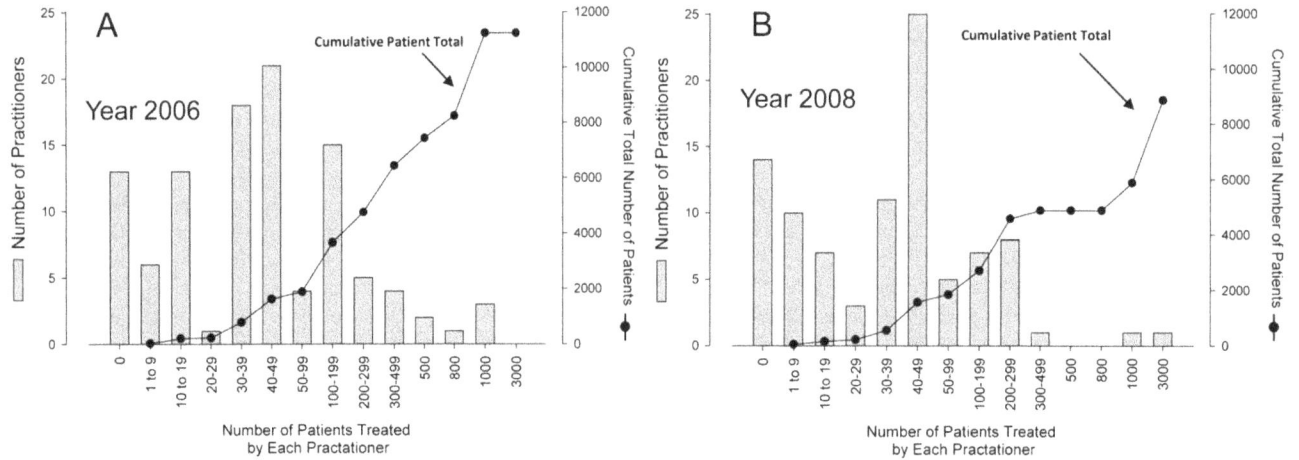

Figure 1. Cumulative total and the distribution of patients treated among the survey respondents. Practitioners were grouped according to the number of patients whom they treated with IV vitamin C in the preceding twelve months. For ease of display, number of patients were divided into arbitrary ranges which are shown on the X axis. The number of practitioners who treated the specified number of patients are shown on the Y axis. Patients were unevenly distributed among survey respondents. In 2006, out of 106 practitioners who responded to the survey, 13 did not use high dose IV vitamin C, 30 respondents treated more than 100 patients each, and 3 treated 1000 or more patients (Fig 1A). For 2008, the corresponding numbers were 93, 14, 18 and 2 respectively (Fig 1B). Cumulative total of patients treated by all practitioners are shown as line diagrams (scaled to Y axis on right).

practitioners), vein irritation (by 9 practitioners), and nausea and vomiting (by 9 practitioners). Other reported side effects are listed in table 3. Less commonly reported adverse effects are listed in Table S2.

Data obtained from the FDA Adverse Events Reporting System database for 20 consecutive quarters indicated that 77 patients treated with 0.2–1.0 gram doses of IV vitamin C had reported adverse events (Table 4). However, all patients either had serious or life-threatening systemic illnesses, and/or were receiving many potentially toxic drugs (i.e. cancer therapeutics) in addition to IV vitamin C (for details, see Table S3). Some individual patients appear to have been reported multiple times (see Table S3). In comparison to CAM practitioners, the dose of vitamin C administered was very low (1 gram or less). In no case could we exclude multiple confounding factors as the cause of the reported adverse effects (Table 4). Whether vitamin C caused or

contributed to these side effects cannot be determined from the available data.

Through searching published literature (see methods for details), 187 papers were found on the use of high dose IV vitamin C, including papers that reported side effects. There were three cases of renal failure, all in patients with pre existing renal impairment [22,23], [24]. Two patients with glucose 6 phosphate dehydrogenase deficiency developed hemolysis [25,26] (Table 5).

Practitioner Demographics

86% of practitioners were physicians (Table 6) and most patients were treated at for-profit centers. Some practitioners did not provide requested demographics data. Therefore, the numbers given in this table do not tally with the total number of survey respondents. (For detailed demographic information, see Table S4).

Table 1. Details of high dose IV vitamin C use by survey respondents for the years 2006 and 2008.

	2006			2008		
	Mean	**Median**	**Range**	**Mean**	**Median**	**Range**
Dose (g/treatment)	28	31	1–200	28	50	1–200
Number of treatments per patient	19	16	1–80	24	16	1–80
Number treated by one practitioner	121	40	1–1150	112	40	1–3000
Duration of treatments (min)	105	90	2–1440	81	90	1–900
Frequency of treatments (once every so many days)	4	3.5	1–7	4	2	1–7
Lowest dose (g/treatment)	12	9	1–60	17	15	1–75
Highest dose (g/treatment)	79	75	5–200	87	95	20–200
Infusion rate (g/min)	0.89	0.5	0.03–25	0.525	0.5	0.028–2.5
Total number of vials of vitamin C used (25g/50ml) (Calculated from survey data)	318,539			354,647		
Total number of vials of vitamin C sold by companies in the US (25g/50 ml)	750,000			855,000		

Vitamin C is supplied in 50 ml bottles containing 25grams. Estimated total number of doses (bottles) used each year was calculated as the cumulative sum of each practitioners' number of patients×that practitioners' average dose in bottles×that practitioner's average number of doses per patient.

Table 2. Indications for treatment with high dose IV vitamin C.

Year		2006	2008
Total number of patients treated		*11233*	*8876*
Number of patients with data available		*9481*	*5928*
Number of Patients with	**Infection**	4587	2264
	Cancer	1379	1509
	Other Conditions	3515	2155

Some respondents did not list the number of patients treated for each of the conditions for which they used intravenous vitamin C treatment. Therefore, the data do not provide indications for treatment for all patients who received IV vitamin C.

Discussion

The data here show that 11,233 and 8876 patients received IV vitamin C over two periods of one year each, with a mean number of infusions per patient of 19–24 and a mean dose of approximately 28 grams per patient. We estimate that survey respondents used approximately 318,539 and 354,647 dosing units of vitamin C each year. These numbers account for less than half of the doses of vitamin C doses sold within the United States for the matching year. Considered together, these data indicate that use of IV vitamin C was both substantial and probably underestimated. This is one of the first papers to document previously unrecognized and widespread use of a CAM agent administered IV. To our knowledge, only two other CAM therapies are used IV. The first, chelation therapy, is also used in standard medical practice [27]. The second, an IV vitamin and mineral mixture termed the Myer's cocktail, has variable components, has had little formal investigation, and contains less than 5 grams of vitamin C [28,29]. Further, there have been few surveys of CAM practitioners, as opposed to surveys of patients. There were minimal adverse effects reported, which was also the case in the published literature. Exceptions were for patients with pre-existing renal insufficiency/failure or glucose 6-phosphate dehydrogenase (G6PD) deficiency, both known to predispose to vitamin C toxicity [30]. Adverse events reported to the FDA could not be interpreted due to confounding factors.

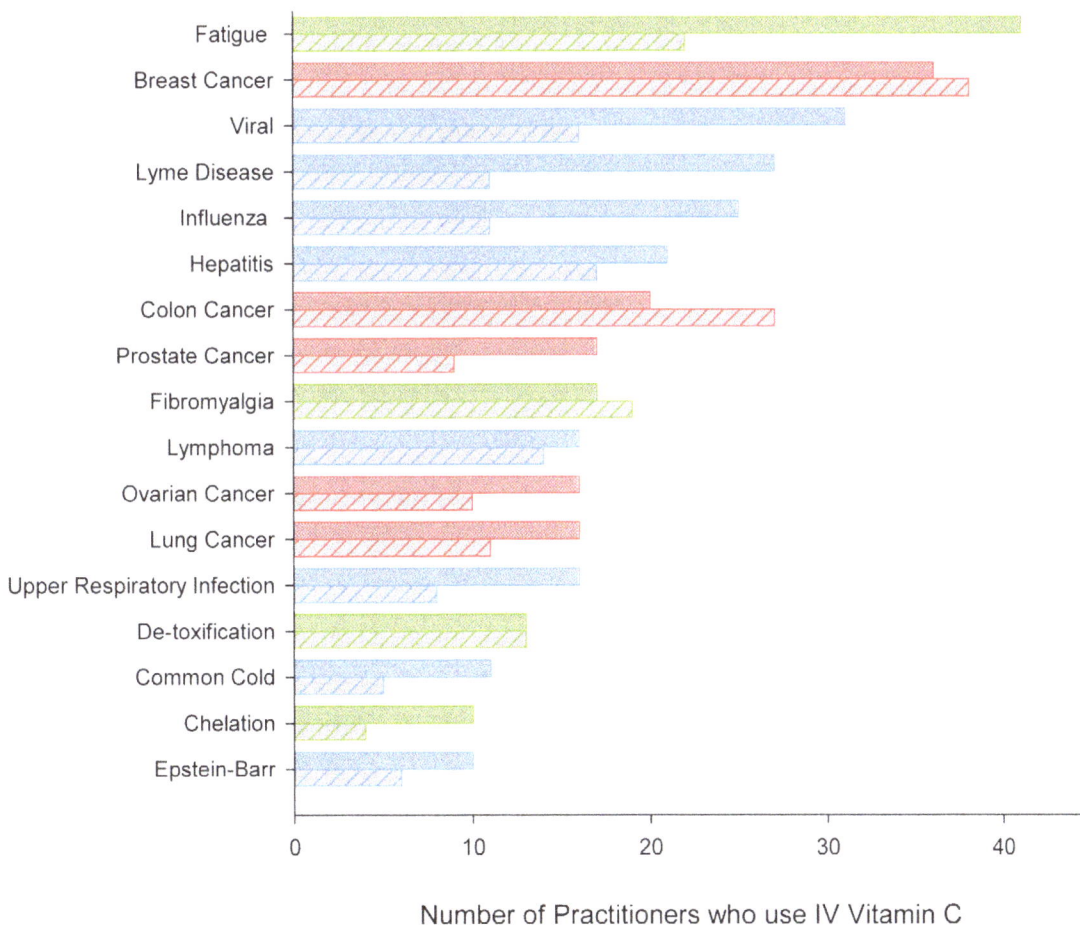

Figure 2. Number of practitioners who used intravenous vitamin C for various conditions. X axis shows the number of practitioners who used intravenous vitamin C to treat each of the conditions listed on the Y axis. Blue bars denote infections, red bars denote cancers, and green bars denote other indications. Data for 2006 (solid bars) and 2008 (hatched bars) show that intravenous vitamin C was most often used to treat infections and cancer. Indications for which less than four practitioners used high dose intravenous vitamin C are listed in Table S1.

Table 3. Adverse events reported with IV vitamin C use in the survey for the years 2006 and 2008.

Complication	Number of Patients	
	2006	2008
None Described	5349	3878
Lethargy/Fatigue	10	49
Local Vein Irritation	3	-
Phlebitis	3	-
Kidney Stone (oxalate)	-	1
Kidney Stone (urate)	-	1
Kidney Stone (unspecified)	2	-
Hemolysis	2	-
Elevated Blood Glucose	2	-
Muscle Cramps	1	-
Headache	1	-
Change in Mental Status	1	20
Nausea/Vomiting	1	-
Flu Like Syndrome	1	-
Renal Failure	-	1*
Syncope	-	1
Pain at Tumor	-	1
No Data	5857	4924

Data included in the table represent only those practitioners who reported exact patient numbers.
*Described as "not confirmed (possible). Patient had partial renal failure and cancer metastases to kidneys."
Data on practitioners who reported adverse events but did not report the number of patients affected are detailed below as: side effect (with the number of practitioners who reported each side effect in parenthesis).
For the year 2006: lethargy/fatigue (9), local vein irritation (3), nausea/vomiting (2), hypoglycemia (2), allergy (2), phlebitis (1), cellulitis (1), hematuria (1), dry mouth (1), Herxheimer reaction (1), localized thrombosis (1), and syncope (1).
For the year 2008: lethargy/fatigue (9), nausea/vomiting (6), local vein irritation (4), headache (3), phlebitis (3), heartburn (1), dizziness (1), venosclerosis (1), mild palpitation (1), and cold (1), dizziness (1), "initiation of mem occasionally" (1), and other (1).

Table 4. Adverse effects reported to the Food and Drug Administration (FDA) in patients treated with IV vitamin C.

Year	Number of Cases reported	Dose Range (g/day)	Can confounders be eliminated?
2004	15	0.5–1	No
2005	7	0.25–1	No
2006	11	0.2–1	No
2007	11	Not Given	No
2008	33	0.5–1	No

When the vitamin C dose was provided as ml, the dose was converted to mg on the basis that vitamin C is supplied as 0.5gram/ml solution. Some practitioners did not mention the dose of vitamin C used. The format of the FDA adverse events database did not permit identification of specific patients, so that the same patient may have been reported multiple times in the same quarter or in several quarters, inflating the number of patients with adverse events.

Pharmacologic doses of vitamin C given IV may produce drug effects in many body tissues, mediated by hydrogen peroxide formation in extracellular fluid but not blood [18–20]. Emerging clinical data are consistent with plausibility [43] and safety [16], but whether there is benefit or harm in humans can only be addressed by rigorous clinical trials.

IV vitamin C administered in gram doses can cause serious side effects in some patients. A metabolic end-product of vitamin C metabolism is oxalate, and oxalate nephropathy has been reported in patients with renal impairment given gram doses of IV vitamin C [22–24]. Prolonged treatment with vitamin C increases plasma oxalate concentrations in patients with renal failure [44] and results in increased urinary oxalate in patients receiving total parenteral nutrition [45], although in these patient groups the consequences of hyperoxalemia are unknown. Patients with glucose 6-phosphate dehydrogenase deficiency can develop intravascular hemolysis when gram doses of vitamin C are given IV [25,26]. Vitamin C, even with oral dosing, might induce hemolysis in patients with Paroxysmal Nocturnal Hemoglobinuria [46,47]. A recent phase one study of high dose IV vitamin C in patients with advanced cancer did not find any serious side effects [16]. Exclusion criteria for the phase I study included renal failure and glucose-6-phosphate dehydrogenase deficiency. Recently, a study in mice reported decreased efficacy of cancer chemotherapeutic agents with parenteral dehydroascorbic acid, a metabolite of vitamin C [48]. Dehydroascorbic acid cannot be detected in human blood or tissues, is not commercially available for parenteral use nor used by CAM practitioners, is toxic at high concentrations [49,50], and should not be administered parenterally in humans.

No definitive serious adverse events were reported by survey respondents. Despite the anonymity of the survey, practitioners may have been reluctant to describe adverse events. Whether IV vitamin C is safe for general use remains to be determined. Because of the possibility of unrecognized side effects or of drug interactions, practitioners should enquire whether their patients, especially those with chronic, intractable or difficult to treat conditions, are receiving high dose IV vitamin C treatment elsewhere. Physicians should be alert to potential interactions of high dose vitamin C not only with conventional medicines but also with CAM treatments. An example is the case of exacerbated, severe cyanide poisoning in a patient on concurrent treatment with high dose oral vitamin C and Amygdalin (laetrile, a metabolic product of which is cyanide) [51].

Soon after its discovery and synthesis in 1932, parenteral vitamin C was shown to significantly decrease polio virus infections in primates [31,32]. Although these findings were not repeatable [33,34], one practitioner treated thousands of patients with parenteral vitamin C, primarily for infections, and popularized its use [2,3,5]. Such reports probably were a basis for continued use of parenteral vitamin C by other CAM practitioners [6,7,35]. Independently, others postulated that vitamin C could be useful in cancer treatment by enhancing or strengthening collagen and intercellular matrix synthesis and thereby decreasing metastases [36,37]. Ewan Cameron, joined by Nobelist Linus Pauling, reported in retrospective case series that oral and IV vitamin C might benefit patients with advanced cancers [9,10]. Placebo-controlled double blinded clinical trials at the Mayo Clinic showed no efficacy [38–40] but CAM practitioners continued to use IV vitamin C [11,13,35], consistent with our survey results. Pharmacokinetics evidence [15,41,42] now reveals that the exclusively oral vitamin C doses used in the Mayo studies would have produced peak plasma concentrations of approximately 0.2 mM, while the same dose given IV would produce peak plasma concentrations approximately 25 fold higher [15].

Table 5. Adverse effects of vitamin C reported in the literature.

#	Type of Side Effect	Patient Details	Vitamin C Dose	Clinical Details Pre Vitamin C Treatment	Post Vitamin C Treatment	Outcome (and reference)
1	Acute Renal Failure	70 M	2.5g IV×1 dose	Creatinine 5.0	Flank pain, hematuria. Creatinine 10.	Permanent renal failure(24)
					Renal biopsy – Calcium oxalate crystals in tubular lumen	
2		58 F	45g IV×1 dose	Nephrotic syndrome	Oliguria. Treated with dopamine and hemodialysis. After first dialysis plasma vitamin C 15.4mg/dl (0.87mM), oxalate 2.3mg/dl. Intractable ventricular fibrillation. Post mortem- intra tubular calcium oxalate crystals.	Died(22)
				Creatinine 0.8		
3		61 M	60g IV×1 dose	Metastatic prostate cancer	Anuric. Creatinine 13.4. Plasma vitamin C 116.2mg/dl (6.6mM). Treated with nephrostomy and forced diuresis. Renal biopsy - acute tubular necrosis and extensive oxalate deposition	Recovered(23)
				Obstructive uropathy		
				Creatinine 0.7		
4	Hemolysis in Patients with Glucose-6-Phosphate Dehydrogenase Deficiency	68 M	80g IV×2 days	Second degree burns of one hand	Hemoglobin 5.8. Retics 5.9%. Anuria, creatinine 13.8. Coma, hemiparesis, possible intravascular coagulation. Supportive treatment and hemodialysis.	Died on day 22(25)
5		32 M	40g IV 3×/wk 20–40g/day oral×1 month then 80g IV×1 dose	HIV	Breathlessness, fever, dark urine. Hemoglobin 6.7 Retics 15.6%. Bilirubin 3.16. Conservative treatment with high fluid intake	Recovered(26)

Normal ranges and units of measurement for laboratory values are: Serum creatinine - mg/dl (normal range 0.6–1.5mg/dl). Hemoglobin g/dl (normal range: male 13–18g/dl, female 12–16g/dl). Reticulocyte count in % (normal range 0.5–2.5% red cells). Plasma bilirubin- mg/dl (normal range <1mg/dl). Plasma vitamin C - mg/dl (normal range 0.6–2 mg/dl).

Our study has limitations that, when considered together, may underestimate use of IV vitamin C. Because our survey was distributed to participants in a CAM conference, the survey excluded the vast majority of CAM practitioners. Respondents who filled in the survey form did so from memory without access to records, so that the information obtained can only be considered approximate. The format of the survey questions may have inadvertently resulted in underestimating vitamin C use, because the survey questions used ranges, for simplicity. For example, the highest value listed for numbers of patients treated in

a calendar year was ">40". If practitioners did not specify precise numbers as requested in subsequent questions, 40 was used as the number of patients treated, although the true number may have been higher. That there was only 24% overlap between survey respondents in 2006 and 2008 provides additional evidence that community use of IV vitamin C was underestimated. Data concerning industry sales of IV ascorbate only give approximations of use. On one hand, because not all units sold would have been used, use may be overestimated. Conversely, other smaller companies and compounding pharmacies may supply parenteral vitamin C but were not included in the survey. Therefore, the total number of vials sold may also be underestimated. The exact number of doses of parenteral vitamin C used in the US per year remains unknown. The survey response rate of approx 35% suggests we underestimated use, and perhaps adverse events. A reduced response rate may have occurred because some conference attendees were not practitioners and therefore did not return survey forms. Because of these uncertainties, the number of US patients treated with IV vitamin C cannot be accurately estimated from survey data. Since a primary aim of the survey was to determine if IV administered vitamin C is in use, and not a census of patients treated, the response rate does not detract from the value of the data.

Data obtained on adverse effects from PUBMED and the FDA also have limitations. Physicians may have not reported complications because they were not recognized, or were delayed, or were not attributed to vitamin C. Most practitioners do not report or publish adverse events. There may be as yet unknown adverse effects or interactions of IV ascorbate with other drugs. Side effects

Table 6. Details of treating practitioners and institutions.

		Number of Practitioners	
		2006	2008
Characteristics of Practitioners	Physician (MD)	66	49
	Doctor of Osteopathy (DO)	11	12
	Doctor of Naturopathy (ND)	8	8
	Nurse	2	1
	Physician's Assistant (PA)	2	2
Type of Institution	For-Profit organization	81	68
	Non-Profit/Other*	7	4

*Other includes an academic medical center and a tribal medical center.

reported to FDA are difficult to interpret because of confounding factors. All reported patients received other potentially toxic drugs and/or had other diagnoses that may have been responsible for the reported adverse effects (see Table S3). Because of the FDA adverse events format, the same patient was likely to have been reported multiple times. Because of the low doses of IV vitamin C in the FDA dataset, it is highly unlikely that any of the reported adverse effects were due to the vitamin. Despite this, and because the information available in the FDA database is limited, it is not possible to accurately determine whether vitamin C caused or contributed to the reported side effects.

IV vitamin C is already in wide use, and physicians should know that their patients may seek IV vitamin C treatment in addition to conventional therapies. Beneficial effects of intravenous vitamin C on the disease conditions for which it is used are unproven, but side effects appear to be minor. Physicians should be cognizant of potential adverse or other unexpected effects, and of unrecognized interactions with drugs used in conventional and alternative medicine. CAM practitioners have an obligation to screen patients and should not administer high dose IV vitamin C to patients with pre existing renal disease, renal insufficiency or renal failure; glucose 6-phosphate dehydrogenase deficiency; a history of oxalate nephrolithiasis; or paroxysmal nocturnal hemoglobinuria. Based on emerging evidence, vitamin C in pharmacologic concentrations appears to be a pro-drug for delivery of hydrogen peroxide to the extravascular space. High dose IV vitamin C appears to have a positive safety profile, favorable pharmacology, evidence for mechanism of action, some anti-cancer effects *in vitro* and in animals, and widespread use outside conventional medicine with minimal harm, but without any proven clinical benefit.

References

1. Nutrition Business Journal (2008) NBJ's Supplement Business Report 2008: An Analysis of Markets, Trends, Competition and Strategy in the U.S. Dietary Supplement Industry. Figure 3–33(Table 1); Figure 4–18. BoulderCO: Penton Media INC. Lifestyle Division. New Hope Natural Media.
2. Klenner FR (1949) The treatment of poliomyelitis and other virus diseases with vitamin C. South Med Surg 111: 209–14.
3. Klenner FR (1951) Massive doses of vitamin C and the virus diseases. South Med Surg 113: 101–7.
4. Calleja HB, Brooks RH (1960) Acute hepatitis treated with high doses of vitamin C. Report of a case. Ohio Med 56: 821–23.
5. Klenner FR (1971) Observations on the dose and administration of ascorbic acid when employed beyond the range of a vitamin in human pathology. Journal of Applied Nutrition 23: 61–88.
6. Cathcart RF (1891) Vitamin C, titrating to bowel tolerance, anascorbemia, and acute induced scurvy. Med Hypotheses 7: 1359–76.
7. Riordan NH, Riordan HD, Meng X, Li Y, Jackson JA (1995) Intravenous ascorbate as a tumor cytotoxic chemotherapeutic agent. Med Hypotheses 44: 207–13.
8. Pauling L (1976) Vitamin C the common cold and the flu. San Francisco: W.H.Freeman and Co.
9. Cameron E, Pauling L (1976) Supplemental ascorbate in the supportive treatment of cancer: Prolongation of survival times in terminal human cancer. Proc Natl Acad Sci U S A 73: 3685–89.
10. Cameron E, Pauling L (1978) Supplemental ascorbate in the supportive treatment of cancer: reevaluation of prolongation of survival times in terminal human cancer. Proc Natl Acad Sci U S A 75: 4538–42.
11. Riordan NH, Riordan HD, Casciari JJ (2000) Clinical and experimental experiences with intravenous vitamin C. J Orthomolecular Med 15: 201–3.
12. Levy TE (2002) Vitamin C, Infectious Diseases, and Toxins: Curing the Incurable. Philadelphia: Xlibris.
13. Gonzalez MJ, Miranda-Massari JR, Mora EM, Guzman A, Riordan NH, Riordan HD, et al. (2005) Orthomolecular oncology review: ascorbic acid and cancer 25 years later. Integr Cancer Ther 4: 32–44.
14. Levine M, Espey MG, Chen Q (2009) Losing and finding a way at C: new promise for pharmacologic ascorbate in cancer treatment. Free Radic Biol Med 47: 27–29.
15. Padayatty SJ, Sun H, Wang Y, Riordan HD, Hewitt SM, Katz A, et al. (2004) Vitamin C pharmacokinetics: implications for oral and intravenous use. Ann Intern Med 140: 533–37.
16. Hoffer LJ, Levine M, Assouline S, Melnychuk D, Padayatty SJ, Rosadiuk K, et al. (2008) Phase I clinical trial of i.v. ascorbic acid in advanced malignancy. Ann Oncol 19: 1969–74.
17. Padayatty SJ, Levine M (2000) Reevaluation of ascorbate in cancer treatment: emerging evidence, open minds and serendipity. J Am Coll Nutr 19: 423–25.
18. Chen Q, Espey MG, Krishna MC, Mitchell JB, Corpe CP, Buettner GR, et al. (2005) Pharmacologic ascorbic acid concentrations selectively kill cancer cells: action as a pro-drug to deliver hydrogen peroxide to tissues. Proc Natl Acad Sci U S A 102: 13604–9.
19. Chen Q, Espey MG, Sun AY, Lee JH, Krishna MC, Shacter E, et al. (2007) Ascorbate in pharmacologic concentrations selectively generates ascorbate radical and hydrogen peroxide in extracellular fluid in vivo. Proc Natl Acad Sci U S A 104: 8749–54.
20. Chen Q, Espey MG, Sun AY, Pooput C, Kirk KL, Krishna MC, et al. (2008) Pharmacologic doses of ascorbate act as a prooxidant and decrease growth of aggressive tumor xenografts in mice. Proc Natl Acad Sci U S A 105: 11105–9.
21. Verrax J, Calderon PB (2009) Pharmacologic concentrations of ascorbate are achieved by parenteral administration and exhibit antitumoral effects. Free Radic Biol Med 47: 27–9.
22. Lawton JM, Conway LT, Crosson JT, Smith CL, Abraham PA (1985) Acute oxalate nephropathy after massive ascorbic acid administration. Arch Intern Med 145: 950–951.
23. Wong K, Thomson C, Bailey RR, McDiarmid S, Gardner J (1994) Acute oxalate nephropathy after a massive intravenous dose of vitamin C. Aust N Z J Med 24: 410–411.
24. McAllister CJ, Scowden EB, Dewberry FL, Richman A (1984) Renal failure secondary to massive infusion of vitamin C. JAMA 252: 1684.
25. Campbell GD, Jr., Steinberg MH, Bower JD (1975) Ascorbic acid-induced hemolysis in G-6-PD deficiency. Ann Intern Med 82: 810.
26. Rees DC, Kelsey H, Richards JD (1993) Acute haemolysis induced by high dose ascorbic acid in glucose-6- phosphate dehydrogenase deficiency. BMJ 306: 841–42.
27. Barnes PM, Powell-Griner E, McFann K, Nahin RL (2004) Complementary and alternative medicine use among adults: United States 2002. Adv Data. 1–19.
28. Gaby AR (2002) Intravenous nutrient therapy: the "Myers' cocktail". Altern Med Rev 7: 389–403.
29. Ali A, Njike VY, Northrup V, Sabina AB, Williams AL, Liberti LS, et al. (2009) Intravenous micronutrient therapy (Myers' Cocktail) for fibromyalgia: a placebo-controlled pilot study. J Altern Complement Med 15: 247–57.
30. Levine M, Rumsey SC, Daruwala R, Park JB, Wang Y (1999) Criteria and recommendations for vitamin C intake. JAMA 281: 1415–23.
31. Jungeblut CW (1935) Inactivation of poliomyelitis virus in vitro by crystalline vitamin C (ascorbic acid). Journal of Experimental Medicine 62: 517–21.

Acknowledgments

We thank CAM practitioners for their cooperation in completing the surveys, and Dr. Jill Norris, University of Colorado Health Sciences Center, for advice on preparing the survey.

Author Contributions

Conceived and designed the experiments: SJP AYS QC MGE JD ML. Performed the experiments: SJP AYS QC MGE JD ML. Analyzed the data: SJP AYS QC MGE JD ML. Contributed reagents/materials/analysis tools: SJP AYS QC MGE JD ML. Wrote the paper: SJP AYS QC MGE JD ML.

32. Jungeblut CW (1937) Further observations on vitamin C therapy in experimental poliomyelitis. Journal of Experimental Medicine 66: 459–77.

33. Sabin AB (1939) Vitamin C in relation to experimental poliomyelitis. Journal of Experimental Medicine 69: 507–16.

34. Jungeblut CW (1939) A further contribution to vitamin C therapy in experimental poliomyelitis. Journal of Experimental Medicine 70: 315–32.

35. Riordan HD, Jackson JA, Schultz M (1990) Case study: high-dose intravenous vitamin C in the treatment of a patient with adenocarcinoma of the kidney. J Orthomolecular Med 5: 5–7.

36. McCormick WJ (1954) Cancer: the preconditioning factor in pathogenesis; a new etiologic approach. Arch Pediatr 71: 313–22.

37. Cameron E, Rotman D (1972) Ascorbic acid, cell proliferation, and cancer. Lancet 1: 542.

38. Moertel CG, Fleming TR, Creagan ET, Rubin J, O'Connell MJ, Ames MM (1985) High-dose vitamin C versus placebo in the treatment of patients with advanced cancer who have had no prior chemotherapy. A randomized double-blind comparison. N Engl J Med 312: 137–41.

39. Creagan ET, Moertel CG, O'Fallon JR, Schutt AJ, O'Connell MJ, Rubin J, et al. (1979) Failure of high-dose vitamin C (ascorbic acid) therapy to benefit patients with advanced cancer. A controlled trial. N Engl J Med 301: 687–90.

40. Wittes RE (1985) Vitamin C and cancer. N Engl J Med 312: 178–79.

41. Levine M, Conry-Cantilena C, Wang Y, Welch RW, Washko PW, Dhariwal KR, et al. (1996) Vitamin C pharmacokinetics in healthy volunteers: evidence for a Recommended Dietary Allowance. Proc Natl Acad Sci U S A 93: 3704–9.

42. Levine M, Wang Y, Padayatty SJ, Morrow J (2001) A new recommended dietary allowance of vitamin C for healthy young women. Proc Natl Acad Sci U S A 98: 9842–46.

43. Padayatty SJ, Levine M (2006) Vitamins C and E and the prevention of preeclampsia. N Engl J Med 355: 1065.

44. Canavese C, Petrarulo M, Massarenti P, Berutti S, Fenoglio R, Pauletto D, et al. (2005) Long-term, low-dose, intravenous vitamin C leads to plasma calcium oxalate supersaturation in hemodialysis patients. Am J Kidney Dis 45: 540–549.

45. Pena dl V, Lieske JC, Milliner D, Gonyea J, Kelly DG (2004) Urinary oxalate excretion increases in home parenteral nutrition patients on a higher intravenous ascorbic acid dose. JPEN J Parenter Enteral Nutr 28: 435–38.

46. Iwamoto N, Kawaguchi T, Horikawa K, Nagakura S, Hidaka M, Kagimoto T, et al. (1994) Haemolysis induced by ascorbic acid in paroxysmal nocturnal haemoglobinuria. Lancet 343: 357.

47. Iwamoto N, Nakakuma H, Ota N, Shimokado H, Takatsuki K (1994) Ascorbic acid-induced hemolysis of paroxysmal nocturnal hemoglobinuria erythrocytes. Am J Hematol 47: 337–38.

48. Heaney ML, Gardner JR, Karasavvas N, Golde DW, Scheinberg DA, Smith EA, et al. (2008) Vitamin C antagonizes the cytotoxic effects of antineoplastic drugs. Cancer Res 68: 8031–38.

49. Patterson JW (1950) The diabetogenic effect of dehydroascorbic and dehydroisoascorbic acids. J Biol Chem 183: 81–88.

50. Patterson JW (1951) Course of diabetes and development of cataracts after injecting dehydroascorbic acid and related substances. Am J Physiol 165: 61–65.

51. Bromley J, Hughes BG, Leong DC, Buckley NA (2005) Life-threatening interaction between complementary medicines: cyanide toxicity following ingestion of amygdalin and vitamin C. Ann Pharmacother 39: 1566–69.

17

Efficacy of Short-Term High-Dose Statin in Preventing Contrast-Induced Nephropathy

Yongchuan Li ⁹, Yawei Liu ⁹, Lili Fu, Changlin Mei*, Bing Dai*

Division of Nephrology, Nephrology Institute of PLA, Shanghai Changzheng Hospital, Second Military Medical University, Shanghai, China

Abstract

Background: A few studies focused on statin therapy as specific prophylactic measures of contrast-induced nephropathy have been published with conflicting results. In this meta-analysis of randomized controlled trials, we aimed to assess the effectiveness of shor-term high-dose statin treatment for the prevention of CIN and clinical outcomes and re-evaluate of the potential benefits of statin therapy.

Methods: We searched PubMed, OVID, EMBASE, Web of science and the Cochrane Central Register of Controlled Trials databases for randomized controlled trials comparing short-term high-dose statin treatment versus low-dose statin treatment or placebo for preventing CIN. Our outcome measures were the risk of CIN within 2–5 days after contrast administration and need for dialysis.

Results: Seven randomized controlled trials with a total of 1,399 patients were identified and analyzed. The overall results based on fixed-effect model showed that the use of short-term high-dose statin treatment was associated with a significant reduction in risk of CIN (RR = 0.51, 95% CI 0.34–0.76, p = 0.001; I^2 = 0%). The incidence of acute renal failure requiring dialysis was not significant different after the use of statin (RR = 0.33, 95% CI 0.05–2.10, p = 0.24; I^2 = 0%). The use of statin was not associated with a significant decrease in the plasma C-reactive protein level (SMD −0.64, 95% CI: −1.57 to 0.29, P = 0.18, I^2 = 97%).

Conclusions: Although this meta-analysis supports the use of statin to reduce the incidence of CIN, it must be considered in the context of variable patient demographics. Only a limited recommendation can be made in favour of the use of statin based on current data. Considering the limitations of included studies, a large, well designed trial that incorporates the evaluation of clinically relevant outcomes in participants with different underlying risks of CIN is required to more adequately assess the role for statin in CIN prevention.

Editor: Nick Ashton, The University of Manchester, United Kingdom

Funding: This work was supported by grants from the National Natural Science Foundation of China (30900692, 81000283, 30971368) and Shanghai Leading Academic Discipline Project (B902). The funders had no role in study design, data collection and analysis, decision to publish, or preparation of the manuscript.

Competing Interests: The authors have declared that no competing interests exist.

* E-mail: daibin105@yahoo.com.cn (BD); chlmei1954@yahoo.com.cn (CM)

⁹ These authors contributed equally to this work.

Introduction

Contrast-induced nephropathy (CIN), characterized by the development of acute renal failure after exposure to radiocontrast, is the third leading cause of hospital-acquired acute renal injury, accounting for 11% of all cases [1]. It is defined as an increase in baseline serum creatinine level of 25% or an absolute increase of 44 μmol/L (0.5 mg/dL). Although CIN is generally benign in most instances, it is associated with lengthened hospital stays, increased health care costs, and higher risk of death [2–4]. Several strategies, including using iso-osmolar contrast, limiting the amount of administered contrast media and volume expansion have become well established methods for the prevention of CIN.

The pathophysiological mechanisms of CIN is not well known. However, multiple studies have suggested that renal vasoconstriction, oxidative stress, inflammation and direct tubular cell damage by contrast media may play crucial important roles in the renal injury process [5–8]. Statins, drugs primarily associated with low-density lipoprotein cholesterol-lowering effects, have been shown to possess pleiotropic effects that include enhancement of endothelial nitric oxide production [9–11], anti-inflammatory and antioxidative actions [12,13]. Therefore, statins are considered as promising candidate agents for the prevention of CIN.

A few studies focused on statin therapy as specific prophylactic measures of CIN have been published with conflicting results [14–22]. In this meta-analysis of randomized controlled trials (RCTs), we aimed to assess the effectiveness of short-term high-dose statin treatment for the prevention of CIN and clinical outcomes and re-evaluate of the potential benefits of statin therapy.

Table 1. Characteristics of included studies.

Author, year	Patients,n		Inclusion criteria	Statin protocol	Control	Contrast type	Median contrast volume,ml		Hydration procedure
	Statin	Control					Statin	Control	
Sang-Ho Jo et al,2008	118	118	CAG;SCr≥1.1 mg/dL or CrCl≤60 mL/min	Simvastatin,40 mg every 12 hours, 1 day pre-procedure and 1 day post-procedure	Placebo	Iodixanol	173	191	Isotonic saline,1 mg/kg/hour for 12 h before and 12 h after procedure
Anna Toso et al,2009	152	152	CAG and/or PCI. CrCl<60 ml/min	Atorvastatin,80 mg/day 2 days pre-procedure and 2 days post-procedure+NAC,1200 mg bid from 1 day before to 1 day post-procedure	Placebo+NAC, 1200 mg bid from 1 day before to 1 day post-procedure	Iodixanol	151	164	NS,1 ml/kg/hour for 12 h before and after the procedure
Xinwei et al,2009	113	115	PCI	Simvastatin, 80 mg/day from admission to the day before, 20 mg/day after procedure	Simvastatin, 20 mg/day from admission to the end	Iodixanol for CKD,iohexol for others	227	240	NS, 1 ml/kg/hour for 6 to 12 hours before and 12 hours after procedure
Zhou Xia et al,2009	50	50	CAG or PCI	Atorvastatin,80 mg/day before for 1day,10 mg/day for 6days after procedure	Atorvastatin, 10 mg/ day for 7 days	Iopamidol	119	113	1000 mL saline infusion, for 12 hours before and 12 hours after intervention
Sadik Acikel et al,2010	80	80	CAG,eGFR>60 ml/min per 1.73 m^2	Atorvastatin,40 mg/day,3 days pre-procedure and 2 days post-procedure	Nothing	Iohexol	105	103	Isotonic saline,1 ml/kg/hour starting 4 h before and continuing until 24 h after procedure
Hakan Ozhan et al,2010	60	70	CAG,SCr≤1.5 mg/dl or eGFR≥70 ml/min per 1.73 m^2	Atorvastatin,80 mg 1 day pre-procedure and 2 days post-procedure+600 mg NAC bid pre-procedure	600 mg NAC bid pre-procedure	Iopamidol	97	93	1000 ml saline infusion during 6 h after procedure
Giuseppe Patti et al,2011	120	121	CAG and/or PCI. SCr≤3 mg/dl	Atorvastatin,80 mg(12 hs before)+40 mg(2 hs before), 40 mg for 2days after procedure	Placebo+40 mg atorvastatin for 2days after procedure	Iobitridol	209	213	For patients CrCl<60 ml/min,1 ml/hour/ kg for 12 h before and 24 h after intervention

Statin = statin-treated group(high-dose);Control = control group(low-dose or non-statin);CAG = coronary angiography;PCI = percutaneous coronary intervention;CrCl = creatinine clearance;Scr = serum creatinine;eGFR = estimated glomerular filtration rate;NAC = N-acetylcysteine;NS = 0.9% sodium chloride.

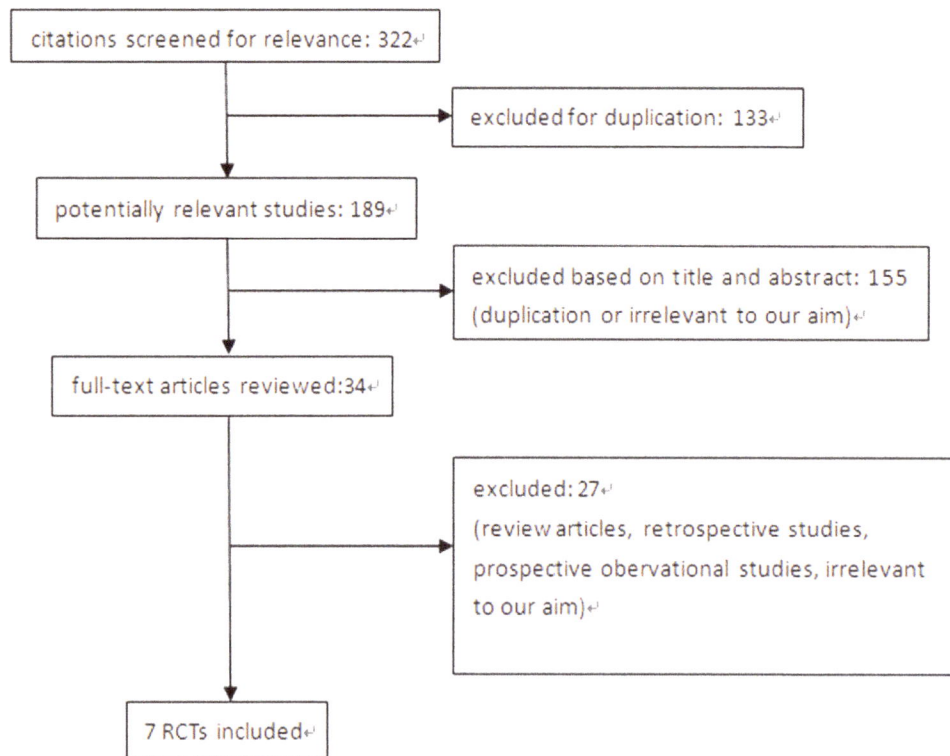

Figure 1. Study selection diagram.

Materials and Methods

Search strategy

The literature search was performed on PubMed (1966-October 2011), OVID (1966 to October 2011), EMBASE (1966-October 2011), Web of science (1986- October 2011) and the Cochrane Central Register of Controlled Trials (1996 to October 2011). We derived three comprehensive search themes that were then combined using the Boolean operator "AND". For the theme "contrast media", we used combinations of MeSH, entry terms and text words: contrast, radiocontrast, contrast medium, contrast media, contrast dye, radiographic contrast, radiocontrast media, radiocontrast medium and contrast agent. For the theme "renal insufficiency", we used: renal insufficiency, renal failure, diabetic nephropathies, nephritis, nephropathy, nephrotoxic, (impair or injury or damage or reduce) and (renal or kidney), contrast-induced nephropathy and contrast-associated nephropathy. For the theme "statin", statin, atorvastatin, rosuvastatin, cerivastatin, simvastatin, pravastatin, lovastatin, Hydroxymethylglutar-yl(HMG)-CoA reductase inhibitors and HMG-CoA reductase inhibitors were used. Appendix S1 shows the detailed search method. We did not restrict by language or type of article. To identify other relevant studies, we manually scanned reference lists from identified trials and review articles, and we also searched conference proceedings. We requested original data by directly contacting authors.

Study selection

We included studies when the following criteria were met: (1) randomized, controlled trials assessing preventive strategies for CIN; (2) the intervention was high-dose statin (defined as a daily dose of 80 mg or 40 mg) versus low-dose statin treatment (defined as a daily dose of 20 mg or 10 mg) or placebo. Studies that incorporated NAC were included only if both arms were administered NAC; (3) studies reported the incidence of contrast-induced nephropathy in both arms. We did not restrict eligibility according to kidney function. The primary outcome measure was the development of contrast-induced nephropathy, defined as an increase in baseline serum creatinine level of 25% or an absolute increase of 44 μmol/L (0.5 mg/dL) within 2 to 5 days after the exposure to contrast medium. Secondary outcome measures were need for dislysis, in-hospital mortality and length of hospital stay.

Data extraction and quality assessment

Data were collected independently by 2 reviewers. Extracted data included patient characteristics (mean age, diabetes status, mean baseline creatinine level and postprocedural change in C-reactive protein level); inclusion criteria; type and dose of contrast media; protocol for the treatment of statins; periprocedural hydration protocol and specific definition of CIN. Quality assessment was judged on concealment of treatment allocation; similarity of both groups at baseline regarding prognostic factors; eligibility criteria; blinding of outcome assessors, care providers, and patients; completeness of follow-up; and intention-to-treat analysis [23]. We quantified study quality by using the Jadad score [24]. A third reviewer adjudicated any disagreement about extracted data. Then data were checked and entered into the Review Manager (Version 5.0. Copenhagen: The Nordic Cochrane Centre, The Cochrane Collaboration, 2008) database for further analysis.

Table 2. Characteristics of included studies-continued.

Author, year	Mean age,y		Diabetic patients,%		Mean baseline sCr level,μmol/L (mg/dL)		Postprocedural changes in CRP levels, mg/L (Mean±SD)		Definition of CIN	Events,n	
	Statin	Control	Statin	Control	Statin	Control	Statin	Control		Statin	Control
Sang-Ho Jo et al,2008	65	66	28.2%	23.6%	114(1.286)	110(1.248)	1.25±1.25	1.27±1.79	Increase of Scr>0.5 mg/dL or >25% within 48 hours	3	4
Anna Toso et al,2009	75	76	20%	22%	106(1.2)	104(1.18)	NS	NS	Increase of Scr≥0.5 mg/dl within 5 days.	15	16
Xinwei et al,2009	65	66	20%	22%	72(0.82)	73(0.83)	1.9±0.5	3.4±1.2	Increase of Scr>0.5 mg/dL or >25% within 48 hours	6	18
Zhou Xia et al,2009	60	61	22%	18%	92(1.04)	95(1.08)	NS	NS	Increase of Scr>0.5 mg/dL or >25% within 72 hours	0	3
Sadik Acikel et al,2010	59	61	23.8%	25.0%	74(0.84)	75(0.85)	NS	NS	Increase of Scr>0.5 mg/dL within 48 hours	0	1
Hakan Ozhan et al,2010	54	55	15.00%	17.14%	77.8(0.88)	77.8(0.88)	NS	NS	Increase of Scr>0.5 mg/dL or >25% within 48 hours	2	7
Giuseppe Patti et al,2011	65	66	30%	25%	92(1.04)	92(1.04)	8.4±10.5	13.1±20.8	Increase of Scr>0.5 mg/dL or >25% within 48 hours	6	16

Statin = statin-treated group (high-dose);Control = control group (low-dose or non-statin);CAG = coronary angiography;PCI = percutaneous coronary intervention;CrCl = creatinine clearance;Scr = serum creatinine;CRP = C-reactive protein;eGFR = estimated glomerular filtration rate;NAC = N-acetylcysteine;NS = 0.9% sodium chloride; NS = not specified or available.

Table 3. Quality of included RCTs.

Author, Year	Jadad Score	Allocation Concealment	Similarity of Baseline Characteristics	Eligibility Criteria	Blinding			Completeness of Follow-up	Intention-to-Treat Analysis
					Outcome Assessor	Care Provider	Patient		
Sang-Ho Jo et al,2008	5	YES	YES	YES	NS	YES	YES	YES	YES
Anna Toso et al,2009	5	YES	YES	YES	NS	YES	YES	YES	YES
Xinwei et al,2009	3	YES	YES	YES	NO	NO	NO	YES	NS
Zhou Xia et al,2009	3	NS	YES	YES	NS	NS	NS	YES	NS
Sadik Acikel et al,2010	1	NS	NO	YES	NO	NO	NO	YES	NS
Hakan Ozhan et al,2010	2	NS	YES	YES	NO	NO	NO	YES	NS
Giuseppe Patti et al,2011	5	YES	YES	YES	YES	YES	YES	YES	YES

NS = not specified or available.

| | High-dose | | Low-dose or non-statin | | | Risk Ratio | | Risk Ratio |
Study or Subgroup	Events	Total	Events	Total	Weight	M-H, Fixed, 95% CI	Year	M-H, Fixed, 95% CI
Sang-Ho Jo et al 2008	3	118	4	118	6.1%	0.75 [0.17, 3.28]	2008	
Zhou 2009	0	50	3	50	5.4%	0.14 [0.01, 2.70]	2009	
Anna Toso et al 2009	15	152	16	152	24.5%	0.94 [0.48, 1.83]	2009	
Xinwei 2009	6	113	18	115	27.3%	0.34 [0.14, 0.82]	2009	
Sadik Acikel et al 2010	0	80	1	80	2.3%	0.33 [0.01, 8.06]	2010	
Hakan Ozhan et al 2010	2	60	7	70	9.9%	0.33 [0.07, 1.54]	2010	
Patti G 2011	6	120	16	121	24.4%	0.38 [0.15, 0.93]	2011	
Total (95% CI)		693		706	100.0%	0.51 [0.34, 0.76]		
Total events	32		65					

Heterogeneity: Chi² = 5.78, df = 6 (P = 0.45); I² = 0%
Test for overall effect: Z = 3.28 (P = 0.001)

0.01   0.1   1   10   100
Favours experimental   Favours control

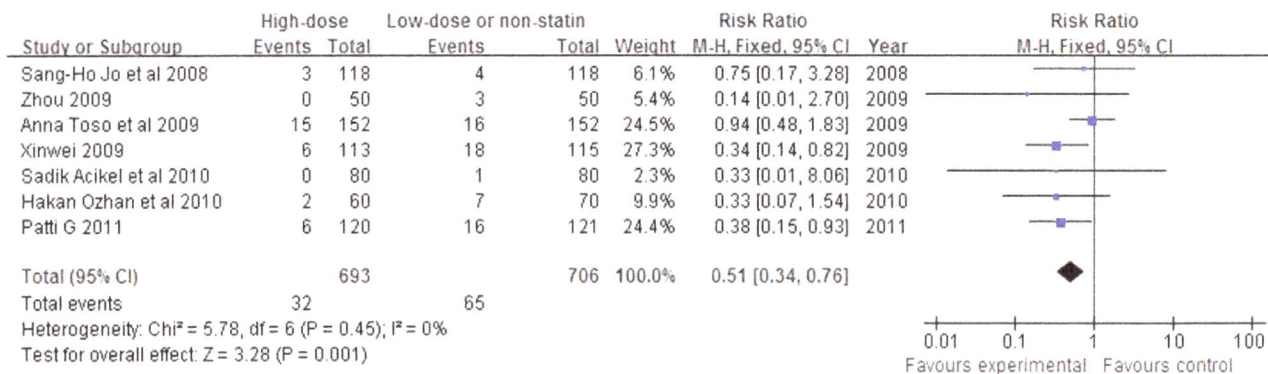

Figure 2. Forest plot of risk ratios and 95% confidence intervals (CI) for the incidence of contrast induced nephropathy among patients assigned to statin therapy versus control.

Statistical analysis

Dichotomous data (contrast-induced nephropathy and need for dialysis) were analyzed using the risk ratio (RR) measure and its 95% confidence interval (CI). Moreover, heterogeneity across trials was evaluated with I^2 statistic, which defined as $I^2 > 50\%$. If heterogeneity existed, a random-effect model was used to assess the overall estimate. Otherwise, a fixed-effect model was chosen. We assessed for potential publication bias by using Begg funnel plots of the natural log of the relative risk versus its standard error [25]. To further detect and evaluate clinically significant heterogeneity, we also a priori decided to perform several subgroup analyses to identify potential differences in treatment across the trials. Subgroup analysis was conducted based on renal function in participants at baseline (with or without renal impairment), the control group property (low dose of statin or control), the addition of NAC (with or without NAC), and Jadad study quality score (Jadad>3 or Jadad≤3). All tests were two-tailed and a P value less than 0.05 was regarded as significant in this meta-analysis.

Results

Selected studies and characteristics

We identified 322 potentially relevant citations from the initial literature search. After independently reviewing the title and abstract of all potential articles, 34 articles were considered of interest and reviewed in full-text. Of these, 27 were excluded from the meta-analysis (review articles, retrospective studies, prospective obervational studies, irrelevant to our aim). Although the study carried out by Acikel Sadik et al [20] did not provide data on the incidence of CIN, we requested it by directly contacting the author. Therefore, seven randomized controlled studies with a total of 1,399 patients with undergoing radiocontrast-related procedures were identified and analyzed [16–22]. Our search strategy is outlined in Figure 1.

Table 1 and table 2 summarizes the characteristics of the included studies. All of them had been reported since 2008. 693 subjects were assigned to short-term high-dose statin treatment group and 706 subjects were assigned to short-term low-dose or non-statin treatment group. The proportion of patients lost to follow-up was less than 5% in all studies. CIN was defined

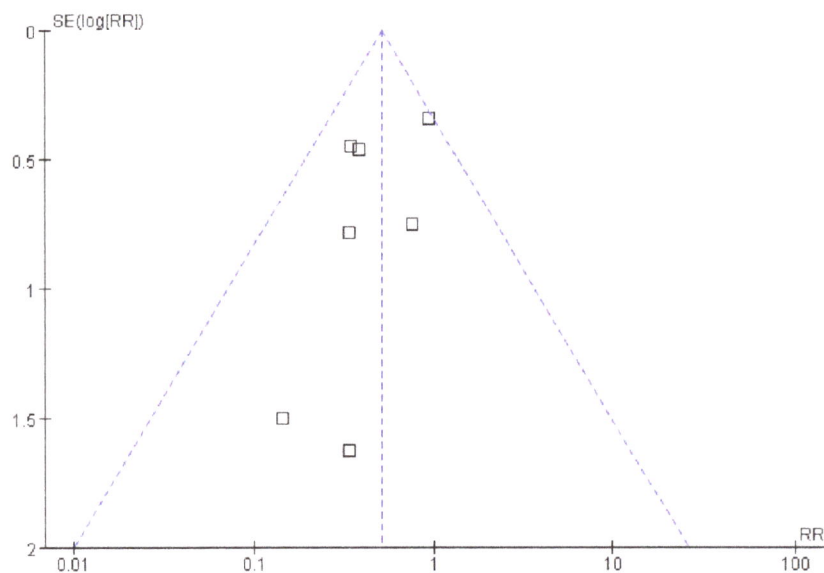

Figure 3. Funnel plot with 95% confidence intervals (CI) to assess for evidence of publication bias.

Study or Subgroup	High-dose Events	Total	Low-dose or non-statin Events	Total	Weight	Risk Ratio M-H, Fixed, 95% CI	Risk Ratio M-H, Fixed, 95% CI
1.4.1 high-dose vs. low-dose statin							
Zhou 2009	0	50	3	50	5.4%	0.14 [0.01, 2.70]	
Xinwei 2009	6	113	18	115	27.3%	0.34 [0.14, 0.82]	
Subtotal (95% CI)		163		165	32.7%	0.31 [0.13, 0.72]	
Total events	6		21				
Heterogeneity: Chi² = 0.31, df = 1 (P = 0.58); I² = 0%							
Test for overall effect: Z = 2.74 (P = 0.006)							
1.4.2 high-dose statin vs. non-statin							
Sadik Acikel et al 2010	0	80	1	80	2.3%	0.33 [0.01, 8.06]	
Hakan Ozhan et al 2010	2	60	7	70	9.9%	0.33 [0.07, 1.54]	
Patti G 2011	6	120	16	121	24.4%	0.38 [0.15, 0.93]	
Sang-Ho Jo et al 2008	3	118	4	118	6.1%	0.75 [0.17, 3.28]	
Anna Toso et al 2009	15	152	16	152	24.5%	0.94 [0.48, 1.83]	
Subtotal (95% CI)		530		541	67.3%	0.61 [0.38, 0.97]	
Total events	26		44				
Heterogeneity: Chi² = 3.48, df = 4 (P = 0.48); I² = 0%							
Test for overall effect: Z = 2.10 (P = 0.04)							
Total (95% CI)		693		706	100.0%	0.51 [0.34, 0.76]	
Total events	32		65				
Heterogeneity: Chi² = 5.78, df = 6 (P = 0.45); I² = 0%							
Test for overall effect: Z = 3.28 (P = 0.001)							

0.01 0.1 1 10 100
Favours experimental Favours control

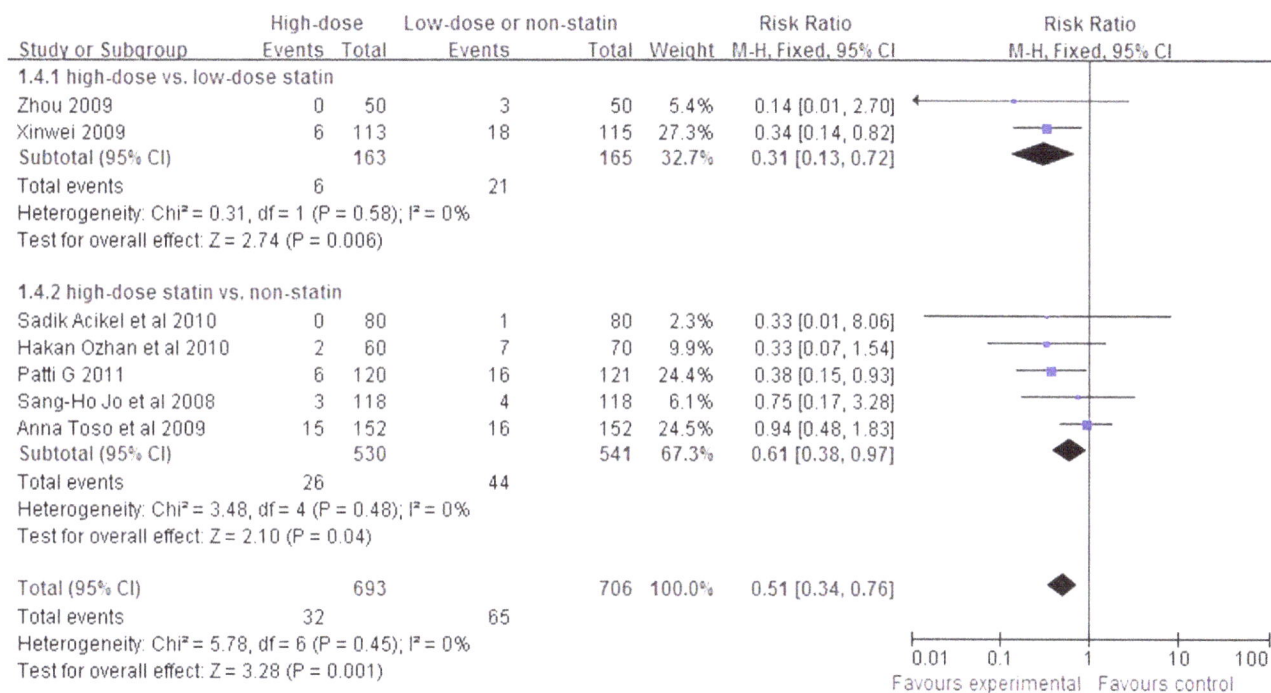

Figure 4. Forest plot of risk ratios and 95% confidence intervals (CI) for the incidence of CIN among patients assigned to short-term high-dose statin treatment versus low-dose or non-statin.

differently among the included studies. Six studies [16,17,19–22] used an increase in serum creatinine of >0.5 mg/dL or >25% from baseline within 48–72 h after radiocontrast exposure as their definition, whereas the other study [18] regarded an absolute increase in serum creatinine of >0.5 mg/dl within 5 days as their primary definition of CIN. Two studies [17,18] involved patients with creatinine clearance rate less than 60 ml/min; four studies [16,20–22] enrolled patients with creatinine clearance rate or estimated glomerular filtration rate>60 ml/min and there was no restriction according to renal function but patients with creatinine level >3 mg/dl were excluded in the study by Patti G et al [19]. All studies evaluated patients undergoing coronary angiography or

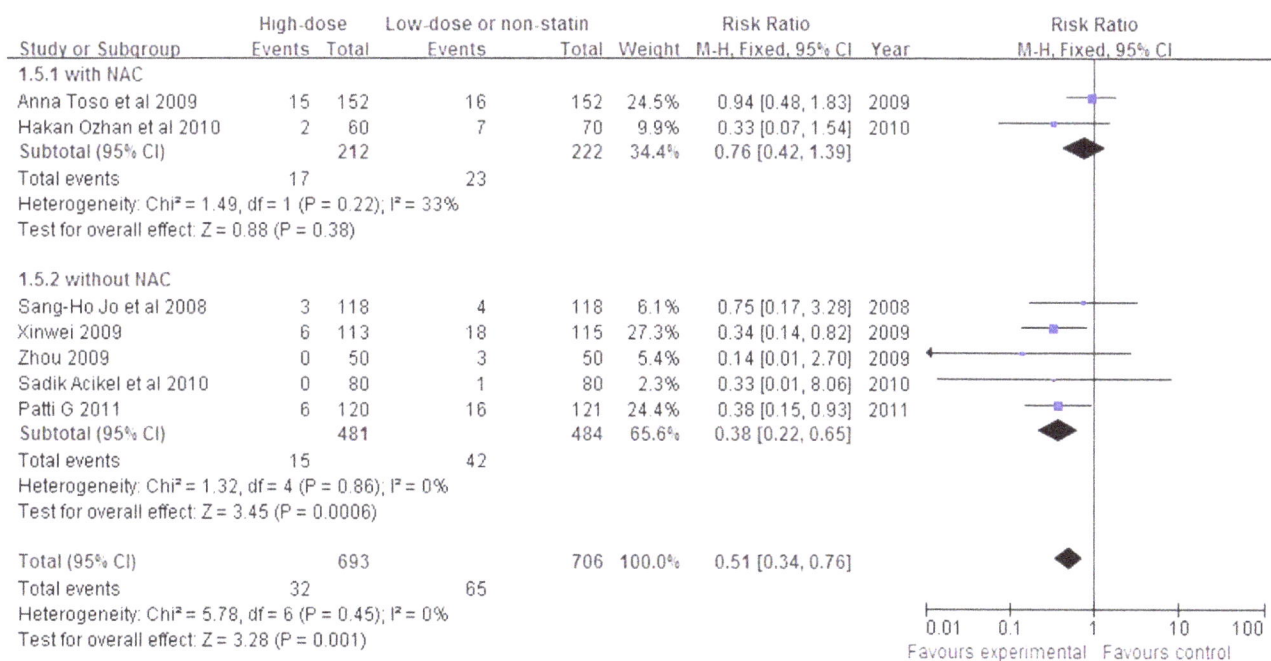

Study or Subgroup	High-dose Events	Total	Low-dose or non-statin Events	Total	Weight	Risk Ratio M-H, Fixed, 95% CI	Year	Risk Ratio M-H, Fixed, 95% CI
1.5.1 with NAC								
Anna Toso et al 2009	15	152	16	152	24.5%	0.94 [0.48, 1.83]	2009	
Hakan Ozhan et al 2010	2	60	7	70	9.9%	0.33 [0.07, 1.54]	2010	
Subtotal (95% CI)		212		222	34.4%	0.76 [0.42, 1.39]		
Total events	17		23					
Heterogeneity: Chi² = 1.49, df = 1 (P = 0.22); I² = 33%								
Test for overall effect: Z = 0.88 (P = 0.38)								
1.5.2 without NAC								
Sang-Ho Jo et al 2008	3	118	4	118	6.1%	0.75 [0.17, 3.28]	2008	
Xinwei 2009	6	113	18	115	27.3%	0.34 [0.14, 0.82]	2009	
Zhou 2009	0	50	3	50	5.4%	0.14 [0.01, 2.70]	2009	
Sadik Acikel et al 2010	0	80	1	80	2.3%	0.33 [0.01, 8.06]	2010	
Patti G 2011	6	120	16	121	24.4%	0.38 [0.15, 0.93]	2011	
Subtotal (95% CI)		481		484	65.6%	0.38 [0.22, 0.65]		
Total events	15		42					
Heterogeneity: Chi² = 1.32, df = 4 (P = 0.86); I² = 0%								
Test for overall effect: Z = 3.45 (P = 0.0006)								
Total (95% CI)		693		706	100.0%	0.51 [0.34, 0.76]		
Total events	32		65					
Heterogeneity: Chi² = 5.78, df = 6 (P = 0.45); I² = 0%								
Test for overall effect: Z = 3.28 (P = 0.001)								

0.01 0.1 1 10 100
Favours experimental Favours control

Figure 5. Forest plot of risk ratios and 95% confidence intervals (CI) for the incidence of CIN among patients assigned to statin therapy versus control with NAC using or not.

Study or Subgroup	High-dose Events Total		Low-dose or non-statin Events	Total	Weight	Risk Ratio M-H, Fixed, 95% CI	Year	Risk Ratio M-H, Fixed, 95% CI
1.6.1 Without renal impairment								
Zhou 2009	0	50	3	50	5.4%	0.14 [0.01, 2.70]	2009	
Xinwei 2009	6	113	18	115	27.5%	0.34 [0.14, 0.82]	2009	
Hakan Ozhan et al 2010	2	60	7	70	10.0%	0.33 [0.07, 1.54]	2010	
Sadik Acikel et al 2010	0	80	1	80	2.3%	0.33 [0.01, 8.06]	2010	
Patti G 2011	1	85	6	82	9.4%	0.16 [0.02, 1.31]	2011	
Subtotal (95% CI)		388		397	54.6%	0.29 [0.15, 0.57]		
Total events	9		35					
Heterogeneity: Chi² = 0.69, df = 4 (P = 0.95); I² = 0%								
Test for overall effect: Z = 3.59 (P = 0.0003)								
1.6.2 With renal impairment								
Sang-Ho Jo et al 2008	3	118	4	118	6.2%	0.75 [0.17, 3.28]	2008	
Anna Toso et al 2009	15	152	16	152	24.7%	0.94 [0.48, 1.83]	2009	
Patti G 2011	5	35	10	39	14.6%	0.56 [0.21, 1.47]	2011	
Subtotal (95% CI)		305		309	45.4%	0.79 [0.47, 1.32]		
Total events	23		30					
Heterogeneity: Chi² = 0.75, df = 2 (P = 0.69); I² = 0%								
Test for overall effect: Z = 0.90 (P = 0.37)								
Total (95% CI)		693		706	100.0%	0.52 [0.35, 0.77]		
Total events	32		65					
Heterogeneity: Chi² = 6.51, df = 7 (P = 0.48); I² = 0%								
Test for overall effect: Z = 3.25 (P = 0.001)								

0.01   0.1   1   10   100
Favours experimental   Favours control

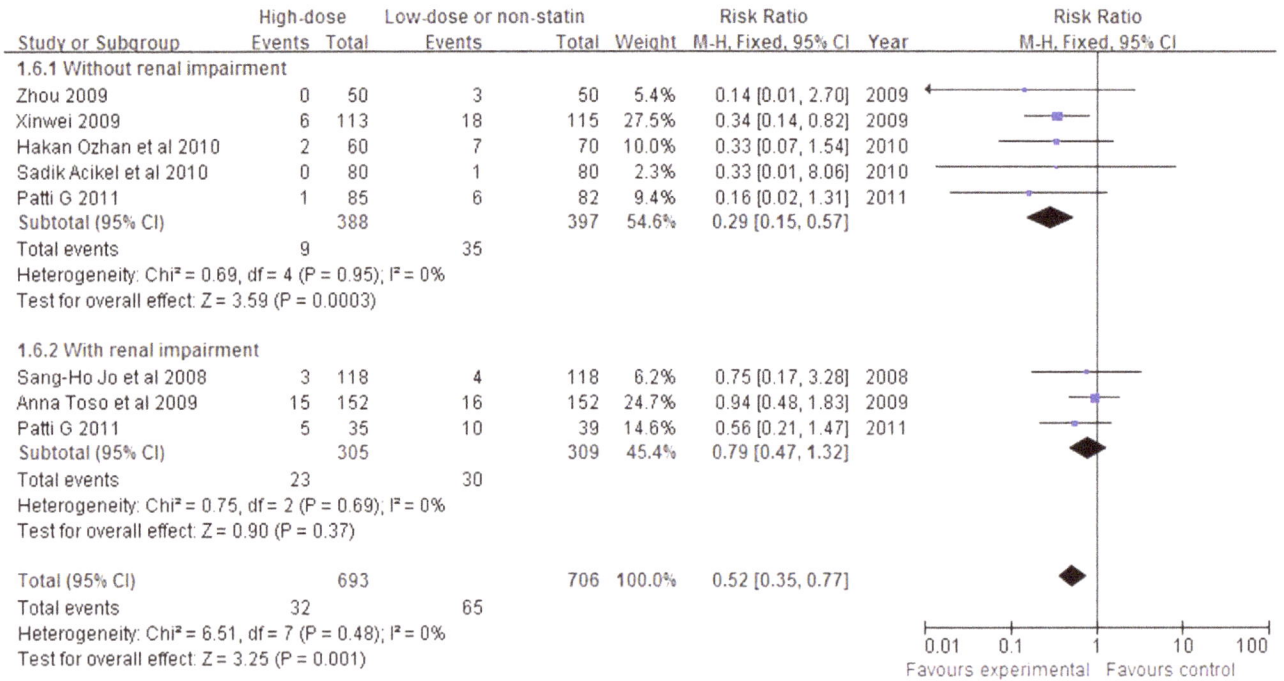

Figure 6. Forest plot of risk ratios and 95% confidence intervals (CI) for the incidence of CIN among patients assigned to statin therapy versus control according to renal function.

other intervention, for example, percutaneous coronary intervention (PCI). All of the patients received low-osmolar or iso-osmolar contrast media and median contrast volume ranged from 93 ml to 240 ml. Periprocedural hydration was used in every one, except the patients without pre-existing renal failure in the study by Patti

G et al [19]. Five studies [16,18–20,22] used atorvastatin and simvastatin was used in the other two studies [17,21]. The duration of statin treatment ranged from 3 to >7 days and the total dose ranged from 140 mg to >460 mg in the high-dose statin treatment group. Two of the included studies [16,18] also used

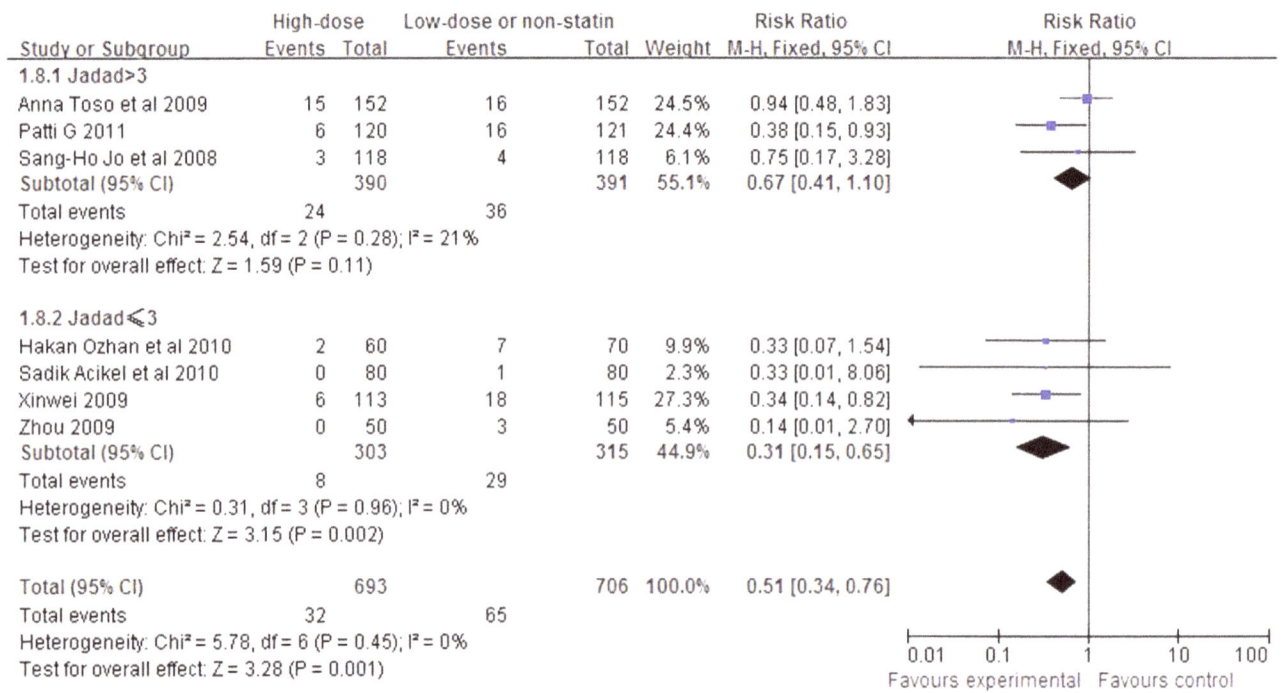

Study or Subgroup	High-dose Events Total		Low-dose or non-statin Events	Total	Weight	Risk Ratio M-H, Fixed, 95% CI	Risk Ratio M-H, Fixed, 95% CI
1.8.1 Jadad>3							
Anna Toso et al 2009	15	152	16	152	24.5%	0.94 [0.48, 1.83]	
Patti G 2011	6	120	16	121	24.4%	0.38 [0.15, 0.93]	
Sang-Ho Jo et al 2008	3	118	4	118	6.1%	0.75 [0.17, 3.28]	
Subtotal (95% CI)		390		391	55.1%	0.67 [0.41, 1.10]	
Total events	24		36				
Heterogeneity: Chi² = 2.54, df = 2 (P = 0.28); I² = 21%							
Test for overall effect: Z = 1.59 (P = 0.11)							
1.8.2 Jadad⩽3							
Hakan Ozhan et al 2010	2	60	7	70	9.9%	0.33 [0.07, 1.54]	
Sadik Acikel et al 2010	0	80	1	80	2.3%	0.33 [0.01, 8.06]	
Xinwei 2009	6	113	18	115	27.3%	0.34 [0.14, 0.82]	
Zhou 2009	0	50	3	50	5.4%	0.14 [0.01, 2.70]	
Subtotal (95% CI)		303		315	44.9%	0.31 [0.15, 0.65]	
Total events	8		29				
Heterogeneity: Chi² = 0.31, df = 3 (P = 0.96); I² = 0%							
Test for overall effect: Z = 3.15 (P = 0.002)							
Total (95% CI)		693		706	100.0%	0.51 [0.34, 0.76]	
Total events	32		65				
Heterogeneity: Chi² = 5.78, df = 6 (P = 0.45); I² = 0%							
Test for overall effect: Z = 3.28 (P = 0.001)							

0.01   0.1   1   10   100
Favours experimental   Favours control

Figure 7. Forest plot of risk ratios and 95% confidence intervals (CI) for the incidence of CIN among patients assigned to statin therapy versus control according to Jadad score.

oral N-acetylcysteine (600 mg or 1200 mg) twice daily in both arms, started the day before the procedure. Allocation concealment and blinding were used in three studies [17–19] and the quality characteristics of the studies were shown in table 3.

Effects of statin treatment on clinical outcomes

The overall results based on fixed-effect model showed that the use of short-term high-dose statin treatment was associated with a significant reduction in risk of CIN (RR = 0.51, 95% CI 0.34–0.76, p = 0.001; I^2 = 0%; Figure 2). The incidence of acute renal failure requiring dialysis was very low and was not significant different after the use of statin (3 studies [17–19], RR = 0.33, 95% CI 0.05–2.10, p = 0.24; I^2 = 0%).

In-hospital mortality was observed in only one patient who died from acute heart failure aggravated by major bleeding in these seven studies [18]. Although the study carried out by Zhou Xia et al [22] reported incidence of cardiovascular event in short-term high-dose treatment group (5/50) and low-dose group (2/50), it didn't give any details. The total length of hospital stay were reported only in two studies. There was no difference between statin-treated group and control group in length of hospital stay in the study [17] by Jo SH et al. However, length of stay after intervention was shorter in patients randomized to atorvastatin (2.9±0.9 vs 3.2±0.8 days, P = 0.007) in the other study [19].

Figure 3 demonstrates that there was no evidence to suggest publication bias according to the relative symmetry in the Begg funnel plot.

Postprocedural changes in C-reactive protein (CRP) levels were analyzed in three trials [17,19,21]. The use of statin was not associated with a significant decrease in the plasma CRP level (SMD −0.64, 95% CI: −1.57 to 0.29, P = 0.18, I^2 = 97%).

Subgroup analysis

Classified according to low-dose statin-treated or not in control group, studies [16–20] comparing short-term high-dose statin treatment with non-statin treatment showed a significant protective trend toward decreased incidence of CIN (RR = 0.61, 95%CI 0.38–0.97, P = 0.04; Figure 4) and the same effect was seen in other two studies [21,22] which compared short-term high-dose with low-dose statin treament (RR = 0.31, 95%CI 0.13–0.72, P = 0.006).

In all five studies in which statin was compared with control without the addition of NAC, the risk of CIN was significantly decreased (RR = 0.38, 95%CI 0.22–0.65, P = 0.0006; Figure 5). In contrast, the risk of CIN did not significantly differ in the two studies in which statin plus NAC versus NAC only (RR = 0.76, 95%CI 0.42–1.39, P = 0.38).

In studies that included patients without renal impairment at baseline (creatinine clearance rate or estimated glomerular filtration rate>60 ml/min), RR was 0.29 (95%CI 0.15–0.57, P = 0.0003; Figure 6). A reduced risk of CIN was not found in studies that included patients with pre-existing renal impairment (creatinine clearance rate ≤60 ml/min). RR for CIN associated with the use of statin was 0.79 (95%CI 0.47–1.32, P = 0.37).

Classified according to the Jadad score >3 or not, studies whose Jadad score≤3 showed a significant reduction of CIN (RR = 0.31, 95%CI 0.15–0.65, P = 0.002; Figure 7). However, the risk of CIN did not significantly differ in the studies whose Jadad score>3 (RR = 0.67, 95%CI 0.41–1.10, P = 0.11).

Discussion

In the past two decades, although hydration has been well recognized and widely performed to prevent the CIN, the incidence of CIN did not decrease. So the efficacy of many other interventions are still under testing. From 2004 to 2011, a few studies focused on using statin as a specific prophylactic measure of CIN prevention have been published. In this meta-analysis of 7 randomized controlled trials (RCTs), we found that statin could significantly reduce the risk of CIN without decreasing the incidence of death or need for dialysis. However, there was marked clinical heterogeneity among these studies, indicating the need for a large definitive RCT.

In addition to their intended impact on blood cholesterol levels, statins have been found to have multiple nonlipid-lowering effects, which include enhancement of endothelial nitric oxide production [9–11], anti-inflammatory and antioxidative actions [12,13]. Given their pleiotropic effects, statins could decrease acute renal injury after iodinated contrast administration through two major pathways. Firstly, statins may modulate the kidney hypoperfusion after contrast administration by downregulation of angiotensin receptors and decreased synthesis of endothelin-1 [26,27]. Secondly, toxic damage on the tubular cells by oxygen-free radicals and proinflammatory cytokines may be decreased by anti-inflammatory effects of statins that inhibit tissue factor expression by macrophages and prevent the activation of nuclear factor-κB [28]. Moreover, its nonlipid-lowering effect could be demonstrated within a few hours after statin therapy initiation [29,30]. Although many clinical trials [31,32] have shown that high-dose statins provide more clinical benefits, such as atorvastatin 80 mg can further reduce vascular risks compared with low-dose statin therapy, the threshold of statins to reduce the risks of CIN remains unknown. In this meta-analysis, all of the included trials were short-term high-dose statin therapy, two of which compared two different doses of statin in preventing CIN. We found that high-dose statin therapy significantly lowered the incident of CIN compared with low-dose statin therapy. These results were consistent with the previous studies that high-dose statin has been shown to be more potent to suppress platelet activity and inflammatory chemokines than low-dose statin therapy [33].

The results of this meta-analysis are not in line with research from Zhang T et al [34], Zhang L et al [35] and Pappy R et al [36] which showed non-statistically significant reduction in the incidence of CIN with statin treatment from the pooled estimate for the randomized trials. In fact, Zhang T et al [34] and Pappy R et al [36] included both randomized and non-randomized trials in their meta-analysis, while the latter might lead to potential bias because it was impossible to completely remove interference of unknown confounding factors. The meta-analysis by Zhang L et al [35] involved only 4 RCTs, which included an abstract that overlapped with participants included in a separate study by the same author. Therefore, to avoid including any individual participant more than once, abstract by the same author was excluded in our meta-analysis [37]. Moreover, all of above three meta-analysis did not include two large scale studies [19,20] published in recent days.

Although the main conclusion in our meta-analysis was similar to that in the recent meta-analysis [38,39], these similar results shall be treated with cautious interpretation. First, in our meta-analysis, we found that statin was able to prevent CIN only in studies with lower quality, especially those which did not use of blinding, but not effective in high quality studies. This indicated that the results from the meta-analysis could not definite the effects of statins in preventing CIN. Second, pre-existing renal dysfunction was known to be an independent predictor of CIN that occured in up to 15% of patients with chronic kidney disease (CKD). However, subgroup analysis in risk group for CIN also weakened our findings. The studies that included patients with pre-existing renal dysfunction found no preventive effect of statins. Multiple nonreversible pathogenetic mechanisms involved in advanced renal failure may attenuate the response for statins, especially for their vasodilatation and anti-inflammatory effects. In addition, although a higher serum level was expected in CKD patients, local drug concentration still might be compromised due to renal scar and structural impairment. So the safety, pharmacokinetics and permeability of various statins in CKD patients should be well evaluated in future studies. Third, N-acetylcysteine, a thiol-containing antioxidant, was a promising agent to prevent contrast induced nephropathy because of its antioxidative and haemodynamic effects in the renal medulla and its general organ-protective effects described in several ischaemia-reperfusion models [40]. In the subgroup analysis of statin plus NAC versus NAC only, the difference were not significant. This could be attributed to that statin and NAC might decrease CIN occurrence through the similar pathways, such as scavenging oxygen free radicals produced after contrast exposure; therefore, the second agent could not exert addictive renal protection if NAC offered full protection available through antioxidants.

There are several potential limitations in this meta-analysis. Firstly, although all included studies reported the incidence of CIN, few trials designed to investigate the effect of statins on hard clinical outcomes such as acute renal failure requiring dialysis, length of hospital stay and in-hospital mortality. Secondly, we did not have access to patient-level data to determine whether the risk factors (eg, diabetes and age) could influence the effect of short-term high-dose statin treatment on the risk of contrast-induced nephropathy. Finally, studies included in this meta-analysis

analyzed the efficacy of statin with different type of statins for varied periods of time. It is possible that dose, duration and type of statin may have differential effect in prevention of CIN. An accepted uniform statin protocol would be helpful in both the clinical and research arenas.

In conclusion, although this meta-analysis supports the use of statin to reduce the incidence of CIN, this result must be considered in the context of variable patient demographics. Only a limited recommendation can be made in favour of the use of statin based on current data. Considering the limitations of included studies, a large, well designed trial that incorporates the evaluation of clinically relevant outcomes in participants with different underlying risks of CIN is required to more adequately assess the role for statin in CIN prevention.

Acknowledgments

We thank Acikel Sadik who provided additional data to conduct this analysis and Shijian Liu for his kind help with statistical methods.

Author Contributions

Conceived and designed the experiments: BD CLM. Performed the experiments: YCL YWL LLF. Analyzed the data: YCL YWL BD. Wrote the paper: YCL YWL BD CLM.

References

1. Nash K, Hafeez A, Hou S (2002) Hospital-acquired renal insufficiency. Am J Kidney Dis 39(5): 930–6.
2. Gruberg L, Mehran R, Dangas G, Mintz GS, Waksman R, et al. (2001) Acute renal failure requiring dialysis after percutaneous coronary interventions. Catheter Cardiovasc Interv 52(4): 409–16.
3. McCullough PA, Wolyn R, Rocher LL, Levin RN, O'Neill WW (1997) Acute renal failure after coronary intervention: incidence, risk factors, and relationship to mortality. Am J Med 103(5): 368–75.
4. Tepel M, Aspelin P, Lameire N (2006) Contrast-induced nephropathy: a clinical and evidence-based approach. Circulation 113(14): 1799–806.
5. McCullough PA (2008) Multimodality prevention of contrast-induced acute kidney injury. Am J Kidney Dis 51(2): 169–72.
6. Katholi RE, Woods WT Jr., Taylor GJ, Deitrick CL, Womack KA, et al. (1998) Oxygen free radicals and contrast nephropathy. Am J Kidney Dis 32(1): 64–71.
7. Goldenberg I, Matetzky S (2005) Nephropathy induced by contrast media: pathogenesis, risk factors and preventive strategies. CMAJ 172(11): 1461–71.
8. Tumlin J, Stacul F, Adam A, Becker CR, Davidson C, et al. (2006) Pathophysiology of contrast-induced nephropathy. Am J Cardiol 98(6A): 14K–20K.
9. John S, Schneider MP, Delles C, Jacobi J, Schmieder RE (2005) Lipid-independent effects of statins on endothelial function and bioavailability of nitric oxide in hypercholesterolemic patients. Am Heart J 149(3): 473.
10. Kaesemeyer WH, Caldwell RB, Huang J, Caldwell RW (1999) Pravastatin sodium activates endothelial nitric oxide synthase independent of its cholesterol-lowering actions. J Am Coll Cardiol 33(1): 234–41.
11. Laufs U, Liao JK (1998) Post-transcriptional regulation of endothelial nitric oxide synthase mRNA stability by Rho GTPase. J Biol Chem 273(37): 24266–71.
12. Ridker PM, Rifai N, Clearfield M, Downs JR, Weis SE, et al. (2001) Measurement of C-reactive protein for the targeting of statin therapy in the primary prevention of acute coronary events. N Engl J Med 344(26): 1959–65.
13. Wagner AH, Kohler T, Ruckschloss U, Just I, Hecker M (2000) Improvement of nitric oxide-dependent vasodilatation by HMG-CoA reductase inhibitors through attenuation of endothelial superoxide anion formation. Arterioscler Thromb Vasc Biol 20(1): 61–9.
14. Attallah N, Yassine L, Musial J, Yee J, Fisher K (2004) The potential role of statins in contrast nephropathy. Clin Nephrol 62(4): 273–8.
15. Khanal S, Attallah N, Smith DE, Kline-Rogers E, Share D, et al. (2005) Statin therapy reduces contrast-induced nephropathy: an analysis of contemporary percutaneous interventions. Am J Med 118(8): 843–9.
16. Ozhan H, Erden I, Ordu S, Aydin M, Caglar O, et al. (2010) Efficacy of short-term high-dose atorvastatin for prevention of contrast-induced nephropathy in patients undergoing coronary angiography. Angiology 61(7): 711–4.
17. Jo SH, Koo BK, Park JS, Kang HJ, Cho YS, et al. (2008) Prevention of radiocontrast medium-induced nephropathy using short-term high-dose simvastatin in patients with renal insufficiency undergoing coronary angiography (PROMISS) trial–a randomized controlled study. Am Heart J 155(3): 499.e1–8.
18. Toso A, Maioli M, Leoncini M, Gallopin M, Tedeschi D, et al. (2010) Usefulness of atorvastatin (80 mg) in prevention of contrast-induced nephropathy in patients with chronic renal disease. Am J Cardiol 105(3): 288–92.
19. Patti G, Ricottini E, Nusca A, Colonna G, Pasceri V, et al. (2011) Short-Term, High-Dose Atorvastatin Pretreatment to Prevent Contrast-Induced Nephropathy in Patients With Acute Coronary Syndromes Undergoing Percutaneous Coronary Intervention (from the ARMYDA-CIN [Atorvastatin for Reduction of MYocardial Damage during Angioplasty-Contrast-Induced Nephropathy] Trial. Am J Cardiol 108(1): 1–7.
20. Acikel S, Muderrisoglu H, Yildirir A, Aydinalp A, Sade E, et al. (2010) Prevention of contrast-induced impairment of renal function by short-term or long-term statin therapy in patients undergoing elective coronary angiography. Blood Coagul Fibrinolysis 21(8): 750–7.
21. Xinwei J, Xianghua F, Jing Z, Xinshun G, Ling X, et al. (2009) Comparison of usefulness of simvastatin 20 mg versus 80 mg in preventing contrast-induced nephropathy in patients with acute coronary syndrome undergoing percutaneous coronary intervention. Am J Cardiol 104(4): 519–24.
22. Zhou X, Jin YZ, Wang Q, Min R, Zhang XY (2009) Efficacy of high dose atorvastatin on preventing contrast induced nephropathy in patients underwent coronary angiography. Zhonghua Xin Xue Guan Bing Za Zhi 37(5): 394–6.
23. Verhagen AP, de Vet HC, de Bie RA, Kessels AG, Boers M, et al. (1998) The Delphi list: a criteria list for quality assessment of randomized clinical trials for conducting systematic reviews developed by Delphi consensus. J Clin Epidemiol 51(12): 1235–41.
24. Jadad AR, Moore RA, Carroll D, Jenkinson C, Reynolds DJ, et al. (1996) Assessing the quality of reports of randomized clinical trials: is blinding necessary. Control Clin Trials 17(1): 1–12.
25. Begg CB, Mazumdar M (1994) Operating characteristics of a rank correlation test for publication bias. Biometrics 50(4): 1088–101.
26. Ichiki T, Takeda K, Tokunou T, Iino N, Egashira K, et al. (2001) Downregulation of angiotensin II type 1 receptor by hydrophobic 3-hydroxy-3-methylglutaryl coenzyme A reductase inhibitors in vascular smooth muscle cells. Arterioscler Thromb Vasc Biol 21(12): 1896–901.
27. Hernandez-Perera O, Perez-Sala D, Navarro-Antolin J, Sánchez-Pascuala R, Hernández G, et al. (1998) Effects of the 3-hydroxy-3-methylglutaryl-CoA

reductase inhibitors, atorvastatin and simvastatin, on the expression of endothelin-1 and endothelial nitric oxide synthase in vascular endothelial cells. J Clin Invest 101(12): 2711–9.

28. Bonetti PO, Lerman LO, Napoli C, Lerman A (2003) Statin effects beyond lipid lowering–are they clinically relevant. Eur Heart J 24(3): 225–48.

29. Davignon J (2004) Beneficial cardiovascular pleiotropic effects of statins. Circulation 109(23 Suppl 1): III39–43.

30. Morikawa S, Takabe W, Mataki C, Kanke T, Itoh T, et al. (2002) The effect of statins on mRNA levels of genes related to inflammation, coagulation, and vascular constriction in HUVEC. Human umbilical vein endothelial cells. J Atheroscler Thromb 9(4): 178–83.

31. Cannon CP, Braunwald E, McCabe CH, Rader DJ, Rouleau JL, et al. (2004) Intensive versus moderate lipid lowering with statins after acute coronary syndromes. N Engl J Med 350(15): 1495–504.

32. LaRosa JC, Grundy SM, Waters DD, Shear C, Barter P, et al. (2005) Intensive lipid lowering with atorvastatin in patients with stable coronary disease. N Engl J Med 352(14): 1425–35.

33. Piorkowski M, Fischer S, Stellbaum C, Jaster M, Martus P, et al. (2007) Treatment with ezetimibe plus low-dose atorvastatin compared with higher-dose atorvastatin alone: is sufficient cholesterol-lowering enough to inhibit platelets. J Am Coll Cardiol 49(10): 1035–42.

34. Zhang T, Shen LH, Hu LH, He B (2011) Statins for the prevention of contrast-induced nephropathy: a systematic review and meta-analysis. Am J Nephrol 33(4): 344–51.

35. Zhang L, Zhang L, Lu Y, Wu B, Zhang S, et at (2011) Efficacy of statin pretreatment for the prevention of contrast-induced nephropathy: a meta-analysis of randomised controlled trials. Int J Clin Pract 65(5): 624–30.

36. Pappy R, Stavrakis S, Hennebry TA, Abu-Fadel MS (2011) Effect of statin therapy on contrast-induced nephropathy after coronary angiography: A meta-analysis. Int J Cardiol 151(3): 348–53.

37. SH Jo, BK Koo, TJ Youn, JY Hahn, YS Kim, et al. (2005) Prevention of contrast induced nephropathy by short-term statin in patients with renal insufficiency undergoing coronary angiography: a randomized controlled trial. Am J Cardiol 96(3): 115H–6H.

38. Zhang BC, Li WM, Xu YW (2011) High-Dose Statin Pretreatment for the Prevention of Contrast-Induced Nephropathy: A Meta-analysis. Can J Cardiol 27(6): 851–8.

39. Zhou Y, Yuan WJ, Zhu N, Wang L (2011) Short-term, high-dose statins in the prevention of contrast-induced nephropathy: a systematic review and meta-analysis. Clin Nephrol 76(6): 475–83.

40. Tepel M, Zidek W (2002) Acetylcysteine and contrast media nephropathy. Curr Opin Nephrol Hypertens 11(5): 503–6.

18

Scoring Systems for Predicting Mortality after Liver Transplantation

Heng-Chih Pan[1], Chang-Chyi Jenq[1,4], Wei-Chen Lee[3,4]*, Ming-Hung Tsai[2,4], Pei-Chun Fan[1], Chih-Hsiang Chang[1], Ming-Yang Chang[1,4], Ya-Chung Tian[1,4], Cheng-Chieh Hung[1,4], Ji-Tseng Fang[1,4], Chih-Wei Yang[1,4], Yung-Chang Chen[1,4]*

1 Kidney Research Center, Department of Nephrology, Chang Gung Memorial Hospital, Taipei, Taiwan, 2 Division of Gastroenterology, Chang Gung Memorial Hospital, Taipei, Taiwan, 3 Laboratory of Immunology, Department of General Surgery, Chang Gung Memorial Hospital, Taipei, Taiwan, 4 Chang Gung University College of Medicine, Taoyuan, Taiwan

Abstract

Background: Liver transplantation can prolong survival in patients with end-stage liver disease. We have proposed that the Sequential Organ Failure Assessment (SOFA) score calculated on post-transplant day 7 has a great discriminative power for predicting 1-year mortality after liver transplantation. The Chronic Liver Failure - Sequential Organ Failure Assessment (CLIF-SOFA) score, a modified SOFA score, is a newly developed scoring system exclusively for patients with end-stage liver disease. This study was designed to compare the CLIF-SOFA score with other main scoring systems in outcome prediction for liver transplant patients.

Methods: We retrospectively reviewed medical records of 323 patients who had received liver transplants in a tertiary care university hospital from October 2002 to December 2010. Demographic parameters and clinical characteristic variables were recorded on the first day of admission before transplantation and on post-transplantation days 1, 3, 7, and 14.

Results: The overall 1-year survival rate was 78.3% (253/323). Liver diseases were mostly attributed to hepatitis B virus infection (34%). The CLIF-SOFA score had better discriminatory power than the Child-Pugh points, Model for End-Stage Liver Disease (MELD) score, RIFLE (risk of renal dysfunction, injury to the kidney, failure of the kidney, loss of kidney function, and end-stage kidney disease) criteria, and SOFA score. The AUROC curves were highest for CLIF-SOFA score on post-liver transplant day 7 for predicting 1-year mortality. The cumulative survival rates differed significantly for patients with a CLIF-SOFA score ≤8 and those with a CLIF-SOFA score >8 on post-liver transplant day 7.

Conclusion: The CLIF-SOFA score can increase the prediction accuracy of prognosis after transplantation. Moreover, the CLIF-SOFA score on post-transplantation day 7 had the best discriminative power for predicting 1-year mortality after liver transplantation.

Editor: Stanislaw Stepkowski, University of Toledo, United States of America

Funding: The authors have no support or funding to report.

Competing Interests: The authors have declared that no competing interests exist.

* Email: cyc2356@gmail.com (Y-CC); weichen@cgmh.org.tw (W-CL)

Introduction

Liver transplantation is a viable treatment option for patients with end-stage liver disease, hepatocellular carcinoma, and fulminant hepatitis. [1–7] Over the past several decades, the immunosuppression, surgical techniques, and experience in managing liver allograft recipients has gradually matured and the outcome of liver transplantation has greatly improved. [8] However, organ shortage has been a new challenge because of a greater treatment demand. The selection of an adequate transplant candidate is important and the decision-making process for allocation of restricted medical resources is complex and difficult. Clinicians and investigators have, therefore, been persistently looking for objective scoring systems capable of providing accurate information on disease severity and predicting post-transplant prognosis. Main scoring systems such as the Child-Pugh score, the model for end-stage liver disease (MELD) score, the RIFLE (risk of renal dysfunction, injury to the kidney, failure of the kidney, loss of kidney function, and end-stage kidney disease) criteria, and the sequential organ failure assessment (SOFA) score, have been applied to predict the outcome after liver transplant.

In our previous report, we had compared the above main scoring systems and documented that the SOFA score calculated on post-transplant day 7 had a greater discriminative power for predicting 3-month and 1-year mortality after liver transplantation. [9] However, the SOFA score was developed from a general ICU population rather than patients with end-stage liver disease. In 2009, a group of European investigators decided to create the Chronic Liver Failure (CLIF) consortium, which was dedicated to

Table 1. The sequential organ failure assessment (SOFA) and chronic liver failure (CLIF)-SOFA scores.

SOFA Score	0	1	2	3	4
Respiration					
PaO2/FiO2	>400	>300–≤400	>200–≤300	>100–≤200 with ventilator	≤100 with ventilator
Coagulation					
Platelets, ×10³/mm³	>150	>100–≤150	>50–≤100	>20–≤50	≤20
Liver					
Bilirubin, mg/dL (μmol/L)	<1.2 (<20)	≥1.2–<2.0 (20–32)	≥2.0–<6.0 (33–101)	≥6.0–<12.0 (102–204)	≥12.0 (>204)
Cardiovascular					
Hypotension	MAP≥70 mm Hg	MAP<70 mm Hg	Dopamine ≤5 or dobutamine (any dose)*	Dopamine >5 or epi ≤0.1 or norepi ≤0.1*	Dopamine >15 or epi >0.1 or norepi >0.1*
CNS					
Glasgow Coma Score	15	13–14	10–12	6–9	<6
Renal					
Creatinine, mg/dL (μmol/L) or urine output	<1.2 (<110)	≥1.2–<2.0 (110–170)	≥2.0–<3.5 (171–299)	≥3.5–<5.0 (300–440) or <500 mL/day	≥5.0 (>440) or <200 mL/day

CLIF-SOFA Score	0	1	2	3	4
Respiration					
PaO2/FiO2 or Sp O2/FiO2	>400>512	>300–<400>357–≤512	>200–≤300>214–≤357	>100–≤200>89–≤214	≤100≤89
Coagulation					
INR	<1.1 Same as SOFA	≥1.1–<1.25	≥1.25–<1.5	≥1.5–<2.5	≥2.5 or platelet ≤20
Liver					
Cardiovascular					
Hypotension	MAP≥70 mm Hg	MAP<70 mm Hg	Dopamine ≤5 or dobutamine (any dose)* or terlipressin	Dopamine >5 or epi ≤0.1 or norepi ≤0.1*	Dopamine >15 or epi >0.1 or norepi >0.1*
CNS					
HE grade	No HE	I	II	III	IV
Renal					
Creatinine, mg/dL	<1.2	≥1.2–<2.0	≥2.0–<3.5	≥3.5–<5.0 or use of RRT	≥5.0

CLIF-C OF Score	1	2	3
Respiration			
PaO2/FiO2 or SpO2/FiO2	>300>357	>200–≤300>214–≤357	≤200**≤214**
Coagulation			
INR	<2.0	≥2.0–<2.5	≥2.5
Liver			
Bilirubin, mg/dL	<6.0	≥6.0–<12.0	≥12.0

Table 1. Cont.

SOFA Score	0	1	2	3	4
Cardiovascular					
Hypotension		MAP≥70 mm Hg	MAP<70 mm Hg	Use of vasopressors	
CNS					
HE grade		No HE	I–II	III–IV	
Renal					
Creatinine, mg/dL		<2.0	≥2.0–<3.5	≥3.5 or use of RRT	

*Abbreviations: CNS, central nervous system; CLIF-C OF: chronic liver failure-consortium organ failure; CLIF-SOFA: chronic liver failure - sequential organ failure assessment; epi, epinephrine; FiO2, fractional inspired oxygen; HE, hepatic encephalopathy; INR, international normalized ratio; MAP, mean arterial pressure; norepi, norepinephrine; PaO2, arterial oxygen tension; RRT, renal replacement therapy; SOFA: sequential organ failure assessment; SpO2, pulse oximetric saturation.

the study of the complication of cirrhosis. The investigators used a modified SOFA score for diagnosis of organ failure, the so-called CLIF-SOFA score. Like the original SOFA score, the CLIF-SOFA score assessed the six organ systems, but it also took into account some specificities of end-stage liver disease (Table 1). [10] The purpose of this investigation was to compare the efficacy of the newly developed CLIF-SOFA score with that of commonly used scoring systems in predicting prognosis after liver transplantation.

Materials and Methods

Ethics statement

The protocol for this clinical study was designed in full compliance with the ethical principles of the Declaration of Helsinki and was consistent with Good Clinical Practice guidelines and with applicable local regulatory requirements. Because this study examined only preexisting data, written informed consent was not obtained from each patient. In its place, we informed patients of their right to refuse enrolment via telephone interview. These procedures for informed consent and enrolment are in accordance with the detailed regulations regarding informed consent described in the guidelines. This study, including the procedure for enrolment, was approved by the Institutional Review Board of Chang Gung Memorial Hospital.

Patient information and data collection

This study was conducted between October 2002 and December 2010 in a 2000-bed tertiary care referral hospital in Taiwan. In this study, we included 323 consecutive patients with end-stage liver disease patients who had undergone liver transplantation. We excluded pediatric patients and patients who had previously undergone liver transplantation.

The following data were collected retrospectively: demographic data, etiologies of liver disease, clinical variables, donor type, intraoperative blood loss, anesthesia time, length of ICU stay and hospitalization, and outcome. The Child-Pugh points, MELD score, SOFA score, and RIFLE criteria were used to assess illness severity on the first day of admission before transplantation and on post-transplantation days 1, 3, 7 and 14. The primary study outcomes were 1-year mortality rates after liver transplantation. Follow-up at 1 year after transplantation was performed via telephone interview or by analyzing the chart records.

Definitions

The severity of the liver disease on admission to the ICU was determined by using the Child–Pugh points and the MELD scoring systems. The MELD score was calculated with the following formula: [11].

$$\text{MELD score} = (0.957 \ln[\text{creatinine}] + 0.378 \ln[\text{bilirubin}] + 1.120 \ln[\text{international normalized ratio of prothrombin}] + 0.643) \times 10.$$

Severity of the illness can also be assessed by using the SOFA score, the CLIF-SOFA score, and the CLIF-C OF score (the CLIF-Consortium Organ Failure score, a simplified version of the CLIF-SOFA Score) based on 6 organ systems [12] (Table 1). The worst physiological and biochemical values determined on the first day of ICU admission were recorded. The RIFLE criteria were also used to group patients according to risk, injury, and failure. [13] No patient met the criteria for loss or end-stage renal disease. The following simple model for mortality was constructed: non–acute renal failure (0 points), RIFLE-R (1 point), RIFLE-I (2 points), and RIFLE-F (3 points) [14].

Table 2. Patient demographic data and clinical Characteristics according to In-hospital mortality.

	All patients (n = 323)	Survivors (n = 281)	Non-survivors (n = 42)	P-value
Age (years)	51 ± 10	51 ± 10	50 ± 14	NS (0.187)
Gender (M/F) (%)	231(72)/92(28)	199(71)/82(29)	32(76)/10(24)	NS (0.583)
BMI (kg/m²)	24.3 ± 4.0	24.7 ± 4.0	21.1 ± 2.4	<0.001
Diabetes mellitus (yes/no) (%)	55(17)/268(83)	46(16)/235(84)	9(21)/33(79)	NS (0.387)
Chronic kidney disease (yes/no) (%)	31(10)/292(90)	22(8)/259(92)	9(21)/33(79)	0.005
Proteinuira on admission (yes/no (%))	45(14)/278(86)	31(11)/250(89)	14(33)/28(67)	<0.001
Variceal bleeding on admission (yes/no) (%)	62(19)/261(81)	50(18)/231(82)	12(29)/30(71)	NS (0.613)
Hemoglobin on admission (g/dL)	10.6 ± 2	10.7 ± 2	9.8 ± 2	0.008
Leukocytes on admission (×10⁹/L)	2.9 ± 3.7	2.8 ± 3.5	3.3 ± 4.9	NS (0.569)
Platelets on admission (×10⁹/L)	73 ± 46	73 ± 46	71 ± 45	NS (0.809)
Prothrombin time INR on admission	1.8 ± 0.7	1.8 ± 0.7	1.9 ± 0.7	NS (0.050)
Serum sodium on admission (mmol/L)	142 ± 69	142 ± 74	137 ± 8	NS (0.650)
AST on admission (U/L)	89 ± 94	87 ± 79	98 ± 168	NS (0.498)
ALT on admission (U/L)	67 ± 120	67 ± 121	66 ± 118	NS (0.938)
Total bilirubin on admission (mg/dL)	8.5 ± 11.9	7.6 ± 10.8	14.3 ± 16.5	0.003
Lactate on admission (mmol/L)	2.1 ± 0.8	1.5 ± 0.8	2.9 ± 0.9	NS (0.064)
A-a gradient on admission	251 ± 413	233 ± 407	316 ± 430	0.039
Urea on admission (mmol/L)	8.3 ± 10.3	7.8 ± 10.7	10.1 ± 8.82	0.007
Serum creatinine on admission (mg/dL)	1.1 ± 1.0	1.1 ± 1.0	1.3 ± 1.1	NS (0.064)
MAP on admission (mmHg)	86 ± 12	86 ± 13	85 ± 10	NS (0.427)
Child-Pugh points on admission	10 ± 3	10 ± 3	11 ± 2	0.010
MELD score on admission	17 ± 10	17 ± 10	21 ± 10	0.025
RIFLE on admission (No AKI/Risk/Injury/Failure)	286/16/9/12	250/13/9/9	36/3/0/3	NS (0.449)
SOFA on admission	5 ± 3	5 ± 2	7 ± 3	0.001
CLIF-SOFA on admission	6 ± 3	5 ± 3	8 ± 4	0.001
Anesthesia time (hours)	12 ± 2	12 ± 2	12 ± 2	NS (0.362)
Donor type (deceased/splint/living)	51/40/232	42/32/207	9/8/25	NS (0.091)
Length of ICU stay (days)	21 ± 23	19 ± 22	34 ± 27	0.002
Length of hospital stay (days)	48 ± 32	47 ± 30	55 ± 39	NS (0.215)
Graft-to-recipient weight ratio (%)	1.04 ± 0.30	1.03 ± 0.26	1.10 ± 0.44	NS (0.125)
Blood loss volume (ml)	3034 ± 3731	2672 ± 3057	4430 ± 5431	0.014
Reimplantation time	42 ± 11	42 ± 11	43 ± 11	NS (0.801)

*Abbreviations: INR, international normalized ratio; AST: aspartate aminotransferase; ALT: alanine aminotransferase; MAP, mean arterial pressure; MELD: model for end-stage liver disease; SOFA: sequential organ failure assessment; CLIF-SOFA: chronic liver failure - sequential organ failure assessment; RIFLE: the risk of renal failure, injury to the kidney, Failure of kidney function, loss of kidney function, and end-stage renal failure; ICU: intensive care unit.

Statistical analysis

Continuous variables were summarized with means and standard derivations unless otherwise stated. All variables were tested for normal distribution with the Kolmogorov–Smirnov test. Student's t-test was employed to compare the means of continuous variables and normally distributed data; otherwise, the Mann–Whitney U test was employed. Categorical data were tested using the chi-square test. Cumulative survival curves as a function of time were constructed with the Kaplan-Meier approach and compared with the log rank test.

Calibration was assessed by the Hosmer–Lemeshow goodness-of-fit test (C statistic) to compare the number of observed and predicted deaths in risk groups for the entire range of death probabilities. Discrimination was examined using the area under the receiver operating characteristic curve (AUROC). An AUROC close to 0.5 indicates that the model performance approximates that of flipping a coin. However, the model nears 100% sensitivity and specificity despite any cutoff point as the area nears 1.0. To compare the areas under the two resulting AUROC curves we used a nonparametric approach. AUROC analysis was also performed to calculate the sensitivity, specificity, and overall correctness of the Child–Pugh points, the MELD score, the RIFLE classification, the SOFA score, and the CLIF-SOFA score. Finally, cutoff points were calculated by obtaining the best Youden index (sensitivity + specificity − 1). [15] The scores calculated at pre-OP, post-OP Day1, Day3, and Day7 were compared between 1-year survival and mortality groups by repeated-measurement analysis of variance (ANOVA) using the general linear model

Table 3. Primary liver disease.

Primary liver disease	All patients (n = 323)
Alcoholic, n (%)	47 (14)
Hepatitis B, n (%)	200 (62)
Hepatitis C, n (%)	84 (26)
Hepatoma, n (%)	88 (27)
Single etiology	
Alcoholic, n (%)	16 (5)
Hepatitis B, n (%)	111 (34)
Hepatitis C, n (%)	31 (10)
Hepatoma, n (%)	3 (1)
Multiple etiologies	
Alcoholic + hepatitis B, n (%)	21 (6)
Alcoholic + hepatitis C, n (%)	5 (2)
Alcoholic + hepatoma, n (%)	3 (1)
Hepatitis B + hepatitis C, n (%)	17 (5)
Hepatitis B + hepatoma, n (%)	49 (15)
Hepatitis C + hepatoma, n (%)	31 (10)
Alcoholic + hepatitis B + hepatoma	2 (1)
Other causes, n (%)*	34 (10)
Total (Single etiology + Multiple etiologies)	323(100)

*Biliary cirrhosis, biliary sclerosis, autoimmune hepatitis, Wilson's disease, polycystic liver disease, drugs, and unknown causes.

procedure. All statistical tests were two-tailed and a value of $P < 0.05$ was considered statistically significant. Data were analyzed with the statistical package SPSS 12.0 for Windows 95 (SPSS, Inc., Chicago, IL, USA).

Results

Patient characteristics

We enrolled 323 patients who underwent liver transplantation between October 2002 and December 2010. The overall 3-month and 1-year survival rates were 86.4% (279/323) and 78.3% (253/323), respectively. Patient data and clinical characteristics of survivors and non-survivors according to in-hospital mortality are listed in Table 2. The median age of the patients was 51 years; 231 patients were men (71%) and 92 were women (29%). The median length of ICU stay was 21 days.

The pre-transplant Child-Pugh points, MELD, SOFA, and CLIF-SOFA scores were statistically significant predictors of in-hospital mortality; the pre-transplant.

RIFLE criteria was not. Fifty-one patients (15.8%) received deceased-donor grafts; there was no significant difference in the age or gender between the survivors and non-survivors. The primary liver diseases are listed in Table 3. In this study, hepatitis B virus infection was observed to be the cause of liver diseases in most of the patients

Calibration, Discrimination, and Severity of the Illness Scoring Systems

We have listed the results of goodness-of-fit as measured by the Hosmer-Lemeshow chi-square statistic denoting the predicted mortality risk, the predictive accuracy of the Child-Pugh points, MELD score, RIFLE criteria, SOFA score, and CLIF-SOFA

score in predicting 1-year mortality in Table 4. The comparison between discriminatory values of the 5 scoring systems has also been included in Table 4. Based on the analysis of the AUROC curves, the discriminatory power of the CLIF-SOFA score was excellent. The AUROC curves of the CLIF-SOFA score calculated on post-transplant day 1, 3, 7, and 14 were significantly superior to those of the Child-Pugh points and RIFLE criteria. Moreover, the AUROC curves of the CLIF-SOFA score calculated on post-transplant day 1 and 7 were significantly superior to those of the MELD and SOFA score. The AUROC curves were highest for the CLIF-SOFA score on post-liver transplant day 7 for predicting 1-year mortality (0.877±0.033).

Indices for predicting short-term prognosis

To assess the validity of the scoring methods, we tested the sensitivity, specificity, and overall correctness of prediction at cut-off points that provided the best Youden index (Table 5). On post-liver transplant day 7, the Youden index and overall correctness for predicting 1-year mortality were higher for the CLIF-SOFA score than those for the Child-Pugh points, MELD score, RIFLE criteria, and SOFA score. Figure 1 illustrates that the cumulative survival rates differed significantly for patients with a CLIF-SOFA score ≤8 and for those with a CLIF-SOFA score >8 on post-liver transplant day 7. Figure 2 shows significant increases in the CLIF-SOFA scores between the periods for the 1-year mortality group but not for the 1-year survival group by repeated-measures analysis of variance.

Data not shown

Only the pre-transplant SOFA score and CLIF-SOFA score were statistically significant predictors of 1-year post-transplant

Table 4. Calibration and discrimination for the scoring methods used in predicting 1-year mortality.

	Calibration			Discrimination		
	Goodness-of-fit (x^2)	df	p	AUROC±SE	95% CI	P
On admission						
Child-Pugh points	13.626	7	0.058	0.576±0.046	0.506–0.687	0.060
MELD score	5.519	8	0.701	0.580±0.050	0.482–0.678	0.119
RIFLE				0.566±0.054	0.460–0.671	0.202
SOFA	3.586	5	0.610	0.618±0.054	0.512–0.724	0.022
CLIF-SOFA	2.542	6	0.864	0.635±0.053	0.531–0.739	0.009
CLIF-C OF	23.315	3	<0.001	0.669±0.039	0.592–0.745	<0.001
Postoperative day 1						
Child-Pugh points	4.400	5	0.493	0.629±0.045	0.541–0.718	0.012
MELD score	5.960	8	0.652	0.637±0.049	0.541–0.734	0.008
RIFLE	1.341	2	0.511	0.591±0.054	0.485–0.696	0.078
SOFA	5.359	7	0.616	0.706±0.050	0.608–0.804	<0.001
CLIF-SOFA	9.516	7	0.218	0.788±0.047	0.695–0.880	<0.001
CLIF-C OF	2.316	4	0.678	0.712±0.039	0.635–0.789	<0.001
Postoperative day 3						
Child-Pugh points	1.271	5	0.938	0.714±0.044	0.627–0.801	<0.001
MELD score	9.404	8	0.309	0.733±0.048	0.639–0.827	<0.001
RIFLE	1.297	1	0.255	0.638±0.054	0.531–0.745	0.007
SOFA	9.968	6	0.126	0.769±0.048	0.625–0.813	<0.001
CLIF-SOFA	10.692	7	0.153	0.808±0.041	0.729–0.888	<0.001
CLIF-C OF	4.217	4	0.377	0.820±0.035	0.752–0.888	<0.001
Postoperative day 7						
Child-Pugh points	6.751	4	0.150	0.726±0.051	0.585–0.786	<0.001
MELD score	10.011	8	0.264	0.758±0.046	0.667–0.849	<0.001
RIFLE	11.967	2	0.003	0.656±0.054	0.550–0.761	0.002
SOFA	1.001	6	0.986	0.813±0.040	0.734–0.892	<0.001
CLIF-SOFA	7.395	7	0.389	0.877±0.033	0.813–0.941	<0.001
CLIF-C OF	6.378	3	0.095	0.850±0.033	0.785–0.915	<0.001
Postoperative day 14						
Child-Pugh points	5.710	3	0.127	0.763±0.040	0.685–0.840	<0.001
MELD score	23.453	8	0.003	0.792±0.047	0.700–0.884	<0.001
RIFLE	5.957	2	0.051	0.625±0.053	0.521–0.730	0.015
SOFA	10.075	7	0.184	0.807±0.042	0.724–0.889	<0.001
CLIF-SOFA	15.193	7	0.034	0.853±0.033	0.788–0.918	<0.001
CLIF-C OF	1.266	3	0.737	0.815±0.038	0.740–0.889	<0.001

*Abbreviations: CLIF-C OF: chronic liver failure-consortium organ failure; CLIF-SOFA: chronic liver failure - sequential organ failure assessment; MELD: model for end-stage liver disease; RIFLE: the risk of renal failure, injury to the kidney, Failure of kidney function, loss of kidney function, and end-stage renal failure; SOFA: sequential organ failure assessment.

mortality; the pre-transplant Child-Pugh points, MELD score, and RIFLE criteria were not.

In the study population, 64 patients with CLIF-SOFA score >8 while 254 patients with CLIF-SOFA score ≤8 on day 7 post-transplantation. The patients with CLIF-SOFA score >8 on day 7 post-transplantation had higher rates of acute rejection (29.7% *vs.* 12.6%, $p = 0.002$), hospital death (51.6% *vs.* 15.0%, $p<0.001$) and 1-year mortality (75.0% *vs.* 7.5%, $p<0.001$) than those with CLIF-SOFA score ≤8 on day 7 post-transplantation.

Discussion

In this study, the overall 3-month and 1-year survival rates were 86.4% (279/323) and 78.3% (253/323), which is consistent with that reported previously. [9,16,17] We found that the SOFA score and CLIF-SOFA score on admission day were independent predictors of in-hospital mortality and 1-year mortality after liver transplantation (Table 2). Our results also show that the CLIF-SOFA score is a good scoring system for predicting patient outcome and that it has better discriminatory power than the Child-Pugh points, MELD score, RIFLE criteria, and SOFA

Table 5. Prediction of subsequent 1-year mortality.

Predictive factors	Cutoff point	Youden index	Sensitivity (%)	Specificity (%)	Overall correctness (%)
Child-Pugh points					
On admission	10	0.15	69	46	58
Postoperative day 1	10	0.25	92	34	63
Postoperative day 3	8	0.37	59	77	67
Postoperative day 7	8	0.37	51	85	68
Postoperative day 14	8	0.33	38	94	66
MELD score					
On admission	10	0.18	85	34	60
Postoperative day 1	22	0.25	85	40	63
Postoperative day 3	20	0.41	62	80	71
Postoperative day 7	20	0.43	59	84	72
Postoperative day 14	20	0.50	64	85	75
SOFA					
On admission	5	0.21	46	75	61
Postoperative day 1	9	0.37	69	68	69
Postoperative day 3	7	0.41	74	74	74
Postoperative day 7	7	0.53	67	82	75
Postoperative day 14	7	0.53	56	93	75
CLIF-SOFA					
On admission	5	0.23	59	64	62
Postoperative day 1	8	0.51	72	79	76
Postoperative day 3	8	0.54	67	87	77
Postoperative day 7	8	0.59	64	95	80
Postoperative day 14	8	0.58	67	88	78
CLIF-C OF					
On admission	6	0.35	76	59	68
Postoperative day 1	8	0.34	43	77	60
Postoperative day 3	8	0.56	78	82	80
Postoperative day 7	8	0.59	69	91	80
Postoperative day 14	8	0.53	76	78	77
RIFLE					
On admission	R category	0.13	23	90	57
Postoperative day 1	R category	0.16	36	80	58
Postoperative day 3	R category	0.24	31	94	63
Postoperative day 7	R category	0.28	46	82	64
Postoperative day 14	R category	0.22	46	76	61

*Abbreviations: CLIF-C OF: chronic liver failure-consortium organ failure; CLIF-SOFA: chronic liver failure - sequential organ failure assessment; MELD: model for end-stage liver disease; RIFLE: the risk of renal failure, injury to the kidney, Failure of kidney function, loss of kidney function, and end-stage renal failure; SOFA: sequential organ failure assessment.

scores (Table 4). Moreover, the CLIF-SOFA score had the best Youden index and the highest overall correctness of prediction (Table 5).

Several studies had tried to find the optimal prognostic scores for critically ill cirrhotic patients. Freire P *et al* showed that SOFA and MELD scores had better overall correctness than Child-Pugh score, APACHE II, and SAPS II scores in predicting ICU mortality [18]. Levesque E *et al* reported that SOFA and SAPS II scores predicted ICU mortality better than Child-Pugh score or MELD scores with or without the incorporation of serum sodium levels [19]. Our previous studies also showed the good discrim-

inative power and independent predictive value of the SOFA score in accurately predicting in-hospital mortality [6,20,21]. Since no extrahepatic parameters are included in the determination of the Child-Pugh points, and no liver-specific prognostic factors are included in the determination of the APACHE II score, their discriminative powers are significantly inferior to that of the SOFA score in predicting prognosis for critically ill cirrhotic patients. The prognosis of cirrhotic patients is grave and liver transplantation is the treatment of choice. Liver transplantation improves survival rate of patients with end-stage liver disease dramatically therefore

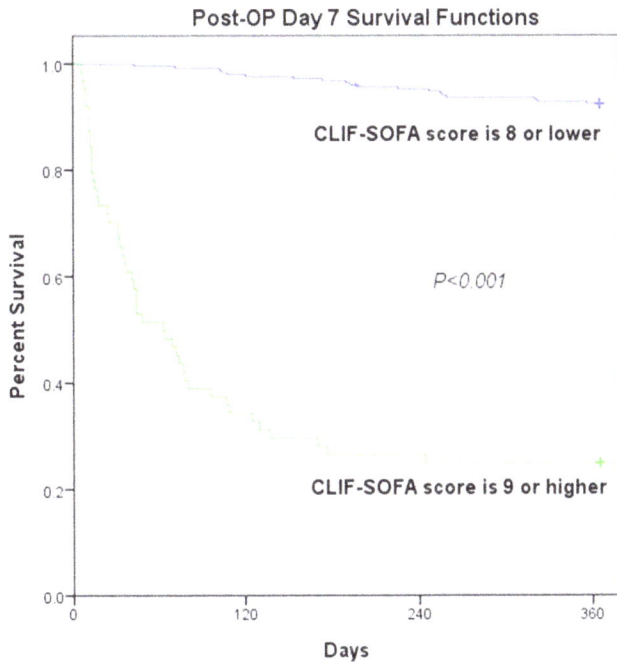

Figure 1. Cumulative survival rate for 323 liver transplant patients according to the CLIF-SOFA scores on day 7 after liver transplantation. *Abbreviations: CLIF-SOFA: chronic liver failure - sequential organ failure assessment.

impacts the capability of pre-transplant scoring systems in predicting short-term prognosis of post-transplant patients.

Theocharidou E *et al* had proposed the Royal Free Hospital (RFH) Score from a cohort of 635 critically ill cirrhotic patients, which included variceal bleeding, bilirubin, INR, lactate, A-a gradient and urea. The AUROC of the pre-transplant RFH score is 0.600 in predicting 1-year survival for liver transplantation

patients in this study, it is even inferior to that of the pre-transplant SOFA (AUROC = 0.618) and CLIF-SOFA (AUROC = 0.635) scores. Based on our clinical experience, we think the 6 parameters of the RFH score are good predictors in predicting short-term prognosis for patients with portal hypertension. However, liver transplantation dramatically turns the course of disease in decompensated cirrhotic patients and post-OP critical care is the key for post- transplant patient survival. Other mortality risk factors are technical problems (especially vascular and biliary anastomoses), rejection, primary graft failure, opportunistic infection, and drug reaction. CLIF-SOFA and SOFA scores could evaluate parameters related to 6 different important organ systems and provide a global assessment of the patient's clinical condition. It might explain the good prediction value of the CLIF-SOFA and SOFA scores. For lacking of CNS and CV parameters, the performance of RFH score is slightly inferior to that of the SOFA and CLIF-SOFA scores in predicting short-term prognosis for patients undergoing liver transplantation.

Similar to other general ICU scores, the SOFA score was developed for the general ICU population. Many studies have reported that the SOFA score could provide a complete representation of illness dynamics, and patients with a higher SOFA score are associated with a lower probability of receiving liver transplantation. [22,23] However, it is possible that some components of the SOFA score could be influenced by the nature of liver disease. For example, platelet counts are always reduced in cirrhotic patients due to hypersplenism, reduced production of thrombopoeitin, alcohol consumption, or antiviral treatment. [24,25] Relatedly, no association has been reported between low platelet level and outcome of cirrhotic patients. [24–26] The CLIF-SOFA score is a newly developed scoring system that is a modified version of the SOFA score (Table 1), and that is exclusively for patients with end-stage liver disease. It replaces platelet count with an international ratio of prothrombin time as the coagulation parameter, and replaces the Glasgow coma scale with hepatoencephalopathy as the CNS parameter. It also takes into account the usage of terlipressin and renal replacement

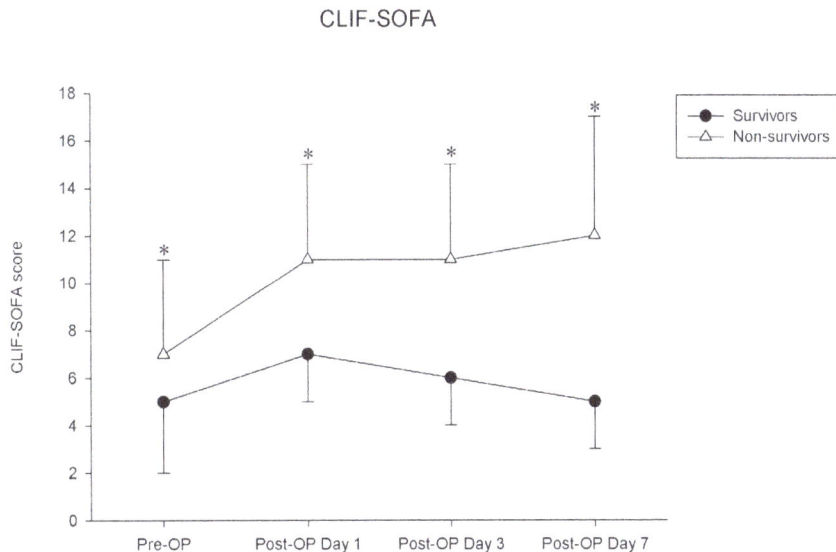

Figure 2. Estimated CLIF-SOFA scores (mean ± standard deviation) for the 1-year survivor group (alive, n = 253) and the 1-year non-survivor group (death, n = 70) during the preoperative period and on postoperative days 1, 3, and 7 (*P<0.05 for survivor group and non-survivor group). By repeated-measures analysis of variance, the CLIF-SOFA scores significantly increased between the period (before transplantation and on postoperative days 1, 3, and 7) in the 1-year non-survivor group but not in the 1-year survivor group. *Abbreviations: CLIF-SOFA: chronic liver failure - sequential organ failure assessment.

therapy in the grading of cardiovascular and renal parameters, respectively. Furthermore, the CLIF-SOFA score added SpO2/FiO2 as an alternative respiration parameter for patients without an A-line. All these modifications were set up especially targeting the disease nature and general treatment protocol of end-stage liver disease [10]. In this study, although both pre-transplant SOFA score and CLIF-SOFA score were statistically significant predictors of 1-year post-transplant mortality, the discriminatory power of CLIF-SOFA score was even superior to that of the SOFA score on post-transplant day 1, 3, 7, and 14 ($p < 0.05$ on post-transplant day 1 and day 7). Both SOFA score and CLIF-SOFA score provided a complete representation of illness dynamics in serial assessment before and after transplantation, but the CLIF-SOFA score showed greater numerical differences between the 1-year survivor group and non-survivor group, especially during the post-transplantation period (Figure 2). Moreover, trends in the CLIF-SOFA score reflect a patient's response to therapeutic strategies, [9,23,27] with a CLIF-SOFA score >8 on post-transplant day 7 indicating a delayed recovery of multiple organ dysfunction from operation that is associated with a higher rate of acute rejection and poor 1-year survival rate (Figures 1–2). Because of implications for graft survival, the diagnosis of acute rejection and its prompt treatment is very important for these patients.

Recentlly, Jalan et al from the CLIF Consortium have generated a simplified version of the CLIF-SOFA Score (the CLIF-Consortium Organ Failure score, CLIF-C OFs, which has only 3-point range per organ system) [12] (Table 1). The performance of the CLIF-C OF score is similar to that of the CLIF-SOFA score and superior to that of the SOFA score significantly (Table 4–5). It is also an excellent scoring system in predicting short-term prognosis for liver transplantation patients. In the same study, Jalan et al also elaborated a specific score for patients with acute-on-chronic liver failure (CLIF-Consortium score for ACLF, CLIF-C ACLFs) that includes the CLIF-C OFs plus age and white-cell count. The accuracy of the CLIF-ACLF score is even superior to that of the CLIF-SOFA and CLIF-C OF scores in the study of Jalan et al. However, the performance of the CLIF-ACLIF is inferior to that of the CLIF-SOFA score in this study (data not shown). There are some explanations for the discrepancy of the study results. First, in this study, age is not significantly associated with in-hospital mortality rate (table 2) and this finding is consistent with our previous reports [6,20,21]. Hepatitis B virus-related liver cirrhosis is the major population in our country, while alcoholic cirrhosis is the major population in Europe. The difference of prediction value of age might be attributed to the different population between our studies and European ones. Second, the usage of prednisolone and other

immunosuppressant might impact the application of white blood cell count in predicting outcome for liver transplantation patients. Above 2 reasons might, at least partially, explain why the CLIF-C ACLF score is not an optimal score in predicting prognosis for patients undergoing liver transplantation in our study. Another well-powered trial is required to examine this issue.

In spite of the encouraging results observed in our study, several potential limitations should be recognized. First, the fact that our study was conducted at a single tertiary medical center limits the generalization of the findings to other hospitals with different patient populations. Second, because of the retrospective nature of this investigation, some clinical variables were unavailable. Third, in our study, given that hepatitis B viral infection was the leading cause of liver cirrhosis, the use of our classification system may not be appropriate for patients in North America and in Europe where liver diseases are mostly attributed to hepatitis C viral infection and alcoholism. The patient population contained a high proportion of hepatitis B (62%) patients and hepatoma (27%) patients (Table 3), and may present as a special subgroup in the cirrhotic patient. Finally, the predictive accuracy of logistic regression models had its own limitations.

Conclusion

In conclusion, the short-term prognosis after liver transplantation is best predicted by the CLIF-SOFA score. Our data suggest that the SOFA and CLIF-SOFA scoring systems were independent predictors of 1-year mortality after liver transplantation. The analytical data also showed the CLIF-SOFA score is superior to the Child-Pugh points, MELD score, RIFLE criteria, and SOFA score in predicting short-term prognosis. We confirmed that the pre-transplant and post-transplant CLIF-SOFA scores are accurate and capable of providing an improved prediction of prognosis along with objective information for clinical decision making for treating this subset of patients. On the basis of the observed results, we recommend that a CLIF-SOFA score >8 on post-transplantation day 7 be considered as high risk of acute rejection and negative short-term outcome. Graft biopsy is suggested for these patients to diagnosis and to guide antirejection therapy.

Author Contributions

Conceived and designed the experiments: YCC HCP WCL MYC JTF CWY. Performed the experiments: WCL HCP YCC MHT CCJ PCF. Analyzed the data: YCC HCP CCJ CHC. Contributed to the writing of the manuscript: HCP. Provided intellectual content of the work: CCJ MHT PCF CHC MYC YCT CCH JTF CWY. Edited and revised the manuscript: CCJ MHT PCF CHC MYC YCT CCH JTF CWY.

References

1. Schrier RW (2010) Primary systemic arterial vasodilation in cirrhotic patients. Kidney Int 78: 619; author reply 619–620.

2. Gines P, Guevara M, Arroyo V, Rodes J (2003) Hepatorenal syndrome. Lancet 362: 1819–1827.

3. Iwakiri Y, Groszmann RJ (2006) The hyperdynamic circulation of chronic liver diseases: from the patient to the molecule. Hepatology 43: S121–S131.

4. Martin PY, Gines P, Schrier RW (1998) Nitric oxide as a mediator of hemodynamic abnormalities and sodium and water retention in cirrhosis. N Engl J Med 339: 533–541.

5. Xu L, Carter EP, Ohara M, Martin PY, Rogachev B, et al. (2000) Neuronal nitric oxide synthase and systemic vasodilation in rats with cirrhosis. Am J Physiol Renal Physiol 279: F1110–1115.

6. Pan HC, Jenq CC, Tsai MH, Fan PC, Chang CH, et al. (2012) Risk models and scoring systems for predicting the prognosis in critically ill cirrhotic patients with acute kidney injury: a prospective validation study. PLoS One 7: e51094.

7. Chen YC, Gines P, Yang J, Summer SN, Falk S, et al. (2004) Increased vascular heme oxygenase-1 expression contributes to arterial vasodilation in experimental cirrhosis in rats. Hepatology 39: 1075–1087.

8. Shellman RG, Fulkerson WJ, DeLong E, Piantadosi CA (1988) Prognosis of patients with cirrhosis and chronic liver disease admitted to the medical intensive care unit. Crit Care Med 16: 671–678.

9. Wong CS, Lee WC, Jenq CC, Tian YC, Chang MY, et al. (2010) Scoring short-term mortality after liver transplantation. Liver Transpl 16: 138–146.

10. Moreau R, Jalan R, Gines P, Pavesi M, Angeli P, et al. (2013) Acute-on-chronic liver failure is a distinct syndrome that develops in patients with acute decompensation of cirrhosis. Gastroenterology 144: 1426–1437, 1437. e1421–1429.

11. Wiesner R, Edwards E, Freeman R, Harper A, Kim R, et al. (2003) Model for end-stage liver disease (MELD) and allocation of donor livers. Gastroenterology 124: 91–96.

12. Jalan R, Saliba F, Pavesi M, Amoros A, Moreau R, et al. (2014) Development and Validation of a Prognostic Score to Predict Mortality in Patients with Acute on Chronic Liver Failure. J Hepatol 17: 00408–00405.

13. Bellomo R, Ronco C, Kellum JA, Mehta RL, Palevsky P, et al. (2004) Acute renal failure - definition, outcome measures, animal models, fluid therapy and information technology needs: the Second International Consensus Conference

of the Acute Dialysis Quality Initiative (ADQI) Group. Critical care 8: R204–R212.

14. Lin CY, Chen YC, Tsai FC, Tian YC, Jenq CC, et al. (2006) RIFLE classification is predictive of short-term prognosis in critically ill patients with acute renal failure supported by extracorporeal membrane oxygenation. Nephrology Dialysis Transplantation 21: 2867–2873.

15. Youden W (1950) Index for rating diagnostic tests. Cancer 3: 32–35.

16. Akyildiz M, Karasu Z, Arikan C, Kilic M, Zeytunlu M, et al. (2004) Impact of pretransplant MELD score on posttransplant outcome in living donor liver transplantation. Transplant Proc 36: 1442–1444.

17. Leppke S, Leighton T, Zaun D, Chen SC, Skeans M, et al. (2013) Scientific Registry of Transplant Recipients: collecting, analyzing, and reporting data on transplantation in the United States. Transplant Rev (Orlando) 27: 50–56.

18. Freire P, Romãozinho JM, Amaro P, Ferreira M, Sofia C (2011) Prognostic scores in cirrhotic patients admitted to a gastroenterology intensive care unit. Revista espanola de enfermedades digestivas: organo oficial de la Sociedad Espanola de Patologia Digestiva 103: 177.

19. Levesque E, Hoti E, Azoulay D, Ichai P, Habouchi H, et al. (2012) Prospective evaluation of the prognostic scores for cirrhotic patients admitted to an intensive care unit. J Hepatol 56: 95–102.

20. Chen Y, Tian Y, Liu N, Ho Y, Yang C, et al. (2006) Prospective cohort study comparing sequential organ failure assessment and acute physiology, age,

chronic health evaluation III scoring systems for hospital mortality prediction in critically ill cirrhotic patients. International journal of clinical practice 60: 160–166.

21. Jenq CC, Tsai MH, Tian YC, Lin CY, Yang C, et al. (2007) RIFLE classification can predict short-term prognosis in critically ill cirrhotic patients. Intensive Care Med 33: 1921–1930.

22. Karvellas CJ, Lescot T, Goldberg P, Sharpe MD, Ronco JJ, et al. (2013) Liver transplantation in the critically ill: a multicenter Canadian retrospective cohort study. Crit Care 17: R28.

23. Jalan R, Gines P, Olson JC, Mookerjee RP, Moreau R, et al. (2012) Acute-on chronic liver failure. J Hepatol 57: 1336–1348.

24. Bleibel W, Caldwell SH, Curry MP, Northup PG (2013) Peripheral platelet count correlates with liver atrophy and predicts long-term mortality on the liver transplant waiting list. Transpl Int 26: 435–442.

25. Galbois A, Das V, Carbonell N, Guidet B (2013) Prognostic scores for cirrhotic patients admitted to an intensive care unit: which consequences for liver transplantation? Clin Res Hepatol Gastroenterol 37: 455–466.

26. Das V, Boelle PY, Galbois A, Guidet B, Maury E, et al. (2010) Cirrhotic patients in the medical intensive care unit: early prognosis and long-term survival. Crit Care Med 38: 2108–2116.

27. Goldhill DR, Sumner A (1998) Outcome of intensive care patients in a group of British intensive care units. Crit Care Med 26: 1337–1345.

19

Intravascular Administration of Mannitol for Acute Kidney Injury Prevention

Bo Yang[1,⁹], Jing Xu[1,⁹], Fengying Xu[2], Zui Zou[2], Chaoyang Ye[1], Changlin Mei[1]*, Zhiguo Mao[1]*

1 Kidney Institute of Chinese People's Liberation Army, Division of Nephrology, Changzheng Hospital, Second Military Medical University, Shanghai, China, **2** Division of Anesthesiology, Changzheng Hospital, Second Military Medical University, Shanghai, China

Abstract

Background: The effects of mannitol administration on acute kidney injury (AKI) prevention remain uncertain, as the results from clinical studies were conflicting. Due to the lack of strong evidence, the KDIGO Guideline for AKI did not propose completely evidence-based recommendations on this issue.

Methods: We searched PubMed, EMBASE, clinicaltrials.gov and Cochrane Controlled Trials Register. Randomized controlled trials on adult patients at increased risk of AKI were considered on the condition that they compared the effects of intravascular administration of mannitol plus expansion of intravascular volume with expansion of intravascular volume alone. We calculated pooled risk ratios, numbers needed to treat and mean differences with 95% confidence intervals for dichotomous data and continuous data, respectively.

Results: Nine trials involving 626 patients were identified. Compared with expansion of intravascular volume alone, mannitol infusion for AKI prevention in high-risk patients can not reduce the serum creatinine level (MD 1.63, 95% CI −6.02 to 9.28). Subgroup analyses demonstrated that serum creatinine level is negatively affected by the use of mannitol in patients undergoing an injection of radiocontrast agents (MD 17.90, 95% CI 8.56 to 27.24). Mannitol administration may reduce the incidence of acute renal failure or the need of dialysis in recipients of renal transplantation (RR 0.34, 95% CI 0.21 to 0.57, NNT 3.03, 95% CI 2.17 to 5.00). But similar effects were not found in patients at high AKI risk, without receiving renal transplantation (RR 0.29, 95% CI 0.01 to 6.60).

Conclusions: Intravascular administration of mannitol does not convey additional beneficial effects beyond adequate hydration in the patients at increased risk of AKI. For contrast-induced nephropathy, the use of mannitol is even detrimental. Further research evaluating the efficiency of mannitol infusions in the recipients of renal allograft should be undertaken.

Editor: Benedetta Bussolati, Center for Molecular Biotechnology, Italy

Funding: Zhiguo Mao is an Outstanding Young Scholar of Second Miliatory Medical University. This work was supported by the National Nature Science Fund of China (No. 81000281), the Chinese Society of Nephrology (No. 13030340419), Major Fundamental Research Program of Shanghai Committee of Science and Technology (No. 12DJ1400300), and Key Projects in the National Science & Technology Pillar Program in the Twelfth Five-year Plan Period (No. 2011BAI10B00). The funders had no role in study design, data collection and analysis, decision to publish, or preparation of the manuscript.

Competing Interests: The authors have declared that no competing interests exist.

* E-mail: maozhiguo93@gmail.com (ZM); chlmei1954@126.com (CM)

⁹ These authors contributed equally to this work.

Introduction

Acute kidney injury (AKI) is defined as an abrupt decrease of renal function. It is a broad clinical syndrome encompassing various etiologies, including sepsis, dehydration, cardiac surgery (especially with cardiopulmonary bypass (CPB)), radiocontrast agents and so on.[1–3] AKI is associated with prolonged length of stay, increased mortality, and high health-care costs.[4–6] Early recognition and management of the patients at increased risk of AKI are paramount.

As a clinical strategy of AKI prevention, the use of diuretics has been well studied. Practice guideline[1] and comprehensive meta-analyses[7,8] recommend not using loop diuretics to prevent AKI. To date, our knowledge on this issue is fairly well evidence-based.

However, the role of osmotic diuretics in the prevention of AKI has not been well established. Mannitol, an osmotic diuretic, has been used in clinical practice for the prevention of AKI because of its potentially renal protective effects: removal of obstructing tubular casts, dilution of nephrotoxic substances in the tubular fluid, and reduction in the swelling of tubular elements via osmotic extraction of water.[9] Additionally, prophylactic mannitol is effective in animal models of AKI.[10,11] On the other hand, potential nephrotoxicity of mannitol raised clinician's concerns. Mannitol may induce extensive isometric renal proximal tubular vacuolization, intense afferent arteriolar constriction (particularly when combined with cyclosporine A) and acute renal failure in higher doses.[12–14] The results of available clinical researches were also conflicting [15–17] and most of the studies are retrospective, underpowered and inconclusive. Due to the lack of strong evidence, the *KDIGO Clinical Practice Guideline for Acute Kidney Injury* published in 2012 did not propose completely evidence-based recommendations on this issue.[1] To answer the question whether mannitol use in high-risk patients can ameliorate renal outcomes and improve the prognosis, we carried out this systematic review and meta-analysis on the efficiency of using mannitol in patients with increased risk of AKI.

Methods

The protocol of this research has been submitted.

Search strategy and study selection

A search of the medical literature was conducted using PubMed (up to May 2013), EMBASE (1980 to May 2013), Cochrane Controlled Trials Register (issue 4, 2013) and the Clinical Trials Registry (http://clinicaltrials.gov/) (date of search: 2, May 2013). Studies on AKI were identified with the terms *acute kidney injury*; *renal failure, acute* and *mannitol* (either as medical subject heading (MeSH) and free text terms. These were combined using the set operator AND. We also searched the reference lists of the original reports, reviews, letters to the editor, case reports, guidelines and meta-analyses of studies involving mannitol and AKI (retrieved through the electronic searches) to identify studies, which had not yet been included in the computerized databases. All potentially relevant papers were obtained and evaluated in detail. There were no language restrictions. Articles were independently assessed by two review authors (BY and JX) using predesigned eligibility criteria: 1) Randomized Controlled Trials (RCTs); 2) Adult patients at risk for AKI, including contrast-induced AKI; 3) Comparing the effects of intravascular administration of mannitol plus expansion of intravascular volume to expansion of intravascular volume alone; 4) Providing data on renal outcomes. Trials using other pharmacotherapies, management of hemodynamic or oxygenation parameters were eligible, as long as these were administered to both the intervention and control groups. All doses of mannitol were considered. Where more than one publication of a trial existed, we used the most complete publication. We excluded trials with the following properties: 1) Enrolled patients undergoing any kinds of dialysis interventions; 2) Patients with volume overload who cannot tolerate expansion of intravascular volume; 3) Acute postrenal obstructive nephropathy; 4) Mannitol administrated via oral; 5) Any other interventions conducted only in the experimental group or in the control group; 6) No control group. We attempted to contact the original investigators in order to obtain further information if necessary. Any disagreement between review authors was resolved by consensus, and adjudicated with the support of a third review author (CY).

Outcome assessment

The primary outcome assessed was change of serum creatinine concentration (SCr) (μmol/L). The secondary outcomes included incidence of renal failure or need of dialysis, and change of urine output (ml/24 h). Where more than one group of data were reported to monitor the progression of kidney injury, we selected the data collected 24 hours after the exposure of the external risk factors of AKI. For the recipients of kidney transplantation, we discarded the baseline SCr value, but extracted the change of SCr concentration between the moment after operation and the third day after operation.

Data extraction

All data were extracted independently by two review authors (BY and JX.) to a predesigned form (Microsoft Office Excel 2007; Microsoft Corp, Redmond, Washington, USA). All data extraction was then checked by a third review author (CY). The following data were extracted for each trial: first author and publication year; number of centers; geographical location of the study; study population; sample size; proportion of female patients; risk factors of AKI (exposures and susceptibilities induced by comorbidities); interventions in the experimental and the control group; targeted dose; duration of study; concomitant medications; renal outcomes; outcome assessment during study; method used to generate the randomization schedule; allocation concealment and blinding. Data were extracted as intention-to-treat analyses, where all drop-outs were assumed to be treatment failures, wherever trial reporting allowed this. The exact mean and standard deviation (SD) may be difficult to decipher in some studies in which results are presented in figures (not tables). In this situation, two review authors independently estimated the exact values presented in the figures in each study using Engauge Digitizer 4.1 and achieve an agreement on the mean $\pm$ SD.

Assessment of risk of bias

Assessment of risk of bias was performed independently by two review authors (BY and JX), with disagreements resolved by discussion. Risk of bias was assessed according to the quality domains of random sequence generation, allocation concealment, blinding of participants and personnel, blinding of outcome assessment, incomplete outcome data, selective reporting and any other potential threats to validity.[18–21] Risk of bias for each domain was rated as high (seriously weakens confidence in the results), low (unlikely to seriously alter the results), or unclear, as reported in the 'Risk of bias' table. A 'Risk of bias summary' figure which details all of the judgments made for all included studies in the review was generated.[18,22]

Data synthesis and statistical analysis

Heterogeneity among studies was assessed using the I^2 statistic and χ^2 test (assessing the P value). If the P value was less than 0.10 and I^2 exceeded 50%, we considered heterogeneity to be substantial. Random effects model was used to combine the data if significant heterogeneity existed (P<0.1; I^2>50%). Dichotomous data were summarized as risk ratio (RR); numbers needed to treat (NNT) and continuous ones as mean difference (MD), along with 95% confidence intervals (CIs), respectively. For continuous data, especially, when the mean values and SDs from the baseline to the point of data collecting were reported, they were retrieved directly. When standard errors (SEs) were reported instead of SDs, SDs were calculated using the formula: $SD = SE*(n)^{0.5}$.[18] If the mean values and SDs were not available, we computed them according to the Cochrane Handbook for Systematic Reviews of Interventions (version 5.1.0).[18]

We conducted prespecified subgroup analyses according to the various risk factors of AKI, including exposures (for example, cardiac surgery with cardiopulmonary bypass, major noncardiac surgery, radiocontrast agents and nephrotoxic drugs) and susceptibilities (such as chronic kidney disease and diabetes mellitus). Sensitivity analyses were planned to assess effects after removal of outlier RCTs identified in funnel plots. These were exploratory analyses only, and may explain some of the observed variability. The results, however, should be interpreted with caution.

Review Manager (RevMan) [Computer program]. Version 5.2. (Copenhagen: The Nordic Cochrane Centre, The Cochrane Collaboration, 2012) was used to generate forest plots for outcomes with 95% CIs, as well as funnel plots. The funnel plots were assessed for evidence of asymmetry, and possible publication bias or other small study effects.

Results

The search strategy initially yielded 416 citations, 76 of which appeared to be relevant to the systematic review and were retrieved for further assessment.(Figure 1) Of these, 67 were excluded for various reasons, leaving a total of nine eligible articles.[23–31] Among the RCTs included, two studies[26,27] contain multiple but no shared intervention groups. We split these two trials into two pairs of eligible comparisons, respectively.

Study characteristics

Table 1 summarizes the characteristics of the included studies. The nine RCTs enrolled 626 adult patients at increased risk of AKI. 262 patients in four trials[25,27,29,30] underwent elective cardiac surgery with CPB[27,29,30] or major noncardiac surgery.[25] 128 participants in two RCTs[24,28] received radiocontrast agents, which had pre-existing renal dysfunction (SCr>140 μmol/L). Gender of participants in three RCTs was unavailable.[24,26,31] One study[23] containing 55 female subjects focused on the patients prescribed nephrotoxic drug (cisplatin), while in the other five trials,[25,27–30] study populations were male-dominated (73.0%). Two trials[26,31] studied 181 recipients of a cadaveric renal allograft. Except for the 181 recipients of a renal allograft, another 178 patients in three RCTs[24,28,30] already have pre-existing renal dysfunction. The targeted dose of mannitol in experimental groups were fixed in five trials[23,24,26,28,31] (range 25 g to 50 g), while in the other four studies, mannitol was administrated according to body weight of the subjects (range 0.3 g/kg to 1 g/kg). The control management in each trial is expansion of intravascular volume using crystalloid fluid (normal saline, Hartmann's solution, etc.). Renal outcomes were reported in each trial, including SCr, creatinine clearance (CCr), plasma urea, urinary volume and need of dialysis or acute renal failure, but the definition of acute renal failure varied across studies, and it was not clear in one study.[26] No clear and definite adverse events can be identified in any of the trials.

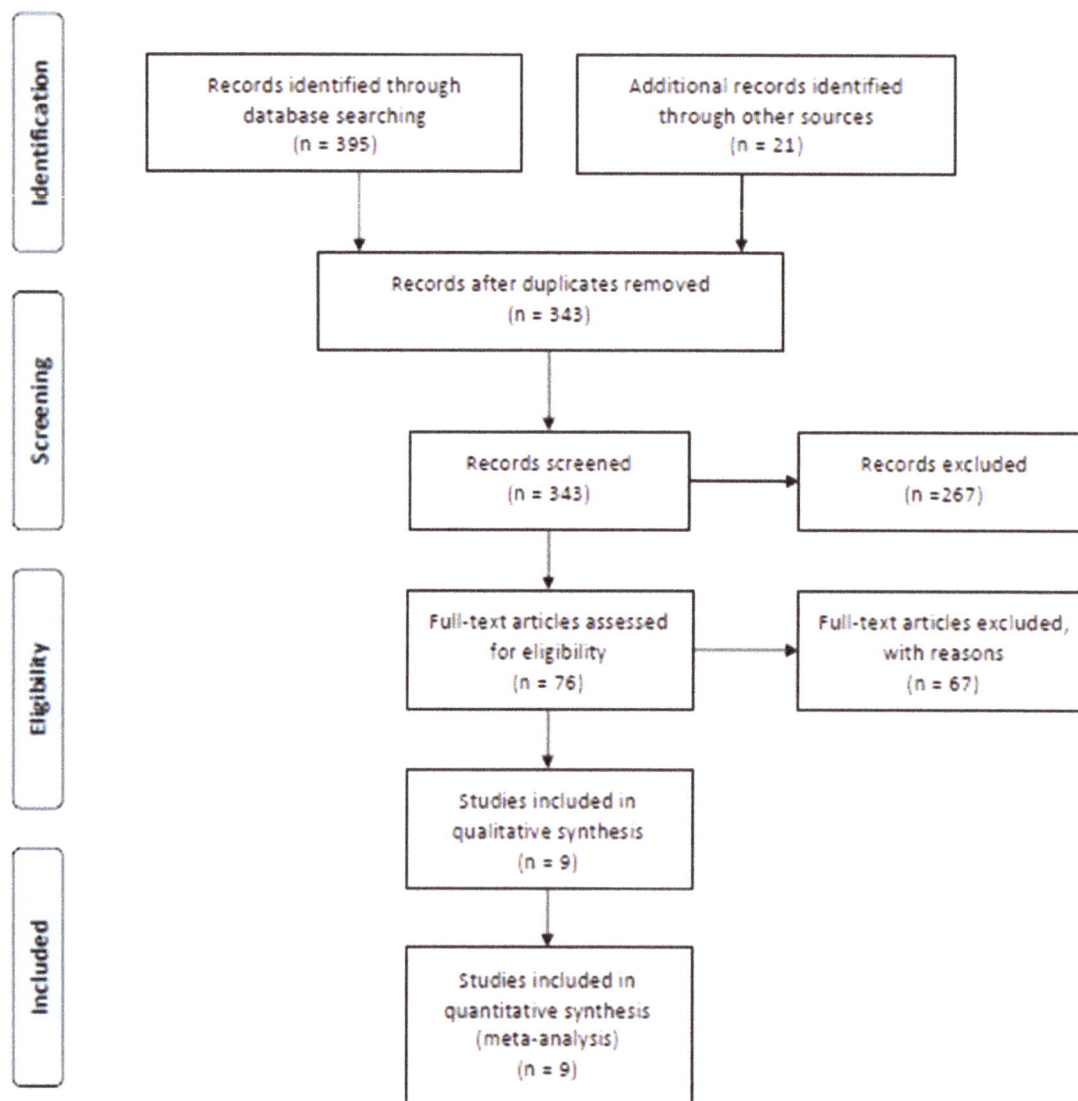

Figure 1. Flow diagram of literature search and study selection. RCT, randomized controlled trial

Table 1. Table of characteristics of included studies.

Study	Study population	Mean age (years)	Sample size (male)	Interventions	Outcomes	Outcome assessment during study
Carcoana 2003[27]	SCr level of <1.5 mg/dL, undergoing elective, primary CABG surgery with CPB	63.3; 64.3; 63.8; 63.4	24(18); 26(19); 25(17); 25(18)	1) placebo, 2) mannitol 1 g/kg added to the CPB prime, 3) DA 2 μg/(kg*min) from the induction of anesthesia to 1 h post-CPB, 4) mannitol plus DA.	β_2M excretion rate at 1 h post-CPB; β_2M excretion rates at 6 and 24 h post-CPB; creatinine clearance; postoperative serum creatinine levels; Urinary output; Length of ICU stay; length of hospitalization; significant clinical events	Urinary output was noted hourly before and after CPB; β_2M excretion rate at 1, 6, and 24 h after CPB; highest postoperative serum creatinine was recorded
Nicholson 1996[25]	Patients undergoing elective aortic aneurysm repair surgery	68; 71	15(13); 13(11)	receive either 1) mannitol 0.3g/kg or 2)an equivalent volume of normal saline given as a rapid intravenous infusion before cross-clamping the aorta.	urine output; creatinine clearance; blood urea; acute renal failure; serum creatinine; urinary albumin; urinary N-acetylglucosaminidase; urinary creatinine	6 h; 24 h; 3d and 7d after surgery
Santoso 2003[23]	be to receive 75 mg/m² of cisplatin alone or in combination with paclitaxel or 5-fluorouracil to treat gynecologic cancers.	49.0; 48.0; 43.7	17(0); 19(0); 19(0)	1)500 mL NS in 2 h and mix cisplatin in 1 L NS; 2)500 mL NS in 2 h and mix cisplatin in 1 L NS with 50 g mannitol; 3) 500 mL NS in 2 h, 40 mg furosemide 30 min before cisplatin and mix cisplatin in 1 L NS	24 h creatinine clearance; SCr; metabolic panel; CA-125 for patients with ovarian cancer	Each clinic visit after cisplatin
Smith 2008[30]	Adult patients having elective cardiac surgery with CPB, and pre-operative renal dysfunction: 130 μmol/L< SCr < 250 μmol/L	74.7; 74.7	23(16); 24(18)	1) 0.5 g/kg of mannitol as a 20% solution in the prime. 2) equivalent volume of Hartmann's solution	Daily urine output and plasma creatinine and urea	1, 2, 3d after surgery
Solomon 1994[28]	Patients scheduled for cardiac angiography who had SCr > 140 μmol/L or CCr< 60 ml/min	67; 60; 63	28(23); 25(19); 25(12)	1) 0.45% NS 1 ml/(kg*h) 2) 0.45% NS 1 ml/(kg*h)+ 25 g mannitol, infused intravenously during the 60 minutes immediately before angiography. 3) 0.45% NS 1 ml/(kg*h)+80 mg furosemide, infused intravenously during the 30 minutes immediately before angiography.	SCr; BUN; urinary sodium; urinary potassium; urinary creatinine	At the time of angiography, 1d,2d
van Valenberg 1987[26]	Recipient of a cadaveric renal allograft	NA	33; 34; 32; 32. Gender: NA	Azathioprine: 1) 20% mannitol 250 ml 2) 5% glucose 250 ml during the last 10 min before the opening of the vascular anastomoses. Cyclosporine: 1) 20% mannitol 250 ml 2) 5% glucose 250 ml during the last 10 min before the opening of the vascular anastomoses.	ARF; SCr postoperatively; graft survival; patient survival	SCr: 1, 2, 3d; graft/ patient survival: 3m, 1y
Weimar 1983[31]	Recipient of a cadaveric renal allograft	Donor:21.5; 20.5. Recipient: 34; 38	22; 22. Gender: NA	1) 20% mannitol 250 ml i.v. before revascularization 2) NS	Patients with immediate renal function; CCr; patients with ATN leading to dialysis	NA
Weisberg 1984[24]	SCr> 1.8 mg/dl, undergoing elective cardiac catheterization	NA	15; 15; 10; 10. Gender: NA	1) saline 100 ml/h; 2) dopamine 2 μg/(kg*min) in NS, 100 ml/h; 3) ANP 50 μg bolus, followed by an infusion of 1 μg/min in NS, 100 ml/h; 4) mannitol 15 g/dl in NS 100 ml/h. the infusions began immediately after full instrumentation for the cardiac catheterization procedure and continued for a total of two hours	RBF; SCr	SCr: 1d, 2d. RBF: baseline, after the drug infusion was begun but before the ventriculogram, immediately after the ventriculogram, after the coronary angiogram
Yallop 2008[29]	Patients scheduled for elective cardiac surgery with CPB	64.1; 62.2	20(14); 20(16)	1) 5 ml/kg of 10% mannitol in the pump prime. 2) Hartmann's solution in the pump prime	Urinary creatinine; microalbumin; SCr; plasma urea; urine output	1, 2, 3, 4, 5d

Abbreviations: NA, not applicable; SCr, serum creatinine; CABG, coronary artery bypass surgery; CPB, cardiopulmonary bypass; DA, dopamine; ICU, intensive care unit; NS, normal saline solution; RBF, renal blood flow; BUN, Blood urea nitrogen; CCr, creatinine clearance; ATN, acute tubular necrosis.

Table 2. Risk of bias.

Study	Random sequence generation	Allocation concealment	Blinding of participants and personnel	Blinding of outcome assessment	Incomplete outcome data	Selective reporting
Carcoana 2003[27]	Computer-generated random-number tables	Patients were randomly allocated by the Department of Investigational Pharmacy	double-blinded	NA	No drop-outs after randomization	The results of all outcomes described in methods were reported
Nicholson 1996[25]	Table of random numbers	Sealed envelope	NA	NA	Unclear bias	The results of all outcomes described in methods were reported
Santoso 2003[23]	Randomized allocation table	NA	NA	NA	Non-intention-to-treat analysis	The results of all outcomes described in methods were reported
Smith 2008[30]	computer-generated random number tables	the anesthetic, theatre and ICU staff were blind to the randomization	NA	NA	No drop-outs after randomization	The results of all outcomes described in methods were reported
Solomon 1994[28]	Random-allocation table	NA	NA	NA	No drop-outs after randomization	The results of all outcomes described in methods were reported
van Valenberg 1987[26]	Randomized controlled trial	NA	NA	NA	Patients with ARF were not analyzed	The results of all outcomes described in methods were reported
Weimar 1983[31]	Random allocated	NA	NA	NA	Intention-to-treat analysis	The results of all outcomes described in methods were reported
Weisberg 1984[24]	Randomized controlled trial	NA	Double-blind	NA	No drop-outs after randomization	The results of all outcomes described in methods were reported
Yallop 2008[29]	computer-generated random number chart	All personnel other than the perfusionist were blinded to the randomization	double-blind	NA	No drop-outs after randomization	The results of all outcomes described in methods were reported

Abbreviations: NA, not applicable; ICU, intensive care unit.

Risk of bias

Risk of bias ratings for each trial (Table 2, Figure S1) were assessed with the Cochrane risk of bias tool.[22] In the domain of random sequence generation, six RCTs were at low risk of bias,[23,25,27–30] while three trials declared as "randomized" but did not report the method of randomization (unclear risk of bias).[24,26,31] No RCTs were at high risk of bias for allocation concealment, however, the method of concealment was unclear (not reported) in five trials.[23,24,26,28,31] None of the studies reported the blinding of outcome assessment, which result in an unclear detection risk of bias in each of the included trials. Additionally, only three RCTs provided the information of blinding of participants and personnel.[24,27,29] In one trial,[26] a high risk of bias was identified in domain of incomplete outcome data. The investigators of this RCT provided SCr levels in cyclosporine-treated patients without acute renal failure who received either mannitol or 5% glucose, but the patients with acute renal failure were excluded from the analysis. Numbers excluded are not balanced across groups, which may introduce attrition bias. According to the data provided in this original study, we can also recognize the direction of bias, which favors the group

prescribed 5% glucose. In the trial conducted by Nicholson, we are not clear whether the patients developing postoperative complications were excluded from the analysis,[25] so we graded the study as unclear risk of bias in this domain. We found no suspect selective reporting in all of the included RCTs.

Effects of interventions

Serum creatinine. Eight studies reported the outcome of SCr change. Overall, there was no significant difference between the experimental group and control group (MD 1.63, 95% CI −6.02 to 9.28; $I^2 = 63\%$, P = 0.008). Statistically non-significant results were identified in three of the subgroup analyses according to the potential etiologies of AKI: 1) cardiac surgery with CPB (MD −2.35, 95% CI −7.46 to 2.75; $I^2 = 0\%$, P = 0.50); 2) major noncardiac surgery (MD −18.00, 95% CI −46.57 to 10.57) and 3) nephrotoxic drugs (MD 7.96, 95% CI −5.49 to 21.41). In the subgroup of radiocontrast agents, a greater increase of SCr in mannitol groups was found (MD 17.90, 95% CI 8.56 to 27.24; $I^2 = 0\%$, P = 0.82), which means the administration of mannitol may exacerbate AKI in patients undergoing radiocontrast agents injection.(Figure 2) Patients in three trials[24,28,30] already had

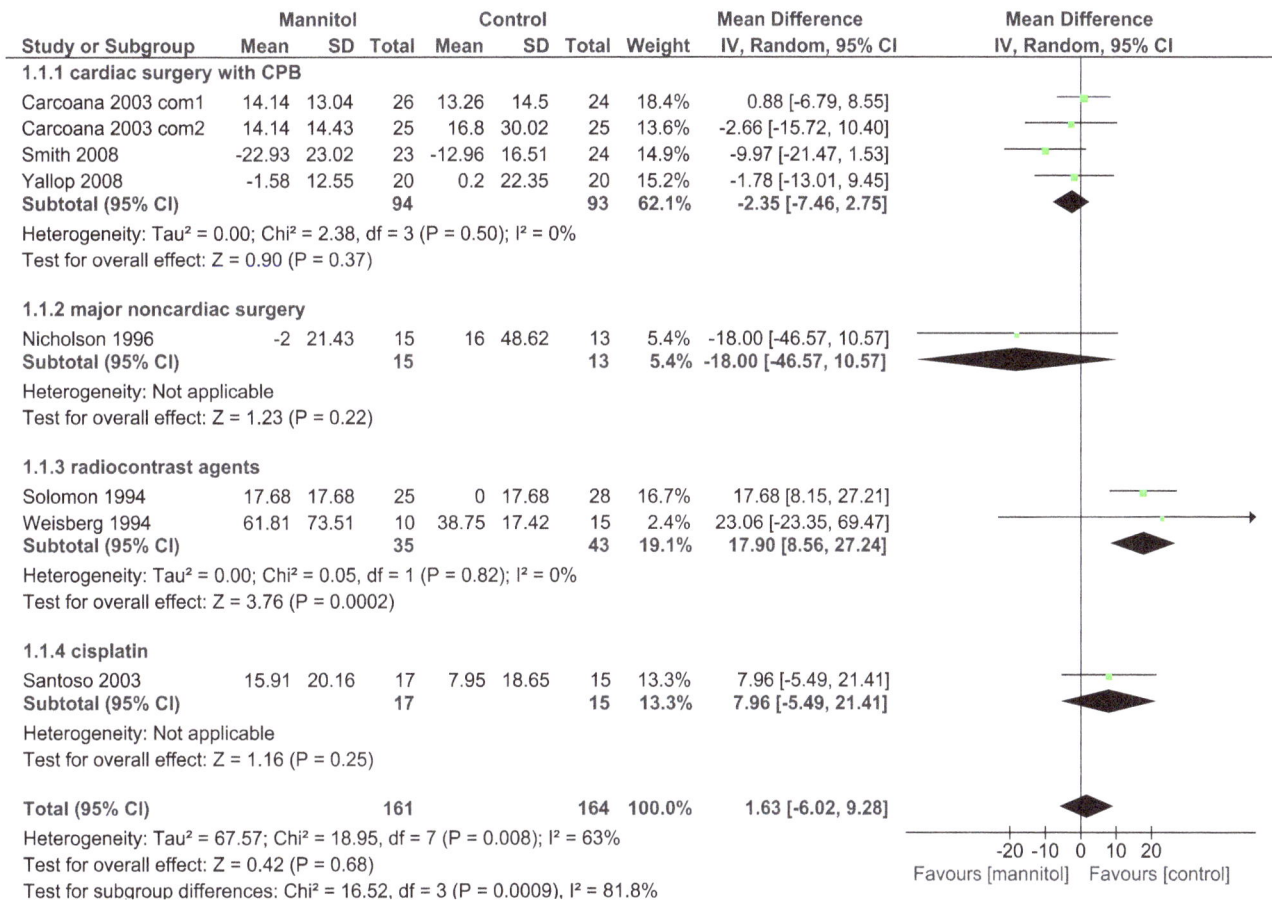

Figure 2. Change of serum creatinine level among participants given mannitol versus control. Note that Carcoana 2003 contain multiple but no shared intervention groups. We split it into two pairs of eligible comparisons (Carcoana 2003 com1 and Carcoana 2003 com2)

pre-existing renal dysfunction, when data of these three RCTs were combined exclusively, no significant difference between mannitol groups and control groups was found (MD 7.18, 95% CI −16.29 to 30.66; $I^2 = 85\%$, P = 0.001). There is also a study focusing on recipients of a cadaveric renal allograft provided the level of SCr, but the result of this trial was not combined with other RCTs', due to the obvious clinical heterogeneity. Analysis of this orphan study shows that compared with the control group, SCr level did not decrease significantly in the mannitol group (MD −141.46, 95% CI −284.93 to 2.01). However, the upper bound of 95% CI is close to "0", which means the results should be interpreted with caution. (Figure S2)

Acute renal failure or need of dialysis. Five comparisons in four studies reported the acute renal failure or need of dialysis. (Figure 3) The overall result indicates that mannitol administration may reduce the incidence of acute renal failure or reduce the need of dialysis (RR 0.34, 95% CI 0.21 to 0.57, NNT 3.45, 95% CI 2.44 to 5.56; $I^2 = 0\%$, P = 0.92), but the statistically significant result is stable only in the subgroup of renal graft (RR 0.34, 95% CI 0.21 to 0.57, NNT 3.03, 95% CI 2.17 to 5.00; $I^2 = 0\%$, P = 0.78). In the subgroup of non-renal graft, we identified no difference between interventions and controls (RR 0.29, 95% CI 0.01 to 6.60).

Urine output. Change of urinary volume can be extracted from five comparisons in four RCTs. (Figure 4) There was no difference in change of urine output (MD −140.56, 95% CI −650.05 to 368.93), but the heterogeneity was significant across

studies ($I^2 = 71\%$, P = 0.008). The funnel plot was generated (not shown), and data in two comparisons from one study[27] were identified as outliers. Then a planned sensitivity analysis was carried out by excluding these two comparisons and the result was stable in sensitivity analysis (MD 2.07, 95% CI −428.54 to 432.67; $I^2 = 73\%$, P = 0.03). (Figure S3)

Publication bias. No evidence of publication bias for the primary outcome was indicated by visual inspection of the funnel plots (not shown). The effect of an outlying study[27] on the outcome of urine output was assessed with a sensitivity analysis. As the results mentioned above, removal of this study did not change the primary result.

Discussion

Summary of results and possible explanations

This systematic review and meta-analysis included nine trials with 626 participants at increased risk of AKI involved. All RCTs were carried out in hospital setting, where the patient's risk factors can be assessed before certain exposures. The patients enrolled were exposed to several common risks of AKI, and this heterogeneity provided a good representativeness of clinical practice. Since the methodological qualities of these studies were relatively high, and no publication bias was identified, we considered the quality of evidence is good and the true effect lies close to that of the estimate of the effect. Our results demonstrated that intravascular administration of mannitol for AKI prevention

Study or Subgroup	Mannitol Events	Mannitol Total	Control Events	Control Total	Weight	Risk Ratio M-H, Fixed, 95% CI	Risk Ratio M-H, Fixed, 95% CI
1.3.1 Renal graft							
van Valenberg 1987 com1	6	33	15	34	32.6%	0.41 [0.18, 0.93]	
van Valenberg 1987 com2	6	32	17	32	37.5%	0.35 [0.16, 0.78]	
Weimar 1983	3	22	12	22	26.4%	0.25 [0.08, 0.77]	
Subtotal (95% CI)		87		88	96.5%	**0.34 [0.21, 0.57]**	
Total events	15		44				
Heterogeneity: Chi² = 0.50, df = 2 (P = 0.78); I² = 0%							
Test for overall effect: Z = 4.13 (P < 0.0001)							
1.3.2 Non-renal graft							
Nicholson 1996	0	15	1	13	3.5%	0.29 [0.01, 6.60]	
Subtotal (95% CI)		15		13	3.5%	**0.29 [0.01, 6.60]**	
Total events	0		1				
Heterogeneity: Not applicable							
Test for overall effect: Z = 0.77 (P = 0.44)							
Total (95% CI)		102		101	100.0%	**0.34 [0.21, 0.57]**	
Total events	15		45				
Heterogeneity: Chi² = 0.52, df = 3 (P = 0.92); I² = 0%							
Test for overall effect: Z = 4.20 (P < 0.0001)							
Test for subgroup differences: Chi² = 0.01. df = 1 (P = 0.92). I² = 0%							

0.02   0.1   1   10   50
Favours [mannitol]   Favours [control]

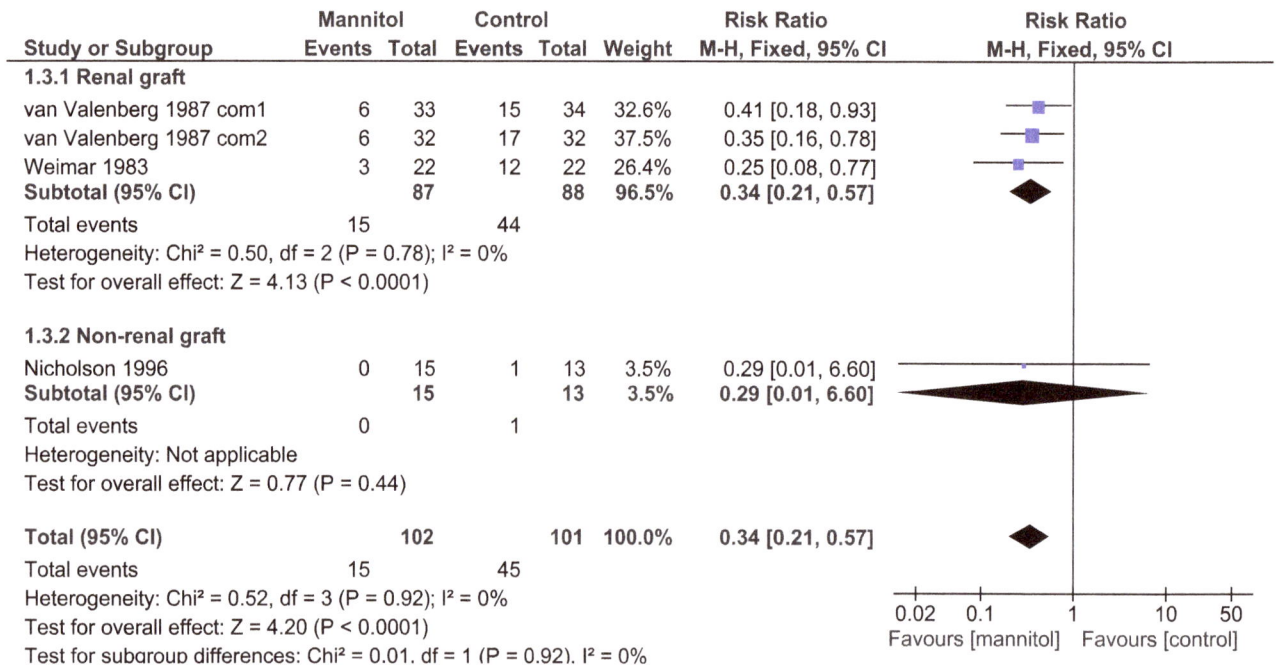

Figure 3. Risk of acute renal failure or need of dialysis intervention among participants given mannitol versus control. Note that van Valenberg 1987 contains multiple but no shared intervention groups. We split it into two pairs of eligible comparisons (van Valenberg 1987 com1 and van Valenberg 1987 com2)

in high-risk patients can not ameliorate the deterioration of renal function. Moreover, SCr level is negatively affected by the use of mannitol in patients undergoing radiocontrast agents injection. In other words, prophylactic mannitol in this kind of patients may be associated with significant toxicity. Although in some animal researches, mannitol provides beneficial effects against contrast-induced nephropathy,[32] the present meta-analysis and former studies based on human concluded the opposite.[33,34] On the other hand, recipients of a cadaveric renal allograft may benefit from the use of mannitol before vessel clamp removal. Recipients prescribed mannitol may experience a greater SCr decrease, smaller chance of acute renal failure and fewer dialysis interventions after transplantation. However, the two included studies[26,31] focusing on the renal transplantation were both conducted in 1980s, and surgical technic, immunosuppressive therapies and other risk factors of AKI have evolved significantly since then.[35,36] Pooling data in the early days alone will damage the completeness and applicability of evidence, and the above results should be interpreted with caution.

The lack of a significant diuretic effect when receiving mannitol is interesting, as showed in this analysis, which seems to be inconsistent with well established knowledge.[37] The first issue to be addressed is clinical heterogeneity. In the trial conducted by Carcoana,[27] urinary output was noted hourly, while in other three RCTs, it was recorded daily. This makes the unit of measurement across studies different (ml/min *vs.* ml/24 h). After the conversion of the ml/min into ml/24 h,[18] heterogeneity (especially in SD value) showed up. The clinical heterogeneity may comes from this kind of nondifferential measurement bias. After excluding this study, we found the result was stable.

Clinically, mannitol has been used to treat fluid overload and cerebral edema. The diuretic effect of mannitol in these non-AKI risk patients was affirmed (although the benefit of its clinical use in decreasing the intracranial pressure is under estimation).[38,39] But according to the results of the present study, the diuretic effect of mannitol was significantly weakened in the patients with increased risk of AKI. It is reasonable to regard the diuretic response as a predictor of renal outcome rather than the

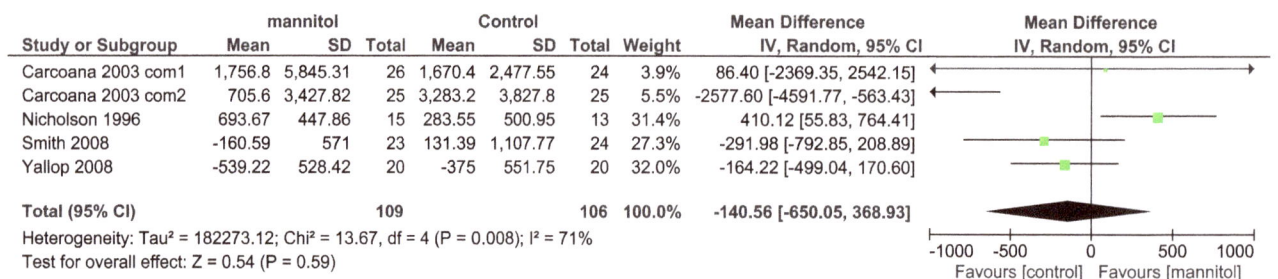

Study or Subgroup	mannitol Mean	mannitol SD	Total	Control Mean	Control SD	Total	Weight	Mean Difference IV, Random, 95% CI	Mean Difference IV, Random, 95% CI
Carcoana 2003 com1	1,756.8	5,845.31	26	1,670.4	2,477.55	24	3.9%	86.40 [-2369.35, 2542.15]	
Carcoana 2003 com2	705.6	3,427.82	25	3,283.2	3,827.8	25	5.5%	-2577.60 [-4591.77, -563.43]	
Nicholson 1996	693.67	447.86	15	283.55	500.95	13	31.4%	410.12 [55.83, 764.41]	
Smith 2008	-160.59	571	23	131.39	1,107.77	24	27.3%	-291.98 [-792.85, 208.89]	
Yallop 2008	-539.22	528.42	20	-375	551.75	20	32.0%	-164.22 [-499.04, 170.60]	
Total (95% CI)			109			106	100.0%	**-140.56 [-650.05, 368.93]**	
Heterogeneity: Tau² = 182273.12; Chi² = 13.67, df = 4 (P = 0.008); I² = 71%									
Test for overall effect: Z = 0.54 (P = 0.59)									

-1000   -500   0   500   1000
Favours [control]   Favours [mannitol]

Figure 4, Change of urine output among participants given mannitol versus control. Note that Carcoana 2003 contains multiple but no shared intervention groups. We split it into two pairs of eligible comparisons (Carcoana 2003 com1 and Carcoana 2003 com2)

therapeutic effect for patients with AKI risk.[40] As four out of five pairs of comparisons in this outcome studied patients undergoing cardiac surgery with CPB, another possible explanation can be reasonable that renal dysfunction after CPB may be induced by micro emboli, in which case mannitol is unlikely to be of diuretic benefit.[41]

Results in relation to other studies

So far, no published systematic review or meta-analyses have assessed the efficiency of mannitol for AKI prevention. A conventional review on this clinical issue published in 2004 summarized the retrospective studies and clinical trials before the year of 2000.[42] In this review, the authors concluded that mannitol has not been proven to be of value for renal protection in humans. This conclusion is consistent with ours, but available evidence at that time was largely underpowered. We included the recently completed well-designed RCTs (Figure S1) and enhanced the strength of the evidence. In accordance with our results, another narrative review of the literature studying the perioperative fluid management in renal transplantation found salutary effects of mannitol infusions in kidney transplantation immediately before opening the vascular anastomoses.[43] The reviewers summarized the results of animal researches, retrospective studies, as well as clinical trials. Due to the nature of narrative review, no clear inclusion criteria and no risk of bias assessment was applied in this study, we considered the strength of the conclusion in that review very low.

Strengths and limitations

Our systematic review and meta-analysis has several strengths. Firstly, most of the trials included in the meta-analysis were of good methodological quality, (Figure S1) which makes the results of meta-analysis less likely to be affected by the biases of the original studies. Secondly, the populations studied varied widely and covered several major risk factors of AKI. Including such a heterogeneous group may increase the generalizability of our review. In addition, we performed appropriate subgroup analyses which fit for investigating heterogeneous results. Finally, since the definition of acute renal failure varied across studies, we chose SCr rather than acute renal failure or need of dialysis as our primary outcome. This design may estimate the efficiency of interventions more exactly.

Our research also has several limitations. First, few RCTs set mortality as their endpoint, which may not be useful when we assess the association between interventions and prognosis. Surrogate endpoints do not always translate into prognosis. Besides, since AKI is a risk factor for chronic kidney disease, it is important to evaluate the long-term renal function of enrolled patients. But the durations of follow-up in these included studies were relatively short. Only an individual study we included reported the renal function after three months and one year of

exposure of AKI risk factor (renal transplantation).[26] The result of this original trial was that the mannitol-induced reduction in the incidence of acute renal failure had no impact on patient or graft survival. In addition, no clear and definite adverse events were reported in any of the RCTs, it is understandable because in this situation, many signs and symptoms can be attributed to either drug side effects or the impaired renal function. Distinguishing these clinical manifestations clearly was impractical.

Conclusions and implications for future research

Intravascular administration of mannitol does not convey additional beneficial effects beyond adequate hydration in the patients at increased risk of AKI. Its use for AKI prevention is not scientifically justified, and for contrast-induced nephropathy prevention is even detrimental. The findings of this review suggest that further research evaluating efficiency of mannitol infusions in the recipients of renal allograft should be undertaken. Besides, the endpoints in studies involved were set as immediate renal function; SCr; and acute renal failure, long term graft and patient survival, and function index should be investigated.

Supporting Information

Figure S1   Risk of bias

Figure S2   Change of serum creatinine level among renal graft recipients given mannitol versus control. Note that van Valenberg 1987 contains multiple but no shared intervention groups. We split it into two pairs of eligible comparisons (van Valenberg 1987 com1 and van Valenberg 1987 com2)

Figure S3   Sensitivity analysis of change of urine output among participants given mannitol versus control. Note that Carcoana 2003 contains multiple but no shared intervention groups. We split it into two pairs of eligible comparisons (Carcoana 2003 com1 and Carcoana 2003 com2)

Checklist S1   PRISMA checklist.

Protocol S1   Study protocol.

Author Contributions

Conceived and designed the experiments: CM ZM. Performed the experiments: BY JX CY. Analyzed the data: BY JX. Contributed reagents/materials/analysis tools: BY JX. Wrote the paper: BY FX ZZ. Checking of data: CY. Critical revision of the manuscript for important intellectual content: ZZ ZM.

References

1. Kidney Disease: Improving Global Outcomes (KDIGO) (2012) Acute Kidney Injury Work Group. KDIGO Clinical Practice Guideline for Acute Kidney Injury. Kidney Int Suppl. 2: 1–138.
2. Harel Z, Chan CT (2008) Predicting and preventing acute kidney injury after cardiac surgery. Curr Opin Nephrol Hypertens 17: 624–628.
3. Venkataraman R (2008) Can we prevent acute kidney injury? Crit Care Med 36: S166–171.
4. Coca SG, Yusuf B, Shlipak MG, Garg AX, Parikh CR (2009) Long-term risk of mortality and other adverse outcomes after acute kidney injury: a systematic review and meta-analysis. Am J Kidney Dis 53: 961–973.
5. Xue JL, Daniels F, Star RA, Kimmel PL, Eggers PW, et al. (2006) Incidence and mortality of acute renal failure in Medicare beneficiaries, 1992 to 2001. J Am Soc Nephrol 17: 1135–1142.
6. Uchino S, Kellum JA, Bellomo R, Doig GS, Morimatsu H, et al. (2005) Acute renal failure in critically ill patients: a multinational, multicenter study. JAMA 294: 813–818.
7. Ho KM, Power BM (2010) Benefits and risks of furosemide in acute kidney injury. Anaesthesia 65: 283–293.
8. Ho KM, Sheridan DJ (2006) Meta-analysis of frusemide to prevent or treat acute renal failure. BMJ 333: 420.
9. Karajala V, Mansour W, Kellum JA (2009) Diuretics in acute kidney injury. Minerva Anestesiol 75: 251–257.
10. Goksin I, Adali F, Enli Y, Akbulut M, Teke Z, et al. (2011) The effect of phlebotomy and mannitol on acute renal injury induced by ischemia/reperfusion of lower limbs in rats. Ann Vasc Surg 25: 1118–1128.

11. Khoury W, Namnesnikov M, Fedorov D, Abu-Gazala S, Weinbroum AA (2010) Mannitol attenuates kidney damage induced by xanthine oxidase-associated pancreas ischemia-reperfusion. J Surg Res 160: 163–168.

12. Dickenmann M, Oetl T, Mihatsch MJ (2008) Osmotic nephrosis: acute kidney injury with accumulation of proximal tubular lysosomes due to administration of exogenous solutes. Am J Kidney Dis 51: 491–503.

13. Visweswaran P, Massin EK, Dubose TD Jr (1997) Mannitol-induced acute renal failure. J Am Soc Nephrol 8: 1028–1033.

14. Gadallah MF, Lynn M, Work J (1995) Case report: mannitol nephrotoxicity syndrome: role of hemodialysis and postulate of mechanisms. Am J Med Sci 309: 219–222.

15. Gubern JM, Sancho JJ, Simo J, Sitges-Serra A (1988) A randomized trial on the effect of mannitol on postoperative renal function in patients with obstructive jaundice. Surgery 103: 39–44.

16. Hayes DM, Cvitkovic E, Golbey RB, Scheiner E, Helson L, et al. (1977) High dose cis-platinum diammine dichloride: amelioration of renal toxicity by mannitol diuresis. Cancer 39: 1372–1381.

17. Al-Sarraf M, Fletcher W, Oishi N, Pugh R, Hewlett JS, et al. (1982) Cisplatin hydration with and without mannitol diuresis in refractory disseminated malignant melanoma: a southwest oncology group study. Cancer Treat Rep 66: 31–35.

18. Higgins J, Green S (2011) Cochrane Handbook for Systematic Reviews of Interventions Version 5.1.0 [updated March 2011]. The Cochrane Collaboration.

19. Kjaergard LL, Villumsen J, Gluud C (2001) Reported methodologic quality and discrepancies between large and small randomized trials in meta-analyses. Ann Intern Med 135: 982–989.

20. Schulz KF, Chalmers I, Hayes RJ, Altman DG (1995) Empirical evidence of bias. Dimensions of methodological quality associated with estimates of treatment effects in controlled trials. JAMA 273: 408–412.

21. Moher D, Pham B, Jones A, Cook DJ, Jadad AR, et al. (1998) Does quality of reports of randomised trials affect estimates of intervention efficacy reported in meta-analyses? Lancet 352: 609–613.

22. Higgins JP, Altman DG, Gotzsche PC, Juni P, Moher D, et al. (2011) The Cochrane Collaboration's tool for assessing risk of bias in randomised trials. BMJ 343: d5928.

23. Santoso JT, Lucci JA 3rd, Coleman RL, Schafer I, Hannigan EV (2003) Saline, mannitol, and furosemide hydration in acute cisplatin nephrotoxicity: a randomized trial. Cancer Chemother Pharmacol 52: 13–18.

24. Weisberg LS, Kurnik PB, Kurnik BR (1994) Risk of radiocontrast nephropathy in patients with and without diabetes mellitus. Kidney Int 45: 259–265.

25. Nicholson ML, Baker DM, Hopkinson BR, Wenham PW (1996) Randomized controlled trial of the effect of mannitol on renal reperfusion injury during aortic aneurysm surgery. Br J Surg 83: 1230–1233.

26. van Valenberg PL, Hoitsma AJ, Tiggeler RG, Berden JH, van Lier HJ, et al. (1987) Mannitol as an indispensable constituent of an intraoperative hydration protocol for the prevention of acute renal failure after renal cadaveric transplantation. Transplantation 44: 784–788.

27. Carcoana OV, Mathew JP, Davis E, Byrne DW, Hayslett JP, et al. (2003) Mannitol and dopamine in patients undergoing cardiopulmonary bypass: a randomized clinical trial. Anesth Analg 97: 1222–1229.

28. Solomon R, Werner C, Mann D, D'Elia J, Silva P (1994) Effects of saline, mannitol, and furosemide to prevent acute decreases in renal function induced by radiocontrast agents. N Engl J Med 331: 1416–1420.

29. Yallop KG, Sheppard SV, Smith DC (2008) The effect of mannitol on renal function following cardio-pulmonary bypass in patients with normal pre-operative creatinine. Anaesthesia 63: 576–582.

30. Smith MN, Best D, Sheppard SV, Smith DC (2008) The effect of mannitol on renal function after cardiopulmonary bypass in patients with established renal dysfunction. Anaesthesia 63: 701–704.

31. Weimar W, Geerlings W, Bijnen AB, Obertop H, van Urk H, et al. (1983) A controlled study on the effect of mannitol on immediate renal function after cadaver donor kidney transplantation. Transplantation 35: 99–101.

32. Seeliger E, Ladwig M, Sargsyan L, Cantow K, Persson PB, et al. (2012) Proof of principle: hydration by low-osmolar mannitol-glucose solution alleviates undesirable renal effects of an iso-osmolar contrast medium in rats. Invest Radiol 47: 240–246.

33. Majumdar SR, Kjellstrand CM, Tymchak WJ, Hervas-Malo M, Taylor DA, et al. (2009) Forced euvolemic diuresis with mannitol and furosemide for prevention of contrast-induced nephropathy in patients with CKD undergoing coronary angiography: a randomized controlled trial. Am J Kidney Dis 54: 602–609.

34. Kelly AM, Dwamena B, Cronin P, Bernstein SJ, Carlos RC (2008) Meta-analysis: effectiveness of drugs for preventing contrast-induced nephropathy. Ann Intern Med 148: 284–294.

35. Lee RA, Gabardi S (2012) Current trends in immunosuppressive therapies for renal transplant recipients. Am J Health Syst Pharm 69: 1961–1975.

36. Garcia GG, Harden P, Chapman J, For the World Kidney Day Steering C (2012) The Global Role of Kidney Transplantation. Nephrol Dial Transplant.

37. Nissenson AR, Weston RE, Kleeman CR (1979) Mannitol. West J Med 131: 277–284.

38. Hankiewicz J, Piotrowski Z (1967) Diuretic properties of mannitol. Pol Med J 6: 563–569.

39. Kamel H, Navi BB, Nakagawa K, Hemphill JC 3rd, Ko NU (2011) Hypertonic saline versus mannitol for the treatment of elevated intracranial pressure: a meta-analysis of randomized clinical trials. Crit Care Med 39: 554–559.

40. Conger JD (1995) Interventions in clinical acute renal failure: what are the data? Am J Kidney Dis 26: 565–576.

41. Sreeram GM, Grocott HP, White WD, Newman MF, Stafford-Smith M (2004) Transcranial Doppler emboli count predicts rise in creatinine after coronary artery bypass graft surgery. J Cardiothorac Vasc Anesth 18: 548–551.

42. Schetz M (2004) Should we use diuretics in acute renal failure? Best Pract Res Clin Anaesthesiol 18: 75–89.

43. Schnuelle P, Johannes van der Woude F (2006) Perioperative fluid management in renal transplantation: a narrative review of the literature. Transpl Int 19: 947–959.

20

Ischemic Acute Kidney Injury Perturbs Homeostasis of Serine Enantiomers in the Body Fluid in Mice: Early Detection of Renal Dysfunction Using the Ratio of Serine Enantiomers

Jumpei Sasabe[1]*, Masataka Suzuki[1], Yurika Miyoshi[2], Yosuke Tojo[3], Chieko Okamura[3], Sonomi Ito[1], Ryuichi Konno[4], Masashi Mita[3], Kenji Hamase[2], Sadakazu Aiso[1]*

1 Department of Anatomy, Keio University School of Medicine, Shinanomachi, Shinjuku-ku, Tokyo, Japan, 2 Graduate School of Pharmaceutical Sciences, Kyushu University, Maidashi, Higashi-ku, Fukuoka, Japan, 3 Innovative Science Research and Development Center, Shiseido Co., Ltd., Fukuura, Kanazawa-ku, Yokohama, Japan, 4 Department of Pharmacological Sciences, International University of Health and Welfare, Kitakanemaru, Ohtawara, Tochigi, Japan

Abstract

The imbalance of blood and urine amino acids in renal failure has been studied mostly without chiral separation. Although a few reports have shown the presence of D-serine, an enantiomer of L-serine, in the serum of patients with severe renal failure, it has remained uncertain how serine enantiomers are deranged in the development of renal failure. In the present study, we have monitored serine enantiomers using a two-dimensional HPLC system in the serum and urine of mice after renal ischemia-reperfusion injury (IRI), known as a mouse model of acute kidney injury. In the serum, the level of D-serine gradually increased after renal IRI in parallel with that of creatinine, whereas the L-serine level decreased sharply in the early phase after IRI. The increase of D-serine was suppressed in part by genetic inactivation of a D-serine-degrading enzyme, D-amino acid oxidase (DAO), but not by disruption of its synthetic enzyme, serine racemase, in mice. Renal DAO activity was detected exclusively in proximal tubules, and IRI reduced the number of DAO-positive tubules. On the other hand, in the urine, D-serine was excreted at a rate nearly triple that of L-serine in mice with sham operations, indicating that little D-serine was reabsorbed while most L-serine was reabsorbed in physiological conditions. IRI significantly reduced the ratio of urinary D−/L-serine from 2.82 ± 0.18 to 1.10 ± 0.26 in the early phase and kept the ratio lower than 0.5 thereafter. The urinary D−/L-serine ratio can detect renal ischemia earlier than kidney injury molecule-1 (KIM-1) or neutrophil gelatinase-associated lipocalin (NGAL) in the urine, and more sensitively than creatinine, cystatin C, or the ratio of D−/L-serine in the serum. Our findings provide a novel understanding of the imbalance of amino acids in renal failure and offer a potential new biomarker for an early detection of acute kidney injury.

Editor: Leighton R. James, University of Florida, United States of America

Funding: This work was supported in part by Grant-in-Aid for Scientific Research (A). No additional external funding received for this study. The funders had no role in study design, data collection and analysis, decision to publish, or preparation of the manuscript.

Competing Interests: A microbore-monolithic ODS column used in this study was provided by Shiseido Co., Ltd. Employees of Shiseido Co., Ltd., provided technical support for the running of a 2D-HPLC system. There are no further employment, consultancy, patents, products in development or marketed products to declare. This does not alter the authors' adherence to all the PLOS ONE policies on sharing data and materials, as detailed online in the guide for authors.

* E-mail: sasabe@a8.keio.jp (JS); aiso@a3.keio.jp (SA)

Introduction

D-Serine is *de novo* synthesized from its enantiomer, L-serine, in mammals [1] and has a pivotal role in glutamatergic neurotransmission in the central nervous system (CNS) [2]. In the peripheral organs, the physiological role or regulation of D-serine remains largely unknown, apart from its regional control in the kidney. D-Serine in the plasma stems from dietary uptake and also from tissues that express the synthetic enzyme of D-serine, and it is excreted by the kidneys for the most part into the urine. Although an uptake carrier of serine in pars recta of renal proximal tubules has a low stereospecificity, only a small portion of filtered D-serine is reabsorbed since L-serine, overwhelming D-serine in primitive urine, competitively inhibits the uptake of D-serine [3]. The reabsorbed D-serine is metabolized by tubular D-amino acid oxidase (DAO) into hydroxypyruvate, hydrogen peroxide, and ammonia. Therefore, the kidney is thought to keep the plasma D-serine at a low level, up to 3% in total plasma serine in humans [4–6].

Several links between deranged D-serine regulation and renal dysfunction have been reported: plasma D-serine level increases up to more than 20% of total serine in patients with highly elevated plasma creatinine [4–6], a high level of DAO is detected in the urine of patients with chronic renal failure [7], and renal ischemia-reperfusion injury (IRI) reduces activity of renal DAO in rats [8]. D-Serine is also known to selectively damage the pars recta of proximal tubules in rats, leading to aminoaciduria and glucosuria [9,10]. Therefore, D-serine has been regarded as both an indicator and an exacerbating factor of renal dysfunction. However, how D-serine is deranged in renal dysfunction remains uncertain.

To monitor alterations of serine enantiomers in the development of renal dysfunction, we used a two-dimensional HPLC (2D-HPLC) system. In the present study, using mice with renal ischemia-reperfusion injury (IRI) as a model of acute kidney injury (AKI), we report that disposition of D-serine in the body fluid after renal IRI is closely correlated with that of creatinine. The alteration of serum D-serine originates from loss of renal DAO activity and reduced glomerular filtration rate (GFR). We also demonstrate that ratios of serine enantiomers in the casual urine may serve as a sensitive biomarker in the early detection of AKI.

Materials and Methods

Ethics Statement

All experiments on animals were carried out in accordance with institutional guidelines. The study protocol was approved by the Animal Experiment Committee of KEIO University.

Materials

The enantiomer of serine and HPLC-grade acetonitrile were obtained from Nacalai Tesque (Kyoto, Japan). Methanol of HPLC grade, trifluoroacetic acid (TFA), citric acid monohydrate, and boric acid were purchased from Wako (Osaka, Japan). Water was purified using a Milli-Q gradient A 10 system (Millipore, Bedford, MA, USA). All other reagents for 2D-HPLC were of the highest reagent grade and were used without further purification.

Human Samples

Human serum samples were obtained from BioServe Biotechnologies (Beltsville, MD, USA), and consisted of four male healthy donors and four male patients with severe renal failure. All of them were Caucasian. None of them had smoking habits or were afflicted with diabetes mellitus. Further clinical information, e.g., the stage of renal failure or pathological diagnosis, was not available. The donors' ages and renal function parameters are listed in Table S1.

Animals

Animals were maintained in a specific pathogen-free environment, housed in a light-controlled room with a 12-h light/dark cycle, and allowed ad libitum access to food and water. C57BL/6J mice were purchased from CLEA Japan (Tokyo, Japan). A mouse line with a C57BL/6J background lacking DAO activity systemically with a natural point mutation of Gly-181-Arg was generated by backcrossing ddY/DAO⁻ mice with C57BL/6J, as described previously [11]. Global serine racemase (SR)-knockout mice were generated as reported previously [12].

IRI Model

Male mice between 12–16 weeks of age underwent experimental procedures for the IRI model. Before induction of IRI, the right kidneys were removed through a small flank incision under pentobarbital. After 12 days, these mice were randomized into two groups: sham-operated (sham-op) control and IRI. The mice were anesthetized with pentobarbital, and the left kidneys were exposed through a small flank incision. Blood flow through the left renal artery and vein was interrupted with a nontraumatic clamp (Schwartz Micro Serrefines; Fine Science Tools Inc., Vancouver, Canada). After 45 min of ischemia, the vessel clamp was removed. The return of the original surface color of the kidneys was confirmed visually, and the abdomen was closed in layers. In sham-operated control mice, the kidneys were treated identically, except for clamping. At 4, 8, 20, or 40 h after reperfusion, mice were anesthetized with diethyl ether; blood and urine were collected from the inferior vena cava and bladder, respectively; and then kidneys were removed with or without perfusion fixation, depending on the subsequent experimental procedure. Sera were separated in a BD microtainer (BD, Franklin Lakes, NJ, USA) by centrifugation at 1500×g for 10 min. The levels of creatinine (Cr) and blood urea nitrogen (BUN) in the sera or urine were determined using a Fuji DRI-CHEM 4000 system (FujiFilm, Tokyo, Japan). Serum cystatin C as well as urinary kidney injury molecule-1 (KIM-1) and neutrophil gelatinase-associated lipocalin (NGAL) were quantified using mouse ELISA kits from R&D Systems (Minneapolis, MN, USA).

Two-dimensional HPLC

Serine enantiomers were determined using a 2D-HPLC system, as previously reported [11,13]. Briefly, amino acids in the serum were derivatized with 4-fluoro-7-nitro-2,1,3-benzoxadiazole (NBD-F) (Tokyo Kasei, Tokyo, Japan); subjected to HPLC (NANOSPACE SI-2 series, Shiseido, Tokyo, Japan); separated into each amino acid by a reversed-phase column (a microbore-monolithic ODS column, 0.53 mm ID×1000 mm, provided by Shiseido); and further separated into enantiomers by an enantio-selective column (Sumichiral OA-2500S, 1.5 mm ID×250 mm, self-packed; material was obtained from Sumika Chemical Analysis Service, Osaka, Japan). The fluorescence intensity was detected at 530 nm with excitation at 470 nm. Representative chromatograms of 2D separation of authentic D−/L-serine and those in mouse serum and urine are shown in Supplementary Fig. S1.

Histological Analysis

Mice were anesthetized with diethyl ether and perfused transcardially with ice-cold phosphate buffer (PB, pH 7.4) and subsequently with 2% paraformaldehyde in PB. Tissues were then cryoprotected in a 20% sucrose solution in PB at 4°C until they sank. They were frozen in Tissue-Tek O.C.T. Compound (Sakura Finetek Japan, Tokyo, Japan). Sections 10 μm thick were sliced on a cryostat at −19°C and stored at −80°C until they were used.

Sections were rinsed in phosphate buffer-saline (PBS, pH 7.4), stained with hematoxylin and eosin (H & E), dehydrated, cleared, and mounted with Entellan new (Merck, Darmstadt, Germany).

For fluorescence staining, sections were rinsed in phosphate buffer-saline (PBS, pH 7.4) and incubated in 20 μg/ml fluorescein-labeled Lotus tetragonolobus lectin (LTL) in PBS for 30 min at room temperature. The sections were washed in PBS and transfered into a DAO-activity staining solution [7 mM pyrophosphate buffer (pH 8.3), 0.1% horseradish peroxidase (Sigma-Aldrich, St. Louis, MO, USA), Cy3-conjugated tyramide (1:400; Perkin-Elmer, Waltham, MA, USA), 0.065% sodium azide, 0.6% nickel ammonium sulfate, 22 mM D-proline, 20 μM FAD] [11], and incubated at room temperature for 7 min under dark conditions. They were washed in PBS and mounted using ProLong Gold Antifade Reagent with DAPI (Invitrogen, Carlsbad, CA, USA).

Sections labeled with fluorescence were imaged using a Zeiss LSM 510 confocal microscope (Carl Zeiss, Oberkochen, Germany). Each section being compared was imaged under identical conditions.

Enzyme Activity Assay of DAO

The activity of DAO was determined as described previously [11]. Briefly, 50 μl of tissue lysate was added to a mixture [150 μl of 100 mM D-alanine, 100 μl of 0.1 mM flavin adenine dinucleotide (FAD), 150 μl of 700 units/ml catalase in 133 mM sodium pyrophosphate (pH8.3), and 50 μl of 70% v/v MeOH], processed with constant agitation at 37°C for 30–60 min, and terminated by adding 500 µl of 10% trichloroacetic acid. To 250 µl of the supernatant solution were added 250 µl of 5 M KOH and 250 µl of 0.5% 4-amino-3-hydrazino-5-mercapto-1,2,4-triazole in 0.5 M HCl. After 15 min incubation at room temperature, 250 µl of 0.75% KIO$_4$ in 0.2 M KOH was added to the mixture with vigorous shaking, and absorbance at 550 nm was measured. DAO activity was calculated as described by Watanabe et al. [14] and expressed as the amount of D-alanine oxidized per minute per milligram of protein.

Statistical Analysis

All values in the text and figures of this study indicate means ± standard error of mean (SEM). Statistical analyses for the experiments were performed with a two-tailed Student's t-test or one-way ANOVA followed by Tukey's multiple comparison test, in which $P<0.05$ was assessed as significant. All analyses were performed using Prism 5 (GraphPad Software, La Jolla, CA, USA).

Results

The D-serine in body fluid is maintained physiologically at low micromolar levels, and its quantitative measurement requires a highly sensitive and selective technique. We measured serine enantiomers using a 2D-HPLC system that enabled us to detect D−/L-serine ranging from 1 fmol to 100 pmol quantitatively with chiral selectivity. Our system was sensitive enough to detect the elevation of D-serine in the serum of patients with severe renal failure (RF) (Fig. S2), and our results were comparable to previous reports [4–6].

Derangement of Serum Serine Enantiomers after Renal IRI

To understand whether such alterations of serine enantiomers might reflect renal dysfunction, we generated renal IRI mice as an experimental model of AKI. Using the 2D-HPLC system, we quantified levels of serine enantiomers in these mice. In C57BL/6J mice, the serum D-serine did not change significantly at 4 or 8 h, was elevated at 20 h, and showed a further increase at 40 h after reperfusion (Sham, 3.7±0.3 µM; IRI 4, 3.4±0.3 µM; IRI 8, 4.3±0.4 µM; IRI 20, 5.5±0.5 µM; IRI 40, 10.6±0.4 µM) (Fig. 1A and B). On the other hand, the level of serum L-serine plunged at 4 h and remained low thereafter (Sham, 106.1±5.0 µM; IRI 4, 46.9±0.9 µM; IRI 8, 61.5±5.6 µM; IRI 20, 70.6±7.5 µM; IRI 40, 64.7±2.2 µM) (Fig. 1A and C). The ratio of D−/L-serine rose at 4 h due to the reduction of L-serine and further increased at 40 h after reperfusion (Sham, 0.036±0.004; IRI 4, 0.074±0.005; IRI 8, 0.073±0.009; IRI 20, 0.082±0.009; IRI 40, 0.164±0.008) (Fig. 1D). Similarly, the levels of serum creatinine fluctuated between 1.0–2.0 mg/dl from 4 h to 20 h and were elevated at 40 h after reperfusion (Sham, 0.59±0.05 mg/dl; IRI 4, 1.108±0.04 mg/dl; IRI 8, 1.89±0.09 mg/dl; IRI 20, 1.14±0.22 mg/dl; IRI 40, 3.73±0.09 mg/dl) (Fig. 1E). Unlike D-serine and creatinine, serum cystatin C, a marker for early detection of renal dysfunction, surged at 4 h and thereafter decreased gradually (Sham, 0.84±0.01 µg/ml; IRI 4, 1.63±0.08 µg/ml; IRI 8, 1.39±0.09 µg/ml; IRI 20, 1.19±0.05 µg/ml; IRI 40, 1.06±0.10 µg/ml) (Fig. 1F). These results show that the level of serum D-serine parallels that of serum creatinine and that a reduction in serum L-serine detects early renal dysfunction, as does an increase of serum cystatin C.

Mechanism Underlying Derangement of Serum Serine Enantiomers through SR and DAO

Regulation of serum serine enantiomers is not well understood, but it is known to be kept in balance by production, degradation, uptake, and excretion. Because SR converts L-serine into D-serine [1] and its expression in the kidney had been reported [15], we next tested whether SR contributes to the derangement of serine enantiomers after IRI. Serine enantiomers in SR knockout (SR-KO) mice were determined using 2D-HPLC. Disruption of SR reduced the basal level of serum D-serine (C57BL/6J wild-type, 3.7±0.3 µM; SR-KO, 2.5±0.2 µM). However, in the same manner as the alterations detected in C57BL/6J wild-type mice, the levels of serum D-serine increased progressively at 20 and 40 h after IRI (Sham, 2.5±0.2 µM; IRI 20, 4.8±0.5 µM; IRI 40, 6.6±0.6 µM) (Fig. 2A), while serum L-serine was significantly reduced at 20 h and remained low at 40 h after reperfusion (Sham, 89.6±9.6 µM; IRI 20, 60.0±4.5 µM; IRI 40, 62.1±5.8 µM) (Fig. 2B). The D−/L-serine ratio was elevated parallel to the increase of D-serine (Sham, 0.029±0.004; IRI 20, 0.082±0.012; IRI 40, 0.110±0.018) (Fig. 2C). These results indicate that SR does not trigger the derangement of serine enantiomers caused by renal IRI.

Serum level of D-serine can be influenced by DAO, a unique degrading enzyme of D-serine, highly expressed in the kidney. Enzyme activity of endogenous renal DAO was detected in frozen tissue sections using enzyme histochemistry (EHC), as described previously [11,16]. DAO enzymatically labeled with Cy3 was colocalized with FITC-labeled LTL, a proximal tubule marker (Fig. 3A and B). DAO was detected in LTL-positive proximal tubular epithelial cells in sham-op controls, and IRI reduced the number of proximal tubules with DAO activity at 40 h after reperfusion (Fig. 3B). In a quantification assay, DAO enzyme activity in the total kidney of C57BL/6J wild-type mice was suppressed to 73% and 67% of that of sham-op controls at 20 and 40 h after IRI, respectively [$F_{(2, 12)} = 10.97$, $P = 0.0020$] (Fig. 3C). Reduced renal DAO enzyme activity was detected also in SR-KO mice after IRI (71% at 20 h and 57% at 40 h compared with sham-op controls)[$F_{(2, 7)} = 11.34$, $P = 0.0064$] (Fig. 3D). To confirm the effect of reduced DAO activity on serum levels of serine enantiomers, we measured serum D−/L-serine in mice lacking DAO activity with a point mutation of G181R (DAO-null mice). Lack of DAO increased the basal level of serum D-serine (C57BL/6J wild-type, 3.7±0.3 µM; DAO-null, 10.8±0.4 µM). In the DAO-null mice, IRI elevated the serum D-serine at 20 h, but did not show a further increase at 40 h after reperfusion (Sham, 10.8±0.4 µM; IRI 20, 16.0±0.6 µM; IRI 40, 15.1±1.5 µM) [$F_{(2, 15)} = 8.866$, $P = 0.0029$] (Fig. 4A). Levels of serum L-serine tended to increase at 20 h and were reduced at 40 h after reperfusion (Sham, 85.5±5.8 µM; IRI 20, 116.6±10.0 µM; IRI 40, 73.3±11.1 µM) [$F_{(2, 15)} = 5.832$, $P = 0.0134$] (Fig. 4B). The ratio of D−/L-serine was unchanged at 20 h and elevated at 40 h after reperfusion compared with sham-op (Sham, 0.132±0.012; IRI 20, 0.142±0.013; IRI 40, 0.225±0.032) [$F_{(2, 15)} = 5.776$, $P = 0.0138$] (Fig. 4C). These results show that lack of DAO activity inhibits the steady increase of serum D-serine or decrease of serum L-serine caused by IRI, suggesting that the loss of DAO activity contributes, at least in part, to the derangement of serine enantiomers.

Impact of Loss of DAO activity on Renal Pathology after IRI

In rats, D-serine is nephrotoxic because of its metabolites produced by DAO. To further evaluate the contribution of DAO

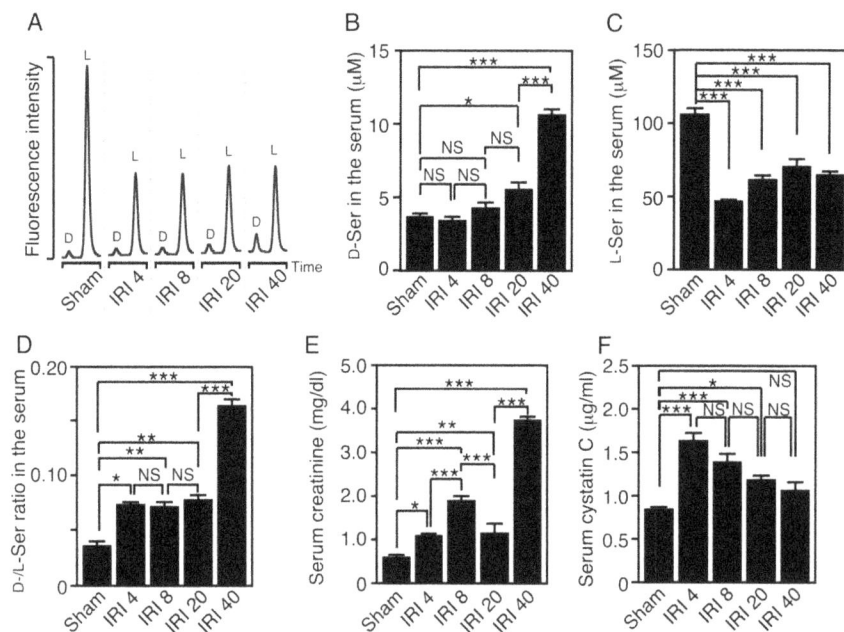

Figure 1. Renal IRI increases D-serine and reduces L-serine in mouse serum. (A) Shown are typical chromatograms of serum D−/L-serine obtained by 2D-HPLC. [Mice with sham-op (Sham); and those at 4, 8, 20, and 40 h after renal IRI (IRI 4, IRI 8, IRI 20, and IRI 40)] (B-F) Concentrations of serum D-serine (B), L-serine (C), creatinine (E), and cystatin C (F) in the C57BL/6J mice were determined, and ratios of D-serine to L-serine concentrations were calculated (D) (Sham, n = 8; IRI 4, n = 5; IRI 8, n = 9; IRI 20, n = 6; and IRI 40, n = 7). *$P < 0.05$, **$P < 0.01$, ***$P < 0.001$ (one-way ANOVA followed by Tukey's multiple comparison test). NS means 'not significant'. Data are plotted as the mean ± SEM.

to the progression of renal damage, we performed histological analysis of the kidney in C57BL/6J wild-type mice and DAO-null mice with or without IRI. The sham-op DAO-null mice showed no obvious difference in the pattern of tubules compared with sham-op wild-type controls as shown in H & E staining (Fig. 5A, upper panels). IRI tended to damage tubules more severely in DAO-null mice than in wild-type animals (Fig. 5A, lower panels) (percentage of damaged tubules: wild-type, 51.7±5.3%; and DAO-null, 65.7±5.8%. n = 5, each), although the ATN score did not differ significantly between wild-type and DAO-null mice (Fig. 5B). The number of intact proximal tubules, which was evaluated using staining with LTL, was significantly lower in DAO-null mice than in wild-type animals after renal IRI (Fig. 5C and D) [Fig. 5D: $F_{(3, 16)} = 89.64$, $P < 0.0001$]. The increase of

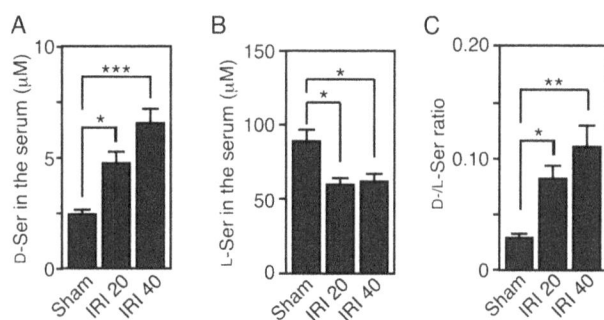

Figure 2. Knockout of SR does not affect alterations of serine enantiomers after IRI. Concentrations of D-serine (A), L-serine (B), and D−/L-serine ratio (C) in the sera of SR-KO mice were determined using 2D-HPLC (Sham, n = 4; IRI 20, n = 4; and IRI 40, n = 4). *$P < 0.05$, **$P < 0.01$, ***$P < 0.001$ (one-way ANOVA followed by Tukey's multiple comparison test). Data are plotted as the mean ± SEM.

serum Cr and BUN triggered by IRI tended to be higher in DAO-null mice than in wild-type controls, with significance at reperfusion time of 20 h for Cr and 40 h for BUN (Fig. 5E and F) [Fig. 5E: $F_{(5, 28)} = 159.4$, $P < 0.0001$; Fig. 5F: $F_{(5, 28)} = 89.3$, $P < 0.0001$]. These results indicated that DAO protects proximal tubules mildly. Therefore, the D-serine metabolites produced by DAO do not seem to exacerbate IRI-induced renal dysfunction in mice, but undegraded D-serine is suggested to do so.

Urinal Excretion of Serine Enantiomers after Renal IRI

Since loss of DAO activity in mice did not nullify the effect of IRI on serine enantiomers, involvement of other factors, such as failure to excrete serine enantiomers in the urine, cannot be excluded. Amounts of D−/L-serine in the urine display a pattern that is the inverse of those in the serum (Fig. 1A and 6A, *see chromatograms of sham-op groups*). Urinary excretion of D-serine is nearly three times greater than that of L-serine, due to preferential reabsorption of L-serine in the proximal tubule in physiological conditions. IRI reduced by half the concentration of D-serine in the casual urine at 4 h after reperfusion, with the concentration fluctuating at low levels thereafter (Sham, 52.0±7.6 μM; IRI 4, 24.5±5.7 μM; IRI 8, 9.9±1.1 μM; IRI 20, 36.9±3.3 μM; IRI 40, 22.4±3.8 μM) [$F_{(4, 22)} = 9.288$, $P = 0.0001$] (Fig. 6A and B). On the other hand, excretion of L-serine in the casual urine began to increase from 8 h and remained high at 20 and 40 h after reperfusion (Sham, 19.0±3.0 μM; IRI 4, 23.6±2.7 μM; IRI 8, 62.6±9.9 μM; IRI 20, 136.1±14.9 μM; IRI 40, 93.8±12.1 μM) [$F_{(4, 22)} = 29.49$, $P < 0.0001$] (Fig. 6A and C). Concentrations of solutes in casual urine are often expressed in terms of urinary creatinine because the excretion of creatinine is constant across individuals. However, creatinine correction is not reliable in renal dysfunction because creatinine excretion itself is disturbed in severe renal dysfunction (Fig. 6D). In this case, the D−/L-serine ratio is reliable for evaluating the urinary excretion of serine

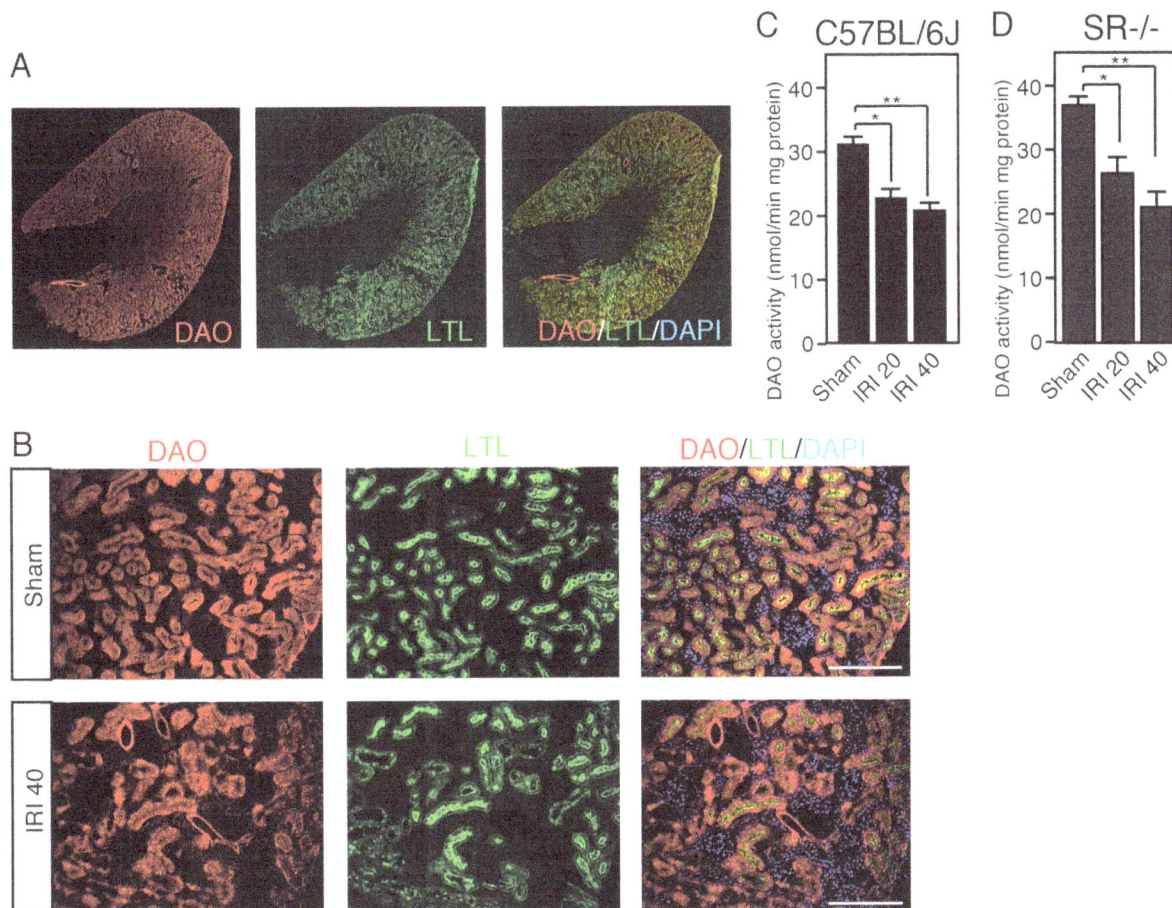

Figure 3. IRI reduces the number of proximal epithelial cells with DAO activity. (A and B) A horizontally sliced section of the kidney in a C57BL/6J wild-type mouse (A) and high magnifications of renal cortex in the mice (Sham or IRI 40) (B) were stained with DAO enzyme histochemistry, a proximal tubular marker (LTL), and a nuclear marker (DAPI). Scale bars, 200 μm. (C and D) DAO activity in the total kidneys of C57BL/6J wild-type mice [Sham, n = 4; IRI 20, n = 5; and IRI 40, n = 6] (C) and SR-KO mice [Sham, n = 3; IRI 20, n = 4; and IRI 40, n = 3] (D) was determined in a quantitative assay. *$P<0.05$, **$P<0.01$ (one-way ANOVA followed by Tukey's multiple comparison test). Data are plotted as the mean ± SEM.

enantiomers because the value is not affected by the level of urine concentration. The ratio of D−/L-serine showed a sharp decline at 4 h and became lower than 0.5 after 8 h (Sham, 2.82±0.18; IRI 4, 1.10±0.26; IRI 8, 0.16±0.01; IRI 20, 0.28±0.02; IRI 40, 0.25±0.04) [$F_{(4, 22)}=62.33$, $P<0.0001$] (Fig. 6E). On the other hand, the levels of urinary KIM-1, a key molecule for early diagnosis of AKI [17], surged at 20 h, but did increase significantly at 4 and 8 h after IRI (Sham, 1.7±0.6 ng/ml; IRI 4, 1.3±0.5 ng/ml; IRI 8, 0.4±0.2 ng/ml; IRI 20, 37.8±1.1 ng/ml; IRI 40, 11.4±4.3 ng/ml) [$F_{(4, 23)}=81.45$, $P<0.0001$] (Fig. 6F). Urinary levels of NGAL, another promising molecule [18], displayed an upward tendency at 4 h, but with no statistical significance, and rose significantly at 8 h after IRI and thereafter (Sham, 34.3±7.3 ng/ml; IRI 4, 51.1±16.3 ng/ml; IRI 8, 119.6±1.2 ng/ml; IRI 20, 119.2±1.5 ng/ml; IRI 40, 119.3±1.5 ng/ml) [$F_{(4, 23)}=31.89$, $P<0.0001$] (Fig. 6G). These results show that the urinary D−/L-serine ratio detects renal ischemia earlier than serum creatinine, urinary KIM-1, or NGAL, and more sensitively than serum cystatin C. And such deranged excretion of serine enantiomers caused by renal IRI may be the main trigger for both accumulation of D-serine and reduction of L-serine in the serum.

DAO is detected in the urine of chronic renal failure, so we further tested whether DAO affects the drop in the urinary D−/L-serine ratio after renal IRI. In DAO-null mice, IRI strikingly reduced the urinary D−/L-serine ratio (Fig. 6H–J). Therefore, non-metabolic factors such as disturbed reabsorption in the proximal tubule may contribute to the decline in the urinary D−/L-serine ratio after IRI.

Discussion

We have shown that renal IRI perturbs homeostasis of serine enantiomers in the serum and urine. In the serum, D-serine accumulates gradually in the late phase after IRI, whereas the level of L-serine falls sharply in the early phase. In the casual urine, the concentration of D-serine is reduced in the early phase after IRI, while that of L-serine is elevated in the late phase. Reduced activity of renal DAO caused by IRI is in part responsible for D-serine accumulation in the serum. Decreased GFR and disturbed proximal reabsorption are suggested to contribute to a large extent to such alterations of serine enantiomers.

The serum level of D-serine is physiologically retained at up to 5 μM, less than 1/20 of that of L-serine, and has little individual variability in humans (Fig. S2) [19,20] or in mice (Fig. 1) [21]. The degree of D-serine accumulation, corresponding to 10–20% of L-serine, in the blood of mice with severe renal dysfunction after renal IRI is similar to that in humans with RF (Fig. 1 and S2) [4–

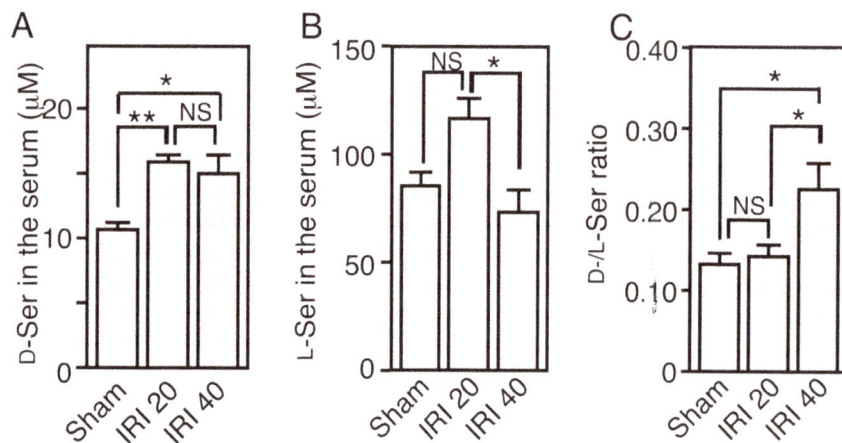

Figure 4. Lack of DAO activity suppresses IRI-induced accumulation of D-serine in serum. (A-C) The serine enantiomers in the sera of DAO-null mice were determined using 2D-HPLC, and their concentrations (D-serine, A; L-serine, B) and ratio (C) are shown (Sham, n = 6; IRI 20, n = 6; and IRI 40, n = 5). *$P<0.05$, **$P<0.01$ (one-way ANOVA followed by Tukey's multiple comparison test). NS is 'not significant'. Data are plotted as the mean $\pm$ SEM.

6], validating this animal model for investigating serine derangement in renal dysfunction. The level of serum D-serine is balanced by food intake, metabolism by SR/DAO, and renal filtration rate. For two reasons, renal reabsorption has little effect on the serum D-serine level under physiological conditions. One is preferential uptake of L-serine by a serine transporter on proximal tubules under the condition that L-serine dominates D-serine in primitive urine [3]. The other is degradation of reabsorbed D-serine by DAO in the proximal tubules. When activity of renal DAO is reduced due to the damage on the proximal tubules, disturbed

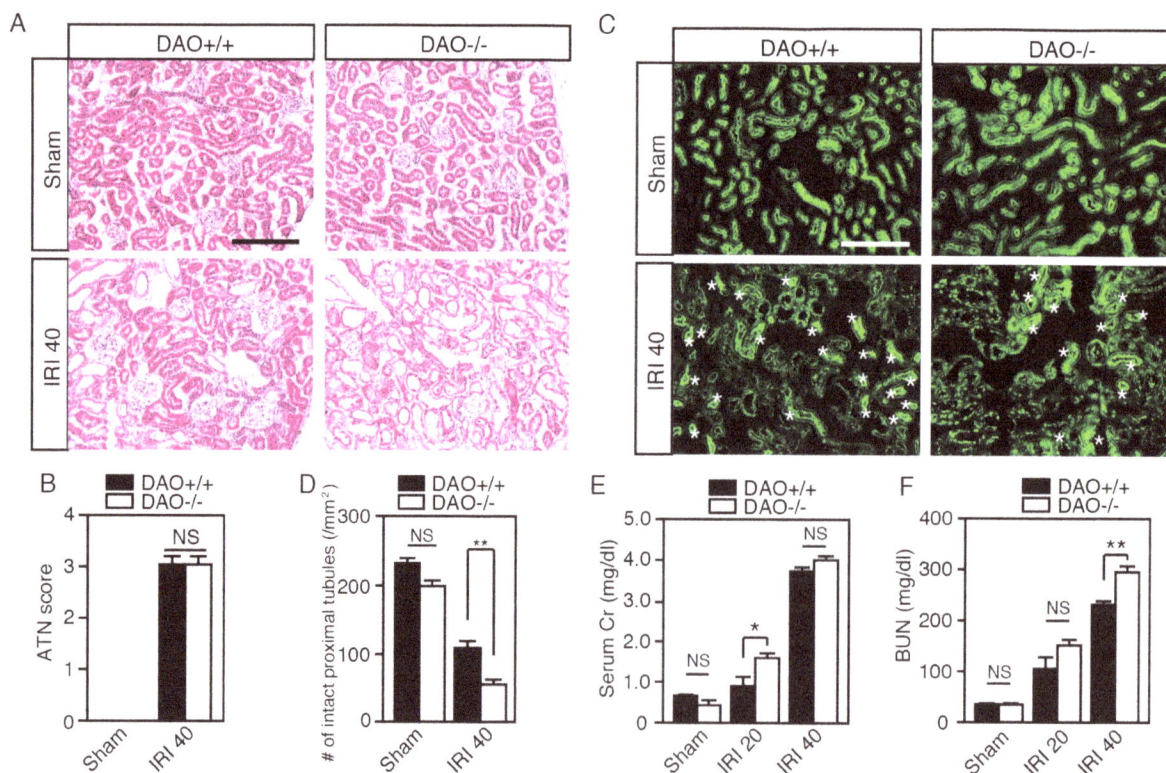

Figure 5. Lack of DAO activity exacerbates loss of intact proximal tubules and renal dysfunction induced by IRI. (A and C) Renal cortices in C57BL/6J wild-type (DAO$^{+/+}$) and DAO-null mice (DAO$^{-/-}$) after sham-op (Sham) or IRI (at 40 h after reperfusion) were stained with H & E (A) or LTL (C). (B) Damaged tubules were evaluated and ATN score was calculated in slices stained with H & E (n = 5, each group). (D) Number of intact proximal tubules was counted in slices stained with LTL (n = 5, each group). (E and F) Serum Cr (E) and BUN (F) in DAO$^{+/+}$ [Sham n = 5; IRI 20, n = 5; and IRI 40, n = 7] and DAO$^{-/-}$ mice [Sham, n = 6; IRI 20, n = 5; and IRI 40, n = 6] were measured. *$P<0.05$, **$P<0.01$, and NS is 'not significant' (one-way ANOVA followed by Tukey's multiple comparison test). Data are plotted as the mean $\pm$ SEM.

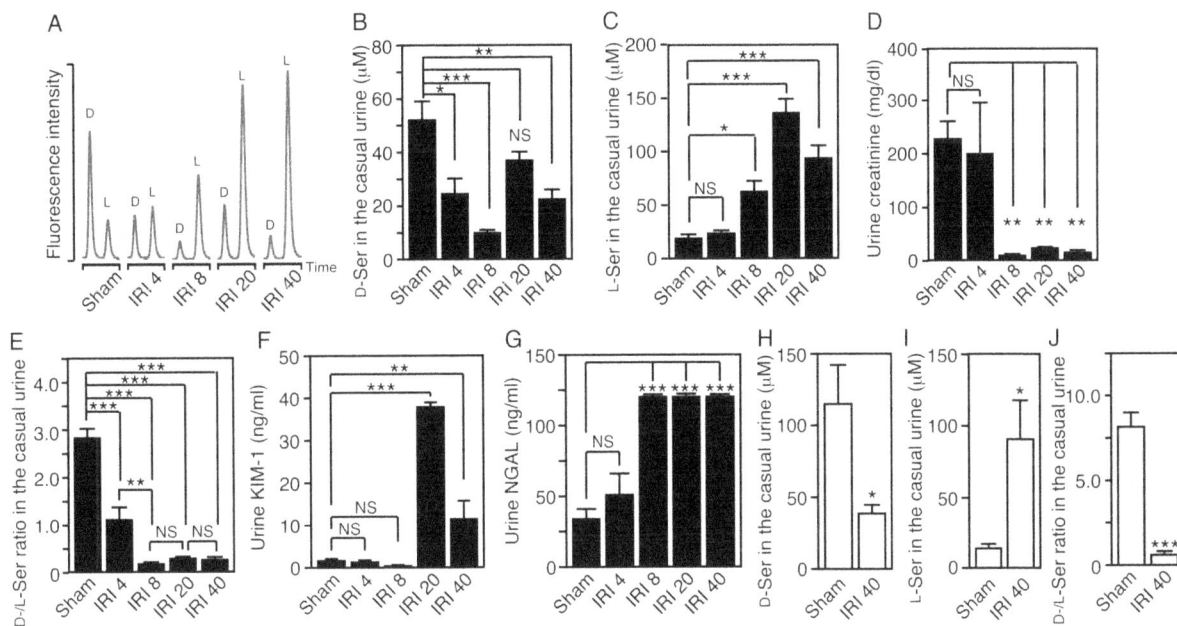

Figure 6. IRI inverts D−/L-serine ratio in urine. Urinary serine enantiomers were analyzed using 2D-HPLC. (A) Typical chromatograms showing urinary D−/L-serine in C57BL/6J wild-type mice with or without renal IRI. (B-G) Concentrations of D-serine (B), L-serine (C), creatinine (D), KIM-1 (F), and NGAL (G), and ratios of D−/L-serine (E) in the urine of the wild-type mice were determined (Sham, n = 7; IRI 4, n = 5; IRI 8, n = 5; IRI 20, n = 5; and IRI 40, n = 5). *$P<0.05$, **$P<0.01$, ***$P<0.001$ (one-way ANOVA followed by Tukey's multiple comparison test). NS means 'not significant'. (H-J) Concentrations of D-serine (H) and L-serine (I), and D−/L-serine ratios (J) in the urine of DAO-null mice were determined. *$P<0.05$, ***$P<0.001$ (two-tailed Student's t test). Data are plotted as the mean ± SEM.

degradation of reabsorbed D-serine increases its influx into systemic circulation. On the other hand, in DAO-null mice, reabsorbed D-serine passes through proximal tubules without degradation by DAO, returns back to systemic circulation, and elevates its levels in the serum. Because DAO activity is absent regardless of renal damage, IRI-induced increase of D-serine is attenuated in DAO-null mice (Fig. 4A). Our finding that loss of DAO or SR in mice could not completely nullify the IRI-induced alteration of D-serine in the serum (Fig. 2A and 4A) indicates that decreased GFR, but not impaired reabsorption, may play a role in D-serine accumulation caused by IRI. This view is supported by our results that the serum D-serine level correlates well with that of serum creatinine (Fig. 1B and E), which is not reabsorbed in tubules. The decrease of D-serine concentration in casual urine after renal IRI parallels that of urinary creatinine (Fig. 6B and D), indicating that the decrease can be explained by reduced renal filtration rate and concentrating ability, but not by impaired proximal reabsorption or degradation by DAO (Fig. 6H-J). Thus, disposition of D-serine in body fluid resembles that of creatinine.

On the other hand, disposition of L-serine is different from that of D-serine or creatinine. Although in this study we did not investigate the renal metabolism of L-serine, it is natural to think that the alterations of L-serine result largely from impairment of proximal reabsorption because the decrease in the serum (Fig. 1C) and increase in the urine (Fig. 6C) occur in the acute phase after renal IRI. In DAO-null mice, such serum L-serine reduction is attenuated although concentration of urinary L-serine is increased as in wild-type mice (Fig. 4B and 6I). Decrease of GFR caused by more-severe renal damage in DAO-null mice than in wild-type mice (Fig. 5E) may reduce urine volume and total urinary L-serine excretion, which might explain the attenuation of L-serine loss in the serum.

D-Serine potentially involves renal pathophysiology. Although high-dose injection of D-serine damages proximal tubules through oxidative stress due to metabolism by DAO in rats [9,10,22,23], our results suggest that D-serine metabolism by DAO does not exacerbate IRI-induced renal pathology in mice, but rather improves it (Fig. 5). D-Serine can affect N-methyl-D-aspartate (NMDA) glutamate receptors in the kidney. The NMDA receptor is a ligand-gated ion channel that belongs to a large family of ionotropic glutamate receptors and requires binding of a coagonist besides glutamate for its full activation. D-Serine is now regarded as an endogenous coagonist of NMDA receptors in the CNS [2,24]. In addition to broad distribution of NMDA receptors in the CNS, it has become evident that functional NMDA receptors are also expressed in various parts of nephrons including the glomeruli, proximal tubules, and collecting ducts, indicating their diverse involvement in the regulation of renal function [25–30]. Moreover, several inhibitors of NMDA receptors have been reported to ameliorate the progression of renal dysfunction in rats with renal IRI [31,32]. Considering that D-serine potentiates NMDA-evoked currents in renal cell culture [25], derangement of serum D-serine after renal IRI may affect the progression of renal pathology through impairing activities of NMDA receptors in the nephrons.

Renal IRI is a common cause of AKI, occurring with hypotension and cardiovascular surgery and inevitably during kidney transplantation. AKI is a critical clinical condition associated with a high degree of mortality, even with best supportive care. In clinical practice, AKI is predominantly detected by changes in serum creatinine. However, because serum creatinine increases only after substantial loss of GFR, the current clinical diagnosis of AKI based on creatinine limits its early detection, and consequently the prompt implementation of preventive measures, in routine clinical care. Recently, numerous new biomarkers – categorized as inflammatory mediators, excreted tubular proteins, and surrogate markers that indicate tubular damage – have been proposed as early detection markers of AKI [33]. Because AKI is multifactorial and heterogeneous in origin, it seems likely that not one single marker but a panel of biomarkers will be required to detect all subtypes of AKI. We have newly shown that the D−/L-serine ratio, especially in casual urine, detects early-stage ischemic AKI more sensitively than other promising biomarkers. Since the urinary D−/L-serine ratio is mostly determined by the rate of proximal reabsorption of L-serine, reduction of the ratio represents damage specific to proximal tubules. The reproducibility of our results in human AKI and their clinical significance, such as diagnostic specificity/ sensitivity and prognostic value of the D−/L-serine ratio, should be verified in future studies.

We conclude from our study that ischemic AKI disrupts the physiological balance of serine enantiomers in the serum and urine. The imbalance of amino acids as total amounts of D- and L-forms has been well characterized in chronic RF [34,35], and the supplementation of lost amino acids is considered important in supportive therapy. Considering that D- and L-serine are imbalanced differently in AKI, the imbalance of total amino acids in chronic RF should also be reevaluated by separating D- and L-amino acids. Thus, our study provides a novel understanding of serine enantiomers in ischemic AKI as well as a new paradigm of amino acid balance in renal physiology and pathology.

Supporting Information

Figure S1 Determination of serine enantiomers by 2D-HPLC. (A-J) Chromatograms show representative 2D-separation of authentic D−/L-serine as their NBD derivatives (A and B), or those in the serum (C-F) or urine (G-J) in wild-type mice with sham-operation (C, D, G, and H) or IRI (E, F, I, and J). (A, C, E, G, and I) Reversed-phase separation of NBD-serine was performed by using a microbore ODS column. The black bars indicate the fractions online collected to a loop and transferred to the enantioselective column, Sumichiral OA-2500S, in which NBD-serine enantiomers were further separated (B, D, F, H, and J).

Figure S2 Serum serine enantiomers are altered in patients with renal failure. D- (A) and L-serine (B) in the serum of healthy volunteers (n = 4) and patients with RF (n = 4) were measured with 2D-HPLC. (C) The ratio of D-serine to L-serine is shown. $*P<0.05$, $**P<0.01$, $***P<0.001$ (Student's t test).

Table S1 Ages and parameters for renal function in human samples. Data are shown as mean ± S.E.M. (N = 4, each).

Acknowledgments

We thank K. Yamashita, N. Suzuki, A. Gotoh, and M. Kato for assistance with animal work and D. Wylie for expert opinion on the manuscript. We appreciate M. Yamamoto for indispensable support.

Author Contributions

Conceived and designed the experiments: JS SA. Performed the experiments: JS MS YM YT CO SI. Analyzed the data: JS KH. Contributed reagents/materials/analysis tools: RK MM KH. Wrote the paper: JS.

References

1. Wolosker H, Sheth KN, Takahashi M, Mothet JP, Brady RO Jr, et al. (1999) Purification of serine racemase: biosynthesis of the neuromodulator D-serine. Proc Natl Acad Sci U S A 96: 721–725.
2. Basu AC, Tsai GE, Ma CL, Ehmsen JT, Mustafa AK, et al. (2009) Targeted disruption of serine racemase affects glutamatergic neurotransmission and behavior. Mol Psychiatry 14: 719–727.
3. Silbernagl S, Volker K, Dantzler WH (1999) D-Serine is reabsorbed in rat renal pars recta. Am J Physiol 276: F857–863.
4. Nagata Y, Akino T, Ohno K, Kataoka Y, Ueda T, et al. (1987) Free D-amino acids in human plasma in relation to senescence and renal diseases. Clin Sci (Lond) 73: 105–108.
5. Brückner H, Hausch M (1993) Gas chromatographic characterization of free D-amino acids in the blood serum of patients with renal disorders and of healthy volunteers. J Chromatogr 614: 7–17.
6. Fukushima T, Santa T, Homma H, Nagatomo R, Imai K (1995) Determination of D-amino acids in serum from patients with renal dysfunction. Biol Pharm Bull 18: 1130–1132.
7. Kawasaka K, Tatsumi N (1998) D-Amino acid oxidase activity in urine obtained from patients with renal disorders. Clin Nephrol 49: 214–220.
8. Zhang H, Qi L, Lin Y, Mao L, Chen Y (2012) Study on the decrease of renal D-amino acid oxidase activity in the rat after renal ischemia by chiral ligand exchange capillary electrophoresis. Amino Acids 42: 337–345.
9. Ganote CE, Peterson DR, Carone FA (1974) The nature of D-serine-induced nephrotoxicity. Am J Pathol 77: 269–282.
10. Kaltenbach JP, Carone FA, Ganote CE (1982) Compounds protective against renal tubular necrosis induced by D-serine and D-2,3-diaminopropionic acid in the rat. Exp Mol Pathol 37: 225–234.
11. Sasabe J, Miyoshi Y, Suzuki M, Mita M, Konno R, et al. (2012) D-Amino acid oxidase controls motoneuron degeneration through D-serine. Proc Natl Acad Sci U S A 109: 627–632.
12. Miyoshi Y, Konno R, Sasabe J, Ueno K, Tojo Y, et al. (2012) Alteration of intrinsic amounts of D-serine in the mice lacking serine racemase and D-amino acid oxidase. Amino Acids 43: 1919–1931.
13. Miyoshi Y, Hamase K, Okamura T, Konno R, Kasai N, et al. (2011) Simultaneous two-dimensional HPLC determination of free D-serine and D-alanine in the brain and periphery of mutant rats lacking D-amino-acid oxidase. J Chromatogr B 879: 3184–3189.
14. Watanabe T, Motomura Y, Suga T (1978) A new colorimetric determination of D-amino acid oxidase and urate oxidase activity. Anal Biochem 86: 310–315.
15. Xia M, Liu Y, Figueroa DJ, Chiu CS, Wei N, et al. (2004) Characterization and localization of a human serine racemase. Brain Res Mol Brain Res 125: 96–104.
16. Horiike K, Tojo H, Arai R, Nozaki M, Maeda T (1994) D-Amino-acid oxidase is confined to the lower brain stem and cerebellum in rat brain: regional differentiation of astrocytes. Brain Res 652: 297–303.
17. Han W, Bailly V, Abichandani R, Thadhani R, Bonventre J (2002) Kidney Injury Molecule-1 (KIM-1): a novel biomarker for human renal proximal tubule injury. Kidney Int 62: 237–44.
18. Mishra J, Ma Q, Prada A, Mitsnefes M, Zahedi K, et al. (2003) Identification of neutrophil gelatinase-associated lipocalin as a novel early urinary biomarker for ischemic renal injury. J Am Soc Nephrol 14: 2534–43.
19. Hashimoto K, Fukushima T, Shimizu E, Komatsu N, Watanabe H, et al. (2003) Decreased serum levels of D-serine in patients with schizophrenia: evidence in support of the N-methyl-D-aspartate receptor hypofunction hypothesis of schizophrenia. Arch Gen Psychiatry 60: 572–576.
20. Grant SL, Shulman Y, Tibbo P, Hampson DR, Baker GB (2006) Determination of D-serine and related neuroactive amino acids in human plasma by high-performance liquid chromatography with fluorimetric detection. J Chromatogr B 844: 278–282.
21. Miyoshi Y, Hamase K, Tojo Y, Mita M, Konno R, et al. (2009) Determination of D-serine and D-alanine in the tissues and physiological fluids of mice with various D-amino-acid oxidase activities using two-dimensional high-performance liquid chromatography with fluorescence detection. J Chromatogr B 877: 2506–2512.
22. Maekawa M, Okamura T, Kasai N, Hori Y, Summer KH, et al. (2005) D-Amino-acid oxidase is involved in D-serine-induced nephrotoxicity. Chem Res Toxicol 18: 1678–1682.
23. Krug AW, Volker K, Dantzler WH, Silbernagl S (2007) Why is D-serine nephrotoxic and alpha-aminoisobutyric acid protective? Am J Physiol Renal Physiol 293: F382–390.
24. Mothet JP, Parent AT, Wolosker H, Brady RO Jr, Linden DJ, et al. (2000) D-Serine is an endogenous ligand for the glycine site of the N-methyl-D-aspartate receptor. Proc Natl Acad Sci U S A 97: 4926–4931.
25. Anderson M, Suh JM, Kim EY, Dryer SE (2011) Functional NMDA receptors with atypical properties are expressed in podocytes. Am J Physiol Cell Physiol 300: C22–32.
26. Gonzalez-Cadavid NF, Ryndin I, Vernet D, Magee TR, Rajfer J (2000) Presence of NMDA receptor subunits in the male lower urogenital tract. J Androl 21: 566–578.

27. Kottgen M, Benzing T (2011) Strangers on a train: atypical glutamate receptors in the kidney glomerulus. Focus on "Functional NMDA receptors with atypical properties are expressed in podocytes". Am J Physiol Cell Physiol 300: C9–10.

28. Leung JC, Travis BR, Verlander JW, Sandhu SK, Yang SG, et al. (2002) Expression and developmental regulation of the NMDA receptor subunits in the kidney and cardiovascular system. Am J Physiol Regul Integr Comp Physiol 283: R964–971.

29. Sproul A, Steele SL, Thai TL, Yu S, Klein JD, et al. (2011) N-methyl-D-aspartate receptor subunit NR3a expression and function in principal cells of the collecting duct. Am J Physiol Renal Physiol 301: F44–54.

30. Deng A, Thomson SC (2009) Renal NMDA receptors independently stimulate proximal reabsorption and glomerular filtration. Am J Physiol Renal Physiol 296: F976–982.

31. Yang CC, Chien CT, Wu MH, Ma MC, Chen CF (2008) NMDA receptor blocker ameliorates ischemia-reperfusion-induced renal dysfunction in rat kidneys. Am J Physiol Renal Physiol 294: F1433–1440.

32. Pundir M, Arora S, Kaur T, Singh R, Singh AP (2013) Effect of modulating the allosteric sites of N-methyl-D-aspartate receptors in ischemia-reperfusion induced acute kidney injury. J Surg Res: 183: 668–677.

33. Obermuller N, Geiger H, Weipert C, Urbschat A (2013) Current developments in early diagnosis of acute kidney injury. Int Urol Nephrol, in press.

34. Furst P (1989) Amino acid metabolism in uremia. J Am Coll Nutr 8: 310–323.

35. Tizianello A, Deferrari G, Garibotto G, Robaudo C, Saffioti S, et al. (1989) Amino acid imbalance in patients with chronic renal failure. Contrib Nephrol 75: 185–193.

The Association between Contrast Dose and Renal Complications Post PCI across the Continuum of Procedural Estimated Risk

Judith Kooiman[1], Milan Seth[2], David Share[3], Simon Dixon[4], Hitinder S. Gurm[2]*

1 Department of Thrombosis and Hemostasis and Department of Nephrology, Leiden University Medical Center, Leiden, Zuid-Holland, The Netherlands, **2** Department of Internal Medicine, Division of Cardiovascular Medicine, University of Michigan, Ann Arbor, Michigan, United States of America, **3** Blue Cross Blue Shield of Michigan, Detroit, Michigan, United States of America, **4** Beaumont Hospital, Royal Oak, Michigan, United States of America

Abstract

Background: Prior studies have proposed to restrict the contrast volume (CV) to <3x calculated creatinine clearance (CCC), to prevent contrast induced nephropathy (CIN) post percutaneous coronary interventions (PCI). The predictive value of this algorithm for CIN and therefore the benefit of this approach in high risk patients has been questioned. The aim of our study was to assess the association between contrast dose and the occurrence of CIN in patients at varying predicted risks of CIN and baseline CCC following contemporary PCI.

Methods: Consecutive patients undergoing PCI between 2010–2012 were included. Baseline risk of CIN was calculated using a previously validated risk tool. High contrast dose was defined as CV/CCC >3. Likelihood ratio tests were used to evaluate whether the effect of a high contrast dose on the risk of CIN and nephropathy requiring dialysis (NRD) varied across the spectrum of baseline predicted risk.

Results: Of the 82,120 PCI included in our analysis, 25% were performed using a high contrast dose. Patients treated with a high compared with a low contrast dose were at increased risks of CIN and NRD, throughout the entire range of baseline predicted risk and CCC in our population. The effect size of a high contrast dose on risks of both outcomes varied significantly with baseline predicted CIN risk and CCC (CIN p = 0.004, NRD p<0.001 for adding interactions), and was largest for patients with predicted CIN risk <10% and pre-existing chronic kidney disease.

Conclusions: The use of a high contrast dose is associated with increased risks of CIN and NRD across the continuum of baseline predicted risk and CCC. Efforts to reduce contrast dose may therefore be effective in preventing renal complications in all patients undergoing PCI.

Editor: Davide Capodanno, Ferrarotto Hospital, University of Catania, Italy

Funding: The BMC2 registry is funded by Blue Cross Blue Shield of Michigan. Hitinder S. Gurm receives research funding from the National Institutes of Health and Agency for Healthcare Research and Quality. The funders had no role in study design, data collection and analysis, decision to publish, or preparation of the manuscript.

Competing Interests: One of the co-authors, Dr. Share is currently employed by Blue Cross Blue Shield of Michigan. Hitinder S. Gurm has, in the interim, consulted for Osprey medical, a company that is developing devices for prevention of contrast induced kidney injury. No compensation was received for this work but the company made a donation to a local non-profit of his choice. This does not alter the authors' adherence to all the PLOS ONE policies on sharing data and materials.

* E-mail: hgurm@med.umich.edu

Introduction

Contrast media induced renal complications are common among patients undergoing percutaneous coronary interventions (PCI) [1]. Contrast induced nephropathy (CIN) and the need for dialysis (NRD) post PCI have been associated with increased early and long-term mortality rates, and add significantly to healthcare expenses [1,2]. Current guidelines support multiple strategies for prophylaxis of CIN including adequate hydration, minimization of contrast dose and the use of iso-osmolar or certain low-osmolar contrast media[3–7].

Use of renal function based contrast dosing with the total contrast volume (CV) restricted to less than thrice the calculated creatinine clearance (CCC) has been suggested as a practical strategy to reduce the risk of CIN [3]. However, the predictive value of this dosing algorithm for CIN and hence the benefit of this approach in patients at high risk of renal complications post PCI has been debated [8].

We recently reported an accurate prediction model for the risk of renal complications in patients undergoing PCI [9]. This model estimates the risk of CIN and NRD based on pre-procedural variables, has a higher discriminative power than other commonly used prediction models, and can therefore be used to study the effect of a high contrast dose on the occurrence of CIN in patients with varying baseline risks of renal complications.

The aim of our current study was to assess the impact of high contrast dose (CV/CCC >3) on the risk of renal complications across the continuum of pre-procedural predicted risk of CIN in a large cohort of patients undergoing contemporary PCI.

Methods

Our study population comprised consecutive patients undergoing PCI between January 2010 and September 2012 across 47 hospitals in Michigan participating in the Blue Cross Blue Shield of Michigan Cardiovascular Consortium (BMC2). Hence, this cohort consists of patients other than the population in which the effect of renal function-based contrast dosing on the risk of renal complications was originally assessed (who underwent PCI between 2007 and 2008) [3]. BMC2 is a quality improvement collaborative that tracks the inpatient outcome of consecutive patients undergoing PCI at all non-federal hospitals in the State of Michigan. The details of the BMC2 and its data collection and auditing process have been described previously [10,11]. Procedural data on all consecutive patients undergoing PCI at participating hospitals are collected using standardized data collection forms. Collected data include clinical and demographic patient characteristics, procedural, and angiographic characteristics, as well as medications used before, during, and after PCI, and in-hospital outcomes. All data elements have been prospectively defined, and the protocol is approved by local institutional review boards at each of the participating hospitals. In addition to a random audit in 2% of all PCI procedures, medical records of all patients undergoing multiple procedures or coronary artery bypass grafting and of patients who died in the hospital are reviewed routinely to ensure data accuracy.

Patients who were already on dialysis at the time of PCI, those with missing serum creatinine values pre or post procedurally, and those who died in the catheterization laboratory were excluded from outcome analysis. Patients with missing values for weight, gender, or CV were also excluded as these variables were needed to determine whether a patient received a high contrast dose. The type and volume of contrast media and hydration protocols used were as per the operator preference guided by institutional policy and practice.

Study Endpoints

CIN was defined as an acute decline in renal function post PCI resulting in an absolute increase in serum creatinine ≥ 0.5 mg/dL from baseline [12]. Baseline creatinine values were collected within a month prior to PCI. Among patients who had multiple assessments of serum creatinine in the month prior to PCI, the value closest to the time of the procedure was considered as the baseline value. Peak creatinine was defined as the highest value of creatinine in the week following the procedure or during the hospitalization following PCI and was ascertained as per local clinical practice. Time between PCI and peak creatinine was at least 1 day, and varied depending on length of hospital stay. The secondary endpoint for the study was NRD defined as a new, unplanned need for dialysis during hospitalization due to progression of chronic kidney disease post PCI.

High contrast dose was defined as administration of a CV thrice the CCC. CCC was calculated using the Cockgroft-Gault equation [13].

Statistical Analyses

Continuous variables are presented as mean with standard deviation and categorical variables as percentages, with standardized differences between groups presented for both types of variables as percentages. Unless otherwise stated, student t-tests for continuous and Chi-squared tests for categorical variables were utilized for univariate comparisons.

Baseline estimated risk of CIN was calculated using the BMC2 CIN prediction tool [9]. Multivariate logistic regression models with CIN and NRD as outcomes were developed including high contrast dose, baseline estimated CIN risk, CCC, and other baseline clinical covariates as main effect terms. To investigate potential effect modification of baseline predicted CIN risk on CIN and NRD rates associated with a high contrast dose, regression models adding two and three way interaction terms involving baseline estimated CIN risk (logit transformed linear and quadratic terms) and CCC with high contrast dose were fitted to the data. A stepwise selection algorithm optimizing the Akaike Information Criteria was used to select an optimal model. The selected models including interactions were then compared to the base model using likelihood ratio tests to assess whether inclusion of interactions significantly improved the fit of the model.

Model predicted relative risks for CIN and NRD comparing high with low contrast dosages were plotted over a range of CCC and baseline predicted risk of CIN, to demonstrate the extent and implications of effect modification.

All analyses were performed in R version 2.14.1 using freely distributed contributed packages [14,15].

Results

Our study cohort comprised 82,120 (85%) of the 96,753 PCI procedures performed across Michigan between January 2010 through December 2012. Of the 14,633(15%) procedures that were excluded from the analysis, 2,251 (15%) patients were already on dialysis at the time of the procedure, 11,997 (82%) had missing serum creatinine values prior to (n = 2,229 (15%)) or following PCI (n = 9,907 (68%)), with 139 patients missing both pre and post procedural creatinine values. Additionally, 466 patients lacked information on CV, 99 on bodyweight, and 1 patient on gender. As all of these variables were needed to determine whether a patient received a high contrast dose, patients missing one or more of these data elements were excluded.

Table 1 reports characteristics at baseline of study patients categorized to the use of either a low or a high contrast dose at time of PCI (CV/CCC < = 3 and CV/CCC >3). In this cohort, 20,915(25.3%) patients received a high contrast dose who had a greater burden of comorbidities, a higher baseline estimated CIN risk, and were more likely to have preexisting chronic kidney disease.

The median predicted risk of CIN of the cohort was 0.54% (range = 0–80.4%, IQR = 0.08%–2.43%), and 90% of patients had a predicted risk of less than 7.92%. Patients at higher predicted risk of CIN were more likely to be treated with a high contrast dose (p<0.001, Figure 1).

CIN occurred in 2,146/82,120 (2.61%, 95% CI 2.51–2.72%) patients, and NRD in 308/82,120 (0.37%, 95% CI 0.33–0.42%). The median baseline CIN risk estimate, calculated using the risk tool, was 11.6% (IQR 3.1–25.5%) among patients developing CIN, and 24.9% (10.9–36.6%) among those with NRD. Of patients with CIN, 1,144/2,146 (53.3%, 95% CI 51.2–55.4%) received a high contrast doses, as did 211/308 (68.5%, 95% CI 63.0–73.7%) patients with NRD.

In regression models adjusting for baseline predicted CIN risk and CCC, high contrast dose was significantly associated with increased rates of both CIN (OR = 1.61, 95% CI 1.46–1.79, P< .001) and NRD (OR = 1.65, 95% CI 1.24–2.21, P<.001), indicating that high contrast dose is an independent predictor of these outcomes. Within a multivariate model adjusting for baseline

Table 1. Baseline characteristics of patients treated with high versus low contrast dose.

Characteristic	CV/CCC ≤3	CV/CCC >3	P-value	Standardized difference (%)
N (procedures)	61.205 (74.5%)	20.915 (25.5%)	NA	NA
BMI	31.48±7.83	27.89±5.63	<0.001	52.54
Age	62.16±11.36	73.26±10.53	<0.001	101.28
Creatinine clearance (CCC)	106.24±42.83	59.10±22.87	<0.001	137.31
Contrast volume (ml)	171.84±63.15	248.90±88.46	<0.001	100.28
Predicted CIN risk (%)	2.10±4.99	5.23±8.91	<0.001	43.32
Female gender	18.838/61.205 (30.8%)	9.039/20.915 (43.2%)	<0.001	25.98
Race - White	53.502/61.205 (87.4%)	17.725/20.915 (84.7%)	<0.001	7.71
Race - Black or African American	6.189/61.205 (10.1%)	2.655/20.915 (12.7%)	<0.001	8.13
Current/recent smoker (w/in 1 year)	20.138/61.178 (32.9%)	4.099/20.906 (19.6%)	<0.001	30.60
Hypertension	51.108/61.185 (83.5%)	18.726/20.905 (89.6%)	<0.001	17.79
Prior MI	20.910/61.196 (34.2%)	7.645/20.910 (36.6%)	<0.001	5.01
Prior heart failure	7.924/61.185 (13.0%)	4.696/20.907 (22.5%)	<0.001	25.11
Prior PCI	27.440/61.200 (44.8%)	9.087/20.913 (43.5%)	<0.001	2.79
Prior CABG	9.642/61.187 (15.8%)	5.668/20.912 (27.1%)	<0.001	27.92
Cerebrovascular disease	7.821/61.187 (12.8%)	4.652/20.907 (22.3%)	<0.001	25.11
Peripheral arterial disease	8.447/61.190 (13.8%)	4.937/20.909 (23.6%)	<0.001	25.35
Diabetes mellitus	22.697/61.198 (37.1%)	7.715/20.912 (36.9%)	0.614	0.40
CAD presentation/Evaluation				
No symptom. no angina	4.172/61.185 (6.8%)	1.329/20.906 (6.4%)	0.021	1.86
Symptom unlikely ischemic	1.352/61.185 (2.2%)	494/20.906 (2.4%)	0.197	1.03
Stable angina	9.701/61.185 (15.9%)	3.215/20.906 (15.4%)	0.102	1.31
Unstable angina	24.129/61.185 (39.4%)	7.957/20.906 (38.1%)	<0.001	2.82
Non-STEMI	12.223/61.185 (20.0%)	4.619/20.906 (22.1%)	<0.001	5.20
STEMI or equivalent	9.608/61.185 (15.7%)	3.292/20.906 (15.7%)	0.881	0.12
Cardiogenic shock w/in 24 hours	759/61.187 (1.2%)	592/20.909 (2.8%)	<0.001	11.28
Cardiac arrest w/in 24 hours	1.037/61.166 (1.7%)	460/20.901 (2.2%)	<0.001	3.66
PCI Indication				
Immediate PCI for STEMI	8.451/61.195 (13.8%)	2.912/20.909 (13.9%)	0.672	0.34
PCI for STEMI (unstable. >12 hrs from Sx onset)	421/61.195 (0.7%)	223/20.909 (1.1%)	<0.001	4.06
PCI for STEMI (Stable. >12 hrs from Sx onset)	218/61.195 (0.4%)	85/20.909 (0.4%)	0.301	0.82
Staged PCI	4.222/61.195 (6.9%)	870/20.909 (4.2%)	<0.001	12.00

Data are presented as mean (SD), or N (%) unless stated otherwise.
Abbreviations: BMI = body mass index, CIN = contrast induced nephropathy, CV/CCC = contrast volume/calculated creatinine clearance, MI = myocardial infarction, PCI = percutaneous coronary intervention, CABG = coronary artery bypass graft, CAD = coronary artery disease, STEMI = ST-elevation myocardial infarction.

clinical covariates (age, gender, recent heart failure, cardiogenic shock, cardiac arrest, CAD presentation, PCI status and indications), the effect of high contrast dose on the risk of CIN and NRD was consistent for both outcomes (CIN OR = 1.77, 95% CI 1.58–1.98, P<.001, NRD OR = 1.92, 95% CI 1.13–2.16, P<0.01).

Regression models were developed to investigate potential effect modification of baseline predicted CIN risk and baseline CCC on the association between high contrast dose and the risks of CIN and NRD. The fit of the models were significantly improved compared with the base models after adding of interaction terms involving baseline estimated CIN risk and CCC (Likelihood ratio test: LR 28 on 11 df, p = 0.004 for CIN,LR = 29 on 6 df, p<0.001 for NRD). This indicates that the effect of high contrast dose on

the risks of both CIN and NRD varied significantly across the spectrum of predicted CIN risk and baseline CCC.

Figure 2 depicts the model predicted relative risk of CIN (Figure 2A) and NRD (Figure 2B) for high versus a low contrast dose across the spectrum of baseline predicted risk and CCC. Both figures demonstrate an increased risk of renal complications post PCI associated with a high contrast dose regardless of a patient's baseline predicted risk or CCC, although the effect of a high contrast dose was most pronounced in those at lower predicted risk. The points on the graphed surfaces highlighted in red represent the estimated relative risks of high versus a low contrast dose at the median baseline risk and creatinine clearance values for patients with CIN (risk: 11.6%, CCC: 57 ml/min) and NRD (risk: 24.9%, CCC: 42.6 ml/min). The relative risk associated with

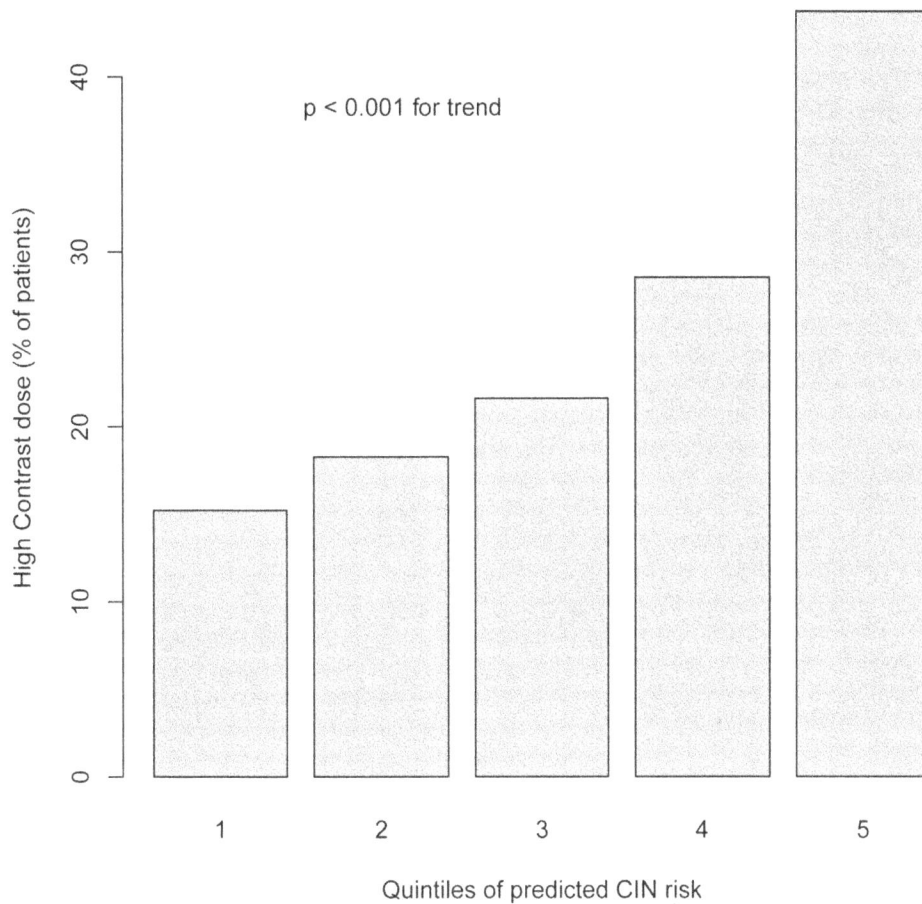

Figure 1. Proportions of patients treated with high dose contrast (Contrast volume/calculated creatinine clearance >3) across the quintiles of predicted risk of contrast induced nephropathy.

high a contrast dose at this point is 1.56 (95% CI 1.37–1.76) for CIN, and 2.05 (95% CI 1.35–2.75) for NRD.

Discussion

The key finding of our study is that the use of a high contrast dose is associated with increased risks of CIN and NRD across the

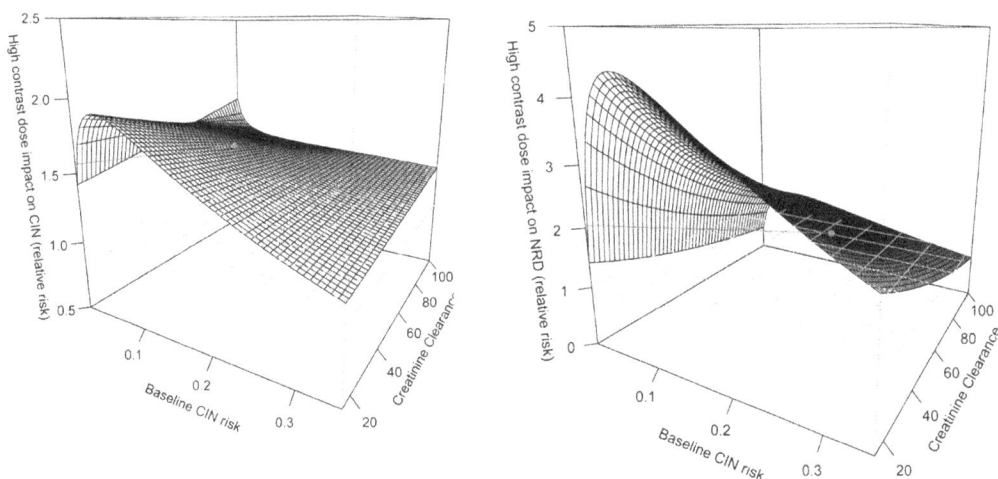

Figure 2. A. The relative risk of contrast induced nephropathy in association with high contrast dose across the continuum of predicted risk of contrast induced nephropathy among patients undergoing PCI. **B.** The relative risk of nephropathy requiring dialysis in association with high contrast dose across the continuum of predicted risk of contrast induced nephropathy among patients undergoing PCI.

continuum of predicted risk and CCC. Efforts to reduce the contrast dose may therefore be effective in preventing renal complications in all patients undergoing PCI. Especially in patients with pre-existing renal failure, restricting the contrast dose might result in lower rates of NRD.

Our findings significantly add to extend prior observations in this field. Work from many groups including ours has highlighted the role of high contrast dose as a risk factor for CIN and NRD in patients undergoing invasive cardiac procedures [3,16,17]. We have now demonstrated that regardless of baseline CCC and predicted risk of renal complications, the use of a high contrast dose is associated with increased risks of CIN and NRD post PCI. These results are in line with the results of two previous smaller studies concluding a high contrast dose to be associated with an increased risk of CIN throughout the continuum of baseline renal function [18,19]. These studies however, did not analyze the effect of baseline predicted risk on the association between a high contrast dose and renal complications post PCI. Our results demonstrated the effect of a high contrast dose on the risk of CIN and NRD to be most pronounced in those at lower predicted risk.

Efforts to improve outcomes of patients undergoing PCI for acute myocardial infarction or cardiogenic shock have traditionally focused on enhancing myocardial perfusion and hemodynamic support [20,21]. Restriction of contrast dose might be another important strategy to improve patient outcome after PCI, as our study findings suggest that the use of high contrast dosages is associated with an increased risk of CIN in all patients undergoing PCI. Limiting the CV to less than thrice the CCC may be even more important in patients at high risk of CIN, in terms of an absolute risk reduction, but also in those with pre-existing chronic kidney disease (i.e. eGFR <60 ml/min) in whom the effect of a high contrast dose on the risks of CIN was more profound compared to those without renal impairment. Our study findings also suggest that efforts to limit contrast dose in patients undergoing PCI may be helpful in reducing the risk of NRD, a complication which although rare, has not declined in the last few years among patients undergoing PCI, regardless of the introduction of less nephrotoxic contrast agents.

Patients at high predicted risk of CIN were more likely to receive a high contrast dose in our study. These patients might more frequently have comorbidity than patients receiving a low contrast dose, like peripheral artery disease, or an altered coronary vasculature due to prior PCI or prior coronary artery bypass graft resulting in more complex PCI procedures, requiring higher contrast volumes. Additionally, as a high contrast dose (CV/CCC >3) is also driven by impaired renal function, the frequent use of a high contrast dose in patients at high risk might also be explained by comorbidity associated with chronic kidney disease, increasing the baseline predicted risk of CIN. Measures to reduce contrast dose are well recognized in literature but most of the work on contrast preservation has been performed in elective or stable patients, not those with acute myocardial infarction. Therefore, further research of the preventive effect of contrast preservation on the risk of renal complications in patients undergoing emergent PCI is warranted [22].

Our study findings must, however, be interpreted with certain qualifications. Our study associations, while strong do not support causality. However, it is unlikely that a randomized trial would ever be performed to evaluate the impact of high versus low contrast dose on the risk of renal complications. Since the findings appear biologically plausible and statistically robust, measures to limit contrast dose especially in high risk patients should be considered to reduce the risk of CIN and NRD. We have used the term CIN, although the role of contrast media in all patients who develop acute kidney injury after PCI remains debatable. It is likely that acute kidney injury after PCI is multifactorial and it may be preferable to use terms that do not assume that all renal dysfunction after PCI is secondary to contrast media. However, regardless of the term used, our study suggests that there is strong association between a high contrast dose and acute renal failure post PCI, even in high risk patients, implying that contrast media have an important contributory role towards the development of acute renal failure post PCI observed in this population. Only one post–procedure creatinine value was available and no follow up beyond the initial hospitalization was performed. Moreover, we lacked information on the timing of post-procedure serum creatinine measurements. No data on the type and amount of hydration used were available and this likely varied across institutions. However, we believe this makes our findings more generalizable to routine clinical care since it reflects observations from contemporary practice across multiple institutions.

To conclude, the use of a high contrast dose at time of PCI is associated with increased risks of CIN and NRD in all patients, regardless of their baseline predicted risk of these complications and renal function. Future research is needed to study whether the use of CV restricting measures decrease the risk of renal complications post PCI in patients with acute myocardial infarction. Until then, efforts to reduce CVs to less than thrice a patient's CCC should be encouraged for all patients undergoing PCI.

Author Contributions

Conceived and designed the experiments: HG JK MS. Analyzed the data: MS. Wrote the paper: JK. Provided critical review on study design and revision of the manuscript: SD DS.

References

1. Rihal CS, Textor SC, Grill DE, Berger PB, Ting HH, et. al. Incidence and prognostic importance of acute renal failure after percutaneous coronary intervention. Circulation 105: 2259–2264.

2. Gupta R, Gurm HS, Bhatt DL, Chew DP, Ellis SG (2005) Renal failure after percutaneous coronary intervention is associated with high mortality. Catheter Cardiovasc Interv 64: 442–448. 10.1002/ccd.20316 [doi].

3. Gurm HS, Dixon SR, Smith DE, Share D, Lalonde T, et al. (2011) Renal function-based contrast dosing to define safe limits of radiographic contrast media in patients undergoing percutaneous coronary interventions. J Am Coll Cardiol 58: 907–914. S0735-1097(11)02052-3 [pii];10.1016/j.jacc.2011.05.023 [doi].

4. Meier P, Ko DT, Tamura A, Tamhane U, Gurm HS (2009) Sodium bicarbonate-based hydration prevents contrast-induced nephropathy: a meta-analysis. BMC Med 7: 23. 1741-7015-7-23 [pii];10.1186/1741-7015-7-23 [doi].

5. Reed M, Meier P, Tamhane UU, Welch KB, Moscucci M, et al. (2009) The relative renal safety of iodixanol compared with low-osmolar contrast media: a meta-analysis of randomized controlled trials. JACC Cardiovasc Interv 2: 645–654. S1936-8798(09)00322-7 [pii];10.1016/j.jcin.2009.05.002 [doi].

6. Reed MC, Moscucci M, Smith DE, Share D, Lalonde T, et al. (2010) The relative renal safety of iodixanol and low-osmolar contrast media in patients undergoing percutaneous coronary intervention. Insights from Blue Cross Blue Shield of Michigan Cardiovascular Consortium (BMC2). J Invasive Cardiol 22: 467–472.

7. Stacul F, van der Molen AJ, Reimer P, Webb JA, Thomsen HS, et al. (2011) Contrast induced nephropathy: updated ESUR Contrast Media Safety Committee guidelines. Eur Radiol 21: 2527–2541. 10.1007/s00330-011-2225-0 [doi].

8. Kalra N, Fenster P (2012) Is renal function-based contrast dosing of radiographic contrast media in patients undergoing percutaneous coronary intervention sufficient to delineate safe limits of contrast dose? J Am Coll Cardiol 59: 432–433. S0735-1097(11)04825-X [pii];10.1016/j.jacc.2011.09.060 [doi].

9. Gurm HS, Seth M, Kooiman J, Share D (2013) A novel tool for reliable and accurate prediction of renal complications in patients undergoing percutaneous coronary intervention. J Am Coll Cardiol 61: 2242–2248. S0735-1097(13)01348-X [pii];10.1016/j.jacc.2013.03.026 [doi].

10. Kline-Rogers E, Share D, Bondie D, Rogers B, Karavite D, et al. (2002) Development of a multicenter interventional cardiology database: the Blue Cross Blue Shield of Michigan Cardiovascular Consortium (BMC2) experience. J Interv Cardiol 15: 387–392.

11. Moscucci M, Rogers EK, Montoye C, Smith DE, Share D, et.al. (2006) Association of a continuous quality improvement initiative with practice and outcome variations of contemporary percutaneous coronary interventions. Circulation 113: 814–822. CIRCULATIONAHA.105.541995 [pii];10.1161/CIRCULATIONAHA.105.541995 [doi].

12. Slocum NK, Grossman PM, Moscucci M, Smith DE, Aronow HD, et al. (2012) The changing definition of contrast-induced nephropathy and its clinical implications: insights from the Blue Cross Blue Shield of Michigan Cardiovascular Consortium (BMC2). Am Heart J 163: 829–834. S0002-8703(12)00095-6 [pii];10.1016/j.ahj.2012.02.011 [doi].

13. Cockcroft DW, Gault MH (1976) Prediction of creatinine clearance from serum creatinine. Nephron 16: 31–41.

14. Liaw A, Wiener M (2002) Classification and Regression by random Forest. R News 2: 18–22.

15. Robin X, Turck N, Hainard A, Tiberti N, Lisacek F, et.al. (2011) pROC: an open-source package for R and S+ to analyze and compare ROC curves. BMC Bioinformatics 12: 77. 1471-2105-12-77 [pii];10.1186/1471-2105-12-77 [doi].

16. Marenzi G, Assanelli E, Campodonico J, Lauri G, Marana I, et al. (2009) Contrast volume during primary percutaneous coronary intervention and subsequent contrast-induced nephropathy and mortality. Ann Intern Med 150: 170–177. 150/3/170 [pii].

17. Freeman RV, O'Donnell M, Share D, Meengs WL, Kline-Rogers E, et al. (2002) Nephropathy requiring dialysis after percutaneous coronary intervention and the critical role of an adjusted contrast dose. Am J Cardiol 90: 1068–1073. S0002914902027716 [pii].

18. Nyman U, Bjork J, Aspelin P, Marenzi G (2008) Contrast medium dose-to-GFR ratio: a measure of systemic exposure to predict contrast-induced nephropathy after percutaneous coronary intervention. Acta Radiol 49: 658–667. 792395239 [pii];10.1080/02841850802050762 [doi].

19. Brown JR, Robb JF, Block CA, Schoolwerth AC, Kaplan AV, et. al. (2010) Does safe dosing of iodinated contrast prevent contrast-induced acute kidney injury? Circ Cardiovasc Interv 3: 346–350. CIRCINTERVENTIONS.109.910638 [pii];10.1161/CIRCINTERVENTIONS.109.910638 [doi].

20. Mehran R, Aymong ED, Nikolsky E, Lasic Z, Iakovou I, et.al. (2004) A simple risk score for prediction of contrast-induced nephropathy after percutaneous coronary intervention: development and initial validation. J Am Coll Cardiol 44: 1393–1399. S0735-1097(04)01445-7 [pii];10.1016/j.jacc.2004.06.068 [doi].

21. McCullough PA (2008) Contrast-induced acute kidney injury. J Am Coll Cardiol 51: 1419–1428. S0735-1097(08)00353-7 [pii];10.1016/j.jacc.2007.12.035 [doi].

22. Nayak KR, Mehta HS, Price MJ, Russo RJ, Stinis CT, et al. (2010) A novel technique for ultra-low contrast administration during angiography or intervention. Catheter Cardiovasc Interv 75: 1076–1083. 10.1002/ccd.22414 [doi].

Persistent Catheter-Related *Staphylococcus aureus* Bacteremia after Catheter Removal and Initiation of Antimicrobial Therapy

Ki-Ho Park[1,2], Yu-Mi Lee[1,2], Hyo-Lim Hong[1,2], Tark Kim[1,2], Hyun Jung Park[1,2], So-Youn Park[1,2], Song Mi Moon[1,2], Yong Pil Chong[1,2], Sung-Han Kim[1,2], Sang-Oh Lee[1,2], Sang-Ho Choi[1,2], Jin-Yong Jeong[1,2,3], Mi-Na Kim[4], Jun Hee Woo[1,2], Yang Soo Kim[1,2]*

1 Department of Infectious Diseases, Asan Medical Center, University of Ulsan College of Medicine, Seoul, Republic of Korea, 2 Center for Antimicrobial Resistance and Microbial Genetics, University of Ulsan, Seoul, Republic of Korea, 3 Asan Institute of Life Sciences, Asan Medical Center, University of Ulsan College of Medicine, Seoul, Republic of Korea, 4 Department of Laboratory Medicine, Asan Medical Center, University of Ulsan College of Medicine, Seoul, Republic of Korea

Abstract

Objectives: Catheter-related *Staphylococcus aureus* bacteremia (CRSAB) occasionally persists despite catheter removal and initiation of appropriate antimicrobial therapy. The aim of this study was to determine the incidence, risk factors, and outcomes of persistent CRSAB after catheter removal and initiation of antimicrobial therapy.

Methods: Consecutive patients with CRSAB were prospectively included from over a 41-month period. We compared the clinical features, 40 bacterial virulence genes, and outcomes between patients with persistent CRSAB (i.e., bacteremia for >3 days after catheter removal and initiation of appropriate antimicrobial therapy) and non-persistent CRSAB.

Results: Among the 220 episodes of CRSAB, the catheter was kept in place in 17 (6%) and removed in 203 (94%) cases. In 43 (21%) of the 203 episodes, bacteremia persisted for >3 days after catheter removal and initiation of antimicrobial therapy. Methicillin resistance (Odds ratio [OR], 9.01; 95% confidence interval [CI], 3.05–26.61; $P<0.001$), non-catheter prosthetic devices (OR, 5.37; 95% CI, 1.62–17.80; $P=0.006$), and renal failure (OR, 3.23; 95% CI, 1.48–7.08; $P=0.003$) were independently associated with persistent CRSAB. Patients with persistent CRSAB were more like to experience complication than were those with non-persistent CRSAB (72% vs. 15%; $P<0.001$). Among all episodes due to methicillin-resistant *S. aureus*, persistent CRSAB isolates were associated with accessory gene regulator (*agr*) group II ($P=.04$), but presence of other bacterial virulence genes, distribution of vancomycin minimum inhibitory concentration distribution, and frequency of vancomycin heteroresistance did not differ between the groups.

Conclusions: In patients with CRSAB, bacteremia persisted in 21% of cases despite catheter removal and initiation of antimicrobial therapy. Methicillin resistance, renal failure, and non-catheter prosthetic devices were independent risk factors for persistent CRSAB, which was associated with a higher rate of complications.

Editor: Patrick M. Schlievert, University of Iowa Carver College of Medicine, United States of America

Funding: This research was supported by Future-based Technology Development Program (Bio Fields) through the National Research Foundation of Korea (NRF) funded by the Ministry of Education, Science and Technology (grant numbers: 2011-0029936).

Competing Interests: The authors have declared that no competing interests exist.

* E-mail: yskim@amc.seoul.kr

Introduction

Staphylococcus aureus bacteremia (SAB) is one of the most common serious bacterial infections worldwide, and intravascular catheters are the most common source of these infections, especially in hospitalized patients [1]. Catheter-related *S. aureus* bacteremia (CRSAB) is a severe healthcare-associated infection that may result in endocarditis, septic thrombophlebitis, metastatic infection, and death [1–3]. Bacteremia may persist and complication may develop during the course of therapy if an infected catheter is not removed or if the initiation of antimicrobial therapy is delayed [4,5]. Thus, catheter removal and initiation of appropriate antimicrobial therapy are essential steps for the optimal treatment of CRSAB.

In practice, however, CRSAB occasionally persists despite catheter removal and initiation of appropriate antimicrobial therapy. There is limited literature evaluating the clinical characteristics and outcomes of patients with persistent CRSAB despite initiation of appropriate therapy. A previous study of 37 patients with CRSAB showed that fever and/or bacteremia that persisted for >3 days after catheter removal and/or initiation of antimicrobial therapy was associated with development of early complications [4]. Furthermore, there is little known about the microbiological and genotypic characteristics of *S. aureus* isolates causing persistent CRSAB. The aim of this study was to determine the incidence, risk factors, and outcomes of persistent CRSAB after catheter removal and initiation of appropriate antimicrobial

Table 1. Clinical characteristics and outcomes of 220 patients with catheter-related *Staphylococcus aureus* bacteremia according to catheter retention or removal.

Variable	Catheter retained (n = 17)	Catheter removed (n = 203)	P value
Age, median (IQR)	50 (46–61)	62 (50–70)	0.02
Male sex	11 (65)	128 (63)	0.89
Community-onset of infection	0 (0)	27 (13)	0.24
Methicillin resistance	9 (53)	122 (60)	0.56
Comorbidity			
Underlying malignancy	14 (82)	108 (53)	0.02
Renal failure	3 (18)	56 (28)	0.57
Diabetes mellitus	0 (0)	56 (28)	0.008
Liver cirrhosis	2 (12)	34 (17)	0.75
Type of catheter			
Central venous catheter	16 (94)	160 (79)	0.21
Long-term intravascular catheters[1]	12 (71)	42 (21)	<0.001
External signs of catheter infection	2 (13)	40 (20)	0.74
Presence of non-catheter prosthetic devices[2]	1 (6)	17 (8)	>0.99
APACHE II score, median (IQR)	18 (15–23)	17 (12–21)	0.38
Pitt bacteremia score, median (IQR)	1 (1–3)	1 (0–3)	0.48
Intensive care unit stay	3 (18)	59 (29)	0.41
Mechanical ventilation	1 (6)	36 (18)	0.32
Prescription of immunosuppressive therapy[3]	5 (29)	43 (21)	0.54
Prescription of cancer chemotherapy[3]	8 (47)	33 (16)	0.005
Recent surgery[3]	2 (12)	57 (28)	0.25
Outcome			
Complicated *S. aureus* bacteremia	9 (53)	55 (27)	0.047
Complicated infection	5 (29)	34 (17)	0.19
Septic thrombophlebitis	1 (6)	19 (9)	>0.99
Infective endocarditis	2 (12)	6 (3)	0.12
Septic emboli to lungs	2 (12)	8 (4)	0.18
Deep tissue abscess	1 (6)	6 (3)	0.44
Septic arthritis	0 (0)	1 (1)	>0.99
Osteomyelitis	0 (0)	1 (1)	>0.99
Attributable mortality	7 (41)	23 (11)	0.003
Late complication	1 (6)	6 (3)	0.44
No complication due to *S. aureus* bacteremia	8 (47)	148 (73)	0.047
Uncomplicated *S. aureus* bacteremia	7 (41)	123 (61)	0.12
Death not-related *S. aureus* bacteremia	1 (6)	25 (12)	0.70

NOTE: Data are no. (%) of patients, unless otherwise indicated. IQR, interquartile range; APACHE II, Acute Physiology and Chronic Health Evaluation II.
[1] Includes perm catheter (n = 31), Hickman catheter (n = 18), and subcutaneous port catheters (n = 5).
[2] Includes prosthetic valve (n = 7), synthetic vascular graft (n = 6), and orthopedic device (n = 5).
[3] Within previous one month.

therapy. We also evaluated the microbiological and genotypic characteristics of isolates associated with persistent CRSAB.

Methods

Ethics Statement

Informed consent was waived given that no interventions were planned and collected data were stored anonymously. The Asan Medical Center Institutional Review Board approved the study and waiver of informed consent (IRB number: 2008-0274).

Study Populations

From August 2008 to December 2011, data were collected as part of a prospective cohort study of *S. aureus* bloodstream infections at Asan Medical Center, Seoul, Korea. During the study period, patients with CRSAB, as defined below, were included. Patients with CRSAB, as defined below, were identified by a daily search of the microbiology laboratory database. Patients younger than 16 years or who had polymicrobial infections were excluded. Only the first episode of bacteremia was included in the analysis to ensure independent observations. During the study period,

Table 2. Clinical characteristics, management, and outcomes of 203 patients with non-persistent and persistent catheter-related *S. aureus* bacteremia after catheter removal and initiation of appropriate antimicrobial therapy.

Variable	Non-persistent CRSAB (n = 160)	Persistent CRSAB (n = 43)	Univariate analysis		Multivariate analysis	
			P value	OR (95% CI)	P value	OR (95% CI)
Age, median (IQR)	62 (49–70)	64 (53–72)	0.16			
Male sex	101 (63)	27 (63)	0.97			
Community-onset of infection	20 (13)	7 (16)	0.52			
Methicillin resistance	84 (53)	38 (88)	<0.001	6.88 (2.57–18.37)	<0.001	9.01 (3.05–26.61)
Comorbidity						
Underlying malignancy	86 (54)	22 (51)	0.76			
Renal failure	35 (22)	21 (49)	<0.001	3.41 (1.68–6.90)	0.003	3.23 (1.48–7.08)
Diabetes mellitus	46 (29)	10 (23)	0.47			
Liver cirrhosis	29 (18)	5 (12)	0.31			
Type of catheter						
Central venous catheter	120 (75)	40 (93)	0.01	4.44 (1.30–15.15)		
Long-term intravascular catheters[1]	31 (19)	11 (26)	0.37			
External signs of catheter infection	32 (20)	8 (19)	0.84			
Presence of non-catheter prosthetic devices[2]	8 (5)	9 (21)	0.003	5.03 (1.81–13.98)	0.006	5.37 (1.62–17.80)
APACHE II score, median (IQR)	17 (12–21)	19 (13–23)	0.13			
Pitt bacteremia score, median (IQR)	1 (0–3)	1 (0–3)	0.76			
Intensive care unit stay	44 (28)	15 (35)	0.34			
Mechanical ventilation	29 (18)	7 (16)	0.78			
Prescription of immunosuppressive therapy[3]	36 (23)	7 (16)	0.38			
Prescription of cancer chemotherapy[3]	28 (18)	5 (12)	0.35			
Recent surgery[3]	45 (28)	12 (28)	0.98			
Clinical management						
Catheter removal within 48 hrs	120 (75)	38 (88)	0.06			
Initiation of appropriate antibiotics within 48 hrs	141 (88)	37 (86)	0.71			
Initial vancomycin use (to MSSA isolates)	31/76 (41)	5/5 (100)	0.02			
Duration of antibiotic therapy	15 (11–21)	27 (20–47)	<0.001			
Outcome						
Complicated *S. aureus* bacteremia	24 (15)	31 (72)	<0.001			
Complicated infection	7 (4)	27 (63)	<0.001			
Septic thrombophlebitis	6 (4)	13 (30)	<0.001			
Infective endocarditis	0 (0)	6 (14)	<0.001			
Other metastatic seeding of infection[4]	1 (1)	15 (35)	<0.001			
Attributable mortality	13 (8)	10 (23)	0.01			
Late complication	4 (3)	2 (5)	0.61			
No complications due to *S. aureus* bacteremia	136 (85)	12 (28)	<0.001			
Uncomplicated *S. aureus* bacteremia	113 (71)	10 (23)	<0.001			
Death not-related *S. aureus* bacteremia	23 (14)	2 (5)	0.09			

NOTE: Data are no. (%) of patients, unless otherwise indicated. CRSAB, catheter-related *Staphylococcus aureus* bacteremia; OR, odds ratio; CI, confidence interval; IQR, interquartile range; MSSA, methicillin-susceptible *S. aureus*; APACHE II, Acute Physiology and Chronic Health Evaluation II.
[1]Includes perm catheter (n = 30), Hickman catheter (n = 10), and subcutaneous port catheters (n = 2).
[2]Includes prosthetic valve (n = 7), synthetic vascular graft (n = 5), and orthopedic device (n = 5).
[3]Within previous one month.
[4]Includes septic emboli to lungs (n = 8), deep tissue abscess (n = 6), septic arthritis (n = 1), and osteomyelitis (n = 1).

antibiotic lock therapy and antibiotic-impregnated catheters were not used.

Definitions

CRSAB was classified as definite or probable according to current IDSA criteria guidelines [6]. CRSAB was considered "definite" (1) if a semiquantitative culture of the removed catheter tip revealed ≥15 colony-forming units by the roll plate technique, and the same organism (by both species and antibiogram) was isolated from the catheter tip and peripheral blood; or (2) indicative differential time to positivity (i.e., the blood culture obtained through catheter became positive at least 2 h earlier than a positive simultaneous blood culture obtained from a peripheral vein) [6,7]. CRSAB was considered "probable" if the patient had a catheter with at least one positive blood culture for S. aureus with compatible clinical presentation and absence of other identifiable source of infection.

CRSAB was considered "persistent" if bacteremia persisted for >3 days after initiation of appropriate therapy. Appropriate therapy was considered to have been initiated if the catheter was removed and if at least one intravenous antibiotic to which the isolate was susceptible was started. CRSAB was considered "non-persistent (1) if bacteremia cleared within 3 days after initiation of appropriate therapy or (2) if follow-up blood cultures were not performed because of resolution of signs and symptoms of the catheter infection after initiation of appropriate therapy.

All surviving patients were followed up 12 weeks after the onset of SAB. Complicated SAB was defined as the presence of (1) attributable mortality, (2) complicated infection present at the time of the initial hospitalization, or (3) late complication. Death was attributable to SAB if blood cultures were positive for S. aureus at the time of death or if death occurred before resolution of the signs and symptoms of SAB without another explanation [8]. Complicated infection included infective endocarditis, septic thrombophlebitis, osteomyelitis, septic arthritis, deep tissue abscess, and septic emboli to lungs [2–4]. Late complication was defined as the isolation of S. aureus from the bloodstream or other sterile body site with the same antibiogram as the initial isolate during the 12-week post-treatment follow-up period [3,4]. Uncomplicated SAB was defined as no evidence of death due to SAB, complicated infection, or late complication within 12-weeks follow-up period. Designa-

tion of death due to a cause other than SAB was based on investigator evaluation during hospitalization and on the death certificate records after discharge.

Laboratory and Molecular Method

All blood cultures were analyzed using by the BACTEC 9240 (Becton Dickinson, Spark, MD, USA) and all S. aureus isolates were identified by standard methods. All blood cultures were analyzed using by the BACTEC 9240 (Becton Dickinson, Spark, MD, USA) and all S. aureus isolates were identified by standard methods. Catheter tip cultures were processed by the semiquantitative roll plate culture method [9]. The minimum inhibitory concentration (MIC) of vancomycin was determined using the Etest (AB Biodisk, Solna, Sweden) according to the manufacturer's instructions. Methicillin-resistant S. aureus (MRSA) blood isolates were assessed by the population analysis profiling-area under the curve (PAP-AUC) method, using the technique of Wootton et al [10]. An isolate was identified as hVISA if the ratio of the AUC of the test isolate to the reference strain (Mu3; ATCC 700698) was ≥0.9. The presence of 40 bacterial virulence factors, including adhesins, toxins, agr subgroups I–IV, and other genes, were examined by multiplex polymerase chain reaction (PCR), as described elsewhere [11–14]. Staphylococcal cassette chromosome (SCCmec) types were identified using a previously described method [15].

Statistical Analysis

Results were analyzed using a commercially available software package (SPSS software, version 14.0 K for Windows; SPSS, Inc., Chicago, IL). Categorical variables were evaluated using the chi-square or Fisher exact test. Continuous variables were compared using the Student t test or the Mann-Whitney U test, where appropriate. All variables that were significant in univariate analysis were included in a logistic regression model for multivariate analysis. Time to complication was described by the Kaplan-Meier method and compared using the log-rank test. All tests of significance were two-tailed, and a P value <0.05 was considered statistically significant.

Results

Patients

During the 41-month study period, 239 episodes of CRSAB occurred in 237 adult patients. Two patients had two episodes of CRSAB; only the first episode was included in the analysis. Twelve patients with polymicrobial bacteremia excluded and five patients were lost to follow-up. As a result, 220 patients were included in the analysis. Among them, 135 (61%) were found to have definite CRSAB, and the other 85 (39%) had probable CRSAB.

The source of bacteremia was presumed to be a temporary central venous catheter in 117 (53%), a tunneled cuffed intravascular catheter (e.g., Permcath or Hickman catheter) in 49 (23%), a peripheral vascular catheter in 42 (19%), a peripheral inserted central venous catheter in 5 (2%), a subcutaneous port catheter in 5 (2%), and an arterial catheter in 2 (1%). One hundred and sixty-one patients (73%) had an echocardiogram during the course of therapy; 143 patients (89%) had only transthoracic echocardiogram, and 18 patients (11%) had both transthoracic and transesophageal echocardiogram.

Of the 220 episodes of CRSAB, the catheter was removed from 203 patients (94%), and kept in place in 17 patients (6%). Among the latter 17 patients, 9 recovered, 7 died of SAB, and 1 recovered from SAB but died due to progression of malignancy. Catheter retention group was more likely to have underlying malignancy and long-term intravascular catheters, and to have been received

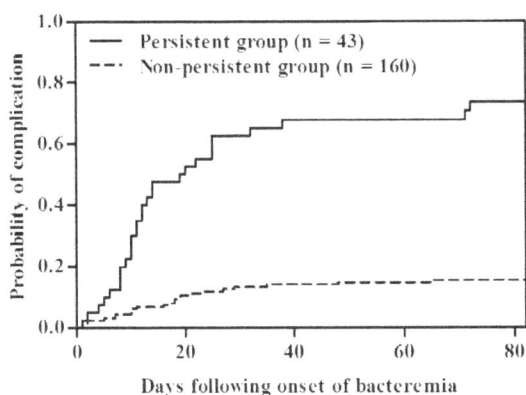

Figure 1. Kaplan-Meier plot showing time to development of complication among patients with catheter-related *Staphylococcus aureus* bacteremia. Complications were more common in patients who had persistent bacteremia for >3 days after catheter removal and initiation of appropriate antimicrobial therapy than in those who did not have persistent bacteremia (log-rank test, *P*<0.001).

Table 3. Univariate and multivariate analyses of risk factors for development of complication in 203 patients with catheter-related *Staphylococcus aureus* bacteremia.

Variable	No SAB-related complication (n = 148)	SAB-related complication (n = 55)	Univariate analysis P value	Univariate analysis OR (95% CI)	Multivariate analysis P value	Multivariate analysis OR (95% CI)
Age, median (IQR)	61 (49–70)	64 (54–71)	0.29	1.01 (0.99–1.04)		
Male sex	91 (62)	37 (67)	0.45	1.29 (0.67–2.48)		
Community-onset of infection	18 (12)	9 (16)	0.43	1.41 (0.59–3.37)		
Methicillin resistance	81 (55)	41 (75)	0.01	2.42 (1.22–4.82)		
Underlying malignancy	74 (50)	34 (62)	0.13	1.62 (0.86–3.05)		
Renal failure	31 (21)	25 (46)	0.001	3.15 (1.62–6.10)		
Diabetes mellitus	42 (28)	14 (26)	0.68	0.86 (0.43–1.74)		
Liver cirrhosis	27 (18)	7 (13)	0.35	0.65 (0.27–1.60)		
Central venous catheter	112 (76)	48 (87)	0.07	2.20 (0.92–5.30)		
Long-term intravascular catheters	28 (19)	14 (26)	0.31	1.46 (0.70–3.05)		
External signs of catheter infection	27 (18)	13 (24)	0.39	1.39 (0.66–2.93)		
Presence of non-catheter prosthetic device	6 (4)	11 (20)	0.001	5.92 (2.07–16.92)	0.052	3.50 (0.99–12.40)
APACHE II score, median (IQR)	16 (11–21)	20 (15–24)	0.001	1.06 (1.02–1.11)	<0.001	1.07 (1.02–1.12)
Pitt bacteremia score, median (IQR)	1 (0–3)	1 (0–4)	0.48	1.03 (0.91–1.18)		
Intensive care unit stay	44 (30)	15 (27)	0.73	0.89 (0.44–1.79)		
Mechanical ventilation	28 (19)	8 (15)	0.47	0.73 (0.31–1.72)		
Prescription of immunosuppressive therapy[1]	29 (20)	14 (26)	0.36	1.40 (0.68–2.91)		
Prescription of cancer chemotherapy[1]	24 (16)	9 (16)	0.98	1.01 (0.45–2.34)		
Recent surgery[1]	41 (28)	16 (29)	0.85	1.07 (0.54–2.12)		
Persistent CRSAB	12 (8)	31 (56)	<0.001	14.64 (6.61–32.42)	<0.001	13.84 (5.98–32.06)
Catheter removal >48 hrs after onset of bacteremia	115 (78)	43 (78)	0.94	1.03 (0.49–2.17)		
Inappropriate antibiotic therapy within 48 hrs	14 (10)	11 (20)	0.04	2.39 (1.01–5.66)	0.03	3.04 (1.09–8.45)
Vancomycin MIC by Etest[2]	(n = 81)	(n = 41)				
≤1.0 mg/L	25 (31)	15 (37)	NA	reference		
1.5 mg/L	38 (47)	19 (46)	0.67	0.83 (0.36–1.94)		
≥2.0 mg/L[3]	18 (22)	7 (17)	0.43	0.65 (0.22–1.91)		
hVISA[2]	27 (33)	18 (44)	0.25	1.57 (0.72–3.38)		

NOTE: Data are no. (%) of patients, unless otherwise indicated. SAB, *Staphylococcus aureus* bacteremia; OR, odds ratio; CI, confidence interval; IQR, interquartile range; Acute Physiology and Chronic Health Evaluation II; CRSAB, catheter-related *S. aureus* bacteremia; MIC, minimum inhibitory concentration; NA, not applicable; hVISA, heteroresistant vancomycin-intermediate *S. aureus*.
[1]Within previous one month.
[2]Analysis was restricted to 122 MRSA cases.
[3]Two isolates had vancomycin MICs of 3 mg/L.

chemotherapy than catheter removal group. Catheter removal group was more likely to be old and to have diabetes mellitus. The complication rate was significantly higher in catheter retained group than catheter removal group (53% [9/17] vs. 27% [55/203], *P* = 0.047) (Table 1).

Risk Factors Associated with Persistent CRSAB

Of the 203 episodes of CRSAB in which the catheters were removed, bacteremia persisted for >3 days after catheter removal and initiation of appropriate antimicrobial therapy in 43 patients (21%). Clinical characteristics of 203 patients with persistent and non-persistent CRSAB are shown in Table 2. Using univariate analysis, baseline clinical characteristics that were associated with persistent CRSAB included methicillin resistance (*P*<0.001), renal failure (*P*<0.001), central venous catheter (*P* = 0.01), and presence of non-catheter prosthetic devices (*P* = 0.003). Using multivariate

analysis, methicillin resistance (odds ratio [OR], 9.01; 95% CI, 3.05–26.61; *P*<0.001), presence of non-catheter prosthetic devices (OR, 5.37; 95% CI, 1.62–17.80; *P* = 0.006), and renal failure (OR, 3.23; 95% CI, 1.48–7.08; *P* = 0.003) were significantly associated with persistent CRSAB. Similar risk estimates were also observed when analyses were restricted to 125 patients with confirmed CRSAB. However, no significant risk factors were observed when analyses were restricted to 78 patients with probable CRSAB (data not shown).

Clinical Management and Outcomes of Patients with Persistent CRSAB

Catheter was removed within 48 hrs in 120 patients (75%) with non-persistent CRSAB and in 38 patients (88%) with persistent CRSAB (*P* = 0.06). Appropriate antimicrobial therapy was started within 48 hrs in 141 patients (88%) with non-persistent CRSAB

Table 4. Microbiological and genotypic characteristics of 122 methicillin-resistant *Staphylococcus aureus* isolates causing persistent and non-persistent catheter-related bacteremia.

Characteristic	Non-persistent CRSAB (n = 84)	Persistent CRSAB (n = 38)	*P* value
Vancomycin MIC by Etest			0.16
≤1.0 mg/L	23 (27)	17 (45)	
1.5 mg/L	43 (51)	14 (37)	
≥2.0 mg/L[1]	18 (22)	7 (18)	
hVISA	29 (35)	16 (42)	0.42
Adhesin genes			
clfA	84 (100)	38 (100)	NA
clfB	84 (100)	38 (100)	NA
cna	0 (0)	0 (0)	NA
ebps	82 (98)	36 (95)	0.59
fnbA	84(100)	38 (100)	NA
fnbB	82 (98)	38 (100)	>0.99
map/eap	3 (4)	2 (5)	0.65
sdrC	72 (86)	30 (79)	0.35
sdrD	77 (92)	36 (95)	0.72
sdrE	81 (96)	36 (95)	0.65
Toxin genes			
edin	0 (0)	0 (0)	NA
Eta	0 (0)	0 (0)	NA
Etb	0 (0)	0 (0)	NA
Hla	82 (98)	35 (92)	0.17
Hlb	51 (61)	25 (66)	0.59
Hld	80 (95)	37 (97)	>0.99
Hlg	0 (0)	0 (0)	NA
hlg-2	81 (96)	38 (100)	0.55
lukE-lukD	81 (96)	38 (100)	0.55
lukM	0 (0)	0 (0)	NA
Pvl	0 (0)	0 (0)	NA
Sea	7 (8)	1 (3)	0.43
Seb	0 (0)	0 (0)	NA
Sec	56 (67)	31 (82)	0.09
Sed	0 (0)	0 (0)	NA
See	0 (0)	0 (0)	NA
Seg	75 (89)	37 (97)	0.17
She	0 (0)	0 (0)	NA
Sei	76 (91)	36 (95)	0.72
Sej	0 (0)	0 (0)	NA
Sek	5 (6)	1 (3)	0.66
Sel	66 (79)	34 (90)	0.15
Sem	74 (88)	35 (92)	0.75
Sen	75 (89)	36 (95)	0.50
Seo	75 (89)	37 (97)	0.17
Sep	2 (2)	0 (0)	>0.99
Seq	5 (6)	1 (3)	0.66
Tst	61 (73)	32 (84)	0.16
Other virulence genes			
icaA	84 (100)	38 (100)	NA
agr subgroup[2]			

Table 4. Cont.

Characteristic	Non-persistent CRSAB (n = 84)	Persistent CRSAB (n = 38)	P value
Subgroup I	21 (26)	4 (10)	0.06
Subgroup II	60 (73)	34 (90)	0.04
Subgroup III	1 (1)	0 (0)	>0.99
SCCmec type[3]			
Type II	63 (76)	34 (89)	0.08
Type III	6 (7)	1 (3)	0.43
Type IV	14 (17)	3 (8)	0.19

NOTE: Data are no. (%) of isolates, unless otherwise indicated. CRSAB, catheter-related *Staphylococcus aureus* bacteremia; MIC, minimum inhibitory concentration; hVISA, heteroresistant vancomycin-intermediate *S. aureus*; NA, not applicable; SCCmec, staphylococcal chromosomal cassette mec.
[1]Two isolates had vancomycin MICs of 3 mg/L.
[2]Includes 120 isolates: 2 isolates was nontypeable.
[3]Includes 121 isolates: 1 isolate was nontypeable.

and in 37 patients (86%) with persistent CRSAB ($P = 0.71$). Among patients with bacteremia due to methicillin-susceptible *S. aureus*, all of five patients with persistent bacteremia received vancomycin as the initial antibiotic, but 31 (41%) of 76 patients with non-persistent bacteremia received vancomycin as the initial antibiotic ($P = 0.02$). Patients with persistent CRSAB received more prolonged antibiotic therapy than did those with non-persistent CRSAB (median 27 vs. 15 days; $P < 0.001$) (Table 2).

Complications occurred in 31 patients (72%) with persistent CRSAB and in 24 patients (15%) with non-persistent CRSAB ($P < 0.001$) (Table 2). A Kaplan-Meier plot also showed that the cumulative incidence curves for complications were significantly different between patients with persistent and non-persistent CRSAB ($P < 0.001$) (Figure 1). Patients with persistent CRSAB were significantly more like to have complicated infection than those with non-persistent CRSAB (63% [27/43] vs. 4% [7/160], $P < 0.001$). Infection-attributable morality was higher in patients with persistent CRSAB than in those with non-persistent CRSAB (23% [10/43] vs. 8% [13/160]; $P = 0.01$). Late complication rates were similar between both groups (5% [2/43] vs. 3% [4/160]; $P = 0.61$) (Table 2). To determine whether persistent CRSAB was independently associated with complications, we performed univariate and multivariate analyses of risk factors associated with the development of complication. Using multivariate analysis, APACHE II score (OR, 1.07; 95% CI, 1.02–1.12; $P < 0.001$), persistent status (OR, 13.84; 95% CI, 5.98–32.06; $P < 0.001$), and initial inappropriate antimicrobial therapy (OR, 3.04; 95% CI, 1.09–8.45; $P = 0.03$) were independently associated with the development of complications. Among 122 patients infected with MRSA, complication rates were similar according to vancomycin MIC and presence of hVISA phenotype (Table 3).

Microbiological and Genotypic Characteristics of MRSA Isolates Associated with Persistent Catheter-related Bacteremia

Because most episodes (88%) of persistent CRSAB were caused by MRSA, we further evaluated the microbiological and genotypic characteristics of 122 MRSA isolates associated with persistent and non-persistent CRSAB. There were no significant differences in the distribution of vancomycin MIC and frequency of hVISA phenotype. Accessory gene regulator (*agr*) subgroup II was more common in persistent CRSAB isolates than non-persistent CRSAB isolates (90% vs. 73%; $P = 0.04$). Other bacterial virulence genes did not differ between the groups (Table 4).

Discussion

Optimal management of CRSAB includes early catheter removal and initiation of appropriate antimicrobial therapy [2,6,16]. In practice, however, physicians occasionally encounter patients with persistent CRSAB despite catheter removal and initiation of appropriate antimicrobial therapy. We found that 21% of CRSAB cases persisted for ≥3 days after catheter removal and initiation of appropriate antimicrobial therapy. Methicillin resistance, presence of non-catheter prosthetic devices, and renal failure were independently associated with persistent catheter-related bacteremia, which adversely affect patient outcomes.

Persistent bacteremia was more common in episodes caused by MRSA (31% [38/122]) than in those caused by MSSA (6% [5/81]). These results are in line with a prior report documenting the significant association between methicillin resistance and hematogenous complications of CRSAB [2]. One of the possible explanations for these findings may be that glycopeptides are less active against staphylococci than are antistaphylococcal beta-lactams [17–20]. In addition, MRSA stains with decreased susceptibility to glycopeptide have emerged, and glycopeptide failure to treat these strains have been reported in various MRSA infection [21]. A recent meta-analysis showed that vancomycin MIC value at the higher end of susceptible range (≥1.5 mg/L) was significantly associated with mortality and treatment failure [22]. Some portion of these failures may be due to unrecognized heterogeneously resistant *S. aureus* (hVISA) which is readily not detected by standard clinical laboratory methods [23]. However, no study stratified MIC data by source of bacteremia, thus it remains unclear whether a high MIC line-related BSI (low risk) has similar implications to a high MIC endovascular BSI (high risk). Among our patients with CRSAB, whose catheters were removed, high vancomycin MIC and hVISA phenotype were not associated with persistent CRSAB and complication. Therefore, our data suggests that when interpreting the impact of MRSA strains with decreased susceptibility on clinical outcomes, outcomes should be stratified by the source of bacteremia or by whether source control was adequate (e.g. intravascular catheter removal).

Because most episodes (88%) with persistent CRSAB were caused by MRSA, we evaluated the microbiological and genotypic characteristics of MRSA isolates associated with persistent CRSAB. Our investigation also showed that *agr* group II was associated with persistent CRSAB. Previously, *agr* group II was linked to vancomycin failure in one study [24], but not in another study [20]. We evaluated several bacterial virulence factors, including adhesin and toxin genes, but we could not find any association between these virulence genes and persistent CRSAB.

The presence of non-catheter prosthetic devices was an independent risk factor for persistent CRSAB in this study. This observation is consistent with prior reports documenting high rates of seeding by *S. aureus* in a variety of noncatheter prosthetic devices [25–29]. Noncatheter prosthetic devices can serve as a focus for hematogenous spread of SAB. The current investigation also demonstrated that renal failure was an independent risk factor for persistent CRSAB. This finding is consistent with the report by Fowler et al. who found that renal failure was an independent risk factor for hematogenous complications [2]. A more recent study by Ghanem et al. found that renal failure at the onset of CRSAB was associated with a high risk of early complications [3]. This elevated risk may be related to uremia-associated phagocytic dysfunction [30]. Renal failure may contribute to complication or persistent bacteremia by superantigen-dependent enhancement of endotoxin shock and renal tubular cell injury [31,32].

Persistent bacteremia after catheter removal and initiation of appropriate antimicrobial therapy usually reflects serious complications of CRSAB, such as septic thrombophlebitis, endocarditis, or metastatic foci of infection [4,33]. A previous report showed that acute early complications of CRSAB more frequently occurred during the initial course of therapy in patients in which fever and/or bacteremia persisted for >3 days after catheter removal than in those who responded within 3 days after catheter removal (7/8 [88%] vs. 1/29 [3%]; P<0.001) [4]. Our study included a large number of cases of CRSAB that were prospectively followed; we confirmed the high rate of early

complications in patients with persistent CRSAB compared with non-persistent CRSAB.

The current study has several limitations. First, it was conducted in a single tertiary care institution and referral center. This may have caused a selection bias towards more severe or complicated cases, resulting in limitations on the generation of the results. Second, clearance of bacteremia was not documented for some patients with non-persistent CRSAB in whom clinical symptoms and signs of CRSAB frequently resolved after catheter removal and initiation of appropriate antimicrobial therapy. However, similar observations were made after analysis was restricted to patients in whom clearance of bacteremia was documented (data not shown). Third, we did not use PFGE to type MRSA blood isolates, and we thus could not evaluate the possibility that clonal relationships may exist among some isolates.

Conclusion

Bacteremia persisted for >3 days after catheter removal and initiation of appropriate antimicrobial therapy in 21% of our CRSAB cases. Baseline risk factors for persistent CRSAB were methicillin resistance, presence of non-catheter prosthetic devices, and renal failure. Persistent CRSAB was associated with high rates of acute complications and infection-related mortality, and its optimal management remains challenging for clinicians.

Author Contributions

Conceived and designed the experiments: KHP YSK. Performed the experiments: TK SMM JYJ. Analyzed the data: KHP YPC. Contributed reagents/materials/analysis tools: YML HLH TK HJP SYP SHK SOL SHC MNK JHW. Wrote the paper: KHP YSK.

References

1. Fowler VG Jr, Olsen MK, Corey GR, Woods CW, Cabell CH, et al. (2003) Clinical identifiers of complicated *Staphylococcus aureus* bacteremia. Arch Intern Med 163: 2066–2072.
2. Fowler VG Jr, Justice A, Moore C, Benjamin DK Jr, Woods CW, et al. (2005) Risk factors for hematogenous complications of intravascular catheter-associated *Staphylococcus aureus* bacteremia. Clin Infect Dis 40: 695–703.
3. Ghanem GA, Boktour M, Warneke C, Pham-Williams T, Kassis C, et al. (2007) Catheter-related *Staphylococcus aureus* bacteremia in cancer patients: high rate of complications with therapeutic implications. Medicine (Baltimore) 86: 54–60.
4. Raad, II, Sabbagh MF (1992) Optimal duration of therapy for catheter-related *Staphylococcus aureus* bacteremia: a study of 55 cases and review. Clin Infect Dis 14: 75–82.
5. Malanoski GJ, Samore MH, Pefanis A, Karchmer AW (1995) *Staphylococcus aureus* catheter-associated bacteremia. Minimal effective therapy and unusual infectious complications associated with arterial sheath catheters. Arch Intern Med 155: 1161–1166.
6. Mermel LA, Allon M, Bouza E, Craven DE, Flynn P, et al. (2009) Clinical practice guidelines for the diagnosis and management of intravascular catheter-related infection: 2009 Update by the Infectious Diseases Society of America. Clin Infect Dis 49: 1–45.
7. Raad I, Hanna HA, Alakech B, Chatzinikolaou I, Johnson MM, et al. (2004) Differential time to positivity: a useful method for diagnosing catheter-related bloodstream infections. Ann Intern Med 140: 18–25.
8. Lodise TP, McKinnon PS, Swiderski L, Rybak MJ (2003) Outcomes analysis of delayed antibiotic treatment for hospital-acquired *Staphylococcus aureus* bacteremia. Clin Infect Dis 36: 1418–1423.
9. Maki DG, Weise CE, Sarafin HW (1977) A semiquantitative culture method for identifying intravenous-catheter-related infection. N Engl J Med 296: 1305–1309.
10. Wootton M, Howe RA, Hillman R, Walsh TR, Bennett PM, et al. (2001) A modified population analysis profile (PAP) method to detect hetero-resistance to vancomycin in *Staphylococcus aureus* in a UK hospital. J Antimicrob Chemother 47: 399–403.
11. Jarraud S, Mougel C, Thioulouse J, Lina G, Meugnier H, et al. (2002) Relationships between *Staphylococcus aureus* genetic background, virulence factors, agr groups (alleles), and human disease. Infect Immun 70: 631–641.
12. Diep BA, Carleton HA, Chang RF, Sensabaugh GF, Perdreau-Remington F (2006) Roles of 34 virulence genes in the evolution of hospital- and community-associated strains of methicillin-resistant *Staphylococcus aureus*. J Infect Dis 193: 1495–1503.
13. Peacock SJ, Moore CE, Justice A, Kantzanou M, Story L, et al. (2002) Virulent combinations of adhesin and toxin genes in natural populations of *Staphylococcus aureus*. Infect Immun 70: 4987–4996.
14. Campbell SJ, Deshmukh HS, Nelson CL, Bae IG, Stryjewski ME, et al. (2008) Genotypic characteristics of *Staphylococcus aureus* isolates from a multinational trial of complicated skin and skin structure infections. J Clin Microbiol 46: 678–684.
15. Oliveira DC, de Lencastre H (2002) Multiplex PCR strategy for rapid identification of structural types and variants of the mec element in methicillin-resistant *Staphylococcus aureus*. Antimicrob Agents Chemother 46: 2155–2161.
16. Hawkins C, Huang J, Jin N, Noskin GA, Zembower TR, et al. (2007) Persistent *Staphylococcus aureus* bacteremia: an analysis of risk factors and outcomes. Arch Intern Med 167: 1861–1867.
17. Kim SH, Kim KH, Kim HB, Kim NJ, Kim EC, et al. (2008) Outcome of vancomycin treatment in patients with methicillin-susceptible *Staphylococcus aureus* bacteremia. Antimicrob Agents Chemother 52: 192–197.
18. Small PM, Chambers HF (1990) Vancomycin for *Staphylococcus aureus* endocarditis in intravenous drug users. Antimicrob Agents Chemother 34: 1227–1231.
19. Chang FY (2000) *Staphylococcus aureus* bacteremia and endocarditis. J Microbiol Immunol Infect 33: 63–68.
20. Fowler VG, Jr., Sakoulas G, McIntyre LM, Meka VG, Arbeit RD, et al. (2004) Persistent bacteremia due to methicillin-resistant *Staphylococcus aureus* infection is associated with agr dysfunction and low-level in vitro resistance to thrombin-induced platelet microbicidal protein. J Infect Dis 190: 1140–1149.
21. Howden BP, Davies JK, Johnson PD, Stinear TP, Grayson ML (2010) Reduced vancomycin susceptibility in *Staphylococcus aureus*, including vancomycin-intermediate and heterogeneous vancomycin-intermediate strains: resistance mechanisms, laboratory detection, and clinical implications. Clin Microbiol Rev 23: 99–139.
22. van Hal SJ, Lodise TP, Paterson DL (2012) The Clinical Significance of Vancomycin Minimum Inhibitory Concentration in *Staphylococcus aureus* Infections: A Systematic Review and Meta-analysis. Clin Infect Dis 54: 755–771.
23. van Hal SJ, Paterson DL (2011) Systematic review and meta-analysis of the significance of heterogeneous vancomycin-intermediate *Staphylococcus aureus* isolates. Antimicrob Agents Chemother 55: 405–410.
24. Moise-Broder PA, Sakoulas G, Eliopoulos GM, Schentag JJ, Forrest A, et al. (2004) Accessory gene regulator group II polymorphism in methicillin-resistant *Staphylococcus aureus* is predictive of failure of vancomycin therapy. Clin Infect Dis 38: 1700–1705.

25. Sendi P, Banderet F, Graber P, Zimmerli W (2011) Periprosthetic joint infection following *Staphylococcus aureus* bacteremia. J Infect 63: 17–22.

26. Chamis AL, Peterson GE, Cabell CH, Corey GR, Sorrentino RA, et al. (2001) *Staphylococcus aureus* bacteremia in patients with permanent pacemakers or implantable cardioverter-defibrillators. Circulation 104: 1029–1033.

27. Murdoch DR, Roberts SA, Fowler Jr VG, Jr., Shah MA, Taylor SL, et al. (2001) Infection of orthopedic prostheses after *Staphylococcus aureus* bacteremia. Clin Infect Dis 32: 647–649.

28. Chang FY, MacDonald BB, Peacock JE, Jr., Musher DM, Triplett P, et al. (2003) A prospective multicenter study of *Staphylococcus aureus* bacteremia: incidence of endocarditis, risk factors for mortality, and clinical impact of methicillin resistance. Medicine (Baltimore) 82: 322–332.

29. Fang G, Keys TF, Gentry LO, Harris AA, Rivera N, et al. (1993) Prosthetic valve endocarditis resulting from nosocomial bacteremia. A prospective, multicenter study. Ann Intern Med 119: 560–567.

30. Vanholder R, De Smet R, Jacobs V, Van Landschoot N, Waterloos MA, et al. (1994) Uraemic toxic retention solutes depress polymorphonuclear response to phagocytosis. Nephrol Dial Transplant 9: 1271–1278.

31. Keane WF, Gekker G, Schlievert PM, Peterson PK (1986) Enhancement of endotoxin-induced isolated renal tubular cell injury by toxic shock syndrome toxin 1. Am J Pathol 122: 169–176.

32. Schlievert PM (1982) Enhancement of host susceptibility to lethal endotoxin shock by staphylococcal pyrogenic exotoxin type C. Infect Immun 36: 123–128.

33. Verghese A, Widrich WC, Arbeit RD (1985) Central venous septic thrombophlebitis-the role of medical therapy. Medicine (Baltimore) 64: 394–400.

Terlipressin versus Norepinephrine in the Treatment of Hepatorenal Syndrome

Antonio Paulo Nassar Junior[1]*****, **Alberto Queiroz Farias**[2], **Luiz Augusto Carneiro d' Albuquerque**[3], **Flair José Carrilho**[2], **Luiz Marcelo Sá Malbouisson**[1]

1 Intensive Care Unit, Department of Gastroenterology, University of Sao Paulo. Sao Paulo, SP, Brazil, **2** Discipline of Gastroenterology, Department of Gastroenterology. University of Sao Paulo. Sao Paulo, SP, Brazil, **3** Liver and Gastrointestinal Transplant Division, Department of Gastroenterology. University of São Paulo, São Paulo, SP, Brazil

Abstract

Background: Hepatorenal syndrome (HRS) is a severe and progressive functional renal failure occurring in patients with cirrhosis and ascites. Terlipressin is recognized as an effective treatment of HRS, but it is expensive and not widely available. Norepinephrine could be an effective alternative. This systematic review and meta-analysis aimed to evaluate the efficacy and safety of norepinephrine compared to terlipressin in the management of HRS.

Methods: We searched the Medline, Embase, Scopus, CENTRAL, Lilacs and Scielo databases for randomized trials of norepinephrine and terlipressin in the treatment of HRS up to January 2014. Two reviewers collected data and assessed the outcomes and risk of bias. The primary outcome was the reversal of HRS. Secondary outcomes were mortality, recurrence of HRS and adverse events.

Results: Four studies comprising 154 patients were included. All trials were considered to be at overall high risk of bias. There was no difference in the reversal of HRS (RR = 0.97, 95% CI = 0.76 to 1.23), mortality at 30 days (RR = 0.89, 95% CI = 0.68 to 1.17) and recurrence of HRS (RR = 0.72; 95% CI = 0.36 to 1.45) between norepinephrine and terlipressin. Adverse events were less common with norepinephrine (RR = 0.36, 95% CI = 0.15 to 0.83).

Conclusions: Norepinephrine seems to be an attractive alternative to terlipressin in the treatment of HRS and is associated with less adverse events. However, these findings are based on data extracted from only four small studies.

Editor: Helge Bruns, University Hospital Heidelberg, Germany

Funding: The authors have no support or funding to report.

Competing Interests: The authors have declared that no competing interests exist.

* Email: paulo_nassar@yahoo.com.br

Introduction

Hepatorenal syndrome (HRS) is a severe functional renal failure occurring in patients with cirrhosis and ascites. It develops as a consequence of the severe reduction in the renal perfusion secondary to splanchnic arterial vasodilation. Arterial vasodilation leads to a decrease in the effective blood volume, homeostatic activation of vasoactive systems (renin-angiotensin-aldosterone system [RAAS], antidiuretic hormone [ADH] and sympathetic nervous system) and, consequently, renal vasoconstriction [1].

HRS is sub-classified into types 1 and 2. Type 1 HRS is characterized by rapid progressive renal failure, usually accompanied by multiorgan failure. Type 2 HRS manifests itself as a slowly progressive functional renal failure associated with refractory ascites [1]. A 40% premature mortality rate has been reported in type 1 HRS [2], but may be as high as 83% [3]. Mortality associated with type 2 HRS ranges from 20% to 60% [2,3]. Since the arterial vasodilation seems to be a key mechanism in the

pathogenesis of HRS, vasoconstrictors have been used as a bridging therapy leading up to the definitive treatment; liver transplantation. The vasopressin analog terlipressin is the most widely studied drug, especially in type 1 HRS [4]. However, it is expensive and unavailable in many countries. Norepinephrine, a catecholamine with predominantly alpha-adrenergic activity, is widely available, inexpensive and has been used for the treatment of HRS type 1 since 2002 [5].

With the ominous prognosis of HRS and the high cost associated with terlipressin in mind, we performed a systematic review and meta-analysis to evaluate the efficacy and safety of norepinephrine compared to terlipressin in the treatment of HRS.

Methods

Literature Search

Studies were identified through a search of the Medline, EMBASE, Scopus, Cochrane Central Register of Controlled

Trials (CENTRAL), Lilacs (*Literatura Latino-Americana e do Caribe em Ciências da Saúde*) and Scielo (*Scientific Eletronic Library Online*) databases. A sensitive search strategy was used, combining the following Medical Subject Headings and keywords: "terlipressin" and "norepinephrine" or "noradrenalin" in combination with "hepatorenal syndrome". References of the included studies were also searched. The search strategy was restricted to randomized clinical trials performed on adult subjects and published before 14 January 2014. There was no language restriction. Titles and abstracts were assessed for eligibility and full-text copies of all articles deemed to be potentially relevant were retrieved. A standardized eligibility assessment was performed independently by two reviewers (APNJ and LMSM). Disagreements were resolved by consensus.

The PRISMA statement was used for guidance [6] and the meta-analysis was registered on the PROSPERO database (CRD42013006723).

Study selection

Studies that fulfilled the following criteria were included:

1. Compared terlipressin to norepinephrine in the treatment of type 1 or type 2 HRS;
2. Reported at least one of the following outcomes: reversal of HRS, effect on mortality, recurrence rates after cessation of the treatment or assessment of adverse events on both arms of the study.

Data extraction and quality assessment

A data extraction sheet was developed. Two authors (APNJ and LMSM) independently extracted the following data from included studies, as available: year of publication, number of patients designated to terlipressin or norepinephrine, methods of randomization, allocation concealment, blinding method, age, type of HRS, etiology of cirrhosis and duration of treatment. Child-Pugh and MELD scores, serum creatinine and mean arterial pressure (MAP) were recorded at baseline. Authors of the included studies were contacted by email to complete the missing data that was required for characterizing the studies.

Two authors (APNJ and LMSM) assessed the risk of bias of individual trials using the Cochrane risk of bias tool [7]. For the outcomes in each included trial, the risk of bias was reported as 'low risk', 'unclear risk', or 'high risk' in the following domains: random sequence generation; allocation concealment; blinding of participants and personnel; blinding of outcome assessment; incomplete outcome data; selective reporting; or other bias. Disagreements were resolved by consensus.

Outcome measurements

The primary outcome was the reversal of HRS, defined as a decrease in the serum creatinine value to 133 µmol/l (1.5 mg/dl) or lower during the treatment. Secondary outcomes were mortality, recurrence of HRS and adverse effects.

Statistical Analysis

Heterogeneity was assessed by the I^2 statistic. A random-effects model was employed due to the anticipated variability between trials in terms of patient populations, interventions, and concomitant interventions. The effect of the treatment on the defined outcome measures was calculated from the raw data using random effects models. Differences observed between the treatment groups were expressed as the pooled risk ratio (RR) with a 95% confidence interval (CI). *A priori* subgroup analysis was performed to assess reversal, mortality and recurrence of type 1 and type 2 HRS. All analyses were performed using STATA version 13.0 (STATA Corporation, College Station, TX, USA) and Open Meta Analyst [8].

Results

Trial identification

The search yielded 77 publications. Four randomized controlled trials were selected for the analysis (Figure 1) [9,10,11,12].

Trial characteristics

Table 1 summarizes the details of included studies. One study was performed in Italy [9] and the remaining three were performed at the same center in India [10,11,12]. Two studies included patients with type 1 HRS [10,11], one with type 2 HRS [12] and one with both types of HRS [9]. The studies performed by Singh et al. [11] and Ghosh et al. [12] were actually a single center trial which randomized patients with HRS type 1 and HRS type 2 to terlipressin or norepinephrine and the results to each condition were published in separated papers. Two studies [9,10] classified the patients according to the first version of the International Ascites Club criteria [13] and the remaining [11,12] by the updated criteria [14].

In all studies, the norepinephrine infusion was adjusted to reach an increase of at least 10 mmHg in MAP. In three studies, norepinephrine infusion was also adjusted in order to reach a urine output of over 200 ml [10,11,12]. Norepinephrine infusion was increased every 4 h to reach these targets in all studies. Terlipressin was administered in fixed doses which could be increased every 3 days to decrease basal value of creatinine by at least 25% [9] or at least 1 mg/dl [10,11,12]. Norepinephrine and terlipressin were administered until the reversal of HRS or for a maximum of 15 days. In all studies, patients were administered intravenous albumin and had central venous pressure (CVP) measurements. Albumin was used to maintain a CVP of 10–15 cm H_2O in the Italian study [9]. In the Indian studies, patients were given 20–40 g of albumin per day, which was discontinued if CVP was more than 18 cm H_2O [10,11,12].

Table 2 shows the characteristics of the patients in each study.

Risk of bias

In table 3, the methodology of the quality assessment for each trial is reported using the Cochrane risk of bias tool. All studies were unblinded and eventually met the overall criteria for high risk of bias.

Outcomes

Reversal of HRS was assessed in 154 patients. There was no difference in the reversal of HRS between norepinephrine or terlipressin (RR = 0.97, 95% CI = 0.76 to 1.23; p = 0.800; $I^2 = 0\%$) (Figure 2). Ninety-five patients with type 1 HRS were included in three studies. There was also no difference in the reversal of HRS between norepinephrine and terlipressin in these patients (RR = 1.01, 95% CI = 0.69 to 1.49; p = 0.943; $I^2 = 0\%$). Fifty-nine patients with type 2 HRS were included in two trials and no difference between treatments could be demonstrated (RR = 0.95, 95% CI = 0.70 to 1.28; p = 0.717; $I^2 = 0\%$).

Since all studies reported the mortality rate at 30 days, this end-point was chosen to perform a pooled estimate. No difference in mortality at 30 days between norepinephrine and terlipressin could be found (RR = 0.89, 95% CI = 0.68 to 1.17; p = 0.404; $I^2 = 0\%$) (Figure 3). There were also no differences in mortality among subgroups of type 1 (RR = 0.88, 95% CI = 0.66 to 1.15;

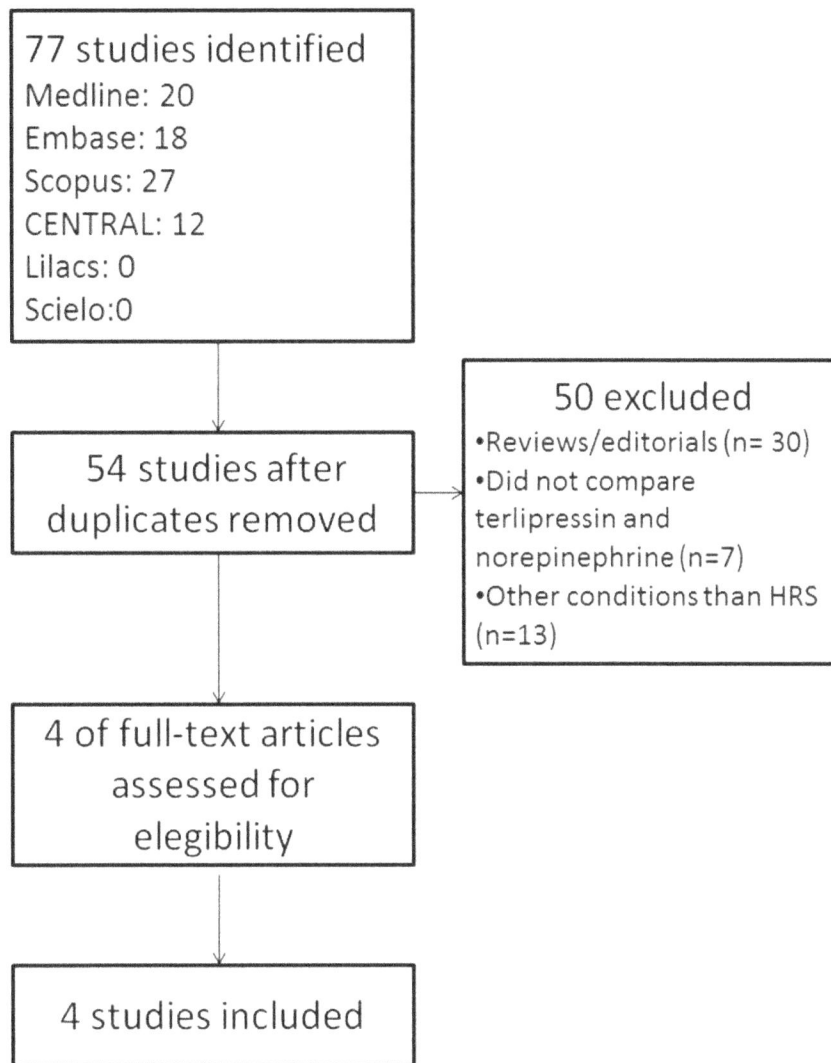

Figure 1. Search strategy.

p = 0.345; $I^2 = 0$%) and type 2 HRS patients (RR = 1.12, 95% CI = 0.44 to 2.83; p = 0.808; $I^2 = 0$%).

Three studies reported recurrence rates of HRS after the cessation of the treatment [9,11,12]. There was no difference in these rates between norepinephrine and terlipressin (RR = 0.72; 95% CI = 0,36 to 1,15; p = 0.357; $I^2 = 0$%) nor was among the subgroups of type 1 (RR = 0.71, 95% CI = 0.13 to 3.82; p = 0.688; $I^2 = 0$%) and type 2 HRS patients (RR = 0.82, 95% CI = 0.036 to 1.84; p = 0.63; $I^2 = 0$%).

Adverse events were less common with norepinephrine (OR = 0.36, 95% CI 0.15 to 0.83; p = 0.017; $I^2 = 0$%) (Figure 4), although all adverse events were of minor importance (Norepinephrine: three episodes of chest pain without electrocardiogram changes or troponin elevation, two episodes of ventricular extrasystoles, one episode of ST segment depression reversed after titration of the dose; terlipressin: 17 episodes of abdominal cramps and increased frequency of stools, two episodes of cyanosis, two episodes of extrasystoles and one episode of ST segment depression reversed after a titration of dose).

Table 1. Included studies.

Study	Design	Screened patients	Included patients	Terlipressin dosage	Norepinephrine dosage
Alessandria,2007 [9]	Single center, unblinded	36	20	1–2 mg every 4 h	0.05–0.7 mcg/kg/min
Sharma, 2008 [10]	Single center, unblinded	49	40	0.5–2 mg every 6 h	0.5–3 mg/h
Singh, 2012 [11]	Single center, unblinded	60	46	0.5–2 mg every 6 h	0.5–3 mg/h
Ghosh, 2013 [12]	Single center, unblinded	58	46	0.5–2 mg every 6 h	0.5–3 mg/h

Table 2. Characteristics of the included patients.

Study	Alessandria et al., 2007 [9]		Sharma et al., 2008 [10]		Singh et al., 2012 [11]		Ghosh et al., 2013 [12]	
	Norepinephrine (n=10)	Terlipressin (n=12)	Norepinephrine (n=20)	Terlipressin (n=20)	Norepinephrine (n=23)	Terlipressin (n=23)	Norepinephrine (n=23)	Terlipressin (n=23)
Age (years)	56±3	55±2	48.2±13.4	47.8±9.8	51.4±11.6	48.3±11.6	45.8±9.2	48.2±10.5
Etiology, Alcohol	2 (20.0%)	4 (33.3%)	12 (60.0%)	14 (70.0%)	10 (43.4%)	12 (52.1%)	15 (65.2%)	16 (69.6%)
Child Pugh score	10±1	11±1	11.0±0.9	10.6±0.8	10.70±2.01	10.43±1.72	10.0±1.77	10.5±2.35
MELD score	26±1	26±2	31.6±6.0	29.6±6.2	26.39±3.13	24.65±5.31	21.3±2.79	21.0±3.28
Serum creatinine (md/dl)	2.3±0.2	2.5±0.3	3.3±1.3	3.0±0.5	3.27±0.71	3.10±0.66	2.15±0.21	2.05±0.22
MAP (mmHg)	71±2	74±3	78.2±5.3	81.4±11.4	64.7±11.9	65.2±10.2	65.3±7.2	66.2±9.5

Data are mean ± standard deviation or number (%) of patients; MELD, model for end-stage liver disease; MAP, mean arterial pressure.

Table 3. Risk of bias assessment.

Study	Sequence generation	Allocation concealment	Blinding of participants, personnel and outcome assessors	Incomplete outcome data	Selective outcome reporting	Other source of bias	Overall risk of bias
Alessandria, 2007 [9]	Unclear	Low	High	Low	Low	Unclear	High
Sharma, 2008 [10]	Low	Unclear	High	Low	Low	Unclear	High
Singh, 2012 [11]	Low	Low	High	Low	Low	Low	High
Ghosh, 2013 [12]	Low	Low	High	Low	Low	Low	High

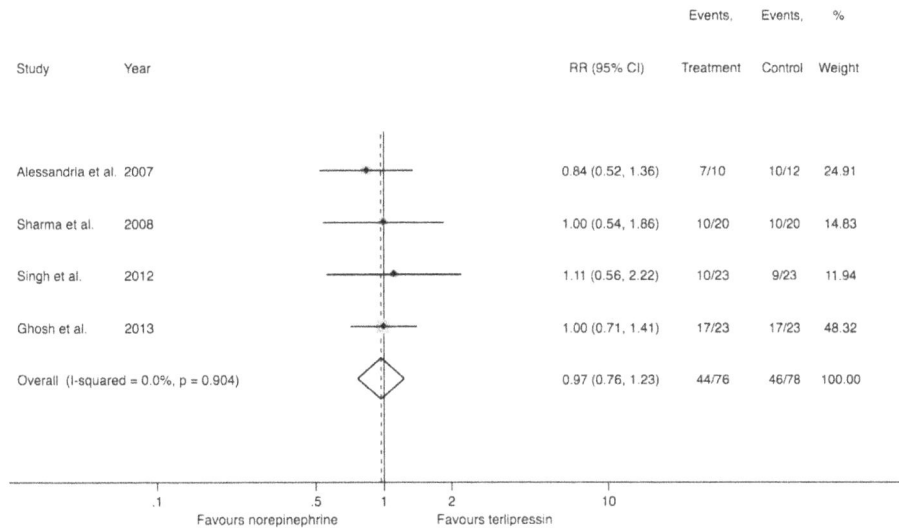

Figure 2. Reversal of hepatorenal syndrome. P values presented are for heterogeneity. P value for overall effect = 0.792. Chi-square = 0.536 (degrees of freedom = 3).

Discussion

The results of this review suggest that in patients with HRS, treatment with norepinephrine is as effective as terlipressin when used in conjunction with albumin. Additionally, norepinephrine seems to be associated with less adverse events than terlipressin. However, these results are based on few trials with a reduced number of patients included.

In patients with cirrhosis, functional kidney failure is caused by a severe reduction of the effective circulating volume due to splanchnic arterial dilation and a reduction in the renal blood flow due to marked multifactorial intrarenal vasoconstriction [15]. This particular form of renal dysfunction develops in the later phases of liver failure and is characterized by low arterial pressure, intense activation of the renin-angiotensin and sympathetic nervous systems with an increase in the plasma levels of renin, norepinephrine, water retention due to increased anti-diuretic hormone and lowering glomerular filtration rates [1]. Without

treatment, short-term mortality exceeds 50% with a median survival time of only 2 weeks [16].

Therapy with systemic vasoconstrictors and albumin is a bridging option to ameliorate renal dysfunction and to improve survival of patients while waiting for definitive treatment with liver transplantation. The rationale of associating these two therapies is to reduce the discrepancy between circulatory capacitance and intravascular volume, thereby increasing the effective arterial blood volume. Terlipressin promotes vasoconstriction in both systemic and splanchnic circulation through activation of V1 receptors of the vascular smooth muscle cells and is reported to reduce portal inflow, portal systemic shunting [17]; and to dilate intrahepatic vessels, consequently reducing intrahepatic resistance to portal inflow [18]. The overall results of the use of terlipressin in conjunction with albumin in the treatment of HRS are an improvement in renal function and an increase in the median survival time as demonstrated in clinical trials and confirmed by at

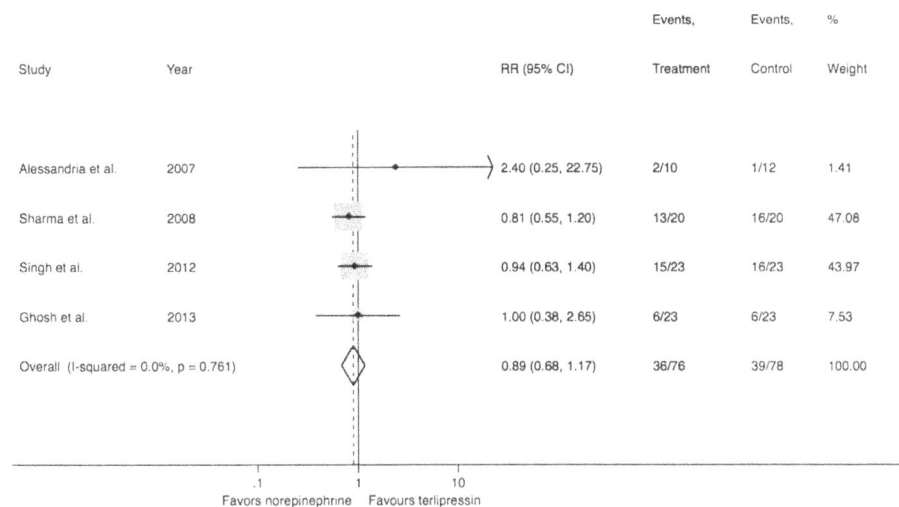

Figure 3. Mortality rates at 30 days. P values presented are for heterogeneity. P value for overall effect = 0.618. Chi-square = 1.077 (degrees of freedom = 3).

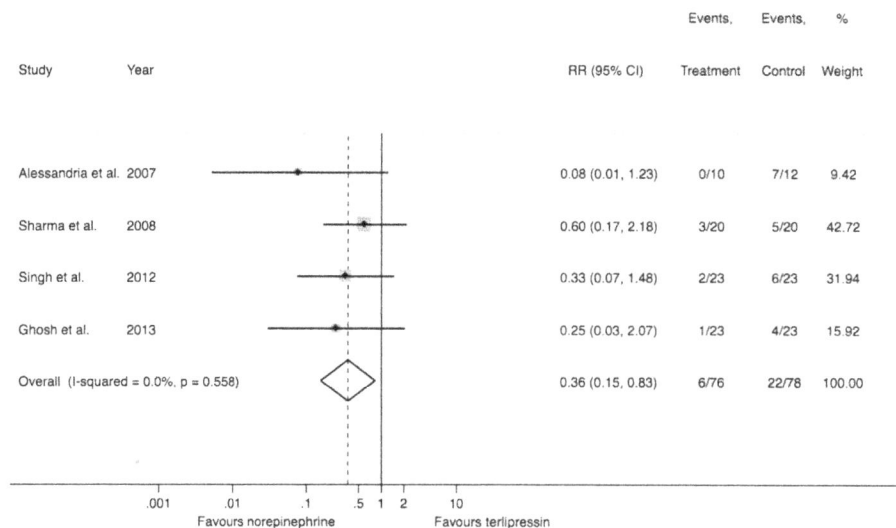

Figure 4. Adverse events. P values presented are for heterogeneity. P value for overall effect = 0.004. Chi-square = 1.901 (degrees of freedom = 3).

least three meta-analyses [4,19,20]. Although terlipressin has become the vasoactive drug of choice where available, a Cochrane meta-analysis has pointed out that all randomized controlled studies that addressed the efficacy of terlipressin were underpowered and at high risk of bias [4]. Additionally, the evidence on the use of terlipressin in type 2 HRS is scarce since these patients were included in only one trial [21].

Norepinephrine, an inexpensive α-adrenergic receptor agonist available worldwide, is a possible alternative treatment for HRS because its intense vasoconstriction action may increase the effective arterial blood volume. A pilot single-center study with 12 patients demonstrated the reversal of HRS in 10 (83%) patients [5]. Since then, according to our literature search, four studies that aimed to compare norepinephrine and terlipressin in treatment of HRS have been published [9,10,11,12].

Reversal of HRS occurred in 58% (Figure 2) of type 1 HRS patients treated with norepinephrine. These figures are very similar to the response rates reported on terlipressin arms of randomized controlled trials of this drug compared to placebo [4], but higher than those found in clinical practice [2,3]. The trial of Ghosh et al. [12] was the first to randomize type 2 HRS patients exclusively. Response rates in this trial (74%) were higher than those found in type 1 HRS patients [12].Type 2 HRS patients included in the study published by Alessandria et al. also had a similar response (77%) to both vasoconstrictors [9].

Thirty day-mortality rates were around 50%. Two studies that included only type 1 HRS patients found a 30 day-mortality rate of over 65% [10,11], which is similar to the ones reported in randomized controlled trials of terlipressin compared with a placebo [4,19], but lower than clinical survey data [2,3]. Recurrence rates were around 30%, similar to those found in observational studies [2,22], but higher than those reported in the largest study which compared terlipressin and placebo [23].

Norepinephrine was associated with less adverse events than terlipressin. This difference was related to the frequency of abdominal cramps and diarrhea found in patients who were given terlipressin (17 cases in 78 patients). These are common adverse events related to terlipressin and are usually self-limiting, but were more common in our meta-analysis than in the Cochrane meta-analysis of terlipressin compared to placebo [4]. Norepinephrine and terlipressin both have a safe cardiovascular profile. Only nine

cardiovascular events were found in the included trials and only two of them (episodes of segment ST depression) led to a change in therapy (a titration of dose) (10). Cardiovascular adverse effect rates were lower than those reported for terlipressin in the meta-analysis previously cited [4].

Although it was not among the outcomes of this review, we observed all included trials reported lower costs with norepinephrine than with terlipressin. However, all of them were performed in specialized units with a high level of surveillance and only costs related to the drugs were reported. Although more expensive, terlipressin has some advantages over norepinephrine. It is given as an intravenous bolus in a peripheral vein. This means that terlipressin can be safely used in regular wards. Norepinephrine is given intravenously as a continuous infusion in a central venous catheter, usually in the setting of intensive care unit. Therefore, a comparison of costs between these two treatments must also take into account intensive care costs.

In spite of an extensive literature search without language restriction that was conducted, we were not able to identify any studies published in non-indexed journals or as conference proceedings. Although included studies had no evidence of significant heterogeneity, and used similar treatment protocols, they had small sample sizes and were single-centered. Three of them were performed at a same center [10,11,12] and they included patients with different HRS criteria, as these were updated from 1996 to 2007 [13,14]. Therefore, the first two studies adopted the first criteria [9,10] and the remaining, the updated criteria [11,12]. Undoubtedly, these findings reduce external validity of the results of this meta-analysis. Additionally, it would be questionable to combine data from patients with patients with type 1 and type 2 HRS since these two conditions have a different course and different responses to vasoconstrictors [1,2,3]. Similar limitations were also acknowledged in the meta-analyses of terlipressin compared to a placebo or other drugs in the treatment of HRS [4,19]. In order to better address the question of efficacy and safety of terlipressin and norepinephrine in the treatment of type 1 and type 2 HRS, we have performed subgroup analysis on each condition.

Since the largest randomized study published with HRS patients included only 112 patients [23], a collaborative research network would be necessary to perform a large clinical trial comparing norepinephrine to terlipressin in the treatment of HRS.

In conclusion, norepinephrine and terlipressin had similar response rates for the treatment of type 1 or 2 HRS. However, norepinephrine was associated with less adverse events than terlipressin. Nevertheless, these findings are based on small studies, with a total of only 154 patients. A larger randomized controlled trial would be needed to draw firm conclusions on the choice of the vasoconstrictor to treat HRS.

Author Contributions

Conceived and designed the experiments: APNJ AQF LMSM. Performed the experiments: APNJ LMSM. Analyzed the data: APNJ AQF LMSM. Contributed to the writing of the manuscript: APNJ AQF LACDA FJC LMSM.

References

1. Arroyo V, Fernandez J (2011) Management of hepatorenal syndrome in patients with cirrhosis. Nat Rev Nephrol 7: 517–526.
2. Salerno F, Cazzaniga M, Merli M, Spinzi G, Saibeni S, et al. (2011) Diagnosis, treatment and survival of patients with hepatorenal syndrome: a survey on daily medical practice. J Hepatol 55: 1241–1248.
3. Carvalho GC, Regis Cde A, Kalil JR, Cerqueira LA, Barbosa DS, et al. (2012) Causes of renal failure in patients with decompensated cirrhosis and its impact in hospital mortality. Ann Hepatol 11: 90–95.
4. Gluud LL, Christensen K, Christensen E, Krag A (2012) Terlipressin for hepatorenal syndrome. Cochrane Database Syst Rev 9: CD005162.
5. Duvoux C, Zanditenas D, Hezode C, Chauvat A, Monin JL, et al. (2002) Effects of noradrenalin and albumin in patients with type I hepatorenal syndrome: a pilot study. Hepatology 36: 374–380.
6. Liberati A, Altman DG, Tetzlaff J, Mulrow C, Gotzsche PC, et al. (2009) The PRISMA statement for reporting systematic reviews and meta-analyses of studies that evaluate healthcare interventions: explanation and elaboration. BMJ 339: b2700.
7. Higgins JP, Altman DG, Gotzsche PC, Juni P, Moher D, et al. (2011) The Cochrane Collaboration's tool for assessing risk of bias in randomised trials. BMJ 343: d5928.
8. Wallace BC, Schmid CH, Lau J, Trikalinos TA (2009) Meta-Analyst: software for meta-analysis of binary, continuous and diagnostic data. BMC Med Res Methodol 9: 80.
9. Alessandria C, Ottobrelli A, Debernardi-Venon W, Todros L, Cerenzia MT, et al. (2007) Noradrenalin vs terlipressin in patients with hepatorenal syndrome: a prospective, randomized, unblinded, pilot study. J Hepatol 47: 499–505.
10. Sharma P, Kumar A, Shrama BC, Sarin SK (2008) An open label, pilot, randomized controlled trial of noradrenaline versus terlipressin in the treatment of type 1 hepatorenal syndrome and predictors of response. Am J Gastroenterol 103: 1689–1697.
11. Singh V, Ghosh S, Singh B, Kumar P, Sharma N, et al. (2012) Noradrenaline vs. terlipressin in the treatment of hepatorenal syndrome: a randomized study. J Hepatol 56: 1293–1298.
12. Ghosh S, Choudhary NS, Sharma AK, Singh B, Kumar P, et al. (2013) Noradrenaline vs terlipressin in the treatment of type 2 hepatorenal syndrome: a randomized pilot study. Liver Int 33: 1187–1193.
13. Arroyo V, Gines P, Gerbes AL, Dudley FJ, Gentilini P, et al. (1996) Definition and diagnostic criteria of refractory ascites and hepatorenal syndrome in cirrhosis. International Ascites Club. Hepatology 23: 164–176.
14. Salerno F, Gerbes A, Gines P, Wong F, Arroyo V (2007) Diagnosis, prevention and treatment of hepatorenal syndrome in cirrhosis. Gut 56: 1310–1318.
15. Angeli P, Gines P (2012) Hepatorenal syndrome, MELD score and liver transplantation: an evolving issue with relevant implications for clinical practice. J Hepatol 57: 1135–1140.
16. Gines A, Escorsell A, Gines P, Salo J, Jimenez W, et al. (1993) Incidence, predictive factors, and prognosis of the hepatorenal syndrome in cirrhosis with ascites. Gastroenterology 105: 229–236.
17. Narahara Y, Kanazawa H, Taki Y, Kimura Y, Atsukawa M, et al. (2009) Effects of terlipressin on systemic, hepatic and renal hemodynamics in patients with cirrhosis. J Gastroenterol Hepatol 24: 1791–1797.
18. Kiszka-Kanowitz M, Henriksen JH, Hansen EF, Moller S, Bendtsen F (2004) Effect of terlipressin on blood volume distribution in patients with cirrhosis. Scand J Gastroenterol 39: 486–492.
19. Dobre M, Demirjian S, Sehgal AR, Navaneethan SD (2011) Terlipressin in hepatorenal syndrome: a systematic review and meta-analysis. Int Urol Nephrol 43: 175–184.
20. Hiremath SB, Srinivas LD (2013) Survival benefits of terlipressin and non-responder state in hepatorenal syndrome: a meta-analysis. Indian J Pharmacol 45: 54–60.
21. Martin-Llahi M, Pepin MN, Guevara M, Diaz F, Torre A, et al. (2008) Terlipressin and albumin vs albumin in patients with cirrhosis and hepatorenal syndrome: a randomized study. Gastroenterology 134: 1352–1359.
22. Nazar A, Pereira GH, Guevara M, Martin-Llahi M, Pepin MN, et al. (2010) Predictors of response to therapy with terlipressin and albumin in patients with cirrhosis and type 1 hepatorenal syndrome. Hepatology 51: 219–226.
23. Sanyal AJ, Boyer T, Garcia-Tsao G, Regenstein F, Rossaro L, et al. (2008) A randomized, prospective, double-blind, placebo-controlled trial of terlipressin for type 1 hepatorenal syndrome. Gastroenterology 134: 1360–1368.

Permissions

List of Contributors

Tsuyoshi Takashima, Motoaki Miyazono, Makoto Fukuda, Tomoya Kishi, Mai Yoshizaki, Sae Sato and Yuji Ikeda
Department of Nephrology, Faculty of Medicine, Saga University, Saga, Japan

Hugh Bostock
Department of Neurology, Inselspital, Bern University Hospital and University of Bern, Bern, Switzerland
Sobell Department of Motor Neuroscience and Movement Disorders, Institute of Neurology, University College London, London, United Kingdom

Werner J. Z'Graggen
Department of Neurology, Inselspital, Bern University Hospital and University of Bern, Bern, Switzerland
Department of Neurosurgery, Inselspital, Bern University Hospital and University of Bern, Bern, Switzerland

Sian E. Piret, Caroline M. Gorvin, Nellie Y. Loh and Rajesh V. Thakker
Nuffield Department of Clinical Medicine, Oxford Centre for Diabetes, Endocrinology and Metabolism, University of Oxford, Oxford, United Kingdom

Christopher T. Esapa and Rosie Head
Nuffield Department of Clinical Medicine, Oxford Centre for Diabetes, Endocrinology and Metabolism, University of Oxford, Oxford, United Kingdom
Mammalian Genetics Unit, MRC Harwell, Harwell Science and Innovation Campus, United Kingdom

Matthew Brown
Nuffield Department of Clinical Medicine, Oxford Centre for Diabetes, Endocrinology and Metabolism, University of Oxford, Oxford, United Kingdom
The University of Queensland Diamantina Institute, Princess Alexandra Hospital, Woolloongabba, Queensland, Australia

Steve D. M. Brown and Roger Cox
Mammalian Genetics Unit, MRC Harwell, Harwell Science and Innovation Campus, United Kingdom

Olivier Devuyst
Institute of Physiology, Zurich Center for Integrative Human Physiology, University of Zurich, Zurich, Switzerland

Gethin Thomas
The University of Queensland Diamantina Institute, Princess Alexandra Hospital, Woolloongabba, Queensland, Australia

Peter Croucher
Garvan Institute for Medical Research, Sydney, Australia

Felix Jansen, Anja Mieth, Andrea Babelova and Ralf P. Brandes
Institut für Kardiovaskuläre Physiologie, Fachbereich Medizin der Goethe-Universität, Frankfurt am Main, Germany

Oliver Jung and Rainer U. Pliquett
Medizinische Klinik III, Klinikum der Goethe-Universität, Frankfurt am Main, Germany

Eduardo Barbosa-Sicard
Institute for Vascular Signalling, Klinikum der Goethe-Universität, Frankfurt am Main, Germany

Christophe Morisseau, Sung H. Hwang, Cindy Tsai and Bruce D. Hammock
Department of Entomology and Cancer Center, University of California Davis, Davis, California, United States of America

Liliana Schaefer
Pharmazentrum Frankfurt/ZAFES/Institut für Allgemeine Pharmakologie, Klinikum der Goethe-Universität, Frankfurt am Main, Germany

Gerd Geisslinger
Pharmazentrum Frankfurt/ZAFES/Institut für Klinische Pharmakologie, Klinikum der Goethe-Universität, Frankfurt am Main, Germany

Kerstin Amann
Department of Pathology, Nephropathology, Friedrich-Alexander University, Erlangen-Nürnberg, Germany

Alessandro Achilli and Hovirag Lancioni
Dipartimento di Biologia Cellulare e Ambientale, Università di Perugia, Perugia, Italy

Anna Olivieri, Maria Pala, Baharak Hooshiar Kashani, Valeria Carossa, Francesca Gandini, Vincenza Battaglia, Viola Grugni and Antonio Torroni
Dipartimento di Genetica e Microbiologia, Università di Pavia, Pavia, Italy

Ugo A. Perego
Dipartimento di Genetica e Microbiologia, Università di Pavia, Pavia, Italy
Sorenson Molecular Genealogy Foundation, Salt Lake City, Utah, United States of America

Ornella Semino
Dipartimento di Genetica e Microbiologia, Università di Pavia, Pavia, Italy
Centro Interdipartimentale "Studi di Genere", Università di Pavia, Pavia, Italy

Aurelia Santoro and Claudio Franceschi
Dipartimento di Patologia Sperimentale, Università di Bologna, Bologna, Italy
CIG-Interdepartmental Center for Biophysics and Biocomplexity Studies, Università di Bologna, Bologna, Italy

Cristina Sirolla and Liana Spazzafumo
Department of Gerontology Research, Statistic and Biometry Center, Italian National Research Center on Aging (INRCA), Ancona, Italy

Anna Rita Bonfigli, Massimo Boemi, Ivano Testa, Maurizio Marra and Roberto Testa
Metabolic and Nutrition Research Center on Diabetes, Italian National Research Center on Aging, INRCA-IRCCS, Ancona, Italy

Antonella Cormio and Maria Nicola Gadaleta
Dipartimento di Biochimica e Biologia Molecolare "E. Quagliariello", Università di Bari, Bari, Italy

Antonio Ceriello
Institut d'Investigacions Biomèdiques August Pi Sunyer (IDIBAPS) and Centro de Investigacion Biomedica en Red de Diabetes y Enfermedades Metabolicas Asociadis (CIBERDEM), Barcelona, Spain

Yongchuan Li, Yawei Liu, Lili Fu, Changlin Mei and Bing Dai
Division of Nephrology, Nephrology Institute of PLA, Shanghai Changzheng Hospital, Second Military Medical University, Shanghai, China

Zhengxiu Su, Hongguo Zhu, Menghuan Zhang, Liangliang Wang, Hanchang He, Shaoling Jiang, Fan Fan Hou and Aiqing Li
Division of Nephrology, Nanfang Hospital, Southern Medical University, State Key Laboratory of Organ Failure Research, National Clinical Research Center of Kidney Disease, Guangzhou, Guangdong, China

Nikolaos Pagonas, Joachim Jankowski, Walter Zidek and Timm H. Westhoff
Deparment of Nephrology, Charité – Campus Benjamin Franklin, Berlin, Germany

Wolfgang Vautz, Luzia Seifert and Rafael Slodzinski
Leibniz-Institut für Analytische Wissenschaften ISAS – e.V., Dortmund, Germany

Hong-Mei Zhang
Department of Clinical Oncology, Xijing Hospital, The Fourth Military Medical University, Xi'an, China
Department of Medicine, Health Science Center, University of Texas, San Antonio, Texas, United States of America

Amrita Kamat
Department of Medicine, Health Science Center, University of Texas, San Antonio, Texas, United States of America
Audie L. Murphy Division, Geriatric Research, Education and Clinical Center, South Texas Veterans Health Care System, San Antonio, Texas, United States of America

Bin-Xian Zhang
Department of Medicine, Health Science Center, University of Texas, San Antonio, Texas, United States of America
Department of Comprehensive Dentistry, Health Science Center, University of Texas, San Antonio, Texas, United States of America
Audie L. Murphy Division, Geriatric Research, Education and Clinical Center, South Texas Veterans Health Care System, San Antonio, Texas, United States of America

Howard Dang
Department of Comprehensive Dentistry, Health Science Center, University of Texas, San Antonio, Texas, United States of America

Chih-Ko Yeh
Department of Comprehensive Dentistry, Health Science Center, University of Texas, San Antonio, Texas, United States of America
Audie L. Murphy Division, Geriatric Research, Education and Clinical Center, South Texas Veterans Health Care System, San Antonio, Texas, United States of America

Ki-Ho Park, Yu-Mi Lee, Hyo-Lim Hong, Tark Kim, Hyun Jung Park, So-Youn Park, Song Mi Moon, Yong Pil Chong, Sung-Han Kim, Sang-Oh Lee, Sang-Ho Choi, Jun Hee Woo and Yang Soo Kim
Department of Infectious Diseases, Asan Medical Center, University of Ulsan College of Medicine, Seoul, Republic of Korea
Center for Antimicrobial Resistance and Microbial Genetics, University of Ulsan, Seoul, Republic of Korea

Jin-Yong Jeong
Department of Infectious Diseases, Asan Medical Center, University of Ulsan College of Medicine, Seoul, Republic of Korea

Center for Antimicrobial Resistance and Microbial Genetics, University of Ulsan, Seoul, Republic of Korea
Asan Institute of Life Sciences, Asan Medical Center, University of Ulsan College of Medicine, Seoul, Republic of Korea

Mi-Na Kim
Department of Laboratory Medicine, Asan Medical Center, University of Ulsan College of Medicine, Seoul, Republic of Korea

Ankita Varshney, Gulam Rabbani and Rizwan Hasan Khan
Interdisciplinary Biotechnology Unit, Aligarh Muslim University, Aligarh, India

Mohd Rehan and Naidu Subbarao
School of Information Technology, Centre for Computational Biology and Bioinformatics, Jawaharlal Nehru University, New Delhi, India

Patricia Keiko Saito, Roger Haruki Yamakawa and Sueli Donizete Borelli
Department of Basic Health Sciences, Universidade Estadual de Maringá, Maringá, Paraná, Brazil

Erica Pereira Aparecida
Histogene Laboratory of Histocompatibility and Genetics, Maringá, Paraná, Brazil

Waldir Verissimo da Silva Júnior
Department of Statistics, Universidade Estadual de Maringá, Maringá, Paraná, Brazil

Stephen E. Roberts, Lori A. Button and John G. Williams
College of Medicine, Swansea University, Swansea, United Kingdom

Yu-Hao Zhou, Zhi-Chao Jin, Mei-Jing Wu, Jia-Jie Zang, Jin-Fang Xu, Chun-Fang Wu, Ying-Yi Qin, Qing-Bin Gao and Jia He
Department of Health Statistics, Second Military Medical University, Shanghai, China

Shi-Lei Guo
Department of Anatomy, Second Military University, Shanghai, China

Qing Cai
Department of Rheumatology and Immunology, Changhai Hospital, Second Military Medical University, Shanghai, China

Dand-Hui Yu
Academic Journal of Second Military Medical University, Shanghai, China

Li-Gong Tang
Department of Urology, Wuhan General Hospital, Guangzhou Command PLA, Wuhan, China

Shan-Shan Zhang
Tumor Immunology and Gene Therapy Center, Eastern Hepatobiliary Surgery Hospital, Second Military Medical University, Shanghai, China

Sebastian J. Padayatty, Andrew Y. Sun, Michael Graham Espey and Mark Levine
Molecular and Clinical Nutrition Section, National Institute of Diabetes and Digestive and Kidney Diseases, National Institutes of Health, Bethesda, Maryland, United States of America

Qi Chen and Jeanne Drisko
Program in Integrative Medicine, University of Kansas Medical Center, Kansas City, Kansas, United States of America

Maria del Carmen Basualdo and Ruud M. Buijs
Dept. de Biologia Celular y Fisiologia, Instituto de Investigaciones Biomedicas, UNAM, Mexico City, Mexico

Nadia Saderi
Dept. de Biologia Celular y Fisiologia, Instituto de Investigaciones Biomedicas, UNAM, Mexico City, Mexico
NEF-Lab, Dept. Cytomorphology, University of Cagliari, Monserrato (CA), Italy

Roberto Salgado-Delgado
Dept. de Biologia Celular y Fisiologia, Instituto de Investigaciones Biomedicas, UNAM, Mexico City, Mexico
Facultad de Ciencias, UASLP, San Luis Potosì, Mexico

Gian-Luca Ferri
NEF-Lab, Dept. Cytomorphology, University of Cagliari, Monserrato (CA), Italy

Rafael Avendaño-Pradel and Carolina Escobar
Dept. de Anatomia, Facultad de Medicina, UNAM, Mexico City, Mexico

Laura Chávez-Macías and Juan E. Olvera Roblera
Unidad de Neuropatología, Hospital General de Mexico, Mexico City, Mexico

Gian Paolo Fadini, Saula de Kreutzenberg and Angelo Avogaro
Department of Clinical and Experimental Medicine, University of Padova Medical School, Padova, Italy

Shoichi Maruyama and Takenori Ozaki
Department of Nephrology, Nagoya University Graduate School of Medicine, Nagoya, Japan

Akihiko Taguchi
Department of Cerebrovascular Disease, National Cardiovascular Center, Osaka, Japan

James Meigs
Harvard Medical School and General Medicine Division, Massachusetts General Hospital, Boston, Massachusetts, United States of America

Stefanie Dimmeler and Andreas M. Zeiher
Molecular Cardiology and Internal Medicine III, Wolfgang Goethe University, Frankfurt, Germany

Georg Nickenig and Nikos Werner
Department of Internal Medicine II, Division of Cardiology, Pneumology, and Angiology, University Hospital Bonn, Bonn, Germany

Caroline Schmidt-Lucke
Department of Cardiology and Pneumology, Charitè, Universitätsmedizin Berlin, Campus Benjamin Franklin, Berlin, Germany

Mario Tumbarello and Enrico Maria Trecarichi
Istituto di Clinica delle Malattie Infettive, Università Cattolica del Sacro Cuore, Roma, Italy

Morena Caira and Livio Pagano
Istituto di Ematologia, Università Cattolica del Sacro Cuore, Roma, Italy

Anna Candoni
Clinica di Ematologia, Università di Udine, Udine, Italy

Domenico Pastore
Divisione di Ematologia, Università di Bari, Bari, Italy

Chiara Cattaneo
U. O. Ematologia, Spedali Civili, Brescia, Italy

Rosa Fanci
Unità Operativa di Ematologia, Azienda Ospedaliera Universitaria Careggi, Firenze, Italy

Annamaria Nosari
Divisione di Ematologia e Centro Trapianti Midollo, Ospedale Niguarda Ca' Granda, Milano, Italy

Antonio Spadea
Ematologia, Istituto Regina Elena, Roma, Italy

Alessandro Busca
Divisione di Ematologia, Ospedale le Molinette, Torino, Italy

Nicola Vianelli
Istituto di Ematologia ed Oncologia Clinica "Lorenzo e Ariosto Serágnoli", Ospedale; S.Orsola-Malpighi, Università di Bologna, Bologna, Italy

Teresa Spanu
Istituto di Microbiologia, Università Cattolica del Sacro Cuore, Roma, Italy

Roksana Rodak and Claudia C. Wagner
Division of Internal Medicine, University Hospital Zurich, Zurich, Switzerland

Stefan Markun
Division of Internal Medicine, University Hospital Zurich, Zurich, Switzerland
Institute of General Practice and Health Service Research, University of Zurich, University Hospital of Zurich, Zurich, Switzerland

Barbara M. Holzer, Vladimir Kaplan and Lukas Zimmerli
Division of Internal Medicine, University Hospital Zurich, Zurich, Switzerland
Center of Competence Multimorbidity, University of Zurich, Zurich, Switzerland

Edouard Battegay
Division of Internal Medicine, University Hospital Zurich, Zurich, Switzerland
Center of Competence Multimorbidity, University of Zurich, Zurich, Switzerland
University Research Priority Program Dynamics of Healthy Aging, University of Zurich, Zurich, Switzerland

Jumpei Sasabe, Masataka Suzuki, Sonomi Ito and Sadakazu Aiso
Department of Anatomy, Keio University School of Medicine, Shinanomachi, Shinjuku-ku, Tokyo, Japan

Yurika Miyoshi and Kenji Hamase
Graduate School of Pharmaceutical Sciences, KyushuUniversity, Maidashi, Higashi-ku, Fukuoka, Japan

Yosuke Tojo, Chieko Okamura and Masashi Mita
Innovative Science Research and Development Center, Shiseido Co., Ltd., Fukuura, Kanazawa-ku, Yokohama, Japan

Ryuichi Konno
Department of Pharmacological Sciences, International University of Health and Welfare, Kitakanemaru, Ohtawara, Tochigi, Japan

Ellen Neven, Tineke M. De Schutter, Geert Dams, Patrick C. D'Haese and Geert J. Behets
Laboratory of Pathophysiology, Department of Biomedical Sciences, University of Antwerp, Antwerp, Belgium

Kristina Gundlach, Sonja Steppan and Janine Büchel
Fresenius Medical Care Deutschland GmbH, Bad Homburg, Germany

Jutta Passlick-Deetjen
Department of Nephrology, University of Düsseldorf, Düsseldorf, Germany

Chih-Hsiang Chang, Pei-Chun Fan, Ming-Yang Chang, Ya-Chung Tian, Cheng-Chieh Hung, Ji-Tseng Fang, Chih-Wei Yang and Yung-Chang Chen
Kidney Research Center, Department of Nephrology, Chang Gung Memorial Hospital, Taipei, Taiwan
Chang Gung University College of Medicine, Taoyuan, Taiwan
Chang Gung University College of Medicine, Taoyuan, Taiwan

Bo Yang, Jing Xu, Chaoyang Ye, Changlin Mei and Zhiguo Mao
Kidney Institute of Chinese People's Liberation Army, Division of Nephrology, Changzheng Hospital, Second Military Medical University, Shanghai, China

Fengying Xu and Zui Zou
Division of Anesthesiology, Changzheng Hospital, Second Military Medical University, Shanghai, China

Nuha Mahmoud Hamdi
Immunology Department, Riyadh Regional Laboratory, King Saud Medical Complex, Riyadh, Kingdom of Saudi Arabia

Fadel Hassan Al-Hababi
Virology Department, Riyadh Regional Laboratory, King Saud Medical Complex, Riyadh, Kingdom of Saudi Arabia

Amr Ekhlas Eid
Nephrology Department, Riyadh Medical Complex, King Saud Medical Complex, Riyadh, Kingdom of Saudi Arabia

Heng-Chih Pan, Pei-Chun Fan and Chih-Hsiang Chang
Kidney Research Center, Department of Nephrology, Chang Gung Memorial Hospital, Taipei, Taiwan

Chang-Chyi Jenq, Ming-Yang Chang, Ya-Chung Tian, Cheng-Chieh Hung, Ji-Tseng Fang, Chih-Wei Yang and Yung-Chang Chen
Kidney Research Center, Department of Nephrology, Chang Gung Memorial Hospital, Taipei, Taiwan
Chang Gung University College of Medicine, Taoyuan, Taiwan

Ming-Hung Tsai
Division of Gastroenterology, Chang Gung Memorial Hospital, Taipei, Taiwan
Chang Gung University College of Medicine, Taoyuan, Taiwan

Wei-Chen Lee
Laboratory of Immunology, Department of General Surgery, Chang Gung Memorial Hospital, Taipei, Taiwan
Chang Gung University College of Medicine, Taoyuan, Taiwan

Mary M. Christopher
Department of Pathology, Immunology and Microbiology, University of California Davis, Davis, CA, 95616, United States of America

Michelle G. Hawkins
Department of Medicine and Epidemiology, University of California Davis, Davis, CA, 95616, United States of America

Andrew G. Burton
William R. Pritchard Veterinary Medical Teaching Hospital, University of California Davis, Davis, CA, 95616, United States of America

Marine Livrozet and Sophie Vandermeersch
Sorbonne Universités, UPMC Univ Paris 06, UMR S
702, Paris, France
INSERM, UMR S 702, Paris, France

Jean-Jacques Boffa
Sorbonne Universités, UPMC Univ Paris 06, UMR S
702, Paris, France
INSERM, UMR S 702, Paris, France
Néphrologie, AP-HP, Hôpital Tenon, Paris, France

**Jean-Philippe Haymann, Laurent Baud, Michel
Daudon and Emmanuel Letavernier**
Sorbonne Universités, UPMC Univ Paris 06, UMR S
702, Paris, France

INSERM, UMR S 702, Paris, France
Explorations Fonctionnelles Multidisciplinaires, AP-
HP, Hôpital Tenon, Paris, France

Laurent Mesnard
Department of Physiology and Biophysics, Cornell
University, Ithaca, New York, United States of America

Elizabeth Thioulouse
Biochimie, AP-HP, Hôpital Trousseau, Paris, France

Jean Jaubert
Institut Pasteur, Mouse Functional Genetics Unit,
Paris, France
CNRS URA 2578, Paris, France

Dominique Bazin
CNRSLCMCP-Sorbonne Universités UPMC Univ Paris
06, Collège de France, Paris, France

**Antonio Paulo Nassar Junior and Luiz Marcelo Sa´
Malbouisson**
Intensive Care Unit, Department of Gastroenterology,
University of Sao Paulo. Sao Paulo, SP, Brazil

Index

A

Acute Kidney Injury (AKI), 156

Albuminuria, 36, 53, 80, 82-83, 85, 98-99, 103, 110

Antimicrobial Therapy, 180, 182-184, 186-187

Arachidonic Acid, 80, 82, 85-88

C

C-reactive Protein, 14-15, 21, 40, 62-63, 73, 75, 79, 136, 139, 143-144

Cabg, 55-56, 58-60, 159, 176

Cardiocerebral, 55-59

Cerebrovascular Disease, 14, 39, 56-57, 59-60, 70, 176

Chelation Therapy, 131

Chronic Liver Failure (CLIF), 146-147

Circulating Progenitor Cells (CPC), 14

Cmv Infection, 12

Continuous Renal Replacement Therapy, 38, 41-43

Contrast Induced Nephropathy (CIN), 174

Coronary Artery Disease, 22, 56, 60, 72, 176

Cpb, 156, 158-160, 163

Creatinine, 1-2, 4-6, 15, 23-26, 28-31, 33-37, 40, 42, 45, 47, 56, 70, 74, 76, 78, 81, 91, 93, 97, 99-100, 104, 110, 119, 133, 139, 141, 149, 156-161, 169, 171, 179, 190, 192

Crsab, 180-187

Cryptococcal Meningitis (CM), 118

CSF, 118-119, 121

Cyclosporine, 156, 159-160

D

DAO, 13, 165-171

Diabetic Nephropathy, 53, 62, 72, 88, 98-99, 103-106

Diazepam, 23-25, 31-34

Dsc, 24, 36

E

Ectopic Calcifications, 8

Eets, 80, 85-87

Enalapril, 107-112, 114-116

Endocarditis, 125, 127, 180-183, 187-188

F

Fluconazole Monotherapy, 118, 120-121

Fluorescence Spectroscopy, 26, 29

Furosemide/dihydralazine (f/d), 110-112, 114

G

Geldanamycin Derivative, 98

GO, 47, 49, 116

H

Haart, 118-119, 121-122

HDL, 15, 62-63, 67, 70

Heart Phosphoproteome, 48, 50-51, 53

Hepatorenal Syndrome, 154, 189-190, 193, 195

Hete, 80, 82, 85, 87

Hsp90 Inhibitor, 98-99, 104

Human Motor Axons, 90-91, 97

HUS, 73-74, 77-79

Hyperkalemia, 42, 90, 94, 96-97

I

Intellectual Disability, 123-127

Ischemia-reperfusion Injury (IRI), 165-166

Isothermal Titration Calorimetry, 24, 26, 28

K

Kidney Injury Molecule-1 (KIM-1), 165

Klotho, 2, 4, 6

L

L-serine, 165-172

Lanthanum Carbonate (LA), 1-2

Linoleic Acid, 99, 102, 104, 106

Lithogenic Diseases, 8

M

Mass Spectrometry, 44-46, 82

Metformin-associated Lactic Acidosis, 38, 43

Mitochondrial Dna, 61, 64, 71-72

Model For End-stage Liver Disease (MELD), 146

Morphometry, 81, 107-108

Myocardial Fibrosis, 107-108, 110, 112, 114-116

N

Nerve Excitability, 90-91, 93-97

Norepinephrine, 39, 45, 148, 189-195

P

Percutaneous Coronary Interventions (PCI), 174

Phlebitis, 128, 132, 183

Plasma Therapy, 73-74

Pneumonia, 57, 123-126

Preoperative Aspirin, 55-60

Protein Kinases, 44-45, 47

R

Randomized Controlled Trials (RCTS), 136, 143, 157

Ras, 21, 45, 56-57, 86-87, 107, 110, 112, 114-115

S

Septic Thrombophlebitis, 180-182, 187-188

Serum Creatinine, 1-2, 4-6, 15, 23-24, 36, 47, 56, 74, 91, 97, 99-100, 104, 119, 133, 136-139, 141, 149, 156-157, 161, 163, 167, 169, 171, 175, 190, 192

Statin Therapy, 106, 136, 140-144

String Analysis, 48, 50-51

Systolic Blood Pressure, 4-5, 15, 45, 47-48, 70, 74, 81, 83, 107-108, 110-111

T

T2DM, 61-62, 65, 67-72

Terlipressin, 147, 153, 189-195

Thrombotic Microangiopathies (TMA), 73

TTP, 73-75, 77, 79

U

Uremic Toxins, 23, 36